Study Guide for

Pathophysiology Concepts of Altered Health States

Eighth Edition

Wolters Kluwer | Lippincott Williams & Wilkins
Health
Philadelphia · Baltimore · New York · London
Buenos Aires · Hong Kong · Sydney · Tokyo

Managing Editor: Annette Ferran
Senior Production Editor: Debra Schiff
Director of Nursing Production: Helen Ewan
Senior Managing Editor/Production: Erika Kors
Manufacturing Coordinator: Karin Duffield
Compositor: Aptara

8th Edition

9 8 7 6 5 4 3

Printed in the United States of America

ISBN: 978-0-7817-6913-6

    Care has been taken to confirm the accuracy of the information presented and to describe generally accepted practices. However, the authors, editors, and publisher are not responsible for errors or omissions or for any consequences from application of the information in this book and make no warranty, expressed or implied, with respect to the currency, completeness, or accuracy of the contents of the publication. Application of this information in a particular situation remains the professional responsibility of the practitioner; the clinical treatments described and recommended may not be considered absolute and universal recommendations.

    The authors, editors, and publisher have exerted every effort to ensure that drug selection and dosage set forth in this text are in accordance with the current recommendations and practice at the time of publication. However, in view of ongoing research, changes in government regulations, and the constant flow of information relating to drug therapy and drug reactions, the reader is urged to check the package insert for each drug for any change in indications and dosage and for added warnings and precautions. This is particularly important when the recommended agent is a new or infrequently employed drug.

    Some drugs and medical devices presented in this publication have Food and Drug Administration (FDA) clearance for limited use in restricted research settings. It is the responsibility of the health care provider to ascertain the FDA status of each drug or device planned for use in his or her clinical practice.

LWW.COM

Preface

This Study Guide was written by Brian Kipp, PhD, and Jo Anne Kirk, MSN, RN, to accompany the eighth edition of *Pathophysiology: Concepts of Altered Health States* by Carol Mattson Porth and Glenn Matfin. The Study Guide is designed to help you practice and retain the knowledge you've gained from the textbook, and it is structured to integrate that knowledge and give you a basis for applying it in your practice. The following types of exercises are provided in each chapter of the Study Guide.

ASSESSING YOUR UNDERSTANDING

The first section of each Study Guide chapter concentrates on the basic information of the textbook chapter and helps you to remember key concepts, vocabulary, and principles.

- Fill in the Blanks

Fill-in-the-blank exercises test important chapter information, encouraging you to recall key points.

- Labeling

Labeling exercises are used where you need to remember certain visual representations of the concepts presented in the textbook.

- Matching

Matching questions test your knowledge of the definition of key terms.

- Sequencing

Sequencing exercises ask you to remember particular sequences or orders, for instance of normal or abnormal physiologic processes.

- Short Answers

Short-answer questions cover facts, concepts, procedures, and principles of the chapter. These questions ask you to recall information as well as demonstrate your comprehension of the information.

APPLYING YOUR KNOWLEDGE

The second section of each Study Guide chapter consists of case study–based exercises that ask you to begin to apply the knowledge you've gained from the textbook chapter and reinforced in the first section of the Study Guide chapter. A case study scenario based on the chapter's content is presented, and then you are asked to answer some questions, in writing, related to the case study. The questions could cover lab values, next steps in treatment, anticipated diagnoses, and the like.

PRACTICING FOR NCLEX

The third and final section of the Study Chapters helps you practice NCLEX-style questions while further reinforcing the knowledge you have been gaining and testing for yourself through the textbook chapter and the first two sections of the study guide chapter. In keeping with the NCLEX, the questions presented are multiple-choice and scenario-based, asking you to reflect, consider, and apply what you know and to choose the best answer out of those offered.

ANSWER KEYS

The answers for all of the exercises and questions in the Study Guide are provided at the back of the book, so you can assess your own learning as you complete each chapter.

We hope you will find this Study Guide to be helpful and enjoyable, and we wish you every success in your studies and future profession.

The Publishers

Contents

CHAPTER 1

Concepts of Health and Disease

SECTION I: LEARNING OBJECTIVES

1. State the World Health Organization definition of health

2. State a definition of pathophysiology

3. Characterize the disease process in terms of etiology, pathogenesis, morphology, clinical manifestations, and prognosis

4. Explain the meaning of reliability, validity, sensitivity, specificity, and predictive value as it relates to observations and tests used in the diagnosis of disease

5. Define the term *epidemiology*

6. Compare the meaning of the terms *incidence* and *prevalence* as they relate to measures of disease frequency

7. Compare the sources of information and limitations of mortality and morbidity statistics

8. Characterize the natural history of a disease

9. Differentiate primary, secondary, and tertiary levels of prevention

10. Propose ways in which practice guidelines can be used to improve health care

SECTION II: ASSESSING YOUR UNDERSTANDING

Activity A *Fill in the blanks.*

1. Pathophysiology is the study of _____ and its manifestations via changes in cells, tissues, and organs.

2. The World Health Organization defines the state of _____ as a state of complete physical, mental, and social well-being and not merely the absence of disease and infirmity.

3. The term _____ can be defined as an interruption, cessation, or disorder of a body system or organ structure.

4. The multiple factors that predispose a patient to a particular disease are known as _____ .

5. _____ are present at birth but may not be relevant until later stages of development.

6. Defects or damage that occurs after birth are termed _____ defects.

7. The description as to the nature or cause of a health problem that is arrived at following examination is the _____ .

8. _____ is not clinically apparent and is not destined to become clinically apparent. _____ is manifested by signs and symptoms.

9. _____ is the study of disease occurrence in a population.

10. _____ is a measure of the existing disease in a population, whereas _____ is reflective of the development of new cases.

Activity B *Match the key terms in Column A with their definitions in Column B.*

Column A

____ **1.** Etiology

____ **2.** Mortality

____ **3.** Pathogenesis

____ **4.** Morphology

____ **5.** Cohort

____ **6.** Morbidity

____ **7.** Clinical manifestations

____ **8.** Prognosis

____ **9.** Evidence-based practice

____ **10.** Prevention

Column B

a. Predicted outcome of a disease process

b. Causes of disease

c. Fundamental structure or form of cells or tissues

d. Signs and symptoms of a disease

e. Group of persons that shares certain characteristics

f. Sequence of cellular and tissue events

g. Characteristics of death-producing effects of a disease

h. Effects of disease on patient's life

i. Using current and best information in treatment

j. Halting disease progress or development

Activity C

1. Diagnosing and treating a disease involves a complex set of steps that a clinician must perform in order to provide a patient with the best care possible. Make a flowchart of the evaluation process of the health status of an afflicted patient as a clinician would.

Activity D *Briefly answer the following.*

1. Define the term *pathophysiology*. Compare and contrast that definition with definitions for *physiology* and *pathology*.

_____

_____

_____

2. Explain what is meant by the term *clinical course*. In your answer, address the differences between an acute disorder and chronic disease.

_____

_____

_____

3. Differentiate between a congenital condition and an acquired defect.

_____

_____

_____

4. What is the difference between syndromes and sequelae?

_____

_____

_____

5. What is the importance of risk factors and how they are determined for a given population?

_____

_____

_____

SECTION III: APPLYING YOUR KNOWLEDGE

Activity E *Consider the following scenario and answer the questions.*

A nurse from a local hospital has been asked to present an educational event for a community group. They have asked her to speak on communicable diseases.

1. When presenting to this group, the nurse should include information on what aspects of the topic?

2. One member of the group asks, "The nurse who takes care of my mother said that she uses 'evidence-based guidelines' when she cares for her patients. What does that mean?" How would the nurse answer this question?

SECTION IV: PRACTICING FOR NCLEX

Activity F *Answer the following questions.*

1. A disease agent can affect more than one organ of the body, and more than one disease agent can affect the same organ of the body. Therefore, the majority of diseases
  a. are multifactorial in origin.
  b. are complicated and hard to diagnose.
  c. are simple and easy to diagnose.
  d. have a single cause.

2. Which science is called on to study the risk factors in multifactorial diseases?
  a. Scientology
  b. Morphology
  c. Histology
  d. Epidemiology

3. What do morbidity and mortality statistics refer to?
  a. Long-term consequences and recovery rates of a disease
  b. Cause of death and impact on the family because of a disease
  c. Functional effects and death-producing characteristics of a disease
  d. Effects a disease has on a person's life and treatment

4. Which of the following statements accurately describes clinical practice guidelines, or evidence-based practice guidelines? Mark all that apply.
  a. They are intended to inform practitioners and clients in making decisions about health care for specific clinical circumstances.
  b. They should review various outcomes; weigh various outcomes, both positive and negative; and make recommendations.
  c. They can take the form of algorithms, which are step-by-step methods for solving

a problem; written directives for care; or a combination thereof.
  d. They take the place of both written orders by the doctor and the nursing care plan.

5. There are three fundamental types of prevention used in health care: primary, secondary, and tertiary. Which of the following statements accurately describes secondary prevention?
  a. Secondary prevention detects disease early, and most is done in clinical settings.
  b. Secondary prevention goes beyond treating the problem with which the person presents.
  c. Secondary prevention is often accomplished outside the health care system at the community level.
  d. Secondary prevention takes place within health care systems and involves the services of a number of different types of health care professionals.

6. Why are some diseases termed *syndromes*?
  a. They have complications.
  b. They leave sequelae such as lesions as residual effects.
  c. They are a compilation of signs and symptoms characteristic of a specific disease state.
  d. They are a group of disease states that has the same etiology.

7. Which of the following is the term given to the progression and projected outcome of a disease without medical intervention?
  a. Prognosis
  b. Morbidity
  c. Natural history
  d. Risk factors

8. *Pathogenesis* is the term used to describe the sequence of cellular and tissue events that occurs from the time of first contact with an etiologic agent until the disease becomes evident. What is another way of defining pathogenesis?
  a. What sets the disease process in motion
  b. Multiple factors that predispose to a particular disease
  c. The causes of disease
  d. How the disease process evolves

9. *Signs and symptoms* describe the structural and functional changes that accompany a disease. Symptoms are what the patient describes to the caregiver. Signs are what the caregiver observes. Which of the following would not be considered signs and symptoms?

   a. Headache and dizziness

   b. Elevated white cell count and fever of 101.5°F

   c. Pain and difficulty swallowing

   d. Black eye and green thumb

10. Diagnostic tests are used to gain information about the patient that is pertinent to the presenting signs and symptoms. Diagnostic tests are judged for their validity, reliability, sensitivity, specificity, and predictive value. In the field of clinical laboratory measurements, standardization is aimed at increasing the trueness and reliability of measured values. Standardization relies on which of the following? Mark all that apply.

    a. In vitro laboratory equipment

    b. Reference measurement procedures

    c. Written standards

    d. U.S. Food and Drug Administration approval

Concepts of Altered Health in Children

SECTION I: LEARNING OBJECTIVES

1. Characterize the use of percentiles to describe growth and development during infancy and childhood

2. Describe the major events that occur during prenatal development from fertilization to birth

3. Define the terms *low birth weight, small for gestational age,* and *large for gestational age*

4. Identify reasons for abnormal intrauterine growth

5. Describe assessment methods for determination of gestational age

6. Describe the use of the Apgar score in evaluating infant well-being at birth

7. Describe the causes and manifestations of neonatal hypoglycemia

8. List three injuries that can occur during the birth process

9. Describe physical growth and organ development during the first year of life

10. Explain how the common health care needs of the premature infant differ from the health care needs of the term newborn or infant

11. Differentiate between organic and nonorganic failure to thrive syndrome

12. Define *early childhood*

13. Describe the growth and development of early childhood

14. Discuss the common health problems of early childhood

15. Define *middle to late childhood*

16. Characterize the growth and development that occurs during middle to late childhood

17. Discuss the common health problems of middle to late childhood

18. Define what is meant by the period known as *adolescence*

19. Characterize the physical and psychosocial changes that occur during adolescence

20. Cite the developmental tasks that adolescents need to fulfill

21. Describe common concerns of parents regarding their adolescent child

22. Discuss how the changes that occur during adolescence can influence the health care needs of the adolescent

SECTION II: ASSESSING YOUR UNDERSTANDING

Activity A *Fill in the blanks.*

1. The phrase _____ describes a process whereby a fertilized ovum becomes an adult person.

2. The development of an embryo to a fetus progresses through three distinct phases. In the first phase, _____ occurs as a process of increasing cell numbers and elaboration of cell material. In the second stage, _____ cells interact, move, and form organs and tissues. During the third stage, the tissues _____ into functional organs capable of adult function.

3. The _____ is a system of evaluating an infant's well-being at birth.

4. Cranial injuries, skull fractures, and broken clavicles are all _____.

5. The leading complication in newborn infants is _____. It is caused by a lack of surfactant production.

6. _____ is defined as paroxysmal abdominal pain manifested by loud crying, retraction of legs, and extreme irritability.

7. During middle to late childhood, children typically gain approximately _____ and grow an average of _____ per year.

8. In adolescence, the risk of infection _____ due to the competency level of the immune system.

9. Skin infections are much more common in adolescence due to increased frequency of _____.

10. The causes of childhood _____ are undoubtedly multifactorial, but ultimately reflect an imbalance between the amount of calories the child consumes in food and beverages and the calories that the child uses.

Activity B *Consider the following figure and answer the questions.*

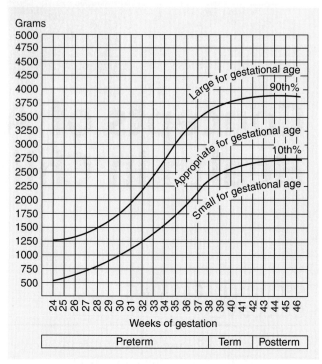

1. Using this chart, determine whether a child born at 37 weeks and weighing 1,750 g is large, appropriate, or small for gestational age.

2. Using this chart, determine whether a child born at 40 weeks and weighing 2,700 g is large, appropriate, or small for gestational age.

Activity C *Match the key terms in Column A with their definitions in Column B.*

Column A	Column B
_____ 1. Low birth weight	a. Use of six external physical signs and six neuromuscular signs to evaluate the development of an infant at term
_____ 2. Development	
_____ 3. Physical growth	
_____ 4. Morphogenesis	

_____ **5.** Neurulation

_____ **6.** Ballard method

_____ **7.** Fontanels

_____ **8.** Infantile hypoglycemia

_____ **9.** Jaundice

_____ **10.** Small for gestational age

b. Unossified membranous tissue in the fetal skull

c. Changes in the body as a whole

d. Fetal undergrowth or below the 10th percentile

e. Blood sugar level below 40 to 45 mg/dL

f. Formation of the neural plate, neural folds, and their closure

g. Sign of excessive circulating levels of unconjugated, lipid-soluble bilirubin

h. Weight of 2500 g or less at birth

i. Changes in body function and psychosocial behavior

j. Development of form

Activity D *Briefly answer the following.*

1. Prior to birth, fetuses, and following birth, infants, are checked for growth and development. Describe the progression of testing methods and the differing interpretations of data.

_____

_____

_____

2. The clavicle is the most frequently fractured bone in the birth process. Explain why this is true and what would make it more likely to occur.

_____

_____

_____

3. Respiratory distress syndrome is the result of low or absent surfactant production. What is the function of surfactant in the respiratory system?

_____

_____

_____

4. Sudden infant death syndrome (SIDS) affects children younger than 1 year. The actual cause is still unknown, but risk factors have been postulated. List the risk factors for SIDS.

_____

_____

_____

5. Failure to thrive (FTT) refers to inadequate growth due to inability to obtain or use essential nutrients. Nonorganic causes include neglect and abuse. Explain what is meant by an organic cause of FTT.

_____

_____

_____

6. Physiological jaundice is normal for the neonate. When does it become a concern, and why?

_____

_____

_____

SECTION III: APPLYING YOUR KNOWLEDGE

Activity E *Consider the following scenario and answer the questions.*

A 6-year-old girl is brought to the clinic for a well-child examination. While doing your physical assessment, you notice dental caries on and between the teeth.

1. What education would be given to this child and her family pertinent to her developmental stage?

   _____

   _____

   _____

2. What common health concerns should you be aware of when examining a child of this age?

   _____

   _____

   _____

3. What is the major task, as defined by Erickson, at this developmental stage?

   _____

   _____

   _____

SECTION IV: PRACTICING FOR NCLEX

Activity F   *Answer the following questions.*

1. A mother brings her 2-year-old son in for a well-child check. After weighing and measuring the toddler, the nurse mentions that the child falls within 1 standard deviation of the mean in both height and weight. What does this mean?

   a. The toddler is the same height and weight as 75% of other toddlers that age and weight.

   b. The toddler is the same height and weight as 68% of other toddlers that age and weight.

   c. The toddler is small and underweight for his age.

   d. The toddler is tall and overweight for his age.

2. A nurse is teaching a class on fetal development to a group of pregnant women. The nurse knows to include in her teaching that the embryonic period in fetal development is from the

   a. moment of conception to the 8th week of pregnancy.

   b. moment of implantation to the 6th week of pregnancy

   c. second week after conception to the 12th week of pregnancy.

   d. second week after fertilization to the 8th week after fertilization.

3. A pregnancy lasts 10 lunar months, or 38 weeks from the date of fertilization. When is an infant considered to be "term"?

   a. When it is born between the beginning of the 38th week and the end of the 41st week

   b. When it is born between the beginning of the 36th week and the end of the 40th week

   c. When it weighs between 2500 and 4500 g

   d. When it weighs between 3000 and 4000 g

4. Common concerns of adolescence include conflicts with parents, conflicts with siblings, concerns about school, and concerns about peers and peer relationships. Of major concern to them is the establishment of a personal identity. This is a time when many of their concerns manifest themselves in psychosomatic illnesses. What are the illnesses reported most by adolescents?

   a. Headache, stomachache, and insomnia

   b. Headache, insomnia, and dental caries

   c. Stomachache, dental caries, and leg pain

   d. Insomnia, skeletal pain, and headache

5. Small for gestational age infants are more prone to episodes of hypoglycemia than infants who are considered appropriate for gestational age. What factor is considered to be the most likely cause of these hypoglycemic episodes?

   a. They are too small for their pancreas to produce the insulin their body requires.

   b. They do not have enough brown fat to maintain their body temperature.

   c. They have depleted glycogen stores in their liver.

   d. Their bodies are so small that their pancreas produces too much insulin for their body requirements.

6. Middle to late childhood, ages 6 to 12 years of age, brings with it a more developed immune system. Yet, this is when acute or chronic conditions can appear for the first time. Which of the following diseases often appears in middle to late childhood?

   a. Pneumonia

   b. Nephrotic syndrome

c. Cerebral palsy

d. Asthma

7. The anterior fontanel of an infant is an area of unossified membranous material that is considered "open" when the infant is born. It is the largest of several areas, or fontanels, in an infant's skull. When does the anterior fontanel close, or ossify?

a. 18 months to 2 years of age

b. 1 to 2 years of age

c. 6 to 9 months of age

d. 2 to 3 years of age

8. Early childhood is the period when the child is from 18 months to 5 years of age. Infectious diseases and injuries are major health problems during this period in a child's life. Which of the following is considered a communicable disease?

a. Diaper rash

b. Chickenpox

c. Urinary tract infection

d. Croup

9. Bacterial infections in newborns have nonspecific signs and symptoms in the early stages. Often, it is the nurse who notes that something "just isn't right" with the newborn. For optimal outcomes of these infections, it is imperative to have early diagnosis and treatment. Maternal group B streptococcus (GBS) infections are transmitted to the infant during birth. When are GBS infections treated?

a. During pregnancy to the mother to prevent transmission of the bacteria to the newborn and after birth to the infant prophylactically

b. During the intrapartal period to the mother to help prevent transmission of the bacteria to the newborn and after birth to the infant prophylactically

c. During postpartum care to the mother and at discharge to the infant

d. During the intrapartal period to the mother to help prevent transmission of the bacteria to the newborn and at discharge to the infant as a prophylactic agent

10. Sudden infant death syndrome (SIDS) is defined as the death of an infant younger than 1 year that remains unexplained even after investigation of the death scene, review of

the history, and autopsy of the body. SIDS accounts for more infant deaths, after the neonatal period, than any other cause. What are the risk factors for SIDS?

a. Being Native American and placing the infant on its back to sleep

b. Being Asian and exposing the infant to environmental cigarette smoke

c. Mother's use of drugs during pregnancy and placing the infant in the prone position to sleep

d. Breast-feeding and placing the infant on its back to sleep

11. Macrosomic infants, or those who are large for gestational age, born to diabetic mothers face which of the following risk factors for complications during the neonatal period? Mark all that apply.

a. Hypoglycemia

b. Polycythemia

c. Birth trauma

d. Birth asphyxia

12. When planning an educational event for a group of women having their first babies, a nurse knows to include which information about intrauterine growth retardation? Mark all that apply.

a. The terms *small for gestational age* and *intrauterine growth retardation* are used interchangeably, but do not mean the same thing.

b. Eighty percent of newborns fall between the 10th and the 90th percentile of the Colorado Growth Curve.

c. Intrauterine growth retardation can occur at any time during the pregnancy.

d. An infant who is "small for gestational age" weighs less then 80% of all other newborns.

13. During adolescence, the anterior pituitary gland produces gonadotropic hormones that affect target organs, causing the secretion of sex hormones. It is the sex hormones that cause the appearance of both primary and secondary sex characteristics. Sex hormones, including androgens, stimulate the body to do other things, such as conclude _____ growth. They cause epiphyseal closure of bones and discontinuation of skeletal growth.

Concepts of Altered Health in Older Adults

SECTION I: LEARNING OBJECTIVES

1. State a definition for *young-old, middle-old,* and *old-old,* and characterize the changing trend in the elderly population

2. State a philosophy of aging that incorporates the positive aspects of the aging process

3. Discuss theories of biologic aging

4. Describe common skin changes that occur with aging

5. Explain how muscle changes that occur with aging affect high-speed performance and endurance

6. Describe the process of bone loss that occurs with aging

7. State the common changes in blood pressure regulation that occur with aging

8. List the changes in respiratory function that occur with aging

9. Relate aging changes in neural function to the overall function of the body

10. Briefly discuss the effects of aging on vision, hearing, taste, and smell

11. Describe changes that occur in the gastrointestinal tract with aging

12. State the significance of decreased lean body mass on interpretation of the glomerular filtration rate using serum creatinine levels

13. Compare information obtained from functional assessment with that obtained from a physical examination used to arrive at a medical diagnosis

14. Cite the differences between chronic and transient urinary incontinence

15. State four risk factors for falls in older individuals

16. List five symptoms of depression in older adults

17. Name a tool that can be used for assessing cognitive function

18. State the difference between delirium and dementia

19. Characterize drug therapy in the older adult population

20. List five factors that contribute to adverse drug reactions in the elderly

21. Cite cautions to be used in prescribing medications for the elderly

SECTION II: ASSESSING YOUR UNDERSTANDING

Activity A *Fill in the blanks.*

1. Because there is great diversity in the health of older adults, they are categorized into subgroups of *young-old,* from _____ years of age; *middle-old,* from _____ years of age; and *old-old,* from _____ years of

age to reflect more accurately the changes in function that occur over time.

2. Developmental or genetic theories of aging are termed _____.

3. _____ theories maintain that the changes result from an accumulation of random events or damage from environmental agents or influences.

4. Cellular aging resides with an enzyme called _____ that is believed to govern chromosomal aging.

5. The _____ theory of aging holds that aging results partially from oxidative metabolism and the effects of free radical damage.

6. Areas of the skin that are repeatedly exposed to the sun experience changes in the dermis. _____ fibers rearrange and degenerate, resulting in decreased skin strength and elasticity.

7. Decreases in height as a person ages can be attributed to compression of the _____.

8. In elderly individuals, stiffening of the arteries results in a chronic elevation of _____ pressure.

9. A progressive loss of _____ in the lung is caused by changes in the amount of elastin and composition of collagen fibers and results in decreased Vo_2 max.

10. _____, or hearing loss, occurs as a result of aging plus auditory stressors, trauma, environmental influences, otologic diseases, and genetic influences.

11. _____, or dry mouth, is a common affliction of the elderly and is caused by decreased salivary secretions.

12. The age-associated loss of parietal cells in the stomach results in _____, a decrease in hydrochloric acid secretion.

13. Age-related decreases in renal blood flow result in a decreased _____ rate, which can confuse a diagnosis.

14. The _____ index is commonly used to assess the mental and biological status of an elderly patient.

15. A decrease in bladder capacity, in bladder and sphincter tone, and in the ability to _____ detrusor muscle contractions are common causes of incontinence.

16. The signature symptom of depression is a _____ mood.

17. Major depression is a common consequence of _____ and occurs in about one-third of afflicted patients.

18. _____ is a syndrome of acquired, persistent impairment in several domains of intellectual function.

19. _____ is defined as an organic mental syndrome featuring a cognitive impairment, disturbances of attention, reduced level of consciousness, increased or decreased psychomotor activity, and a disorganized sleep-wake cycle.

20. Drug toxicity is common in elderly patients due to decreases in _____ and decreases in lean muscle mass.

Activity B *Match the key terms in Column A with their definitions in Column B.*

Column A

____ 1. Telomerase

____ 2. Stochastic theory of aging

____ 3. Superoxide

____ 4. Osteoporosis

____ 5. Sedatives

____ 6. Dementia

____ 7. Orthostatic hypotension

____ 8. Lipofuscin

____ 9. Wear and tear theory of aging

____ 10. Alzheimer disease

Column B

a. Yellow insoluble deposits of intracellular material

b. Govern chromosomal aging through its action on telomeres

c. Decreased bone mass

d. Key component of oxidative stress-related aging

e. Mitochondrial damage is one example of this type of aging

f. Accumulated damage to vital parts of the cell leads to aging and death

g. Associated with an increased prevalence of falling

h. A syndrome of acquired, persistent impairment in several domains of intellectual function

i. Significant drop in systolic pressure on assumption of the upright position

j. Chronic, progressive neurologic disorder of unknown cause with symptoms of dementia

Activity C *Briefly answer the following.*

1. The process of aging is one of slow steady decline. Using the oxidative free radical theory of aging as a guide, describe the changes as they develop in the circulatory system to result in higher blood pressure.

_____

_____

_____

2. The process of aging is often likened to a disease state. Explain how disease and aging are different.

_____

_____

_____

3. There are numerous theories of how humans age. One such class of theories is the stochastic theory of aging. Explain the concept of DNA repair and how it fits into this theory.

_____

_____

_____

4. As humans age, muscular strength declines. Provide a rational for why we lose our strength as we age.

_____

_____

_____

5. The elderly are more prone to falling. Explain the degeneration of sensory processes behind the increased risk of falling.

_____

_____

_____

6. Explain the differences between dementia and Alzheimer disease.

_____

_____

_____

SECTION III: APPLYING YOUR KNOWLEDGE

Activity D *Consider the following scenario and answer the questions.*

An elderly gentleman is brought to the emergency room by his daughter after she found him lying on the floor of his house. The daughter tells you that she has been afraid that her father would fall and now he has.

1. The daughter asks the nurse what she can do to help prevent her father from falling again. How should the nurse respond?

_____

_____

_____

2. While conducting the physical assessment, the nurse notices that the gentleman's affect is flat, he responds to questions only briefly, and says that he has lost weight over the past few months. For what would the nurse further assess?

_____

_____

_____

SECTION IV: PRACTICING FOR NCLEX

Activity E *Answer the following questions.*

1. With aging, the skin acquires an overall thin and transparent quality while becoming dry and wrinkled. Which of the following skin disorders are common among the older adult population?
   a. Keratoses and skin cancers
   b. Skin cancers and xenobiotic
   c. Dermatitis and xenomas
   d. Xenomas and keratoses

2. There are many factors that determine the effect of aging on cardiac function in normal healthy persons. Which of these statements is *not* true about aging and cardiac function?

   a. There is a decrease in responsiveness to β-adrenergic stimulation and circulating catecholamines.

   b. There is an increase in systemic vascular resistance and left ventricular afterload.

   c. There is a decrease in the maximal heart rate and maximal cardiac output.

   d. There is a decrease in systemic vascular resistance and left ventricular afterload.

3. Hearing loss in the elderly is characterized by a gradual, progressive onset of bilateral and symmetric sensorineural hearing loss of high-frequency tones. This occurs at various rates in different people. Which sign, in the elderly, is indicative of hearing impairment?

   a. Speech discrimination is difficult.

   b. Repetition is more evident.

   c. Speech is slower and softer.

   d. Shouting occurs when it is not necessary.

4. Both the sense of smell and the sense of taste seem to decline in the elderly. However, in many cases, what is perceived as a decline in ability to taste is actually a decline in the ability to smell. With a decline in the sense of taste and smell, the elderly are at risk for which of the following?

   a. Taking the wrong medication

   b. Being unable to smell smoke if there is a fire

   c. Living in unhealthy and unclean conditions

   d. Eating food that is spoiled and not cooked properly

5. A complex and devastating problem in approximately 5% to 10% of the elderly population is dementia. Dementia is a syndrome of acquired, persistent impairment in several domains of intellectual function. Which of the following is *not* affected in a person with dementia?

   a. Ability to interact with others

   b. Visuospatial ability

   c. Physical changes of aging

   d. Problem-solving ability

6. One of the major indexes of kidney function is the serum creatinine level. It is used as an indication of the glomerular filtration rate (GFR), and is often used when prescribing and calculating drug doses for medications that are eliminated through the kidneys. In older adults, why does this have important implications?

   a. Serum creatinine levels progressively increase as a person ages.

   b. GFR increases as a person ages without a corresponding increase in serum creatinine levels.

   c. Both GFR and serum creatinine levels decrease as a person ages.

   d. GFR decreases without an increase in serum creatinine levels as a person ages.

7. As men age, benign prostatic hypertrophy (BPH) becomes common. As the size of the prostate increases, BPH can cause both obstructive and irritative symptoms. All of the following are obstructive symptoms of BPH except for which one?

   a. Urge incontinence

   b. Postvoid dribbling

   c. Hesitancy

   d. Retention

8. In the elderly population, depression is a significant but underestimated health problem. Statistics show that at least 25% of community-dwelling elderly people are believed to have depressive symptoms. Which of the following symptoms are indicative of depression in older people?

   a. Fatigue and loss of energy

   b. Appetite and weight changes

   c. Sleep disturbance and irritable mood

   d. All of the above

9. Although there are many causes contributing to the diagnosis of dementia in the elderly population, it is believed that up to 70% of these cases involve Alzheimer disease. Alzheimer disease is a chronic, progressive, neurologic disorder of unknown etiology. Two changes occur in the brain of Alzheimer patients: plaques that develop between neurons, called senile plaques, and neurofibrillary tangles that develop within the neurons themselves. Which diagnostic test is used to determine specifically if the elderly patient

has Alzheimer disease or another form of dementia?

a. The Mini-Mental State Examination

b. There is no specific test to confirm the diagnosis

c. A complete metabolic panel performed on the patient's blood

d. The auscultation of bruits in the carotid arteries

10. A nurse is preparing an educational event for the elderly population at a local senior center. The nurse knows that it is important to include information on polypharmacy because of which of these factors?

a. Psychotropic drugs administered to older adults with dementia may cause a decrease in any confusion they are experiencing.

b. Polypharmacy increases the risk of drug interactions and adverse drug reactions and has been found to decrease compliance with drug regimens.

c. Nonsteroidal anti-inflammatory medications given to an older adult with hypertension can cause orthostatic hypotension.

d. Beta-blocking agents administered to an individual with chronic obstructive pulmonary disease may reduce the severity of bronchoconstriction.

11. Falls in the elderly are all too common. One of the major causes of falls in the elderly population, although often overlooked, is medication. Match the type of medication with its physiologic result.

Type of Medication	Physiologic Result
____ **1.** Antihypertensive	**a.** Fatigue
____ **2.** Diuretic	**b.** Electrolyte disturbances
____ **3.** Sedative	**c.** Confusion
____ **4.** Hypnotic	**d.** Impaired alertness

12. Several factors come into effect when making decisions about medication use in the elderly, not the least of which is preventing harm. Choose the answer that places the following decision-making factors in the correct order.

a. A careful evaluation of the need to medicate

b. The cost of the drug as compared to a generic drug if it is available

c. Timing of the dose

d. Analysis of the current medication regimen and disease state

e. Providing written and verbal education on the medication

A. a, d, e, c, b
B. e, a, d, c, b
C. a, d, c, b, e
D. d, b, c, a, e

13. Atrophic gastritis and decreased secretion of intrinsic factor are more common with aging and can result in a malabsorption of vitamin B_{12}. A deficiency of vitamin B_{12} can cause which of these to occur? Mark all that apply.

a. Peripheral neuropathy

b. Lack of intrinsic factor

c. Pernicious anemia

d. Improved coordination

14. Depression can occur as a result of many different physical illnesses. Which of these illnesses can cause depression in the elderly? Mark all that apply.

a. Pancreatic cancer

b. Congestive heart failure

c. Hypocholesteremia

d. Hyperthyroidism

15. Changes in the micturition cycle that accompany the aging process make the older adult prone to urinary incontinence. Urinary incontinence can have many contributing causes, including which of the following? Mark all that apply.

a. Increased ability to inhibit detrusor contractions

b. Impaired mobility and a slower reaction time

c. A decrease in bladder capacity

d. Medications, such as long-acting sedatives and hypnotics

CHAPTER 4

Cell and Tissue Characteristics

SECTION I: LEARNING OBJECTIVES

1. State why the nucleus is called the "control center" of the cell

2. List the cellular organelles and state their functions

3. State four functions of the cell membrane

4. Trace the pathway for cell communication, beginning at the receptor and ending with the effector response, and explain why the process is often referred to as *signal transduction*

5. Compare the functions of G-protein–linked, ion-channel–linked, and enzyme-linked cell surface receptors

6. Describe the phases of mitotic cell division

7. Relate the function of ATP to cell metabolism

8. Compare the processes involved in anaerobic and aerobic metabolism

9. Discuss the mechanisms of membrane transport associated with diffusion, osmosis, endocytosis, and exocytosis and compare them with active transport mechanisms

10. Describe the function of ion channels

11. Describe the basis for membrane potentials

12. Explain the relationship between membrane permeability and generation of membrane potentials

13. Explain the process of cell differentiation in terms of development of organ systems in the embryo and the continued regeneration of tissues in postnatal life

14. Explain the function of stem cells

15. Describe the characteristics of the four different tissue types

16. Explain the function of intercellular adhesions and junctions

17. Characterize the composition and functions of the extracellular components of tissue

SECTION II: ASSESSING YOUR UNDERSTANDING

Activity A *Fill in the blanks.*

1. _____ is composed of water, proteins, lipids, carbohydrates, and electrolytes.

2. All _____ cells have a nucleus, whereas _____ cells do not.

3. The nucleus contains _____, which serves as the template for making the _____, which is later used to direct the synthesis of _____ in the cytoplasm.

4. Ribosomes serve as the site for _____ synthesis in the cytoplasm.

5. _____ endoplasmic reticulum is studded with ribosomes attached to specific binding sites on the membrane.

6. The _____ complex modifies proteins and packages them into secretory granules bound for the membrane.

7. _____ contain powerful hydrolytic enzymes that are used to break down excess and worn-out cell parts as well as foreign substances.

8. Peroxisomes contain a special enzyme that degrades _____.

9. Mitochondria are the site of cellular _____, the product of which is the formation of _____.

10. Transport along the axon of neuronal cells takes place along the primary cytoskeletal component _____.

11. Actin and myosin are examples of functional _____ within muscle cells.

12. Integral proteins span the entire lipid bilayer, whereas _____ proteins are bound to one side of the membrane or the other.

13. The four tissues of the body are _____, _____, _____, and _____.

14. The differences in permeability of _____ is responsible for the generation of membrane potential. Permeability is regulated by ion channels.

15. Of the four tissue types, only _____ and _____ tissue is excitable.

Activity B *Match the key terms in Column A with their definitions in Column B.*

1.

Column A	Column B
____ **1.** tRNA	**a.** Site of synthesis of lipid molecules
____ **2.** Cytokinesis	**b.** Transfer RNA
____ **3.** Tubulin	**c.** Hormone or neurotransmitter
____ **4.** *Glycocalyx*	**d.** Second messenger that mediates cellular responses
____ **5.** G protein	
____ **6.** Smooth endoplasmic reticulum	**e.** Separation of the chromosome pairs
____ **7.** Anaphase	**f.** Protein subunit of microtubules
____ **8.** Centrioles	**g.** Used to direct chromosomes in dividing cells
____ **9.** Proteasomes	

____ **10.** First messenger

h. Division of cells following mitosis

i. Organelles that metabolize misfolded proteins

j. Carbohydrate and protein layer that participates in cell recognition

2.

Column A	Column B
____ **1.** Diffusion	**a.** Secondary active transport where substances are moved in the same direction
____ **2.** Osmosis	
____ **3.** Active transport	**b.** Any type of transport across the cell membrane that requires energy as it moves material against the concentration gradient
____ **4.** Passive transport	
____ **5.** Cotransport	
____ **6.** Facilitated diffusion	**c.** Secondary active transport where substances are moved in the opposite direction
____ **7.** Primary active transport	**d.** The coupling of the transport of one solute to a second solute
____ **8.** Secondary active transport	**e.** Transport across the cell membrane through a protein channel that does not require ATP
____ **9.** Countertransport	**f.** The diffusion of water
____ **10.** Symport	**g.** Any type of transport across the cell membrane that does not require energy

h. Direct use of ATP in the transport of a solute

i. Utilization of the energy derived from the primary active transport of one solute for the cotransport of a second solute

j. Passive movement of solute down the concentration gradient

Activity C *Put the phases of the cell cycle in the correct order, starting with the beginning of interphase.*

1. G2 phase

2. Anaphase

3. Telophase

4. S phase

5. Prophase

6. Metaphase

7. G1 phase

Activity D *Consider the following figure.*

1.

Extracellular fluid

Cytosol

In this figure, label phospholipid by layer, an individual phospholipid, an integral protein, a peripheral protein, a channel protein, a glycoprotein, and a glycolipid.

Activity E *Briefly answer the following.*

1. The cell cycle is regulated by three protein complexes and their interactions. List each protein type and describe how it influences the progression through the cell cycle.

_____

_____

_____

2. In many diseases, the root cause is ischemia (low blood flow) or hypoxia (decreased delivery of oxygen). Using what you know about aerobic metabolism, explain how alterations in oxygen delivery to the tissues are detrimental.

_____

_____

_____

3. Tissues must maintain their shape and integrity in order to function. Explain from the cellular level to the tissue level what is responsible for maintaining tissue shape and structure.

_____

_____

_____

4. Signal transduction is a complex and varied process. Describe the process starting at the first messenger and ending in a physiological response. Be sure to include the various possibilities at both the receptor level and the second messenger level.

_____

_____

_____

5. Large molecules or particles are ingested or released from cells. Describe the basics of ingestion and release.

_____

_____

_____

SECTION III: APPLYING YOUR KNOWLEDGE

Activity F *Consider the following scenario and answer the questions.*

Fourteen-year-old Thomas Kirk is brought to the clinic for a routine physical before starting to play sports in school. He is 77 in. tall and weighs 200 lb. Tom states, "I have tried to lose weight so I can wrestle at a lower weight, and I just don't understand why I still weigh 200 pounds. My science teacher said it's because I have white fat and not brown fat." How would you explain to Tom about the two kinds of adipose tissue in his body?

_____

_____

_____

SECTION IV: PRACTICING FOR NCLEX

Activity G *Answer the following questions.*

1. There are two forms of endoplasmic reticulum (ER) found in a cell. They are the rough and the smooth ER. What does the rough ER do in a cell?
   a. Produces proteins
   b. Combines protein with other components of the cytoplasm
   c. Exports protein from the cell
   d. Destroys ribosomes

2. The Golgi complex, or Golgi bodies, consists of stacks of thin, flattened vesicles or sacs within the cell. These Golgi bodies are found near the nucleus and function in association with the ER. What is one purpose of the Golgi complex?
   a. To produce bile
   b. To receive proteins and other substances from the cell surface by a retrograde transport mechanism
   c. To produce excretory granules
   d. To produce small carbohydrate molecules

3. In Tay-Sachs disease, an autosomal recessive disorder, hexosaminidase A, which is the lysosomal enzyme needed for degrading the GM_2 ganglioside found in nerve cell membranes, is deficient. Although GM_2 ganglioside accumulates in many tissues, where does it do the most harm?
   a. Brain and retinas
   b. Retinas and heart
   c. Nervous system and retinas
   d. Nervous system and brain

4. The mitochondria are literally the "power plants" of the cell because they transform organic compounds into energy that is easily accessible to the cell. What do the mitochondria do?
   a. Make energy
   b. Form proteasomes
   c. Need DNA from other sources to replicate
   d. Extract energy from organic compounds

5. The cell membrane is also called what?
   a. Plasma membrane
   b. Nuclear membrane
   c. Receptor membrane
   d. Bilayer membrane

6. Some messengers, such as thyroid hormone and steroid hormones, do not bind to membrane receptors but move directly across the lipid layer of the cell membrane and are carried to the cell nucleus. What do they do at the cell nucleus?
   a. Transiently open or close ion channels
   b. Influence DNA activity
   c. Stabilize cell function
   d. Decrease transcription of mRNA

7. The Krebs cycle provides a common pathway for the metabolism of nutrients by the body. The Krebs cycle forms two pyruvate molecules. Each pyruvate molecule formed in the cytoplasm from one molecule of glucose yields another molecule of what?
   a. FAD
   b. $NADH + H^+$
   c. ATP
   d. H_2O

8. When cells use energy to move ions against an electrical or chemical gradient, the process is called what?
   a. Passive transport
   b. Neutral transport
   c. Cotransport
   d. Active transport

9. Groups of cells that are closely associated in structure and have common or similar functions are called tissues. What are the types of tissue in the human body?
   a. Connective and muscle tissue
   b. Binding and connecting tissue
   c. Nerve and exothelial tissue
   d. Exothelial and muscle tissue

10. Endocrine glands are epithelial structures that have had their connection with the surface obliterated during development. How are these glands described?
    a. Ductile and produce secretions
    b. Ductless and produce secretions
    c. Ductile and release their glandular products by exocytosis
    d. Ductless and release their glandular products by exocytosis

11. Each skeletal muscle is a discrete organ made up of hundreds or thousands of muscle fibers. Although muscle fibers predominate, substantial amounts of connective tissue, blood vessels, and nerve fibers are also present. What happens during muscle contraction?

    a. When activated by GTP, the cross-bridges swivel in a fixed arc, much like the oars of a boat, as they become attached to the actin filament.

    b. During contraction, each cross-bridge undergoes its own cycle of movement, forming a bridge attachment and releasing it; the same sequence of movement repeats itself when the cross-bridge reattaches to the same cell.

    c. The thick myosin and thin actin filaments slide over each other, causing shortening of the muscle fiber.

    d. Calcium-calmodulin complexes produce the sliding of the filaments that form cross-bridges with the thin actin filaments.

12. The three main parts of a cell are the nucleus, the _____, and the cell membrane.

13. Bilirubin is a normal major pigment of bile; its excess accumulation within cells is evidenced clinically by a yellowish discoloration of the skin and sclera, a condition called _____.

14. Cells in multicellular organisms need to communicate with one another to coordinate their function and control their growth. The human body has several means of transmitting information between cells, what are they? Mark all that apply.

    a. Direct communication between adjacent cells

    b. Express communication between cells

    c. Autocrine and paracrine signaling

    d. Endocrine or synaptic signaling

15. The human body has nondividing cells that have left the cell cycle and are not capable of mitotic division once an infant is born. What are the nondividing cells? Mark all that apply.

    a. Mucous cells

    b. Neurons

    c. Skeletal muscle cells

    d. Cardiac muscle cells

16. Smooth muscle is often called _____ muscle because it contracts spontaneously or through activity of the autonomic nervous system.

CHAPTER 5

Cellular Adaptation, Injury, and Death

SECTION I: LEARNING OBJECTIVES

1. Cite the general purpose of changes in cell structure and function that occur as the result of normal adaptive processes

2. Describe cell changes that occur with atrophy, hypertrophy, hyperplasia, metaplasia, and dysplasia and state general conditions under which the changes occur

3. Cite three sources of intracellular accumulations

4. Compare the pathogenesis and effects of dystrophic and metastatic calcifications

5. Describe the mechanisms whereby physical agents such as blunt trauma, electrical forces, and extremes of temperature produce cell injury

6. Differentiate between the effects of ionizing and nonionizing radiation in terms of their ability to cause cell injury

7. Explain how the injurious effects of biologic agents differ from those produced by physical and chemical agents

8. State the mechanisms and manifestations of cell injury associated with lead poisoning

9. Identify the causes and outcomes of mercury toxicity

10. State how nutritional imbalances contribute to cell injury

11. Describe three types of reversible cell changes that can occur with cell injury

12. Define *free radical* and *reactive oxygen species*

13. Relate free radical formation and oxidative stress to cell injury and death

14. Describe cell changes that occur with ischemic and hypoxic cell injury

15. Relate the effects of impaired calcium homeostasis to cell injury and death

16. Differentiate cell death associated with necrosis and apoptosis

17. Cite the reasons for the changes that occur with the wet and dry forms of gangrene

SECTION II: ASSESSING YOUR UNDERSTANDING

Activity A *Fill in the blanks.*

1. Cells may adapt to the environment by undergoing changes in _____, _____, and _____.

2. There are two types of genes involved in adapting to the environment: the _____ genes that are necessary for normal function of a cell, and the genes that control cellular _____.

3. Atrophy is seen as a decrease in cell _____.

4. Denervation will result in cellular _____.

5. Hypertrophy is an _____ in cell size.

6. An increase in muscle mass associated with exercise is an example of _____.

7. An increase in the number of cells in an organ or tissue is known as cellular _____.

8. Liver regrowth is an example of _____ hyperplasia.

9. _____ or _____ hyperplasia is due to excessive hormonal stimulation or excessive growth factors.

10. _____ represents a reversible change in which one adult cell type is replaced by another adult cell type.

11. Metaplasia usually occurs in response to chronic _____ and _____ and allows for substitution of cells that are better able to survive stressful or harmful conditions.

12. Deranged cell growth of a specific tissue that results in cells that vary in size, shape, and organization is known as _____.

13. Dysplasia is strongly implicated as a precursor of _____.

14. Intracellular _____ represent the buildup of substances that cells cannot immediately use or eliminate.

15. _____ radicals are highly reactive chemical species having an unpaired electron in the outer valence shell of the molecule.

16. _____ deprives the cell of oxygen and interrupts oxidative metabolism and the generation of ATP.

17. Reversible cellular injury is seen as either cellular _____ or _____ accumulation.

18. _____ differs from apoptosis in that it involves unregulated enzymatic digestion of cell components, loss of cell membrane integrity with uncontrolled release of the products of cell death into the intracellular space, and initiation of the inflammatory response.

19. The increased _____ levels may inappropriately activate a number of enzymes with potentially damaging effects.

20. Acidosis develops and denatures the enzymatic and structural proteins of the cell during _____ necrosis.

Activity B *Consider the following figure.*

The figure represents cellular adaptation. Label each adaptation, and state whether it is a physiologic, pathologic, or both.

Activity C *Match the key terms in Column A with their descriptions in Column B.*

Column A

_____ **1.** Metastatic calcification

_____ **2.** Reactive oxygen species (ROS)

_____ **3.** Antioxidants

_____ **4.** Apoptosis

_____ **5.** Dystrophic calcification

_____ **6.** Temperature-induced injury

_____ **7.** Ischemia

_____ **8.** Molecular aging

_____ **9.** Ionizing radiation

_____ **10.** Cellular aging

Column B

a. Macroscopic deposition of calcium salts in injured tissue

b. Oxygen-containing molecules that are highly reactive

c. Ice crystal formation in cytosol

d. Natural and synthetic molecules that inhibit the reactions of ROS with biological structures

e. Occurs in normal tissues as the result of increased serum calcium levels

f. Impaired oxygen delivery

g. Programmed cell death

h. Causes injury due to changes in electron stability

i. Aging focused on mutations and/or changes in gene expression

j. Aging due to shortened telomeres

Activity D *Briefly answer the following.*

1. Why does chronically damaged tissue result in calcification?

_____

_____

_____

2. List the five categories of cellular injury.

_____

_____

_____

3. Lead was recently found in paint used to give children's toys their brilliant colors. Why is this a concern?

_____

_____

_____

4. List and describe the three major mechanisms of cellular injury.

_____

_____

_____

5. Oxidative stress has been implicated as the causative agent in numerous disease states and the cause of physiological aging. Explain how oxidative stress can cause damage and why it is a concern.

_____

_____

_____

6. Explain why one of the complications of hypoxia is the development of acidosis and how acidosis will damage the tissue.

_____

_____

_____

7. Apoptosis occurs under normal stimulation or as the result of cellular injury. There are two pathways for apoptosis to occur. What are they, and what major protein is involved?

_____

_____

_____

SECTION III: APPLYING YOUR KNOWLEDGE

Activity E *Consider the following scenario and answer the question.*

A 50-year-old male is about to receive chemotherapy drugs for a tumor in his liver. He states that he has heard that chemotherapy drugs can hurt normal cells in his body and cells in his tumor. The client asks how this happens.

1. How can chemotherapy drugs injure normal cells?

_____

_____

_____

SECTION IV: PRACTICING FOR NCLEX

Activity F *Answer the following questions.*

1. Many molecular mechanisms mediate cellular adaptation. Some are factors produced by other cells, and some are produced by the cells themselves. These mechanisms depend largely on signals transmitted by chemical messengers that exert their effects by altering the function of a gene. Many adaptive cellular responses alter the expression of "differentiation" genes. What can cells do because of this?

    a. A cell is able to change size or form without compromising its normal function.

    b. A cell incorporates its change in function and passes this change on to other cells like it.

    c. A cell is able to pass its change on to a "housekeeping" cell.

    d. A cell dies once the stimulus to change has been removed.

2. Hypertrophy may occur as the result of normal physiologic or abnormal pathologic conditions. The increase in muscle mass associated with exercise is an example of physiologic hypertrophy. Pathologic hypertrophy occurs as the result of disease conditions and may be adaptive or compensatory. Examples of adaptive hypertrophy are the thickening of the urinary bladder from long-continued obstruction of urinary outflow and the myocardial hypertrophy that results from valvular heart disease or hypertension. What is compensatory hypertrophy?

    a. When the body increases its major organs during times of malnutrition

    b. When one kidney is removed, the remaining kidney enlarges to compensate for the loss

    c. When the body controls myocardial growth by stimulating actin expression to enlarge the heart

    d. When the body stimulates gene expression to begin a progressive decrease in left ventricular muscle mass

3. Metastatic calcification occurs in normal tissues as the result of increased serum calcium levels (hypercalcemia). Anything that increases the serum calcium level can lead to calcification in inappropriate places such as the lung, renal tubules, and blood vessels. What are the major causes of hypercalcemia?

    a. Diabetes mellitus and Paget disease

    b. Hypoparathyroidism and vitamin D intoxication

    c. Hyperparathyroidism and immobilization

    d. Immobilization and hypoparathyroidism

4. Mercury is a toxic substance, and the hazards of mercury-associated occupational and accidental exposures are well known. What is the primary concern for the general public in regard to mercury poisoning today?

    a. Amalgam fillings in the teeth

    b. Mercury from thermometers and blood pressure machines

    c. Mercury found in paint that was made before 1990

    d. Fish such as tuna and swordfish

5. Small amounts of lead accumulate to reach toxic levels in the human body. Lead is found in many places in the environment and is still a major concern in the pediatric population. What would you teach the parents of a child who is being tested for lead poisoning?

    a. Keep your child away from peeling paint.

    b. Keep your child away from anything ceramic.

    c. Do not let your child read newspapers.

    d. Do not let your child tour a mine on a school field trip.

6. In a genetic disorder called xeroderma pigmentosum, an enzyme needed to repair sunlight-induced DNA damage is lacking. This autosomal recessive disorder is characterized by what?

    a. Patches of pink, leathery pigmentation that replace normal skin after a sunburn

    b. Extreme photosensitivity and a greatly increased risk of skin cancer in sun-exposed skin

    c. White, scaly patches of skin that appear on African American people after they have a sunburn

d. Photosensitivity and a decreased risk of skin cancer in sun-exposed skin

7. While presenting a talk to the parents of preschoolers at a local day care center, the nurse is asked about electrical injury to the body. What should she include in her response? Mark all that apply.

a. In electrical injuries, the body acts as a deflector of the electrical current.

b. In electrical injuries, the body acts as a conductor of the electrical current.

c. The most severe damage is caused by lightning and high-voltage wires.

d. When a person touches an electrical source, the current passes through the body and exits to another receptor.

8. A man presents to the emergency room after being out in below zero weather all night. He asks the nurse why the health care team is concerned about his toes and feet. How would the nurse respond?

a. Cold causes injury to the cells in the body by injuring the blood vessels, making them leak into the surrounding tissue.

b. After being out in the cold all night, his toes and feet are frozen, and it will be very painful to warm them again; in addition, the health care team is concerned that he might be a drug addict.

c. "It is obvious that you are a homeless person, and we were wondering how often this has happened to you before and when it will happen again."

d. "Your toes and feet are frozen, and there is a concern about the formation of blood clots as we warm them again."

9. Clinical manifestations of radiation injury result from acute cell injury, dose-dependent changes in the blood vessels that supply the irradiated tissues, and fibrotic tissue replacement. What are these clinical manifestations?

a. Radiation cystitis, dermatitis, and diarrhea from enteritis

b. Dermatitis, diarrhea from enteritis, and hunger

c. Diarrhea from enteritis, hunger, and muscle spasms

d. Radiation cystitis, diarrhea from enteritis, and muscle spasms

10. Biologic agents differ from other injurious agents in that they are able to replicate and can continue to produce their injurious effects. How do gram-negative bacteria cause harm to the cell?

a. Gram-negative bacilli excrete elaborate exotoxins that interfere with cellular production of ATP.

b. Gram-negative bacilli release endotoxins that cause cell injury and increased capillary permeability.

c. Gram-negative bacilli enter the cell and disrupt its ability to replicate.

d. Gram-negative bacilli cannot cause harm to the cell; only gram-positive bacilli can harm the cell.

11. When confronted with a decrease in work demands or adverse environmental conditions, most cells are able to revert to a smaller size and a lower and more efficient level of functioning that is compatible with survival. This decrease in cell size is called _____.

12. Match the pigments (Column A) with their description (Column B).

Column A	Column B
___ 1. Icterus	a. A yellow discoloration of tissue
___ 2. Lipofuscin	b. A blue lead line along the margins of the gum
___ 3. Carbon	c. A brown or dark-brown pigment found in the skin and hair
___ 4. Melanin	d. A yellow-brown pigment that accumulates in neurons

13. Match the type of agent causing cell injury (Column A) to the example (Column B).

Column A	Column B
___ 1. Physical agent	a. Submicroscopic viruses
___ 2. Chemical agent	b. Mechanical forces that produce tissue trauma
___ 3. Biologic agent	c. Free radicals
___ 4. Nutritional factor	d. Vitamin B deficiency

14. You are a nurse preparing an educational event for a group of single parents. You are going to talk about drugs and the damage they can cause to the body. You would know to include which of these? Mark all that apply.

a. Acetaminophen and aspirin

b. Immunosuppressant drugs

c. Alcohol and cigarettes

d. Vitamin supplements and antineoplastic drugs

Genetic Control of Cell Function and Inheritance

SECTION I: LEARNING OBJECTIVES

1. Describe the structure and function of DNA

2. Relate the mechanisms of DNA repair to the development of a gene mutation

3. Describe the function of messenger RNA, ribosomal RNA, and transfer RNA as they relate to protein synthesis

4. Cite the effects of post-translational processing on protein structure and function

5. Explain the role of transcription factors in regulating gene activity

6. Define the terms *autosomes*, *chromatin*, *meiosis*, and *mitosis*

7. List the steps in constructing a karyotype using cytogenetic studies

8. Explain the significance of the Barr body

9. Construct a hypothetical pedigree for a recessive and dominant trait according to Mendel's laws

10. Contrast genotype and phenotype

11. Define the terms *allele*, *locus*, *expressivity*, and *penetrance*

12. Differentiate between genetic and physical genomic maps

13. Briefly describe the methods used in linkage studies, dosage studies, and hybridization studies

14. Describe the goals of the International HapMap Project

15. Describe the process of recombinant DNA technology

16. Characterize the process of RNA interference

SECTION II: ASSESSING YOUR UNDERSTANDING

Activity A *Fill in the blank.*

1. Our genetic information is stored in the structure of _____ acid.

2. _____ acid serves as the template for protein synthesis.

3. The complete set of proteins encoded by the genome is known as the _____.

4. A precise complementary pairing of _____ and _____ bases occurs in the double-stranded DNA molecule.

5. DNA replication is semiconservative, meaning that the parental DNA strands dissociate and pair with _____ strands to complete mitosis.

6. Human somatic cells contain _____ pairs of different chromosomes.

7. In the nucleus, DNA is in the form of _____, and during mitosis, it condenses into _____.

8. The genetic code is _____ repeat of bases.

9. Errors in DNA duplication are known as _____.

10. A _____ represents the variations in the genetic code that are responsible for the differences between individuals.

11. Messenger RNA is formed in the process of _____.

12. The coding sequence of an mRNA molecule is known as _____.

13. MRNA undergoes the process of _____ to form a protein in the cytosol.

14. Molecular _____ assist in the folding of proteins into their three-dimensional conformation.

15. The degree to which a gene or particular group of genes is activated is termed gene _____.

16. Sonic _____ is a gene that participates in the left-to-right axis responsible for the rostral-caudal orientation of the nervous system.

17. Achondroplasia is a condition characterized by short stature with limbs that are disproportionately shorter than the trunk and caused by mutations or altered levels of _____ growth factors.

18. The pattern of gene expression and the outward presentation is the _____.

19. The position of a gene on a chromosome is called its _____, and alternate forms of a gene at the same locus are called _____.

20. A _____ is a graphic method for portraying family history of an inherited trait.

Activity B *Match the key terms in Column A with their definitions in Column B.*

1.

Column A	Column B
____ 1. tRNA	a. Used to align amino acids with ribosomes for the formation of protein
____ 2. Transcription factors	b. Ability of a gene to express its function
____ 3. Penetrance	c. Initiate and regulate transcription
____ 4. mRNA	d. Manner in which the gene is expressed
____ 5. Mitosis	e. Template that is copied from DNA
____ 6. Meiosis	f. Replicating germ cells
____ 7. Expressivity	g. Multiple alleles at different loci affect the outcome
____ 8. Chromosomes	h. Organized and condensed DNA
____ 9. Multifactorial inheritance	i. One pair of genes is involved in the transmission of information
____ 10. Single gene inheritance	j. Duplication of somatic cells

2.

Column A	Column B
____ 1. Collaborative genes	a. More than one allele affects the same trait
____ 2. Multiple alleles	b. One gene masks the phenotypic effects of another nonallelic gene
____ 3. Complementary genes	c. Each gene is mutually dependent on the other
____ 4. Epistasis	d. Two different genes influencing the same trait interact to produce a phenotype neither gene alone could produce
____ 5. Alleles	e. Alternate forms of a gene at the same locus

Activity C *Sequencing*

1. The processing of genetic material involves many well-organized steps. Put the following in order starting at transcription and ending with the three-dimensional protein.

    a. Transcription

    b. Translation begins

    c. mRNA moves to cytosol

    d. mRNA is read by ribosome complex

    e. Posttranslational processing

    f. tRNA moves to ribosome

    g. Ribosomal subunits come together

    h. Formation of peptide bonds

    i. Final 3D protein structure

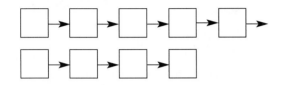

Activity D *Briefly answer the following.*

1. Gregor Mendel was the first to study and characterize inheritance. Explain what he did and what he discovered.

    _____

    _____

    _____

2. Genetic mapping is done to allow us to know the position of certain genes and sequences on the chromosomes. Explain the difference between genetic maps and physical maps. In your explanation, describe the basic methodology used to construct these maps.

    _____

    _____

    _____

3. During meiosis, a process takes place that increases genetic variability. Explain how this occurs. Is it a good or bad thing?

    _____

    _____

    _____

4. Humans have both somatic and sex chromosomes. How many of each do we have, and where do they originate?

    _____

    _____

    _____

5. Only about 2% of the genome encodes instructions for synthesis of proteins. The remainder consists of noncoding regions that serve to determine where, when, and in what quantity proteins are made. Explain how this occurs, and describe its significance.

    _____

    _____

    _____

SECTION III: APPLYING YOUR KNOWLEDGE

Activity E *Consider the following scenario and answer the question.*

Jessica Jones, an adopted child, has been searching for her parents for many years. She believes that she has finally found her father but wants to be 100% sure before she approaches him.

1. Is there any way for her to absolutely identify her father before she meets him? Discuss the use of DNA fingerprinting to identify familial relationships.

    _____

    _____

    _____

SECTION IV: PRACTICING FOR NCLEX

Activity F *Answer the following questions.*

1. It is the proteins that the genes encode that make up the majority of cellular structures and perform most life functions. What is the term used to define the complete set of proteins encoded by a genome?
   a. Proteome
   b. Protogene
   c. Nucleotomics
   d. Chromosome

2. Below are the steps in cell replication. Put them in the correct order.
   a. Complementary molecule is duplicated next to each original strand.
   b. Two strands of DNA separate.
   c. Mitosis occurs.
   d. Two strands become four strands.

   A. a, c, b, d
   B. b, a, d, c
   C. b, d, a, c
   D. d, b, c, a

3. Chromosomes contain all the genetic content of the genome. There are 23 pairs of different chromosomes in each somatic cell, half from the mother and half from the father. One of those chromosomes is the sex chromosome. What are the other 22 pairs of chromosomes called?
   a. Ribosomes
   b. Helixes
   c. Autosomes
   d. Haploids

4. On rare occasions, accidental errors in duplication of DNA occur. What are these called?
   a. Codons
   b. Ribosomes
   c. Endonucleases
   d. Mutations

5. Most human traits are determined by multiple pairs of genes, many with alternate codes accounting for some dissimilar forms that occur with certain genetic disorders. What type of inheritance involves multiple genes at different loci, with each gene exerting a small additive effect in determining a trait?
   a. Polygenic inheritance
   b. Multifactorial inheritance
   c. Monofactorial inheritance
   d. Collaborative inheritance

6. Two syndromes exhibit mental retardation as a common feature. Both disorders have the same deletion in chromosome 15. When the deletion is inherited from the mother, the infant presents with one syndrome; when the same deletion is inherited from the father, Prader-Willi syndrome results. What is the syndrome when the deletion is inherited from the mother?
   a. Turner syndrome
   b. Angelman syndrome
   c. Down syndrome
   d. Fragile X syndrome

7. Homozygotes are what people are called in whom the two alleles of a given pair are the same (AA or aa). Heterozygotes are what people who have different alleles (Aa) at a gene locus are called. What kind of trait is expressed only in homozygous pairing?
   a. Dominant trait
   b. Single-gene trait
   c. Recessive trait
   d. Penetrant trait

8. The International HapMap Project was created with two goals. One is the development of methods for applying the technology of these projects to the diagnosis and treatment of disease. The other is to map which of the many closely related single nucleotide polymorphisms in the human genome?
   a. Codons
   b. Triplet code
   c. Alleles
   d. Haplotypes

9. DNA fingerprinting is based in part on recombinant DNA technology and, in part, on those techniques originally used in medical genetics to detect slight variations in the genomes of different individuals. These techniques are used in forensic pathology to compare specimens from the suspect and the

forensic specimen. What is being compared when DNA fingerprinting is used in forensic pathology?

a. Banding pattern

b. Triplet code

c. Haplotypes

d. Chromosomes

10. There are two main approaches used in gene therapy: Transferred genes can replace defective genes, or they can selectively inhibit deleterious genes. What are the compounds usually used in gene therapy?

a. mRNA sequences

b. Cloned DNA sequences

c. Sterically stable liposomes

d. Single nucleotide polymorphisms

11. The human genome sequence is almost exactly (99.9%) the same in all people. What is believed to account for the differences in each human's behaviors, physical traits, and their susceptibility to disease is the small variation (0.01%) in gene sequence. This is termed a _____.

12. Like DNA, RNA is a long string of nucleotides encased in a large molecule. However, there are three aspects of its structure that makes it different from DNA. What are these aspects? Mark all that apply.

a. RNA's double strand is missing one pair of chromosomes.

b. The sugar in each nucleotide of RNA is ribose.

c. RNA is a single-stranded molecule.

d. RNA's thymine base is replaced by uracil.

13. One of the first products to be produced using recombinant DNA technology was human _____.

14. Cytogenetics is the study of the structure and numeric characteristics of the cell's chromosomes. Chromosome studies can be done on any tissue or cell that grows and divides in culture. What are the characteristics of a chromosomal study? Mark all that apply.

a. The completed picture of a chromosomal study is called karyotyping.

b. Human chromosomes are divided into three types according to the position of the centromere.

c. Special laboratory techniques are used to culture body cell. They are then fixed and stained to display identifiable banding patterns.

d. Complementary genes and collaborative genes are easily recognized.

15. Genetics has its own set of definitions. Match the word with its definition.

____ 1. Genotype

____ 2. Phenotype

____ 3. Pharmacogenetics

____ 4. Somatic cell hybridization

____ 5. Penetrance

a. Traits, physical or biochemical, associated with a specific genotype that are recognizable

b. How drugs respond to an individual's inherited characteristics

c. Genetic information contained in the base sequence triplet code

d. Ability of a gene to express its function

e. Fusion of human somatic cells with those of a different species to yield a cell containing the chromosomes of both species

CHAPTER 7

Genetic and Congenital Disorders

SECTION I: LEARNING OBJECTIVES

1. Define the terms *congenital, allele, gene locus, gene mutation, genotype, phenotype, homozygous, heterozygous, polymorphism, gene penetrance,* and *gene expression*

2. Describe three types of single-gene disorders and their patterns of inheritance

3. Explain the genetic abnormality responsible for the fragile X syndrome

4. Contrast disorders due to multifactorial inheritance with those caused by single-gene inheritance

5. Describe three patterns of chromosomal breakage and rearrangement

6. Trace the events that occur during meiosis and explain the events that lead to trisomy or monosomy

7. Describe the chromosomal and major clinical characteristics of Down, Turner, and Klinefelter syndromes

8. State the primary mechanism of altered body function in mitochondrial gene disorders and relate it to the frequent involvement of neural and muscular tissues

9. Cite the most susceptible period of intrauterine life for development of defects due to environmental agents

10. State the cautions that should be observed when considering use of drugs during pregnancy, including the possible effects of alcohol abuse, vitamin A derivatives, and folic acid deficiency on fetal development

11. List four infectious agents that cause congenital defects

12. Describe the process of genetic assessment

13. Cite the rationale for prenatal diagnosis

14. Describe methods used in arriving at a prenatal diagnosis, including ultrasonography, amniocentesis, chorionic villus sampling, percutaneous umbilical fetal blood sampling, and laboratory methods to determine the biochemical and genetic makeup of the fetus

SECTION II: ASSESSING YOUR UNDERSTANDING

Activity A *Fill in the blanks.*

1. _____ defects, also known as birth defects, are abnormalities of structure, function, or metabolism that are present at birth.

2. Genetic disorders are caused either by an alteration in _____ that disrupts the single-gene sequence or _____ rearrangements.

3. Genes are expressed in an individual as dominant, recessive, or _____ pairs of alleles.

4. A gene _____ is a biochemical event, such as nucleotide change, deletion, or insertion, that produces a new allele.

5. Genetic disorders arise in two ways: _____ from parents or _____ due to an acquired mutation.

6. Someone who carries a gene responsible for a disease but who does not manifest the disease is said to be a _____.

7. _____ syndrome is an autosomal dominant disorder of connective tissue.

8. X-linked inheritance patterns are predominantly _____.

9. Specific chromosomal abnormalities can be linked to more than _____ identifiable syndromes.

10. Chromosomal disorders may take the form of alterations in the _____ of one or more chromosomes or in an _____ number of chromosomes.

11. _____ occurs when there are simultaneous breaks in two chromosomes from different pairs, with exchange of chromosome parts. In the reciprocal type, there is no loss of information.

Activity B *Consider the following figures.*

1.

In the figure, label the abnormality (deletion, ring formation, isochromosomal translocation, Robertsonian translocation, inversion, balanced translocation).

2.

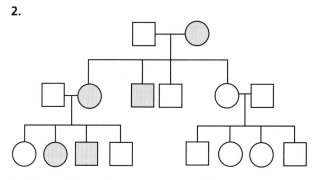

Is this pedigree for an autosomal dominant, autosomal recessive, or sex-linked disease?

Activity C *Match the key concepts in Column A with their descriptions in Column B.*

Column A

_____ 1. Single-gene disorders

_____ 2. Multifactorial inheritance

_____ 3. Autosomal dominant disorder

_____ 4. Haploid

_____ 5. Chromosomal abnormality

_____ 6. Autosomal recessive

_____ 7. Polymorphism

_____ 8. Phenotype

_____ 9. Mutation

_____ 10. Mitochondrial disorders

Column B

a. Single set of chromosomes

b. Disorders are manifested only when both members of the gene pair are affected

c. Traits carried by multiple genes and influenced by the environment

d. Outward expression of a gene

e. Affected parent has a 50% chance of transmitting the disorder to each offspring

f. Follow a non-Mendelian pattern of inheritance

g. Trisomy

h. Disorders caused by a defective or mutant allele at a single-gene locus

i. Biochemical event such as nucleotide change, deletion, or insertion

j. Genes have more than one normal allele at the same locus

Activity D *Briefly answer the following questions.*

1. Inheritance of a genetic disease depends on the location of the mutation within the karyotype. What are the potential methods of inheritance? What will determine the likelihood of the offspring developing the disease? Does the sex of the offspring make any difference?

_____

_____

_____

2. Multifactorial inheritance patterns involve many different genes and their interactions with the environment. Predicting such disorders is difficult, but they do display several characteristics. Explain these characteristics.

_____

_____

_____

3. Chromosomal abnormalities are among the most common reasons for first trimester spontaneous abortions as well as more than 60 different diseases. Structural changes are a common form of chromosomal abnormalities. Explain what a structural change is and list the potential causes.

_____

_____

_____

4. Why are alterations in sex chromosomes better tolerated than alterations of autosomal chromosomes?

_____

_____

_____

5. Mitochondrial genetic abnormalities are not transmitted via Mendelian genetics. In addition, they tend to affect the brain and muscle tissue. Explain why these two characteristics of mtDNA inheritance are true.

_____

_____

_____

SECTION III: APPLYING YOUR KNOWLEDGE

Activity E *Consider the following scenario and answer the questions.*

A 37-year-old woman is 2 months pregnant and has a history of alcohol intake of one to two drinks per day. She states, "My coworker told me that drinking alcohol can harm my baby."

1. She asks you how having a drink or two every day can harm her baby. What would you respond?

   _____

   _____

   _____

2. Discuss the effects of fetal alcohol syndrome.

   _____

   _____

   _____

SECTION IV: PRACTICING FOR NCLEX

Activity F *Answer the following questions.*

1. Chromosomes carry 46 genes, 23 from the mother and 23 from the father. These genes are paired, and if both members of the gene pair are identical, the person is considered homozygous. What is the person considered if both members of the gene pair are not identical?
   a. Heterozygous
   b. Phenotypic
   c. Codominant
   d. Mutant

2. An adolescent presents at the clinic with complaints of pedunculated lesions projecting from the skin on his trunk area. The nurse knows that this is a sign of what?
   a. Marfan syndrome
   b. Neurofibromatosis type 1
   c. Down syndrome
   d. Klinefelter syndrome

3. The parents of an infant boy ask the nurse why their son was born with a cleft lip and palate. The nurse responds that cleft lip and palate are defects that are caused by many factors. The defect may also be caused by teratogens. Which teratogens can cause cleft lip and palate?
   a. Mumps
   b. Pertussis
   c. Rubella
   d. Measles

4. Sometimes an individual that developed from a single zygote is found to have two or more kinds of genetically different cell populations. These individuals are called what?
   a. Mutants
   b. Monosomies
   c. Aneuploidy
   d. Mosaic

5. With increasing age, there is a greater chance of a woman being exposed to damaging environmental agents such as drugs, chemicals, and radiation. These factors may act on the aging oocyte to cause what in a fetus?
   a. Down syndrome
   b. Marfan syndrome
   c. Patau syndrome
   d. Turner syndrome

6. From 15 to 60 days after conception, the embryo is most susceptible to adverse influences. This period is referred to as what?
   a. Period of susceptibility
   b. Period of organogenesis
   c. Period of fetal anomalies
   d. Period of hormonal imbalance

7. Teratogenic substances cause abnormalities during embryonic and fetal development. These substances are divided into three classes. These classes are called what?
   a. Period of organogenesis, third trimester, second month
   b. Outside environmental substances, inside environmental substances, internal environmental substances
   c. Radiation, drugs and chemical substances, infectious agents
   d. Drugs and chemical substances, smoking, bacteria and viruses

8. Infections with the TORCH agents are reported to occur in 1% to 5% of newborn infants in the United States and are among the major causes of neonatal morbidity and mortality. Which of these are clinical and pathologic manifestations of TORCH?

   a. Microcephaly, hydrocephalus, spina bifida

   b. Pneumonitis, myocarditis, macrocephaly

   c. Hydrocephalus, macrocephaly, thrombocytopenia

   d. Microcephaly, hydrocephalus, thrombocytopenia

9. The birth of a child with a defect brings with it two issues that must be resolved quickly. The traumatized parents need emotional support from the nurse and guidance in how to resolve these two issues. What are these issues?

   a. The immediate and future care of the affected child and the possibility of future children in the family having a similar defect

   b. The immediate and future care of the affected child and the possibility of the child's death

   c. The possibility of future children having a similar defect and the possibility of this child's death

   d. The need for financial resources and the possibility of this child's death

10. Genetic counseling and prenatal screening are tools both for the parents of a child with a defect and for those couples who want a child but are at high risk for having a child with a genetic problem. What are the objectives of prenatal screening?

    a. To detect fetal abnormalities and to provide information on where they can have the pregnancy terminated if they so choose

    b. To detect fetal abnormalities and to provide parents with information needed to make an informed choice about having a child with an abnormality

    c. To provide parents with information needed to make an informed choice about having a child with an abnormality and to assure the prospective parents that any defect in their hoped for child can be identified

    d. To allow parents at risk for having a child with a specific defect to begin a pregnancy with the assurance that knowledge about the presence or absence of the disorder in the fetus can be confirmed by testing and to provide information on where they can have the pregnancy terminated if they so choose

11. Match the genetic disorder (Column A) with its kind of disorder (Column B).

Column A	Column B
____ 1. Marfan syndrome	a. Single-gene disorder
____ 2. Huntington's chorea	b. Autosomal dominant
____ 3. Tay-Sachs disease	c. Autosomal recessive disorders
____ 4. Fragile X syndrome	d. Sex-linked disorders

12. Although multifactorial traits cannot be predicted with the same degree of accuracy as the Mendelian single-gene mutations, characteristic patterns exist. What are these characteristic patterns? Mark all that apply.

    a. Multifactorial congenital malformations tend to involve a single organ or tissue derived from the same embryonic developmental field.

    b. The risk of recurrence in future pregnancies is for the same or a similar defect.

    c. The risk increases with increasing incidence of the defect among relatives.

    d. Multifactorial congenital malformations are always present at birth.

13. _____ is a rare metabolic disorder that affects approximately 1 in every 15,000 infants in the United States. The disorder is caused by a deficiency of the liver enzyme phenylalanine hydroxylase. Without a special diet, these children will die.

14. After conception, development is influenced by the environmental factors that the embryo shares with the mother. Some of these factors can act on the developing fetus and cause defects. These factors include which of the following? Mark all that apply.

   a. Drugs

   b. Weather

   c. Air pollution

   d. Radiation

15. The U.S. Food and Drug Administration passed a law in 1983 classifying drugs according to their proven teratogenicity. Listed as follows are the classes of drugs in random order. Put them in order according to their teratogenicity.

   a. Class X   **A.** b, d, c, e, a

   b. Class A   **B.** a, b, c, d, e

   c. Class C   **C.** b, c, d, a, e

   d. Class B   **D.** a, e, b, c, d

   e. Class D

CHAPTER 8

Neoplasia

SECTION I: LEARNING OBJECTIVES

1. Define *neoplasm* and explain how neoplastic growth differs from the normal adaptive changes seen in atrophy, hypertrophy, and hyperplasia

2. Distinguish between cell proliferation and differentiation

3. Describe the phases of the cell cycle

4. Explain the function of cyclins, cyclin-dependent kinases, and cyclin-dependent kinase inhibitors in terms of regulating the cell cycle

5. Describe the properties of stem cells

6. Cite the method used for naming benign and malignant neoplasms

7. State at least five ways in which benign and malignant neoplasms differ

8. Relate the properties of cell differentiation to the development of a cancer cell clone and the behavior of the tumor

9. Trace the pathway for hematologic spread of a metastatic cancer cell

10. Use the concepts of growth fraction and doubling time to explain the growth of cancerous tissue

11. Describe various types of cancer-associated genes and cancer-associated cellular and molecular pathways

12. Describe genetic events and epigenetic factors that are important in tumorigenesis

13. State the importance of cancer stem cells, angiogenesis, and the cell microenvironment in cancer growth and metastasis

14. Explain how host factors such as heredity, levels of endogenous hormones, and immune system function increase the risk for development of selected cancers

15. Relate the effects of environmental factors such as chemical carcinogens, radiation, and oncogenic viruses to the risk of cancer development

16. Identify concepts and hypotheses that may explain the processes by which normal cells are transformed into cancer cells by carcinogens

17. Describe the many possible ways by which cancer acts to disrupt organ function

18. Characterize the mechanisms involved in the anorexia and cachexia, fatigue and sleep disorders, anemia, and venous thrombosis experienced by patients with cancer

19. Define the term *paraneoplastic syndrome* and explain its pathogenesis and manifestations

20. Cite three characteristics of an ideal screening test for cancer.

21. Describe the four methods that are used in the diagnosis of cancer

22. Differentiate between the methods used for grading and staging of cancers.

23. Explain the mechanism by which radiation exerts its beneficial effects in the treatment of cancer

24. Describe the adverse effects of radiation therapy

25. Differentiate between the action of direct DNA-interacting and indirect DNA-interacting chemotherapeutic agents and cell cycle–specific and cell cycle–independent drugs

26. Describe the three mechanisms whereby biotherapy exerts its effects

27. Describe three examples of targeted therapy used in the treatment of cancer

28. Cite the most common types of cancer affecting infants, children, and adolescents

29. Describe how cancers that affect children differ from those that affect adults.

30. Discuss possible long-term effects of radiation therapy and chemotherapy on adult survivors of childhood cancer

SECTION II: ASSESSING YOUR UNDERSTANDING

Activity A *Fill in the blanks.*

1. Cancer is a disorder of altered cell _____ and _____.

2. The process of cell division results in cellular _____.

3. _____ is the process of specialization whereby new cells acquire the structure and function of the cells they replace.

4. Proteins called _____ control entry and progression of cells through the cell cycle.

5. Kinases are enzymes that _____ proteins.

6. Continually renewing cell populations rely on _____ cells of the same lineage that have not yet differentiated to the extent that they have lost their ability to divide.

7. _____ cells remain incompletely undifferentiated throughout life.

8. _____ stem cells are pluripotent cells derived from the inner cell mass of the blastocyst stage of the embryo.

9. The term _____ refers to an abnormal mass of tissue in which the growth exceeds

and is uncoordinated with that of the normal tissues.

10. _____ tumors do not usually cause death unless the location interferes with the function of a vital organ.

11. Malignant neoplasms are less well _____ and have the ability to break loose, enter the circulatory or lymphatic systems, and form secondary malignant tumors at other sites.

12. Tumors are usually named by adding the suffix _____ to the parenchymal tissue type from which the growth originated.

13. A _____ is growth that projects from a mucosal surface.

14. The term _____ is used to designate a malignant tumor of epithelial tissue origin.

15. There are two categories of malignant neoplasms, _____ and _____ cancers.

16. The term _____ is used to describe the loss of cell differentiation in cancerous tissue.

17. A characteristic of cancer cells is the ability to proliferate even in the absence of _____.

18. The _____ complex acting with other proteins has been proposed to be involved with cell migration, apoptosis, and cell cycle regulation.

19. The types of genes involved in cancer are numerous, with two main categories being the _____, which control cell growth and replication, and tumor _____ genes, which are growth-inhibiting regulatory genes.

20. _____ is the only known retrovirus to cause cancer in humans.

21. Tumor cells must double _____ times before a palpable mass is formed.

22. A common manifestation of solid tumors is the cancer _____ syndrome.

23. As cancers grow, they compress and erode blood vessels, causing _____ and _____, along with frank bleeding and sometimes hemorrhage.

24. _____ is a common side effect of many cancers. It is related to blood loss, hemolysis, impaired red cell production, or treatment effects.

25. A tissue _____ involves the removal of a tissue specimen for microscopic study.

26. _____ therapy uses high-energy particles or waves to destroy or damage cancer cells.

27. _____ is a systemic treatment that enables drugs to reach the site of the tumor and other distant sites.

Activity B *Consider the following figure.*

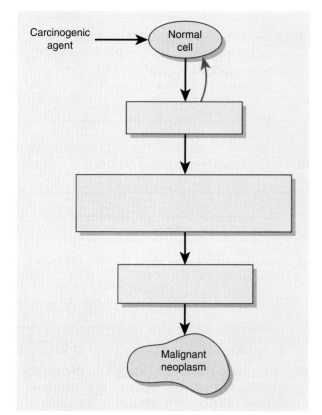

1. In the flowchart, fill in the missing steps using the following terms: *DNA damage, alterations in genes that control apoptosis, unregulated cell differentiation and growth, inactivation of tumor suppressor genes, activation of growth-promoting oncogenes, DNA repair, failure of DNA repair.*

Activity C *Match the key terms in Column A with their definitions in Column B.*

1.

Column A	Column B
___ 1. Malignant mass	a. Defines the differentiation potential of stem cells
___ 2. Cellular potency	b. Undefined or less differentiated cellular mass
___ 3. Renewal	c. Mass of cells due to overgrowth
___ 4. Proliferation	d. Process that removes senescent and/or damaged cells
___ 5. Tumor-initiating cells	e. Stem cells undergoing numerous mitotic divisions while maintaining an undifferentiated state
___ 6. Tumor	f. Cancer stem cells
___ 7. Apoptosis	g. Process of cell specialization
___ 8. Benign mass	h. Well-differentiated mass of cells
___ 9. Differentiation	i. Study of tumors and their treatment
___ 10. Oncology	j. Process of cell division

2.

Column A	Column B
___ 1. Protooncogene	a. Loss of cell differentiation
___ 2. Growth fraction	b. Changes in gene expression without DNA mutation
___ 3. Tumor suppressor gene	c. Variations in size and shape of both the cell and the nucleus
___ 4. Genetic instability	d. Normal gene that can cause cancer if mutated
___ 5. Epigenetic effects	e. Promote cancer when less active
___ 6. Anaplasia	f. Ratio of dividing cells to resting cells
___ 7. Anchorage dependence	g. Tumor suppressor gene
___ 8. Doubling time	h. Marked by chromosomal aberrations

_____ **9.** Pleomor-
       phism

_____ **10.** p53

i. Epithelial cells must be anchored to either neighboring cells or the underlying extracellular matrix to live and grow

j. Time it takes for the total mass of cells in a tumor to double

5. Explain how a diminished immune system may play a role in carcinogenesis.

_____

_____

_____

6. Chemical carcinogens act in two distinct ways, what are they?

_____

_____

_____

Activity D

1. Put the following terms for cellular potency in order from the least differentiated to the most differentiated.

a. Pluripotent

b. Totipotent

c. Unipotent

d. Multipotent

Activity E   *Briefly answer the following*

1. Not all cells in the body can reenter the cell cycle, but some will do so continuously. In terms of regeneration and differentiation, which types of cells will or will not reenter the cell cycle?

_____

_____

_____

2. Compare and contrast benign tumors and malignant tumors.

_____

_____

_____

3. List the five factors used to describe benign and malignant neoplasm.

_____

_____

_____

4. Describe the process and routes of metastasis.

_____

_____

_____

7. Cachexia is marked by a hypermetabolic state. Give two reasons for this, and explain the consequences.

_____

_____

_____

8. What is paraneoplastic syndrome?

_____

_____

_____

9. List some of the common methods used for diagnosing cancer.

_____

_____

_____

10. Cancers are graded and staged on their characteristics in order to determine a treatment regimen. Explain the grading and staging system and how it is met.

_____

_____

_____

SECTION III: APPLYING YOUR KNOWLEDGE

Activity F   *Consider the following scenario and answer the questions.*

Eight-year-old Joe Cheapson has been diagnosed with acute lymphocytic leukemia. His treatment plan includes placement of an implanted central venous catheter and multiple administrations of chemotherapy. Joe says, "NO! I don't want to be stuck with needles all the time."

1. What would you tell Joe to decrease his anxiety?

_____

_____

_____

2. How would you explain the way chemotherapy works to Joe's parents?

_____

_____

_____

SECTION IV: PRACTICING FOR NCLEX

Activity G *Answer the following questions.*

1. The nurse has provided an educational session with a 56-year-old man, newly diagnosed with a benign tumor of the colon. The nurse knows that the patient needs further teaching when he makes which remark?
   a. "This tumor I have, will I die from it?"
   b. "Even though benign tumors cannot stop growing, they are not considered to be cancer."
   c. "Benign tumors still produce normal cells different from other cells around them."
   d. "This kind of tumor cannot invade other organs or travel to other places in the body to start new tumors."

2. The nurse on an oncology floor has just admitted a patient with metastatic cancer. The patient asks how cancer moves from one place in the body to another. What would the nurse answer?
   a. "Cancer cells are not able to float around the original tumor in body fluids."
   b. "Cancer cells enter the body's lymph system and thereby spread to other parts of the body."
   c. "Cancer cells are moved from one place in the body to another by transporter cells."
   d. "Cancer cells replicate and form a chain that spreads from the original tumor site to the site of the metastatic lesion."

3. It is well known that cancer is not a single disease. Thus, it follows that cancer does not have a single cause. It seems more likely that the occurrence of cancer is triggered by the interactions of multiple risk factors. What are identified risk factors for cancer?
   a. Body type, age, hereditary
   b. Radiation, cancer-causing viruses, color of skin
   c. Hormonal factors, chemicals, immunologic mechanisms
   d. Immunologic mechanisms, cancer-causing viruses, color of skin

4. Several cancers have been identified as inheritable through an autosomal dominant gene. Generally, people who inherit these genes are only at increased risk for developing the cancer. There is one type of cancer, however, that is almost certain to develop in someone who inherits the dominant gene. Which cancer carries the highest risk of developing in someone who carries the gene?
   a. Retinoblastoma
   b. Osteosarcoma
   c. Acute lymphocytic leukemia
   d. Colon cancer

5. One group of chemical carcinogens is called indirect-reacting agents. Another term for these agents is procarcinogens, which become active only after metabolic conversion. One of the most potent procarcinogens is a group of dietary carcinogens called
   a. Polycyclic aromatic hydrocarbons.
   b. Aflatoxins.
   c. Initiators.
   d. Diethylstilbestrol.

6. In some cancers, the presenting factor is an effusion, or fluid, in the pleural, pericardial, or peritoneal space. Research has found that almost 50% of undiagnosed effusions in people not known to have cancer turn out to be malignant. Which cancers are often found because of effusions?
   a. Colon and rectal cancers
   b. Lung and ovarian cancers
   c. Breast and colon cancers
   d. Ovarian and rectal cancers

7. Tumor markers are used for screening, establishing prognosis, monitoring treatment, and detecting recurrent disease. Which serum tumor markers have been proven to be among the most useful in clinical practice?

   a. Prostate-specific antigen and deoxyribonucleic acid

   b. Deoxyribonucleic acid and carcinoembryonic antigen

   c. Alpha-fetoprotein and human chorionic gonadotropin

   d. Chorionic gonadotropin and cyclin-dependent kinases

8. Cranial radiation therapy (CRT) has been used to treat brain tumors, acute lymphocytic leukemia, head and neck soft tissue tumors, and retinoblastoma in children. Childhood cancer survivors who had CRT as therapy for their cancers are prone to growth hormone deficiency. In adults, with what is growth hormone deficiency associated?

   a. Hypocalcemia

   b. Cardiovascular longevity

   c. Hyperinsulinemia

   d. Dyslipidemia

9. A big difference in the treatment of childhood cancer as opposed to adult cancer is that chemotherapy is the most widely used treatment therapy for childhood cancer. What is the reason for this?

   a. Pediatric tumors are more responsive to chemotherapy than adult cancers.

   b. Children do not tolerate other forms of therapy as well as adults do.

   c. Children do not complain about the nausea and vomiting caused by chemotherapy like adults do.

   d. Children think losing their hair is "cool."

10. The inherent properties of a tumor that determine how the tumor responds to radiation is called radiosensitivity. When radiation is combined with cytotoxic drugs, it has been noted that there is a radiosensitizing effect on tumor cells. Which drug is considered a radiosensitizer?

    a. Doxorubicin

    b. Cisplatin

    c. Vincristine

    d. Docetaxel

11. Cancer is a disorder of altered cell differentiation and growth. The term _____ refers to an abnormal mass of tissue in which the growth exceeds and is uncoordinated with that of the normal tissues.

12. A woman diagnosed with breast cancer asks the nurse how a malignant tumor in her breast could spread to other parts of her body. The nurse answers that a malignant neoplasm is comprised of less well-differentiated cells that have which of the following abilities? Mark all that apply.

    a. They break loose.

    b. They reinvade their original site.

    c. They enter the circulatory or lymphatic system.

    d. They are excreted through the alimentary canal.

    e. They form secondary malignant tumors at other sites.

13. Cancer cells differ from normal cells in many ways. They have lost the ability to accurately communicate with other cells, and they do not have to be anchored to other cells to survive. How else are they different from other cells? Mark all that apply.

    a. Cancer cells have an increased tendency to stick together.

    b. Cancer cells have an unlimited life span.

    c. Cancer cells have lost contact inhibition.

    d. Cancer cells need increased amounts of growth factor to proliferate.

    e. Cancer cells are genetically unstable.

14. Match the following types of cancer with their screening tests.

Type of Cancer	Screening Test
____ 1. Malignant melanoma	a. Mammography
____ 2. Prostatic	b. Self-examination
____ 3. Cervical	c. Pap smear
____ 4. Breast	d. Prostate-specific antigen

15. Childhood cancers are often diagnosed late in the disease process because the signs and symptoms mimic other childhood diseases. However, with the huge strides in treatment methods, increasingly more children survive childhood cancer. These survivors face the uncertainty that the lifesaving treatment they received during their childhood may produce what late effects? Mark all that apply.

a. Cardiomyopathy and pulmonary fibrosis
b. Cognitive dysfunction and hormonal dysfunction
c. Second malignancies and liver failure
d. Impaired growth and second malignancies

Stress and Adaptation

SECTION I: LEARNING OBJECTIVES

1. Cite Cannon's four features of homeostasis

2. Describe the components of a control system, including the function of a negative feedback system

3. State Selye's definition of stress

4. Define *stressor*

5. Cite two factors that influence the nature of the stress response

6. Explain the interactions among components of the nervous system in mediating the stress response

7. Describe the stress responses of the autonomic nervous system, the endocrine system, the immune system, and the musculoskeletal system

8. Explain the purpose of adaptation

9. List at least six factors that influence a person's adaptive capacity

10. Relate experience and previous learning to the process of adaptation

11. Contrast anatomic and physiologic reserve

12. Propose a way by which social support may serve to buffer challenges to adaptation

13. Describe the physiologic and psychological effects of a chronic stress response

14. Describe the three states characteristic of post-traumatic stress disorder

15. List five nonpharmacologic methods of treating stress

SECTION II: ASSESSING YOUR UNDERSTANDING

Activity A *Fill in the blanks.*

1. The ability of the body to function and maintain _____ under conditions of change in the internal and external environments depends on the thousands of _____ control systems that regulate body function.

2. _____ is only achieved through a system of carefully coordinated physiologic processes that oppose change.

3. Most control systems in the body operate by _____ feedback mechanisms.

4. Selye described _____ as a state manifested by a specific syndrome of the body developed in response to any stimuli that made an intense systemic demand on it.

5. Stress may contribute directly to the production or exacerbation of a _____.

6. There is evidence that the _____ axis, the _____ hormonal system, and the _____ nervous system are differentially activated, depending on the type and intensity of the stressor.

7. Humans, because of their highly developed nervous system and intellect, usually have alternative mechanisms for _____ and have the ability to control many aspects of their environment.

8. The means used to attain this balance are called _____.

9. _____ is considered a restorative function in which energy is restored and tissues are regenerated.

10. _____ is commonly used in excess and can suppress the immune system.

Activity B *Consider the following figure.*

1. In this figure, trace the activation of the hypothalamus to the release of corticotrophin to the effect on the adrenal gland and to the final release of cortisol. Also, label the locus ceruleus.

Activity C *Match the key terms in Column A with their definitions in Column B.*

Column A

____ **1.** Conditioning factors

____ **2.** Antidiuretic hormone

____ **3.** Baroreflex

____ **4.** Allostasis

____ **5.** Physiologic reserve

____ **6.** Angiotensin II

____ **7.** Hardiness

____ **8.** Cortisol

____ **9.** ACTH

____ **10.** Coping mechanisms

Column B

a. Personality characteristic that includes a sense of having control over the environment

b. Factors used to create a new balance between a stressor and the ability to deal with it

c. Physiologic changes in the neuroendocrine, autonomic, and immune systems in response to real or perceived challenges to homeostasis

d. Stressor that produces a response

e. Enhances stress-induced release of vasopressin from the posterior pituitary

f. Ability of body systems to increase their function given the need to adapt

g. Regulation of heart rate and vasomotor tone

h. Suppresses osteoblast activity, hematopoiesis, and protein synthesis

i. Stimulates the adrenal gland to synthesize and secrete the glucocorticoid hormones

j. Increases water retention by the kidneys and produces vasoconstriction of blood vessels

Activity D *Briefly answer the following.*

1. How does the body regulate and maintain homeostasis? Give one example.

_____

_____

_____

2. Describe the stages of general adaptation syndrome.

_____

_____

_____

3. Stress will activate numerous body systems. Many are based in neuroendocrine activity. List the effects of neuroendocrine activation in response to stress.

_____

_____

_____

4. Trained athletes use physiologic and anatomic reserves to achieve top-level performance. Explain and give examples of how this is accomplished.

_____

_____

_____

5. What are the physiologic and anatomic causes of post-traumatic stress disorder?

_____

_____

_____

SECTION III: APPLYING YOUR KNOWLEDGE

Activity E *Consider the following scenario and answer the questions.*

Mr. Jones is a 33-year-old patient brought to the emergency room by his brother. He presents with a history of increased irritability, difficulty concentrating, an exaggerated startle reflex, and increased vigilance and concern over his safety. His brother tells the triage nurse, "Ever since he moved here, he keeps asking why he lived and his family didn't."

1. What information should the nurse gather when obtaining the health history of Mr. Jones?

_____

_____

_____

2. What nursing interventions are needed when caring for Mr. Jones?

_____

_____

_____

SECTION IV: PRACTICING FOR NCLEX

Activity F *Answer the following questions.*

1. The control systems of the body act in many ways to maintain homeostasis. These control systems regulate the functions of the cell and integrate the functions of different organ systems. What else do they do?
   a. Control life processes
   b. Feed cells under stress
   c. Act on invading organisms
   d. Shut down the body at death

2. It has long been known that our bodies need a stable internal environment to function optimally. What serves to fulfill this need?
   a. Organ systems
   b. Control systems
   c. Biochemical messenger systems
   d. Neurovascular systems

3. The general adaptation syndrome is what occurs in the body in response to stressors. When the body's defenses are depleted, signs of "wear and tear" or systemic damage appear. Which diseases have been linked to stress and are believed to be encouraged by the body itself when it can no longer adapt to stress in a healthy manner?
   a. Psychotic disorders
   b. Osteogenesis sarcomas
   c. Rheumatic disorders
   d. Infections of the head and neck

4. A number of responses to the release of neurohormones occur when the body encounters stress, including which of the following?
   a. Increase in appetite
   b. Decreased cerebral blood flow
   c. Decrease in awareness
   d. Inhibition of reproductive function

5. Chronic and excessive activation of the stress response has been shown to play a part in the development of long-term health problems. The stress response can also result from chronic illness. Which health problems have been linked to a stress response that is chronic and excessive?

    a. Suicide and immune disorders

    b. Depression and renal disease

    c. Immune disorders and brain tumors

    d. Suicide and thrombosis in the extremities

6. Our body's response to psychologic perceived threats is not regulated to the same degree as our body's response to physiologic perceived threats. The psychologic responses may be

    a. appropriate and limited.

    b. inappropriate and sustained.

    c. regulated by a positive feedback system.

    d. the result of a baroreflex-mediated response.

7. Adaptation implies that an individual has successfully created a new balance between the stressor and the ability to deal with it. The safety margin for adaptation of most body systems is considerably greater than that needed for normal activities. What is the method of adaptation that allows the body to live with only one of a pair of organs (i.e., one lung or one kidney)?

    a. Genetic endowment

    b. Physiologic reserve

    c. Anatomic reserve

    d. Health status

8. Psychosocial factors can impact the body's response to stress either positively or negatively. It has been shown that social networks play a part in the psychosocial and physical integrity of a person. How do social networks affect how the body deals with stress?

    a. By stepping in and making decisions for the person

    b. By reapportioning the finances of the person

    c. By mobilizing the resources of the person

    d. By protecting the person from other internal stressors

9. The acute stress response can be detrimental in people with preexisting physical or mental health problems. In which of these clients could the acute stress response cause further problems?

    a. Client who is post resection of a brain tumor

    b. Client who is schizophrenic and off medication

    c. Client with a broken femur

    d. Client with heart disease

10. Some clients experience chronic activation of the stress response as a result of severe trauma. Which of the following is the disorder that can occur when the stress response is chronically activated?

    a. Post-traumatic stress disorder

    b. Chronic renal insufficiency

    c. Schizophrenia

    d. Post delivery depression

11. In a _____ organism, it is necessary for the composition of the internal environment to be compatible with the survival needs of the individual cells.

12. Selye suggested that stress could have positive influences on the body, and these periods of positive stress are called _____.

13. The first goal of treatment of stress disorders is to aid clients in avoiding those coping mechanisms that cause their health to be at risk. Second, the treatment of stress disorders should engage them in alternative strategies that reduce stress. Which are nonpharmacologic treatments of stress disorders? Mark all that apply.

    a. Lithium therapy

    b. Music therapy

    c. Education therapy

    d. Massage therapy

14. Match the following terms with their definitions.

Term

_____ **1.** Corticotropin-releasing factor

_____ **2.** Fight-or-flight response

_____ **3.** Allostatic load

_____ **4.** Endocrine-immune interactions

Definition

a. Increased corticosteroid production and atrophy of the thymus

b. Endocrine regulator of pituitary and adrenal activity and neurotransmitter involved in autonomic nervous system activity, metabolism, and behavior

c. Physiologic changes in the neuroendocrine, autonomic, and immune systems occurring in response to real or perceived challenges to homeostasis

d. Most rapid of the stress responses, representing the basic survival response

15. It is believed that there is an interaction between the neuroendocrine system and the immune system. It has been postulated that these interactions play a significant role in autoimmune diseases. These systems have what in common? Mark all that apply.

a. They share common signal pathways.

b. Hormones and neuropeptides can change what immune cells do.

c. Mediators of the immune system can modify neuroendocrine function.

d. They are symbiotic systems and cannot work without each other.

CHAPTER 10

Alterations in Temperature Regulation

SECTION I: LEARNING OBJECTIVES

1. Differentiate between body core temperature and skin temperature and relate the differences to methods used for measuring body temperature

2. Describe the physiologic mechanisms that control the gain and loss of heat from the body

3. Define the terms *conduction, radiation, convection,* and *evaporation,* and relate them to the mechanisms for gain and loss of heat from the body

4. Characterize the physiology of fever

5. Describe the four stages of fever

6. Explain what is meant by intermittent, remittent, sustained, and relapsing fevers

7. State the relation between body temperature and heart rate

8. Differentiate between the physiologic mechanisms involved in fever and hyperthermia

9. State the definition of fever of unknown source in children 0 to 36 months of age

10. State the definition for fever in the elderly and cite possible mechanisms for altered febrile response in the elderly

11. Compare the characteristics of fevers caused by infectious agents and drug-related fevers

12. Compare the mechanisms of malignant hyperthermia and neuroleptic malignant syndrome

13. Define *hypothermia*

14. Compare the manifestations of mild, moderate, and severe hypothermia and relate them to changes in physiologic functioning that occur with decreased body temperature

15. Describe the causes of heat loss and hypothermia in the newborn infant and patient undergoing surgery

SECTION II: ASSESSING YOUR UNDERSTANDING

Activity A *Fill in the blanks.*

1. Core body temperature is normally maintained within a range of _____°C.

2. Core body and skin temperatures are sensed and integrated by thermoregulatory regions within the _____.

3. _____ is the body's main source of heat production.

4. Contraction of the _____ muscles of the skin, which raises skin hairs and produces goose bumps, also aids in heat conservation by reducing the surface area available for heat loss.

5. It has been shown that small elevations in temperature, such as those that occur with _____, enhance immune function.

6. PGE$_2$ binds to receptors in the hypothalamus to induce changes in its set-point via the second messenger _____.

7. PGE$_2$ that is produced by the _____ cells is believed to cause an immediate rise in temperature.

8. A fever that has its origin in the central nervous system is sometimes referred to as a _____.

9. An _____ is one in which temperature returns to normal at least once every 24 hours.

10. A 1°C rise in temperature produces a _____ beats/minute increase in heart rate.

11. The _____ syndrome, which is characterized by *p*eriodic *f*ever, *a*phthous, *p*haryngitis, and cervical *a*denopathy occurring every 21 to 28 days, is the most common cause of recurrent fevers in children younger than 5 years.

12. _____ work at the hypothalamus, presumably by blocking the activity of cyclooxygenase, an enzyme that is required for the conversion of arachidonic acid to _____.

13. Slight elevations in temperature in _____ patients should be considered significant.

14. _____ describes an increase in body temperature that occurs without a change in the set-point of the hypothalamic thermoregulatory center.

15. The _____ is the temperature that the body senses when both temperature and humidity are combined.

16. Heat exhaustion is related to a gradual loss of _____ and _____, usually after prolonged and heavy exertion in a hot environment.

17. Systemic _____ may result from exposure to prolonged cold.

18. General _____ agents lower the metabolic rate and decrease vasoconstriction and shivering thresholds, putting the patient at greater risk for _____.

19. A gradual decline in _____ and _____ occurs as hypothermia progresses.

Activity B *Consider the following figure and answer the questions.*

1. On the temperature strip in the figure, mark the following temperature points or ranges:
   a. Where thermoregulation is lost
   b. Where thermoregulation is impaired
   c. Where normal temperature is located
   d. Where regulation is impaired by fever
   e. Threshold for the upper limits of survival

Activity C *Match the key terms in Column A with their definitions in Column B.*

Column A

_____ **1.** Convection

_____ **2.** Radiation

_____ **3.** Subcutaneous tissues

_____ **4.** Shivering

_____ **5.** Thyroid hormone

_____ **6.** Insensible perspiration

_____ **7.** Arteriovenous shunts

_____ **8.** Set-point

_____ **9.** Conduction

_____ **10.** Evaporation

Column B

a. Shift metabolism to heat production

b. Water that diffuses through the skin independent of sweating

c. Point held by hypothalamus relating to normal body temperature

d. Initiated by impulses from the hypothalamus, can produce a three- to fivefold increase in body temperature.

e. Transfer of heat through air

f. Insulate the core from swings in environmental temperature

g. Heat transfer through the circulation of air currents

h. Use of body heat to convert water on the skin to water vapor

i. Allow blood to move directly from the arterial to the venous system to rapidly decrease heat

j. Direct transfer of heat from one molecule to another

Activity D *Put the stages of a fever in the proper order:*

a. Defervescence

b. Prodrome

c. Flush

d. Chill

Activity E *Briefly answer the following.*

1. Blood flow changes in order to maintain core body temperature. Explain how these changes occur in hot and cold environments.

_____

_____

_____

2. Describe the symptoms associated with each stage of a fever.

_____

_____

_____

3. Why do children experience fevers more commonly?

_____

_____

_____

4. List and explain the possible causes of hyperthermia.

_____

_____

_____

5. What are the possible mechanisms of fever produced by drugs?

_____

_____

_____

6. List and describe the conditions that contribute to hypothermia.

_____

_____

_____

7. Explain the mechanisms and steps of rewarming a hypothermic patient.

_____

_____

_____

SECTION III: APPLYING YOUR KNOWLEDGE

Activity F *Consider the following scenario and answer the questions.*

George Collins, 79 years old, is brought to the clinic by his son. He presents with a history of fever and cough. His son states, "I am really worried about my father; he's not eating well, and sometimes he coughs so hard he can't get his breath."

1. What information should the nurse gather when obtaining the health history of Mr. Collins?

_____

_____

_____

2. What physical examination should the nurse perform?

_____

_____

_____

SECTION IV: PRACTICING FOR NCLEX

Activity G *Answer the following questions.*

1. There are two types of stimuli that affect the raising or lowering of body temperature. What are these stimuli?

  a. Innocuous and noxious

  b. Strong and weak

  c. Hot and cold

  d. Unpleasant and pleasant

2. Fever and hyperthermia describe conditions in which body temperature is higher than the normal range. When does hyperthermia occur?

  a. When the body temperature is 39.5°C

  b. When the body's set-point is unchanged, but the temperature goes up

  c. When the body's set-point changes to a higher set-point

  d. When body temperature is greater than 37.6°C

3. Pyrogens are substances that produce fever in the body. Substances such as bacterial products, bacterial toxins, or whole microorganisms enter the body and stimulate the host cells to produce certain mediators. What are these called?

  a. Exogenous pyrogens

  b. Outer pyrogens

  c. Endogenous pyrogens

  d. Set-point pyrogens

4. Neurogenic fevers begin in the central nervous system. By what characteristics are neurogenic fevers known?

  a. High temperatures that respond quickly to antipyretic therapy

  b. Temperatures that go up and down for no apparent reason

  c. Variable temperatures that are associated with sweating

  d. High temperatures that are not associated with sweating

5. The term *submersion hypothermia* is used when cooling follows acute asphyxia, as occurs in cases of near-drowning. Children have been reported to survive after being submerged from 10 to 40 minutes. This situation is believed to be possible because of the rapid cooling process following a particular reflex. What is the name of that reflex?

  a. Diving reflex

  b. Moro reflex

  c. Bainbridge reflex

  d. Oculocephalic reflex

6. Most febrile illnesses are due to common infections and are relatively easy to diagnose. In certain instances, however, it is difficult to establish the cause of a fever. In these instances, the elevation in temperature is referred to as a fever of unknown origin (FUO). What is a common cause of FUO?

   a. Disseminated intravascular coagulation

   b. Malignancies

   c. Pulmonary emboli

   d. Femoral artery emboli

7. Sometimes recurrent fevers occur but do not follow a strictly periodic pattern. Causes of these recurrent fevers include genetic disorders such as familial Mediterranean fever. What are the characteristics of familial Mediterranean fever?

   a. Early age of onset (<20 years) and seizures

   b. Episodic bouts of peritonitis and duration of 1 week

   c. Early age of onset (<20 years) and high fever

   d. Episodic bouts of peritonitis and low fever

8. Antipyretic drugs, such as aspirin, ibuprofen, and acetaminophen, are often used to alleviate the discomforts of fever and protect vulnerable organs, such as the brain, from extreme elevations in body temperature. The use of aspirin is limited in children, however, because it can sometimes cause which of the following diseases?

   a. Münchhausen syndrome

   b. Guillain-Barré syndrome

   c. Angelman syndrome

   d. Reye syndrome

9. Fever in infants and young children is not an uncommon event. Many trips to the pediatrician's office occur because of fever in children ages 1 day to 3 years. Which sign or symptom does not indicate fever in an infant?

   a. Avid feeding

   b. Hypoventilation

   c. Cyanosis

   d. Poor tissue oxygenation

10. The pathophysiology of heat stroke is believed to result from the direct effect of heat on body cells and the release of cytokines (e.g., interleukins, tumor necrosis factor, interferon) from heat-stressed endothelial cells, leukocytes, and epithelial cells that protect against tissue injury. Which of the following conditions cannot be caused by heat stroke?

    a. Disseminated intravascular clotting and acute renal failure

    b. Acute respiratory distress and rhabdomyoma

    c. Rhabdomyolysis and multiorgan failure

    d. Disseminated intravascular clotting and multiorgan failure

11. Drug fever is a fever that can occur with the administration of a specific drug, and then disappear when the drug is discontinued. Which of the following is a way that drugs can induce fever? Mark all that apply.

    a. Drugs can cause heat dissipation.

    b. Drugs can act as direct pyrogens.

    c. Drugs can induce an autoimmune response.

    d. Drugs can injure tissues directly.

12. A sign that the body is losing heat occurs with the contraction of the _____ muscles of the skin. This raises skin hairs and produces goose bumps; it also aids in heat conservation by reducing the surface area available for heat loss.

13. The four successive stages of fever are listed in random order as follows. Choose the answer that places them in correct order.

    a. Prodromal
    b. Defervescence
    c. Chill
    d. Flush

    A. c,d,a,b
    B. a,b,c,d
    C. dcab
    D. a,c,d,b

14. Diagnosing the primary cause is one of several methods used to treat fever. What are some other methods? Mark all that apply.

   a. Modification of external environment to decrease heat transfer to external environment

   b. Support of hypermetabolic state that accompanies fever

   c. Protection of vulnerable body organs and systems

   d. Modification of internal environment to decrease heat transfer to external environment

15. Malignant hyperthermia is a disorder in which the body's core temperature can rise by 1°C every 5 minutes. Although it is often caused by a halogenated anesthetic agent in combination with succinylcholine, there are also nonoperative precipitating factors. What nonoperative factors can precipitate malignant hyperthermia? Mark all that apply.

   a. Trauma

   b. Exercise

   c. Infection

   d. Environmental heat stress

CHAPTER 11

Activity Tolerance and Fatigue

SECTION I: LEARNING OBJECTIVES

1. Differentiate among aerobic, isometric, and flexibility exercises

2. Describe the physiologic and psychological responses to exercise

3. Define the term *maximal oxygen consumption* and state how it is measured

4. Describe methods that can be used to assess a person's activity tolerance and ability to engage in an exercise program

5. Describe the physiologic effects of exercise in the elderly population

6. Define fatigue and describe its manifestations

7. Differentiate acute from chronic fatigue

8. List at least four health problems that are associated with chronic fatigue

9. Define *chronic fatigue syndrome* and describe assessment findings, presenting symptoms, and laboratory values associated with the disorder

10. Discuss treatment modalities for chronic fatigue syndrome

11. Describe the effects of immobility and prolonged bed rest on cardiovascular, pulmonary, renal, metabolic, musculoskeletal, gastrointestinal, and sensory function.

12. Describe the time course events of the physiologic changes associated with immobility and prolonged bed rest.

13. Identify physical assessment findings that are related to the effects of immobility and prolonged bed rest

14. Describe treatment interventions that counteract the negative effects of immobility and prolonged bed rest

SECTION II: ASSESSING YOUR UNDERSTANDING

Activity A *Fill in the blanks.*

1. _____ is defined as the process of energy expenditure for the purpose of accomplishing an effect.

2. _____ exercise involves the body's ability to transport use of oxygen for energy during prolonged strenuous exercise.

3. Although _____ training has long been accepted as a means of developing strength and muscle mass, its beneficial relationship to health factors and chronic diseases has only recently been recognized.

4. _____ is determined by the rate at which oxygen is delivered to the working muscles.

5. Exercise produces an increase in heart rate and stroke volume, which in turn increases _____.

6. An increase in venous return stimulates right atrial stretch receptors, which stimulate the _____ response and increase cardiac output.

7. _____ is defined as the ability of muscle groups to produce force against resistance.

8. _____ fibers are larger and better suited for high-intensity work, but they fatigue more easily.

9. Persons with congestive heart failure typically experience symptoms of breathlessness, exertional fatigue, and exercise intolerance resulting in _____ of skeletal muscles.

10. The enzyme _____ catalyzes the transfer of the high-energy phosphate groups from ATP to creatine-forming creatine phosphate and ADP.

11. During intense physical activity, blood flow is shunted away from the _____ toward the active skeletal muscles.

12. Strenuous exercise also lowers the production of the nonessential amino acid _____, which serves as an energy source for lymphocytes and macrophages.

13. Elevation in body temperature, cytokine release, and increased levels of various _____ hormones may result in a temporary depression of the body's innate immune defenses during intense exercise.

14. Current evidence supports a 5% to 15% _____ per decade in $\dot{V}O_{2max}$ in men and women beginning at age 25 years.

15. Activity _____ can be viewed as not having sufficient physical or psychological energy reserve to endure or complete required or desired daily activities.

16. The physiologic basis of _____ includes factors such as diaphragmatic, motor, or neurologic mechanisms.

17. _____ fatigue has a rapid onset and is quickly relieved on cessation of activity.

18. Once believed to increase the restorative process, prolonged _____ has now shown to hinder healing.

19. The development of _____ is the third major complication of bed rest.

20. Adverse effects of prolonged immobility and bed rest include a decreased _____, orthostatic intolerance, dehydration, and sensory deprivation, as well as the potential for development of thrombophlebitis, _____, _____, and pressure ulcers.

Activity B *Match the key concepts in Column A with their definitions in Column B.*

Column A

____ 1. Phospho-creatine

____ 2. Iometric exercise

____ 3. Venous distention

____ 4. Increased fibrinolysis

____ 5. Sweating

____ 6. Chronic fatigue

____ 7. Human Activity Profile

____ 8. Metabolic equivalents

____ 9. Acute fatigue

____ 10. Ergometry

Column B

a. Common side effect of disease state

b. Effect of epinephrine during exercise to increase blood vessel health

c. Loss of body heat by evaporation

d. Multiples of the basal metabolic rate

e. Complication of bed rest

f. Originally designed for patients with chronic obstructive pulmonary disease

g. Sustained muscle contraction is generated against an immovable load with no change in length

h. Procedure for determining physical performance capacity

i. May serve as a protective function

j. High-energy phosphate bonds and is unique to muscle fibers

Activity C *Briefly answer the following.*

1. What are the physiologic and psychological benefits of exercise?

   _____

   _____

   _____

2. How does exercise increase the functional state of blood vessels?

   _____

   _____

   _____

3. As we age, our ability to perform declines. Explain the role of skeletal muscle degeneration in this age-related decline.

   _____

   _____

   _____

4. Compare and contrast acute and chronic fatigue.

   _____

   _____

   _____

5. The diagnosis of chronic fatigue syndrome (CFS), a debilitating condition faced by many adults, is on the rise. Explain the pathophysiology of CFS and why there are no definitive treatments.

   _____

   _____

   _____

6. What are the mechanisms of orthostatic hypotension following bed rest?

   _____

   _____

   _____

SECTION III: APPLYING YOUR KNOWLEDGE

Activity D *Consider the following scenario and answer the questions.*

James Whitlow, a 75-year-old marathon runner, has suffered a fractured hip in a fall. Postoperatively, Mr. Whitlow sustains complications, including a myocardial infarction and a pulmonary embolus. He is on bed rest at this time.

1. What is the recommended approach to this patient's care? What does it include?

   _____

   _____

   _____

2. Because bed rest affects all systems in the body, what are the concerns of Mr. Whitlow's caregiver?

   _____

   _____

   _____

SECTION IV: PRACTICING FOR NCLEX

Activity E *Answer the following questions.*

1. There are two types of muscle fibers in skeletal muscle. Which type of muscle fiber is affected most by prolonged immobility or bed rest?

   a. Long muscle fibers

   b. Fast-twitch muscle fibers

   c. Short muscle fibers

   d. Slow-twitch muscle fibers

2. People with congestive heart failure need to be on a closely monitored exercise regimen. What is the reason for this?

   a. Fast-twitch muscle fibers are used more than slow-twitch muscle fibers.

   b. Decreased fatigability is caused by early dependence on anaerobic metabolism and excessive intramuscular acidification.

  c. Anaerobic metabolism, coupled with vaso-constrictor response, can cause an increased afterload on the heart.

  d. Anaerobic metabolism inhibits the vasoconstrictor response and decreases afterload on the heart.

3. A treatment plan for people with peripheral vascular disease has been proposed. Which of the following should it include?

  a. Weight training to strengthen the vastus lateralis

  b. Isometric exercise to increase cardiac endurance

  c. Aerobic exercise to decrease respiratory stress

  d. Exercise training to increase angiogenesis

4. The sweat produced by both a trained person and a nontrained person normally contains sodium chloride in large amounts. What happens when sweat is produced in a trained person?

  a. Sweat production begins before the core temperature rises, and the sweat produced is dilute and conserves sodium chloride.

  b. Sweat is produced within 5 to 6 minutes of the start of exercise, and the sweat, being high in sodium chloride, depletes the body of sodium chloride.

  c. Sweat is produced within 1 to 2 minutes of the start of exercise, and the sweat, being high in sodium chloride, depletes the body of sodium chloride.

  d. Sweat production begins after the core temperature rises, and the sweat, being high in sodium chloride, depletes the body of sodium chloride.

5. Elderly people sometimes have decreased cardiac output. What is believed to be the cause of this condition?

  a. Natural decrease in the load the respiratory system can handle as a person ages

  b. Natural decrease in the maximal heart rate as a person ages

  c. Natural occurrence of increased resistance in the major blood vessels as a person ages

  d. Natural destruction in peripheral blood vessels as a person ages

6. Many types of fatigue are reported by clients with a wide variety of disease disorders. What is an identified cause of fatigue in clients with forced immobility, neuromuscular disorders, and wasting syndromes?

  a. Insomnia caused by nocturia and pain

  b. Interference with the oxygen-carrying capacity of the blood

  c. Loss of muscle mass, muscle strength, and endurance

  d. Pain related to extended immobility

7. Bed rest causes deconditioning responses to occur that affect all body systems. What is one important factor to remember when dealing with the inactivity of immobility?

  a. These responses occur slowly and can be quickly overcome.

  b. These responses can be stopped by frequent turning and repositioning.

  c. These responses occur rapidly and can be quickly overcome.

  d. These responses occur rapidly and take a long time to overcome.

8. Disuse of a muscle and muscle atrophy contribute to the weakening and wasting of muscle tissue. What else do they contribute to?

  a. Joint contractures

  b. Gastrointestinal hyperactivity

  c. Venous hyperresponsiveness

  d. Neural decompensation

9. Chronic fatigue syndrome (CFS) is a disease with an unknown etiology and no definitive treatments. Even the diagnosis of CFS is difficult because the diagnostic criteria are many and require concurrent occurrence of specific symptoms. What is a concurrent symptom needed for the clinical diagnosis of CFS?

  a. Multijoint pain with swelling or redness

  b. Muscle pain

  c. Long periods of refreshing sleep

  d. Malaise lasting more than 24 hours unrelated to exertion

10. All systems in the body are affected by bed rest or immobility. For the immune system, research has demonstrated that interleukin (IL)-1, IL-6, and tumor necrosis factor-alpha are increased during immobility or bed rest. What are these mediators associated with?

    a. Hyperresponsiveness in the central nervous system

    b. Reduction in inflammatory reactions and bone wasting

    c. Hyperinflammatory reactions and tissue injury

    d. Tissue wasting and decreasing bone density

11. There are two main types of exercise. Aerobic exercise involves rhythmic changes in large muscle groups. Isometric, or _____, exercise involves a sustained muscle contraction against an immovable load.

12. During exercise, the respiratory system increases the rate of exchange of oxygen and carbon dioxide. This is caused by a series of physiologic responses. Listed as follows in random order are the physiologic responses causing the increased rate of exchange of oxygen and carbon dioxide. Choose the answer that puts these responses in order of occurrence.

    a. Larger volume of blood under increased pressure is delivered to the lungs.

    b. Respiratory rate increases four- to fivefold.

    c. Cardiac output increases.

    d. More pulmonary capillary beds open.

    e. Tidal volume increases five- to sevenfold.

    f. Minute ventilation increases 20 to 30 times its resting value.

    g. Better perfusion of the alveoli occur.

    h. Oxygen and carbon dioxide exchange more efficiently.

    A. a, e, f, g, d, c, b, h
    B. g, h, a, b, d, f, e, c
    C. b, e, f, c, a, d, g, h
    D. d, a, g, b, e, f, c, h

13. There are several ways of assessing activity tolerance and fatigue. One of these is a procedure for determining physical performance capacity called _____.

14. What are the major complications of bed rest? Mark all that apply.

    a. Venous stasis with the potential for development of deep venous thrombosis

    b. Redistribution and change in blood volume

    c. Increased cardiac workload

    d. Increased intestinal function and diarrhea

    e. Orthostatic hypotension

15. There is a direct proportional response between bone density and the stress placed on them according to _____ law.

Blood Cells and the Hematopoietic System

SECTION I: LEARNING OBJECTIVES

1. Describe the composition and functions of plasma

2. Name the formed elements of blood and cite their function and life span

3. Trace the process of hematopoiesis from stem cell to mature blood cell

4. Cite information gained from a complete blood count

5. State the purpose of the erythrocyte sedimentation rate

6. Describe the procedure used in bone marrow aspiration

SECTION II: ASSESSING YOUR UNDERSTANDING

Activity A *Fill in the blanks.*

1. The percentage of packed red blood cells in a given volume of blood is known as the _____.

2. Plasma, being a liquid, is _____ water by weight, _____ proteins by weight, and _____ other small molecular substances.

3. The _____ produces plasma proteins.

4. _____ is the most abundant of the plasma proteins.

5. The blood cells are not all true _____, hence the term "formed elements."

6. Red blood cells contain the protein _____, which is used to transport oxygen.

7. _____ facilitates the formation of carbonic acid from carbon dioxide and water, which, in turn, dissociates into bicarbonate and hydrogen ions.

8. Leukocytes have granules that contain degradative enzymes known as _____.

9. _____ contain complement activators, bactericidal agents, peroxidases, and other hydrolytic enzymes.

10. In parasitic infections, the _____ use surface markers to attach themselves to the parasite and then release hydrolytic enzymes that kill it.

11. The function of lymphocytes in the lymph nodes or spleen is to defend against microorganisms through the _____ response.

12. The T lymphocytes differentiate in the _____.

13. The _____, precursors of the mononuclear phagocyte system, are often referred to as _____ when they enter the tissues.

14. Thrombocytes are circulating cell fragments of the large _____ that are derived from the myeloid stem cell.

15. Under normal conditions, the numbers and total mass for each type of circulating blood cell remain relatively _____.

Activity B *Consider the following figure.*

In the test tube, label the layers as they separate out of whole blood.

- Plasma
- Formed elements
- Erythrocytes
- Buffy coat

Activity C *Match the key terms in Column A with their definitions in Column B.*

Column A

1. ____ Erythrocytes
2. ____ Leukocytes
3. ____ Lymphoid
4. ____ Neutrophils
5. ____ Eosinophils
6. ____ Basophils
7. ____ Lymphocytes
8. ____ Monocytes
9. ____ Thrombocytes
10. ____ Myeloid

Column B

a. Increase during allergic reactions
b. Include granulocytes, lymphocytes, and monocytes
c. Stem cell line of immune cells
d. Immune cells
e. Largest white blood cell
f. Most numerous of formed elements
g. Nuclei in three to five lobes
h. Contain heparin
i. Last 8–9 days in circulation
j. Stem cell line for granulocytes, erythrocytes, and megakaryocytes

Activity D *Put the following stem cells in order from least differentiated (left) to fully committed cells (right).*

a. Macrophage
b. Monoblast
c. Pluripotent stem cell
d. Myeloid stem cell
e. Monocyte colony-forming units

Activity E *Briefly answer the following:*

1. Explain the importance of stem cells and how they contribute to hematopoietic homeostasis.

_____

_____

_____

2. Erythropoiesis is regulated by special receptors in the kidney. Explain how this relates to endurance athletes training at high elevation.

_____

_____

_____

SECTION III: APPLYING YOUR KNOWLEDGE

Activity F *Consider the following scenario and answer the question.*

Sally Moore, 12 years old, is scheduled to have a bone marrow transplant to treat her acute lymphoid leukemia. The nurse explains to Sally that, after she has the transplant, she will get a transfusion of blood that has been specially treated with something called *growth factors*.

1. Sally asks the nurse why she has to have growth factors in the blood. How does the nurse answer Sally?

_____

_____

_____

SECTION IV: PRACTICING FOR NCLEX

Activity G *Answer the following questions.*

1. The globulins that make up part of the plasma of the blood have three distinct purposes. What are the gamma globulins?
   a. Antibodies of the immune system
   b. Transporters of iron and copper
   c. Transporters of bilirubin and steroids
   d. Autoantibodies of the immune system

2. What are the biconcave disks in the blood that carry oxygen?
   a. Neutrophils
   b. Erythrocytes
   c. Eosinophils
   d. Leukocytes

3. Pluripotent stem cells for an invaluable source of reserve cells for the entire hematopoietic system. Between these cells and the unipotential cells are several levels of differentiation. What are these unipotential cells called?
   a. Embryonic stem cells
   b. Immature neural cells
   c. Colony-forming units
   d. Blood cell precursors

4. Stem cell transplantation has been shown to provide potential cures for diseases such as aplastic anemia and the leukemias. What are the sources of stem cells used for transplant?
   a. Peripheral blood cells and immature embryonic cells
   b. Bone marrow and immature neural cells
   c. Umbilical cord blood and yellow bone marrow
   d. Peripheral blood and yellow bone marrow

5. Some cytokines stimulate the growth and production of new blood cells. Other cytokines support the proliferation of stem cells in the human body. Which cytokines support the proliferation of stem cells in the human body?
   a. Interleukins, interferons, and tumor necrosis factor
   b. Granulocytes, B-cell growth factor, and interferons
   c. Interleukins, T-cell growth factor, and colony-stimulating factors
   d. Transforming growth factor, interferons, and tumor necrosis factor

6. The erythrocyte sedimentation rate is a commonly performed blood test used for monitoring the clinical course of a disease. It is a measurement of how rapidly red blood cells will aggregate and drop to the bottom of a tube as a sediment in anticoagulated blood. What influences the rate of fall that would give information about the clinical course of a disease?
   a. The rate of fall is faster in the presence of cytokines that are increased in an inflammatory disease.
   b. The rate of fall is faster in the presence of fibrinogen that is increased in an inflammatory disease.
   c. The rate of fall is faster in the presence of macrophages that are increased in an inflammatory disease.
   d. The rate of fall is faster in the presence of growth factors that are increased in an inflammatory disease.

7. Although the usual site for a bone marrow test is the posterior iliac crest, other sites include the anterior iliac crest and the sternum. What are the dangers of using the sternum for a bone marrow test in children?
   a. Potential for hemorrhage
   b. Danger of perforating the lungs
   c. Danger of perforating the mediastinum
   d. Potential for infection in the chest cavity

8. Normally, there is a relatively constant number of each type of circulating blood cell. What regulates the number of each type of blood cell?
   a. Immune system
   b. Hematopoietic system
   c. Pluripotent stem cells
   d. Cytokines

9. To have stem cells for transplantation, clients are given specific agents to increase the quantity and migration of the cells from the bone marrow. What is the agent used to accomplish this?

   a. Cytokine growth factor
   b. Human leukocyte antigen growth factor
   c. Platelet growth factor
   d. Human growth factor

10. The cloning of the genes for most of the hematopoietic growth factors has been accomplished. The recombinant proteins that are produced are used in a wide range of clinical problems. What diseases have these proteins been used to fight?

    a. AIDS and autoimmune disorders
    b. Aplastic anemia and the anemia of kidney failure
    c. Anemia of cancer and Parkinson disease
    d. Aplastic anemia and the anemia of Huntington disease

11. Plasma, because of its water volume, is the vehicle used by the body to distribute _____. This is one of the means by which the body warms and cools itself.

12. For each plasma protein, fill in its purpose and the percent it makes up of plasma.

Protein	Percent	Purpose
Albumin		
Globulins		
Fibrinogen		

13. There are many components reported on in a complete blood count (CBC). Fill in the following abbreviations' definitions.

Abbreviation	Definition
Hgb	
Hct	
MCV	
MCHC	
MCH	

14. What are the components of blood? Mark all that apply.

    a. Electrolytes
    b. Enzymes
    c. Ascites
    d. Bile

15. Organ, blood, and bone marrow transplants, once an experimental phenomenon in medicine, are now being done every day. Our ability to match the tissues of one client with those of another person is being more finely developed by researchers around the world. Organ, blood, and bone marrow transplants are lifesaving procedures that come from what sources? Mark all that apply.

    a. A histocompatible donor
    b. A heterologous donor
    c. The patients themselves
    d. An autologous donor

Disorders of Hemostasis

SECTION I: LEARNING OBJECTIVES

1. Describe the five stages of hemostasis
2. Explain the formation of the platelet plug
3. State the purpose of blood coagulation
4. State the function of clot retraction
5. Trace the process of fibrinolysis
6. Compare normal and abnormal clotting
7. Describe the causes and effects of increased platelet function
8. State two conditions that contribute to increased clotting activity
9. State the mechanisms of drug-induced thrombocytopenia and idiopathic thrombocytopenia and the differing features of the disorders in terms of onset and resolution
10. Describe the manifestations of thrombocytopenia
11. Characterize the role of vitamin K in coagulation
12. State three common defects of coagulation factors and the causes of each
13. Differentiate between the mechanisms of bleeding in hemophilia A and von Willebrand disease
14. Describe the effect of vascular disorders on hemostasis

15. Explain the physiologic basis of acute disseminated intravascular coagulation

SECTION II: ASSESSING YOUR UNDERSTANDING

Activity A *Fill in the blanks.*

1. The term _____ refers to the stoppage of blood flow.

2. Platelets have a cell membrane, but have no _____ and cannot reproduce.

3. The platelet shape is maintained by microtubules and _____ and _____ filaments that support the cell membrane.

4. The release of _____ from platelets results in the proliferation and growth of vascular endothelial cells, smooth muscle cells, and fibroblasts, and is important in vessel repair.

5. The combined actions of _____ and _____ lead to the expansion of the enlarging platelet aggregate, which becomes the primary hemostatic plug.

6. The _____ is a stepwise process resulting in the conversion of the soluble plasma protein, fibrinogen, into fibrin.

7. Most of the coagulation factors are proteins synthesized in the _____.

8. It has been suggested that some of these natural anticoagulants may play a role in the bleeding that occurs with _____.

9. _____ represents an exaggerated form of hemostasis that predisposes to thrombosis and blood vessel occlusion.

10. _____, elevated levels of blood lipids and cholesterol, hemodynamic stress, diabetes mellitus, and immune mechanisms may cause vessel damage, platelet adherence, and, eventually, thrombosis.

11. The common clinical manifestations of essential _____ are thrombosis and hemorrhage.

12. In persons with inherited defects in factor V, the mutant factor Va cannot be inactivated by _____.

13. Secondary factors that lead to increased _____ and thrombosis are venous stasis due to prolonged bed rest and immobility, myocardial infarction, cancer, hyperestrogenic states, and oral contraceptives.

14. _____ from mucous membranes of the nose, mouth, gastrointestinal tract, and uterine cavity is characteristic of platelet bleeding disorders.

15. A reduction in platelet number is referred to as _____.

16. _____ destruction may be caused by antiplatelet antibodies, resulting in thrombocytopenia.

17. _____ thrombocytopenic purpura results in platelet antibody formation and excess destruction of platelets.

18. _____ may result from inherited disorders of adhesion or acquired defects caused by drugs, disease, or extracorporeal circulation.

19. Hemophilia A is an _____ recessive disorder that primarily affects males.

20. In liver disease, synthesis of these _____ is reduced, and bleeding may result.

21. Vitamin C deficiency, results in _____, where poor collagen synthesis and failure of the endothelial cells to be cemented together properly causes a fragile wall and bleeding.

22. Common clinical conditions that may cause _____ include obstetric disorders, massive trauma, shock, sepsis, and malignant disease.

Activity B *Consider the following figures:*

1. In the above figure, place the activated factors and proteins in their respective places: XIIa, XIa, IXa, Xa, VIIa, thrombin, prothrombin, fibrinogen, and fibrin.

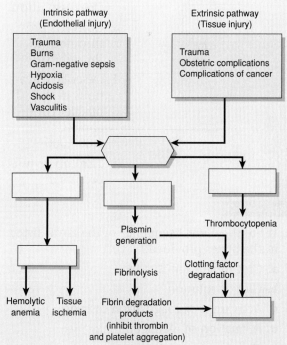

2. In the preceding figure explaining the pathophysiology of disseminated intravascular coagulation, insert the following terms where appropriate: thrombosis, bleeding, thrombin generation, platelet consumption, intravascular fibrin deposition, and plasminogen activation.

Activity C *Match the key terms in Column A with their definitions in Column B.*

Column A

_____ **1.** Thrombin

_____ **2.** Fibrinolysis

_____ **3.** Thrombocytosis

_____ **4.** Thromboxane A$_2$

_____ **5.** Plasmin

_____ **6.** Antiphospholipid syndrome

_____ **7.** Megakaryocytes

_____ **8.** Factor X

_____ **9.** Hemophilia A

_____ **10.** Thrombocytopenia

Column B

a. Breaks down fibrin

b. May be caused by aplastic anemia

c. Enzyme that converts fibrinogen to fibrin

d. Factor VIII deficiency

e. Stimulates vasoconstriction

f. Autoantibodies that result in increased coagulation activity

g. Process of blood clot dissolution

h. Converts prothrombin to thrombin

i. Describe elevations in the platelet count above 1,000,000/μL

j. Thrombocyte precursor

Activity D

1. Write the correct sequence of the terms listed in the boxes provided.
   a. Clot retraction
   b. Clot dissolution
   c. Activation of coagulation cascade
   d. Formation of platelet plug
   e. Vessel spasm

Activity E *Briefly answer the following.*

1. Explain the five stages of hemostasis.

_____

_____

_____

2. Describe the process of platelet activation and plug formation.

_____

_____

_____

3. The coagulation cascade is activated in multiple ways and is integral in maintaining hemostasis. Explain the general stimulation and end results.

_____

_____

_____

4. There are many causes of bleeding disorders. One of the more clinically relevant is drug-induced thrombocytopenia. Explain how drugs such as quinine, quinidine, and certain sulfa-containing antibiotics may induce thrombocytopenia.

_____

_____

_____

5. Disseminated intravascular coagulation is a severe condition that is characterized by widespread coagulation and bleeding. Explain how the disease is initiated, and describe its progression.

_____

_____

_____

SECTION III: APPLYING YOUR KNOWLEDGE

Activity F *Consider the following scenario and answer the questions.*

Parents of a 17-year-old boy with hemophilia have brought him to the emergency department because he is having an exacerbation.

1. What are the two most important nursing objectives when caring for them?

_____

_____

_____

2. In planning teaching for the client and his family, the nurse knows to include what?

_____

_____

_____

SECTION IV: PRACTICING FOR NCLEX

Activity G *Answer the following questions.*

1. Many different proteins, enzymes, and hormones are involved in maintaining hemostasis. Which protein is required for platelet adhesion?
   a. von Willebrand factor
   b. Growth factors
   c. Ionized calcium
   d. Platelet factor 4

2. There are two pathways that can be activated by the coagulation process. One pathway begins when factor XII is activated. The other pathway begins when there is trauma to a blood vessel. What are these pathways?
   a. Clotting and bleeding pathways
   b. Extrinsic and intrinsic pathways
   c. Inner and outer pathways
   d. Factor and trauma pathways

3. Anticoagulant drugs prevent thromboembolic disorders. How does warfarin, one of the anticoagulant drugs, act on the body?
   a. Alters vitamin K, reducing its ability to participate in the coagulation of the blood
   b. Increases prothrombin
   c. Increases vitamin K–dependent factors in the liver
   d. Increases procoagulation factors

4. Heparin is an anticoagulant given by injection to prevent the formation of blood clots. How does heparin work?

   a. Binds to factor X
   b. Promotes the inactivation of clotting factors
   c. Binds to factor Xa
   d. Promotes the inactivation of factor VIII

5. The process of clot retraction squeezes serum from the clot, thereby joining the edges of the broken vessel. Through the action of actin and myosin, filaments in platelets contribute to clot retraction. Failure of clot retraction is indicative of what?
   a. Absence of factor Xa
   b. Low platelet count
   c. Overabundance of factor Xa
   d. High platelet count

6. Thrombocytosis is used to describe elevations in the platelet count above $1,000,000/\mu L$. It is either a primary or a secondary thrombocytosis. Secondary thrombocytosis can occur as a reactive process due to what?
   a. Crohn disease
   b. Lyme disease
   c. Hirschsprung disease
   d. Megacolon

7. A 57-year-old man is diagnosed with thrombocytopenia. The nurse knows that thrombocytopenia refers to a decrease in the number of circulating platelets. The nurse also knows that thrombocytopenia can result from what?
   a. Decreased platelet production
   b. Increased platelet survival
   c. Decreased sequestration of platelets
   d. Increased platelet production

8. A young man has been diagnosed with hemophilia A, and the nurse is planning his discharge teaching. She knows to include what information in her discharge teaching?
   a. Only use NSAIDs for mild pain
   b. Prevent trauma to the body
   c. The client will not be on IV factor VIII therapy at home
   d. It is an X-linked dominant disorder

9. A teenage girl, seen in the clinic, is diagnosed with nonthrombocytopenic purpura. The girl states, "You have taken a lot of blood from me. Which of my tests came back abnormal?" How should the nurse respond?

a. Your complete blood count (CBC) with differential showed a shift to the left.

b. Your CBC with differential showed that you do not have enough iron.

c. Your CBC with differential showed a normal platelet count.

d. Your CBC with differential showed a normal hematocrit.

10. Disseminated intravascular coagulation is a grave coagulopathy resulting from the overstimulation of clotting and anticlotting processes in response to what?

a. Disease or injury

b. Septicemia and acute hypertension

c. Neoplasms and nonpoisonous snakebites

d. Severe trauma and acute hypertension

11. The following five stages of hemostasis are given in random order. Put them into their correct order.

a. Clot dissolution
b. Blood coagulation
c. Vessel spasm
d. Clot retraction
e. Formation of platelet plug

a. c, a, b, e, d
b. a, c, b, d, e
c. c, e, b, d, a
d. e, c, d, b, a

12. The coagulation cascade is the third component of the hemostatic process. It is a stepwise process resulting in the conversion of the soluble plasma protein, fibrinogen, into fibrin. This multistep process ensures that a massive episode of _____ clotting does not occur by chance.

13. _____ is a natural mucopolysaccharide anticoagulant that occurs in the lungs and intestinal mucosa.

14. When platelets adhere to the vessel wall, they release growth factors that cause smooth muscle to grow. This is a major factor in causing atherosclerosis. What are the factors that influence platelets to adhere to the vessel wall? Mark all that apply.

a. Hemodynamic stress

b. High cholesterol

c. Diabetes

d. Low blood lipids

e. Smoking

15. In a client with disseminated intravascular coagulation, microemboli form, causing obstruction of blood vessels and tissue hypoxia. Common clinical signs may be due to what? Mark all that apply.

a. Circulatory failure

b. Immunologic failure

c. Renal failure

d. Right ventricular failure

e. Respiratory failure

CHAPTER 14

Disorders of Red Blood Cells

SECTION I: LEARNING OBJECTIVES

1. Trace the development of a red blood cell from erythroblast to erythrocyte

2. Discuss the function of iron in the formation of hemoglobin

3. Describe the formation, transport, and elimination of bilirubin

4. Explain the function of the enzyme glucose-6-phosphate dehydrogenase in the red blood cell

5. State the meaning of the red blood cell count, percentage of reticulocytes, hemoglobin, hematocrit, mean corpuscular volume, and mean corpuscular hemoglobin concentration as it relates to the diagnosis of anemia

6. Describe the manifestations of anemia and their mechanisms

7. Explain the difference between intravascular and extravascular hemolysis

8. Compare the hemoglobinopathies associated with sickle cell disease and thalassemia

9. Explain the cause of sickling in sickle cell disease

10. Cite common causes of iron-deficiency anemia in infancy, adolescence, and adulthood

11. Describe the relation between vitamin B_{12} deficiency and megaloblastic anemia

12. List three causes of aplastic anemia

13. Compare characteristics of the red blood cells in acute blood loss, hereditary spherocytosis, sickle cell disease, iron-deficiency anemia, and aplastic anemia

14. Differentiate red cell antigens from antibodies in persons with type A, B, AB, or O blood

15. Explain the determination of the Rh factor

16. List the signs and symptoms of a blood transfusion reaction

17. Define the term *polycythemia*

18. Compare causes of polycythemia vera and secondary polycythemia

19. Describe the manifestations of polycythemia

20. Cite the function of hemoglobin F in the neonate and describe the red blood cell changes that occur during the early neonatal period

21. Cite the factors that predispose to hyperbilirubinemia in the infant

22. Describe the pathogenesis of hemolytic disease of the newborn

23. Compare conjugated and unconjugated bilirubin in terms of production of encephalopathy in the neonate

24. Explain the action of phototherapy in the treatment of hyperbilirubinemia in the neonate

25. State the changes in the red blood cells that occur with aging

SECTION II: ASSESSING YOUR UNDERSTANDING

Activity A *Fill in the blanks.*

1. The _____ shape of an erythrocyte provides a larger surface area for oxygen diffusion than would a spherical cell of the same volume, and the thinness of the _____ enables oxygen to diffuse rapidly between the exterior and the innermost regions of the cell.

2. The rate at which hemoglobin is synthesized depends on the availability of _____ for heme synthesis.

3. During its transformation from normoblast to reticulocyte, the red blood cell accumulates hemoglobin as the _____ condenses and is finally lost.

4. Mature red blood cells have a life span of approximately _____ months.

5. The red blood cell relies on the _____ pathway for its metabolic needs.

6. Large doses of nitrites can result in high levels of _____, causing pseudocyanosis and tissue hypoxia.

7. The _____ measures the total number of red blood cells in a microliter of blood.

8. The _____ measures the volume of red blood cell mass in 100 mL of plasma volume.

9. The _____ is the concentration of hemoglobin in each cell.

10. _____ is defined as an abnormally low number of circulating red blood cells or level of hemoglobin.

11. Tissue _____ can give rise to fatigue, weakness, dyspnea, and, sometimes, angina.

12. _____ anemia is characterized by the premature destruction of red blood cells, the retention in the body of iron and the other products of hemoglobin destruction, and an increase in erythropoiesis.

13. Two main types of hemoglobinopathies can cause red blood cell hemolysis: the abnormal substitution of an amino acid in the hemoglobin molecule, as in _____ anemia,

and the defective synthesis of one of the polypeptide chains that form the globin portion of hemoglobin, as in the _____.

14. Hereditary _____ is caused by abnormalities of the spectrin and ankyrin membrane proteins that lead to a gradual loss of the membrane surface.

15. _____ are caused by deficient synthesis of the β chain and _____ by deficient synthesis of the β chain.

16. The most common inherited enzyme defect that results in hemolytic anemia is a deficiency of _____.

17. _____ anemia results from dietary deficiency, loss of iron through bleeding, or increased demands.

18. Iron deficiency in adults in the Western world is usually the result of _____.

19. _____ anemias are caused by impaired DNA synthesis that results in enlarged red blood cells due to impaired maturation and division.

20. _____ anemia is a specific form of megaloblastic anemia caused by atrophic gastritis.

21. _____ describes a disorder of pluripotential bone marrow stem cells that results in a reduction of all three hematopoietic cell lines.

22. _____ is an abnormally high total red blood cell mass with a hematocrit greater than 50%.

23. At birth, changes in the red blood cell indices reflect the transition to extrauterine life and the need to transport _____ from the lungs.

24. Jaundice in infants is the result of increased red blood cell breakdown and the inability of the immature liver to _____ bilirubin.

25. The diagnosis of _____ in the elderly requires a complete physical examination, a complete blood count, and studies to rule out comorbid conditions such as malignancy, gastrointestinal conditions that cause bleeding, and pernicious anemia.

Activity B *Consider the following figure.*

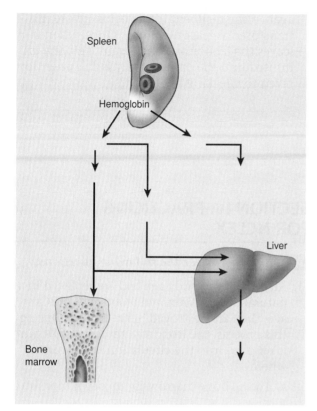

Spleen

Hemoglobin

Liver

Bone marrow

In this figure, fill in the steps associated with red blood cell breakdown and secretion from the body. Begin by labeling where heme and the globin proteins separate. Trace the iron as it is recycled or as it is conjugated by the liver.

Activity C *Match the key terms in Column A with their definitions in Column B.*

Column A

_____ 1. Thalassemia

_____ 2. 2, 3-Diphospho-glycerate

_____ 3. Erythropoietin

_____ 4. Mean corpuscular volume

_____ 5. Transferrin

_____ 6. Autologous donation

Column B

a. Decreases hemoglobin affinity for oxygen

b. Common cause of megaloblastic anemias

c. Measure of size of red blood cell

d. Red blood cell production

_____ 7. B$_{12}$ deficiency

_____ 8. Erythropoiesis

_____ 9. Jaundice

_____ 10. Normochromic cell

e. Caused by deficient globin production

f. Regulator of red blood cell production

g. Normal hemoglobin concentration in red blood cell

h. Yellow discoloration of skin due to high levels of bilirubin

i. Transports iron to plasma

j. Receiving blood from yourself

Activity D *Briefly answer the following.*

1. Hemoglobin is the oxygen-carrying protein found in red blood cells. Describe the molecular structure of hemoglobin. Also, explain how oxygen interacts with hemoglobin.

_____

_____

_____

2. Red blood cells (RBCs) have a finite life span. How long is the life span, and what is the fate of RBCs?

_____

_____

_____

3. What are the three categories of anemic effects?

_____

_____

_____

4. Describe and explain the two consequences of sickle cell disease.

_____

_____

_____

5. Anemia is a common side effect of cancer treatments. Which type of anemia usually develops, and why?

_____

_____

_____

6. Polycythemia vera is a neoplastic disorder of red blood cells. Describe the complications that arise from the rapid increase in hematocrit.

_____

_____

_____

7. Infantile jaundice is caused by the underdeveloped liver being unable conjugate bilirubin. What are the treatment methods for infantile jaundice, and how do they work?

_____

_____

_____

SECTION III: APPLYING YOUR KNOWLEDGE

Activity E   *Consider the following scenario and answer the questions.*

Mrs. McFee, a 62-year-old woman, is in the outpatient procedure area of the hospital. She has a long history of rheumatoid arthritis and is to receive a blood transfusion to treat a chronic disease anemia. She appears very nervous as the nurse begins the transfusion. She states, "My friends have told me that there are serious things that can happen to you because of a transfusion."

1. The nurse would respond that there are several side effects that need to be watched for during a blood transfusion. Together, the nurse and Mrs. McFee will watch for what types of symptoms of a transfusion reaction?

_____

_____

_____

2. The nurse would also explain to Mrs. McFee that two people always check the donor blood against the recipient information before it is transfused at least two times. Once, when it leaves the laboratory, and, again, before it is infused into the patient. Why is this attention given to checking the blood?

_____

_____

_____

SECTION IV: PRACTICING FOR NCLEX

Activity F   *Answer the following questions.*

1. All cells of the body age and are replaced in a natural order. When red blood cells (RBCs) age, they are destroyed in the spleen. During this process, the iron from their hemoglobin is released into the circulation and returned where?

   a. To the bone marrow for incorporation into new RBCs

   b. To the liver to bind with oxygen

   c. To the lungs to bind with oxygen

   d. To the muscles to be stored for strength

2. Bilirubin is the pigment of bile and is made when red blood cells die. There are two types of bilirubin that can be measured in the blood and reported on by the laboratory. What does the laboratory reports them as?

   a. Conjugated and unconjugated

   b. Soluble and insoluble

   c. Positive and negative

   d. Direct and indirect

3. Neonatal hyperbilirubinemia is an increased level of bilirubin in the infant's blood. It is usually a benign condition characterized by what?

   a. A yellow, jaundiced color

   b. Failure to thrive

   c. Brain damage

   d. A reddish, ruddy complexion

4. Anemia resulting from blood loss can be reversed if the blood loss is not so severe that it results in death. How long does it take for the

red blood cell concentration to return to normal?

a. 8 to 10 days

b. 3 to 4 weeks

c. 10 to 14 days

d. 5 to 6 weeks

5. During chronic blood loss, iron-deficiency anemia occurs. Most patients are asymptomatic until their hemoglobin falls below 8 g/dL. The red blood cells that the body does produce have too little hemoglobin. What is the term for the resulting anemia?

a. Macrocytic hyperchromic

b. Macrocytic hypochromic

c. Microcytic hypochromic

d. Microcytic hyperchromic

6. In hemolytic anemia, the red blood cells are destroyed prematurely. What distinguishes almost all types of hemolytic anemia?

a. Normocytic hypochromic cells

b. Microcytic normochromic cells

c. Macrocytic hyperchromic cells

d. Normocytic normochromic cells

7. When hemolytic anemia has intravascular hemolysis, it can be characterized in different ways. Which of the following is not a characterization of hemolytic anemia with intravascular hemolysis?

a. Hemoglobinemia

b. Jaundice

c. Hemosiderinuria

d. Spherocytosis

8. Aplastic anemia is a serious anemia that is a disorder of the pluripotential bone marrow stem cells and causes all three hematopoietic cell lines to be reduced. What is the treatment for aplastic anemia in the young and severely affected client?

a. No treatment

b. Bone marrow transplant

c. Spleen transplant

d. Liver transplant

9. When a client is in chronic renal failure, he or she almost always has anemia because of a deficiency of erythropoietin. What else contributes to the anemia experienced by clients in chronic renal failure?

a. Uremic toxins and retained nitrogen

b. Bleeding tendencies and lack of fibrinogen in blood

c. Hemodialysis and decreased nitrogen

d. Hemolysis of red blood cells and lack of fibrinogen in blood

10. When an Rh-negative mother gives birth to an Rh-positive infant, the mother usually produces antibodies that will attack any subsequent pregnancies in which the fetus is Rh positive. When subsequent babies are Rh positive, erythroblastosis fetalis occurs. What is another name for erythroblastosis fetalis?

a. Microcytic disease of the newborn

b. Hemolytic iron-deficiency anemia

c. Hemolytic disease of the newborn

d. Macrocytic disease of the newborn

11. Pernicious anemia is believed to be an autoimmune disease that destroys the gastric mucosa. This results in chronic atrophic gastritis and the production of antibodies that interfere with _____ binding to intrinsic factor.

12. Sickle cell disease is an inherited disorder seen in African American people. It is marked by the characteristic sickling of red blood cells. This causes both chronic hemolytic anemia and occlusion of blood vessels. Which are considered to be triggers of an episode of sickling? Mark all that apply.

a. Infection

b. Stress

c. Heat

d. Dehydration

e. Alkalosis

13. The indices of the red blood cell (RBC) are used to differentiate the anemias by size and color of cell. Match the term for a RBC with its definition:

Term	Definition
____ 1. Mean corpuscular hemoglobin concentration	**a.** The concentration of hemoglobin in each cell
____ 2. Mean cell hemoglobin	**b.** The mass of the RBC
____ 3. Mean corpuscular volume	**c.** The volume or size of the RBCs

14. A pregnant woman at her first prenatal visit complains to the nurse that she is always tired. The nurse knows that fatigue is one symptom of anemia. What are other symptoms of anemia? Mark all that apply.

    a. Faintness

    b. Dim vision

    c. Ruddy skin

    d. Bradycardia

15. Polycythemia vera most often occurs in men with a median age of 62 years. It is a neoplastic disease of the bone marrow that is characterized by which of the following signs and symptoms? Mark all that apply.

    a. Headache

    b. Dusky red appearance

    c. Ability to concentrate better

    d. Cyanosis of trunk

    e. Hearing difficulty

16. Thalassemia can be classed as major or minor. In thalassemia major, it is necessary to start _____ therapy as early as 6 months of age. If therapy is not started in infants who present with this disease, severe growth retardation will occur.

Disorders of White Blood Cells and Lymphoid Tissues

SECTION I: LEARNING OBJECTIVES

1. Describe the different types of white blood cells and structures of the lymphoid system where they circulate

2. Trace the development of the different white blood cells from their origin in the pluripotent bone marrow stem cell to their circulation in the bloodstream

3. Define the terms *leukopenia, neutropenia, granulocytopenia,* and *aplastic anemia*

4. Cite two general causes of neutropenia

5. Describe the mechanism of symptom production in neutropenia

6. Use the concepts regarding the central and peripheral lymphoid tissues to describe the site of origin of the malignant lymphomas, leukemias, and plasma cell dyscrasias

7. Explain how changes in chromosomal structure and gene function can contribute to the development of malignant lymphomas, leukemias, and plasma cell dyscrasias

8. Contrast and compare the signs and symptoms of non-Hodgkin and Hodgkin lymphomas

9. Describe the measures used in treatment of non-Hodgkin and Hodgkin lymphomas

10. Use the predominant white blood cell type and classification of acute or chronic to describe the four general types of leukemia

11. Explain the manifestations of leukemia in terms of altered cell differentiation

12. Describe the following complications of acute leukemia and its treatment: leukostasis, tumor lysis syndrome, hyperuricemia, and blast crisis

13. Relate the clonal expansion of immunoglobulin-producing plasma cells and accompanying destructive skeletal changes that occur with multiple myeloma in terms of manifestations and clinical course of the disorder

SECTION II: ASSESSING YOUR UNDERSTANDING

Activity A *Fill in the blanks.*

1. The white blood cells include the _____, monocyte/macrophages, and lymphocytes.

2. T lymphocytes mature in the _____.

3. The B lymphocytes differentiate to form immunoglobulin-producing _____ cells.

4. Another population of lymphocytes includes the _____ cells, which do not share

the specificity or characteristics of the T or B lymphocytes, but have the ability to lyse target cells.

5. The granulocyte and monocyte cell lines derive from the _____ stem cells and the lymphocytes from the _____ stem cells.

6. The body's lymphatic system consists of the lymphatic vessels, lymphoid tissue and lymph nodes, _____, and _____.

7. T lymphocytes travel to the thymus, where they differentiate into _____ helper T cells and _____ cytotoxic T cells.

8. In _____ anemia, the myeloid stem cells are affected, resulting in anemia, thrombocytopenia, and agranulocytosis.

9. Alloimmune neonatal neutropenia is neutropenia that occurs after transplacental transfer of maternal _____ directed at an infant's neutrophils.

10. Early signs of infection of _____ include mild skin lesions, stomatitis, pharyngitis, and diarrhea.

11. _____ is a self-limiting lymphoproliferative disorder caused by the Epstein-Barr virus.

12. _____ can involve lymphocytes, granulocytes, and other blood cells.

13. _____ originate in peripheral lymphoid structures such as the lymph nodes, where B and T lymphocytes undergo differentiation and proliferation.

14. _____ cell lymphomas are the most common type of lymphoma in the Western world.

15. Four variants of classical Hodgkin lymphoma have been described: _____ sclerosis, mixed cellularity, _____ rich, and lymphocyte depleted.

16. Persons with _____ are staged according to the number of lymph nodes that are involved; whether the lymph nodes are on one or both sides of the diaphragm; and whether there is disseminated disease involving the bone marrow, liver, lung, or skin.

17. The _____ are malignant neoplasms of cells originally derived from hematopoietic precursor cells.

18. The _____ leukemias involve immature lymphocytes and their progenitors, which originate in the bone marrow but infiltrate the spleen, lymph nodes, central nervous system, and other tissues.

19. Cytogenetic studies have shown that recurrent chromosomal changes occur in more than one-half of all cases of _____.

20. _____ usually have a sudden and stormy onset with signs and symptoms related to depressed bone marrow function.

21. There are two types of acute leukemia: acute _____ and acute _____.

22. _____ are malignancies involving proliferation of more fully differentiated myeloid and lymphoid cells.

23. Chronic lymphocytic leukemia, a clonal malignancy of _____, is the most common form of leukemia in adults in the Western world.

24. The diagnostic hallmark of chronic lymphocytic leukemia is isolated _____.

25. It is generally believed that chronic myelogenous leukemia develops when a single, pluripotential, hematopoietic stem cell acquires a _____ chromosome.

26. _____ are characterized by expansion of a single clone of immunoglobulin-producing plasma cells and a resultant increase in serum levels of a single monoclonal immunoglobulin or its fragments.

27. The development of _____ lesions in multiple myeloma is believed to be related to an increase in expression by osteoblasts of the receptor activator of the nuclear factor-κB.

28. One of the characteristics resulting from the proliferating osteoclasts in multiple myeloma is the unregulated production of a monoclonal antibody referred to as the _____.

Activity B *Match the key terms in Column A with their definitions in Column B.*

Column A

____ 1. Heterophil

____ 2. Leukopoiesis

Column B

a. Neoplasm involving B or T cells

b. Translocation on chromosome 8

_____ **3.** Burkitt lymphoma

_____ **4.** Non-Hodgkin lymphomas

_____ **5.** Neutropenia

_____ **6.** Reed-Sternberg cells

_____ **7.** Kostmann syndrome

_____ **8.** Philadelphia chromosome

_____ **9.** Blast cells

_____ **10.** ZAP-70

c. Found in more than 90% of persons with chronic myelogenous leukemia

d. Production of white blood cells

e. Used for the diagnosis of infectious mononucleosis

f. An abnormally low number of neutrophils

g. Immature precursor cells

h. Definitive marker for Hodgkin lymphoma

i. An arrest in myeloid maturation

j. Normal T cell protein, abnormal in chronic lymphocytic leukemia

Activity C *Briefly answer the following.*

1. Neutrophils are very important as a first line of defense against viral/bacterial infection. Explain what a neutrophil does and the condition that results from a deficiency of neutrophils.

_____

_____

_____

2. Describe the pathogenesis of infectious mononucleosis.

_____

_____

_____

3. Describe the clinical manifestations of non-Hodgkin lymphoma, and relate the symptoms to the pathologic cause.

_____

_____

_____

4. There are two major differences between Hodgkin lymphoma and non-Hodgkin lymphoma. What are they?

_____

_____

_____

5. What are the potential causes of leukemia?

_____

_____

_____

6. Compare and contrast acute lymphocytic leukemia and acute myelocytic leukemia.

_____

_____

_____

7. Describe the progression of chronic myelogenous leukemia through its three stages.

_____

_____

_____

8. What are the potential causes of multiple myeloma?

_____

_____

_____

SECTION III: APPLYING YOUR KNOWLEDGE

Activity D *Consider the following scenario and answer the questions.*

Two-year-old Lucy has been diagnosed with acute lymphocytic leukemia and admitted to your unit for treatment. How would you answer when the parents ask these questions?

1. "What caused Lucy's leukemia?"

_____

_____

_____

2. "What kind of treatment will Lucy have?"

_____

_____

_____

SECTION IV: PRACTICING FOR NCLEX

Activity E *Answer the following questions.*

1. Progenitor cells, or parent cells, for myelopoiesis and lymphopoiesis are derived from which of the following?
   a. Pluripotent stem cells
   b. Unipotent cells
   c. Multipotential progenitor cells
   d. Myeloproliferative cells

2. What is the name of the region of the lymph nodes that contains most of the T cells?
   a. Primary follicles
   b. Paracortex
   c. Secondary follicles
   d. Primary cortex

3. Kostmann syndrome is a severe congenital neutropenia. Which of the following is characteristic of this condition?
   a. Bone marrow disorders
   b. Severe viral infections
   c. Autoimmune disorders
   d. Severe bacterial infections

4. Drug-induced neutropenia is a disease that has significantly increased in incidence over the past several decades. What is the attributing factor in the increased incidence of drug-induced neutropenia?
   a. Treatment of cancer by chemotherapeutic drugs
   b. Decrease in the use of street drugs
   c. Destruction of tissue cells by cocaine
   d. New drugs developed to treat autoimmune diseases

5. Infectious mononucleosis is a lymphoproliferative disorder caused by the Epstein-Barr virus that is usually self-limiting and non-lethal. Which of the following complications can arise during this mostly benign disease?
   a. Peripheral nerve palsies
   b. Rupture of the spleen
   c. Rupture of the lymph nodes
   d. Severe bacterial infections

6. You are presenting an educational event to a group of cancer patients. What would you cite as the most commonly occurring hematologic cancer?
   a. Acute lymphocytic leukemia
   b. Hodgkin lymphomas
   c. Non-Hodgkin lymphomas
   d. Mantle cell lymphoma

7. Endemic Burkitt lymphoma occurs in regions of Africa where what other infections are common?
   a. Herpes zoster and Epstein-Barr virus
   b. Herpes zoster and streptococcal
   c. Malaria and streptococcal
   d. Epstein-Barr virus and malaria

8. Acute lymphoblastic leukemia (ALL) and acute myelogenous leukemia (AML) are two distinct disorders with similar presenting clinical features. What clinical feature do ALL and AML share?
   a. Night sweats
   b. Weight gain
   c. High fever
   d. Polycythemia

9. Definitive diagnosis of multiple myeloma includes the triad of bone marrow plasmacytosis, lytic bone lesions, and what?
   a. Oligoclonal bands in the cerebrospinal fluid
   b. Bence-Jones proteins in the urine
   c. Serum M-protein depression
   d. BCR-ABL fusion protein in serum

10. Chronic lymphocytic leukemia (CLL) commonly causes hypogammaglobulinemia. This makes clients with CLL more susceptible to infection. What are the most common infectious organisms that attack clients with CLL?
    a. Acne rosacea
    b. *Pseudomonas aeruginosa*
    c. *Staphylococcus aureus*
    d. *Escherichia coli*

11. Large granular lymphocytes, or natural killer cells, have the ability to _____ target cells.

12. Which lymphatic tissue is associated with mucous membranes and called mucus-associated lymphatic tissue (or MALT)? Mark all that apply.
    a. Genitourinary systems and central nervous system
    b. Respiratory passages and cardiovascular system
    c. Alimentary canal and genitourinary systems
    d. Cardiovascular system and central nervous system

13. You are speaking to a group of genetic students touring your hospital's laboratory. You talk about the possibility of a genetic predisposition for the leukemias being suggested because of the increased incidence of the disease among a number of congenital disorders. Which congenital disorders are these? Mark all that apply.

a. Cushing syndrome
b. Neurofibromatosis
c. Fanconi anemia
d. Down syndrome
e. Prader-Willi syndrome

14. Tumor lysis syndrome, the massive necrosis of malignant cells that can occur during the initial phase of treatment of acute lymphoblastic leukemia, can lead to metabolic disorders that are life threatening. Which metabolic disorders can occur because of tumor lysis syndrome? Mark all that apply.
    a. Hyperuricemia
    b. Hypokalemia
    c. Acidosis
    d. Alkalosis
    e. Hypocalcemia

15. Secondary malignancies in survivors of Hodgkin lymphoma have been attributed mainly to _____ therapy.

16

Mechanisms of Infectious Disease

SECTION I: LEARNING OBJECTIVES

1. Define the terms *host, infectious disease, colonization, microflora, virulence, pathogen,* and *saprophyte*

2. Describe the concept of host–microorganism interaction using the concepts of commensalism, mutualism, and parasitic relationships

3. Describe the structural characteristics and mechanisms of reproduction for prions, viruses, bacteria, fungi, and parasites

4. Use the concepts of incidence, portal of entry, source of infection, symptomatology, disease course, site of infection, agent, and host characteristics to explain the mechanisms of infectious diseases

5. Differentiate between incidence and prevalence and among endemic, epidemic, and pandemic

6. Describe the stages of an infectious disease after the potential pathogen has entered the body

7. List the systemic manifestations of infectious disease

8. Describe mechanisms and significance of antimicrobial and antiviral drug resistance

9. Explain the actions of intravenous immunoglobulin and cytokines in the treatment of infectious illnesses

10. State the two criteria used in the diagnosis of an infectious disease

11. Explain the differences among culture, serology, and antigen, metabolite, or molecular detection methods for diagnosis of infectious disease

12. Cite three general intervention methods that can be used in treatment of infectious illnesses

13. State four basic mechanisms by which antibiotics exert their action

14. Differentiate *bactericidal* from *bacteriostatic*

15. List the infectious agents considered to pose the highest level of bioterrorism threat

16. Describe the effect of international travel on the spread of infection

17. State an important concept in containment of infections due to bioterrorism and global travel

SECTION II: ASSESSING YOUR UNDERSTANDING

Activity A *Fill in the blanks.*

1. The colonizing bacteria acquire nutritional needs and shelter, and the host is not adversely affected by the relationship; an interaction such as this is called _____.

2. The term _____ describes the presence, multiplication, and subsequent injury within a host by another living organism.

3. A _____ relationship is one in which only the infecting organism benefits from the relationship and the host either gains nothing from the relationship or sustains injury from the interaction.

4. All microorganisms can be _____ pathogens capable of producing an infectious disease when the health and immunity of the host have been severely weakened.

5. The various prion-associated diseases produce very similar symptomatology and pathology in the host and are collectively called _____ diseases.

6. _____ are the smallest obligate intracellular pathogens.

7. Bacteria are autonomously replicating unicellular organisms known as _____ because they lack an organized nucleus.

8. _____ characteristics and microscopic morphology are used in combination to describe bacteria.

9. The _____ are an eccentric category of bacteria that are mentioned separately because of their unusual cellular morphology and distinctive mechanism of motility.

10. The _____ are unicellular prokaryotes capable of independent replication.

11. Serious _____ infections are rare and usually initiated through puncture wounds or inhalation.

12. The fungi can be separated into two groups, _____ and _____, based on rudimentary differences in their morphology.

13. Parasitic infection results from the ingestion of highly resistant cysts or spores that are shed in the _____ of an infected host.

14. The _____ is the initial appearance of symptoms in the host.

15. The period during which the host experiences the maximum impact of the infectious process corresponding to rapid proliferation and dissemination of the pathogen is known as the _____.

16. The _____ is characterized by the containment of infection, progressive elimination of the pathogen, repair of damaged tissue, and resolution of associated symptoms.

17. Inflammation of an anatomic location is usually designated by adding the suffix _____ to the name of the involved tissue in an infection.

18. The suffix _____ is used to designate the presence of a substance in the blood.

19. _____ factors are substances or products generated by infectious agents that enhance their ability to cause disease.

20. In contrast to _____, endotoxins do not contain protein, are not actively released from the bacterium during growth, and have no enzymatic activity.

Activity B *Consider the following figure.*

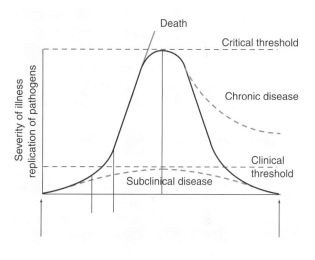

In this figure, label the areas that represent the course through which a disease progresses: resolution, acute phase, convalescent phase, incubation phase, infection, and prodromal phase.

Activity C *Match the key terms in Column A with their definitions in Column B.*

1.

Column A	Column B
____ 1. Microflora	a. Describes the act of establishing an infection
____ 2. Host	
____ 3. Infection	b. Microorganisms that live with a host
____ 4. Disease	

_____ **5.** Colonization

_____ **6.** Virulence

_____ **7.** Pathogens

_____ **8.** Saprophytes

_____ **9.** Prions

_____ **10.** *Rickettsiaceae*

c. Microorganisms so virulent that they are rarely found in the absence of disease

d. Presence, multiplication, and subsequent injury within a host by another living organism

e. Disease-producing potential of a microorganism

f. Any organism capable of supporting the nutritional and physical growth requirements of another

g. Condition of an organism that impairs normal physiologic function

h. Harmless, free-living organisms

i. Disease-causing protein particles that lack a demonstrable genome

j. Organisms combining characteristics of viral and bacterial agents to produce disease in humans

_____ **9.** Facultatively anaerobic bacteria

_____ **10.** *Chlamydia trachomatis*

h. Virus capable of transforming a cell

i. Sexually transmitted genital infections

j. Cannot live long outside strict growth requirements

Activity D *Write the correct sequence of the following in the boxes provided.*

a. Viral DNA copy is integrated into the host chromosome

b. Host cell lysis

c. Reactivation of virus

d. Entry into the host cell

e. Viral RNA genome is first translated into DNA

f. Replication of virus

Activity E *Briefly answer the following.*

1. Explain the general mechanism of cellular viral infection and replication. Differentiate between those that cause lysis and those that do not. Also, explain the concept of a latent virus.

_____

_____

_____

2. Describe the various methods of infiltration taken by organisms that will cause infection, from the organism entering the host to the manifestation of the disease state.

_____

_____

_____

3. Explain the concept of "disease course," and list all the stages that the disease course takes.

_____

_____

_____

2.

Column A

_____ **1.** Plasmids

_____ **2.** Mycoplasmas

_____ **3.** Fastidious bacteria

_____ **4.** Ectoparasites

_____ **5.** *Orthomyxoviridae*

_____ **6.** Enveloped viruses

_____ **7.** *Rickettsiaceae*

_____ **8.** Oncogenic viruses

Column B

a. Organisms are less than one-third the size of bacteria

b. Cause Rocky Mountain spotted fever

c. Flu viruses

d. Herpesvirus and paramyxoviruses

e. Infest external body surfaces

f. Bacterial DNA that may increase virulence

g. Bacteria that can adapt metabolism

4. What is the goal of treatment in regard to infective organisms? Provide the common methods of treatment.

_____

_____

_____

5. Explain the categorization of organisms that carry the potential for bioterrorism.

_____

_____

_____

SECTION III: APPLYING YOUR KNOWLEDGE

Activity F *Consider the following scenario and answer the questions.*

You are a nurse working for a public health agency. You have been asked to give a talk to the local rotary club about infectious diseases. In your presentation, you are going to include information about treatment of these diseases.

1. In discussing the role of antibiotics in the treatment of infectious diseases, you would include definitions of bactericidal and bacteriostatic. What are these definitions?

_____

_____

_____

2. What drugs are used for HIV infections? How are these drugs classified?

_____

_____

_____

SECTION IV: PRACTICING FOR NCLEX

Activity G *Answer the following questions.*

1. What is the term for parasitic relationships between microorganisms and the human body in which the human body is harmed?

a. Infectious disease

b. Mutual disease

c. Communicable disease

d. Commensal disease

2. The infectious agents that cause Rocky Mountain spotted fever and epidemic typhus are transmitted to the human body via vectors such as ticks. What are these infectious agents?

a. Viruses

b. *Rickettsiaceae*

c. *Chlamydiaceae*

d. *Anaplasmataceae*

3. Severe acute respiratory syndrome (SARS), a highly transmissible respiratory infection, crossed international borders in the winter of 2002. What terms are used to describe the outbreak of SARS?

a. Pandemic and nosocomial

b. Regional and endemic

c. Epidemic and pandemic

d. Nosocomial and endemic

4. The clinical picture, or presentation of a disease in the body, is called what?

a. Virulence of the disease

b. Source of the disease

c. Diagnosis of the disease

d. Symptomatology of the disease

5. There are two criteria that have to be met in order for a diagnosis of an infectious disease to occur. What are these two criteria?

a. Recovery of probable pathogen and documentation of signs and symptoms compatible with an infectious process

b. Propagation of a microorganism outside the body and testing to see what destroys it

c. Identification by microscopic appearance and Gram stain reaction

d. Serology and an antibody titer specific to the serology

6. Levels A, B, and C are levels assigned to potential agents of bioterrorism. What are these categorical assignments based on?

a. Safety to terrorist

b. Transmissibility

c. Environmental impact

d. Ease of use to terrorist

7. Global infectious diseases are now being recognized. These diseases, known as endemic to one part of the world, are now being found in other parts of the world due to international travel and a global marketplace. Which of the following is considered a global infectious disease?

   a. Coxsackie disease

   b. Respiratory syncytial disease

   c. West Nile virus

   d. Hand, foot, and mouth disease

8. Which of the following sequences accurately describes the stages of a disease?

   a. Incubation, prodromal, current, recovery, and resolution

   b. Subacute, prodromal, acute, postacute, and convalescent

   c. Prodromal, subacute, acute, postdromal, and resolution

   d. Incubation, prodromal, acute, convalescent, and resolution

9. Sometimes the host's white blood cells are unable to eliminate the microorganism, but the body is able to contain the dissemination of the pathogen. What is this called?

   a. Abscess

   b. Pimple

   c. Lesion

   d. Acne

10. *Escherichia coli* produces an exotoxin called Shiga toxin that enters the body when you eat undercooked hamburger meat and fruit juices that are not pasteurized. What can *E. coli* infection cause?

    a. Nephritic syndrome

    b. Hemorrhagic colitis

    c. Hemolytic thrombocytopenia

    d. Neuroleptic malignant syndrome

11. Transmissible neurodegenerative diseases such as Creutzfeldt-Jakob disease are associated with _____.

12. _____ infections refer to vertically transmitted infections, that is, infections that are transmitted from mother to infant.

13. Match the category of infectious diseases with its source.

Category	Source
____ 1. Zoonoses	a. Passed from mother to child at birth
____ 2. Perinatal infections	
____ 3. Opportunistic	b. Health care facility
____ 4. Nosocomial	c. Passed from animals to humans
	d. Acquired from client's own body

14. Infectious agents produce products or substances called virulence factors that make it easier for them to cause disease. Which of these are virulence factors? Mark all that apply.

    a. Invasive factors

    b. Prodromal factors

    c. Adhesion factors

    d. Toxins

    e. Evasive factors

15. Evasive factors, one type of virulence factor, are factors produced by infectious microorganisms to keep the host's immune system from destroying the microorganism. Which of these are evasive factors? Mark all that apply.

    a. Capsules

    b. Phospholipases

    c. Collagenases

    d. Slime

    e. Mucous layers

Innate and Adaptive Immunity

SECTION I: LEARNING OBJECTIVES

1. Discuss the function of the immune system

2. Contrast and compare the general properties of innate and adaptive immunity

3. Describe the cells of the immune system

4. Characterize the chemical mediators that orchestrate the immune response

5. Characterize the function of the innate immune system

6. Describe components of the innate immune system including epithelial barriers, soluble chemical agents, and cellular components

7. Describe the recognition systems for pathogens in innate immunity

8. State the types and functions of leukocytes that participate in innate immunity

9. Describe the functions of the various cytokines involved in innate immunity

10. Define the role of the complement system in immunity and inflammation.

11. State the properties associated with adaptive immunity

12. Define and describe the characteristics of an antigen

13. Characterize the significance and function of major histocompatibility complex molecules

14. Describe the antigen-presenting functions of macrophages and dendritic cells

15. Contrast and compare the development and function of the T and B lymphocytes

16. State the function of the five classes of immunoglobulins

17. Differentiate between the central and peripheral lymphoid structures

18. Describe the function of cytokines involved in the adaptive immune response

19. Compare passive and active immunity

20. Explain the transfer of passive immunity from mother to fetus and from mother to infant during breast-feeding

21. Characterize the development of active immunity in the infant and small child

22. Describe changes in the immune response that occur with aging

SECTION II: ASSESSING YOUR UNDERSTANDING

Activity A *Fill in the blanks.*

1. The _____ has evolved in multicellular organisms to defend against bacteria, viruses, and other foreign substances.

2. Although the immune response is normally protective, it can also produce undesirable effects such as when the response is excessive, as in _____, or when it recognizes self-tissue as foreign, as in _____ disease.

3. As the first line of defense, _____ immunity consists of the physical, chemical, molecular, and cellular defenses.

4. _____ immunity is the second major immune defense.

5. Substances that elicit adaptive immune responses are called _____.

6. _____ immunity, generated by B lymphocytes, is mediated by molecules called antibodies and is the principal defense against extracellular microbes and toxins.

7. _____ immunity is mediated by specific T lymphocytes and defends against intracellular microbes such as viruses.

8. Dendritic cells and _____ function as antigen-presenting cells for adaptive immunity.

9. The key cells of innate immunity are _____, _____, and natural killer cells.

10. _____ are the early responding cells of innate immunity.

11. During an inflammation response, the monocyte leaves the blood vessel; transforms into a tissue _____; and phagocytoses bacteria, damaged cells, and tissue debris.

12. _____ cells and _____ cells are the only cells in the body capable of specifically recognizing different antigenic determinants of microbial agents and other pathogens.

13. _____ are part of the innate immune system and may be the first line of defense against viral infections.

14. _____ cells are specialized, bone marrow–derived leukocytes found in lymphoid tissue that are important intermediaries between the innate and adaptive immune systems.

15. _____ are cytokines that stimulate the migration and activation of immune and inflammatory cells.

16. Cytokines that stimulate bone marrow pluripotent stem and progenitor or precursor cells to produce large numbers of platelets, erythrocytes, lymphocytes, neutrophils, monocytes, eosinophils, basophils, and dendritic cells are known as _____.

17. The mucous membrane linings of the gastrointestinal, respiratory, and urogenital tracts are protected by sheets of tightly packed _____ cells that block the entry of microbes.

18. The binding of _____ to the pattern recognition receptors on leukocytes initiates the signaling events that lead to innate immunity and tissue changes associated with acute inflammation.

19. _____ is the coating of a microorganism with soluble molecules that tag the microorganism for more efficient recognition by phagocytes.

20. _____ are substances foreign to the host that can stimulate an immune response.

21. Antibodies comprise a class of proteins called _____.

22. _____ immunity depends on maturation of B lymphocytes into plasma cells, which produce and secrete antibodies.

23. The _____ serves as a master regulator for the immune system.

24. _____ T cells suppress immune responses by inhibiting the proliferation of other potentially harmful self-reactive lymphocytes.

25. The central lymphoid organs, the _____ and the _____, provide the environment for immune cell production and maturation.

26. The white pulp layer of the _____ contains concentrated areas of B and T lymphocytes permeated by macrophages and dendritic cells.

Activity B *Consider the following figure.*

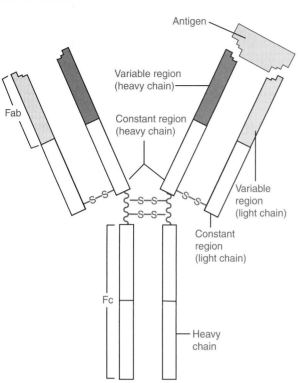

1. What does this figure depict? Discuss the significance of the different parts depicted in the model.

Activity C *Match the key terms in Column A with their definitions in Column B.*

1.

Column A

_____ **1.** Mucins

_____ **2.** Lysozyme

_____ **3.** Epithelial barrier

_____ **4.** Defensins

_____ **5.** Collectins

_____ **6.** Cilia

_____ **7.** Toll-like receptors

_____ **8.** Opsonins

_____ **9.** NF-$\kappa\beta$

_____ **10.** Interferons

Column B

a. Pathogen-associated molecular pattern receptors

b. Renders bacteria and other cells susceptible to phagocytosis

c. Traps and washes away potential invaders

d. Epithelial protrusion that moves mucus to throat

e. Surfactant proteins in respiratory track

f. Physical barrier of skin to infection

g. Disrupts virus infections

h. Small cationic peptides found in the stomach

i. Regulates the production of cytokines and adhesion molecules

j. Hydrolytic enzyme capable of cleaving the walls of bacterial cell

2.

Column A

_____ **1.** Epitopes

_____ **2.** CD4+

_____ **3.** Perforans

_____ **4.** Cell-mediated immunity

_____ **5.** Antigen presentation

_____ **6.** Antibody-mediated immunity

_____ **7.** Major histocompatibility complex

_____ **8.** Haptens

_____ **9.** CD8+

_____ **10.** Tolerance

Column B

a. Processing a complex antigen into epitopes and then displaying the foreign and self-peptides on their membranes

b. Dependent on B cells

c. Self-recognition proteins

d. Type of T helper cell

e. Dependent on T cells

f. Pore-forming molecules

g. Immunologically active sites on antigens

h. Combine with larger protein molecules and serve as antigens

i. Ability of the immune system to be nonreactive to self-antigens

j. Cytotoxic T cells

Activity D *Briefly answer the following.*

1. How do the cells of the immune system communicate with each other?

_____

_____

_____

2. What is the innate immune system, and what is its function?

_____

_____

_____

3. What is the general function of neutrophils and macrophages in the inflammatory response?

_____

_____

_____

4. What are the methods of initiating the complement system, and what are the results of activation?

_____

_____

_____

5. What is the function of MHC proteins, and how are they classified?

_____

_____

_____

6. Explain how a macrophage participates in antigen presentation.

_____

_____

_____

7. How many classes of antibody are there? Give a brief definition of function for each one.

_____

_____

_____

8. Compare and contrast active versus passive immunity.

_____

_____

_____

SECTION III: APPLYING YOUR KNOWLEDGE

Activity E *Consider the following scenario and answer the question.*

A young mother has her 2-week-old infant at the clinic for a well-baby check-up. She is concerned because her baby has been exposed to chickenpox. She states, "What am I going to do? I didn't know my friend's son had just gotten over the chickenpox. Will my baby get chickenpox?"

1. In talking with this mother, the nurse explains passive immunity. What key points will the nurse be sure to mention?

_____

_____

_____

SECTION IV: PRACTICING FOR NCLEX

Activity F *Answer the following questions.*

1. Natural killer cells are specialized lymphocytes that are one of the major parts of which immunity?

   a. Innate

   b. Adaptive

   c. Humoral

   d. Cell mediated

2. Both innate and adaptive immunity have cells that produce cytokines. Cytokines mediate the actions of many cells in both innate and adaptive immunity. How are the actions of cytokines described?

   a. Rapid and self-limiting

   b. Pleiotropic and redundant

   c. Cell specific and targeted

   d. Dendritic and morphologic

3. Stem cells in the bone marrow produce T lymphocytes or T cells, and release them into the vascular system. The T cells then migrate where to mature?

    a. Spleen

    b. Liver

    c. Thymus

    d. Pancreas

4. Cell-mediated immunity is involved in resistance to infectious diseases caused by bacteria and some viruses. It is also involved in cell-mediated hypersensitivity reactions. Which of these does not cause a cell-mediated hypersensitivity reaction?

    a. Latex

    b. Poison ivy

    c. X-ray dye

    d. Blood transfusion

5. Passive immunity is immunity that is transferred from another source and lasts only weeks to months. What is an example of passive immunity?

    a. An injection of gamma-globulin

    b. An immunization

    c. Exposure to poison ivy

    d. Allergy shots

6. An essential property of the immune system is self-regulation. An immune response that is not adequate can lead to immunodeficiency, whereas an immune response that is excessive can lead to conditions from allergic responses to autoimmune diseases. Which of these is *not* an example of a breakdown of the self-regulation of the immune system?

    a. Multiple sclerosis

    b. Huntington disease

    c. Systemic lupus

    d. Fibromyalgia

7. One of the self-regulatory actions of the immune system is to identify self-antigens and be nonreactive to them. What is this ability of the immune system defined as?

    a. Antigen specificity

    b. Nonreactivity

    c. Tolerance

    d. Antigen diversity

8. The laboratory finds IgA in a sample of cord blood from a newborn infant. This finding is important because it signifies what?

    a. Fetal reaction to an infection acquired at birth

    b. Maternal reaction to an infection in the fetus

    c. Maternal exposure to an infection in a sexual partner

    d. Fetal reaction to exposure to an intrauterine infection

9. The daughter of a 79-year-old woman asks the nurse why her mother gets so many infections. The daughter states, "My mother has always been healthy, but now she has pneumonia. Last month she got cellulitis from a bug bite she scratched. The month before that was some other infection. How come she seems to get sick so often now?" What is the nurses' best response?

    a. "As people get older, their immune system doesn't respond as well as it did when they were younger."

    b. "About the time we are 75 or 76 years old, our immune system quits working."

    c. "Your mother just seems to be prone to infections."

    d. "Your mother gets infections frequently because she wants attention from you."

10. The results of recent research suggest that a key role in the origin of some diseases is played by inflammation. Inflammation has a role in the beginnings of which of these diseases?

    a. Osteoporosis

    b. Rheumatoid arthritis

    c. Osteogenesis imperfecta

    d. Hydronephrosis

11. _____, or immunogens, are substances foreign to the host that can stimulate an immune response.

12. Each immunoglobulin has a different role in the immune response. Match each immunoglobulin with its role.

Immunoglobulin   **Role**

____ **1.** IgG

____ **2.** IgA

____ **3.** IgM

____ **4.** IgD

____ **5.** IgE

a. First circulating immunoglobulin to appear in response to an antigen and first antibody type made by a newborn

b. Involved in inflammation, allergic responses, and combating parasitic infections

c. Serves as an antigen receptor for initiating the differentiation of B cells

d. Protects against bacteria, toxins, and viruses in body fluids and activates the complement system

e. Primary defense against local infections in mucosal tissues

13. The mucous membrane linings of the gastrointestinal, respiratory, and urogenital tracts are protected by sheets of tightly packed _____ cells that block the entry of microbes and destroy them by secreting antimicrobial enzymes, proteins, and peptides.

14. In both innate and adaptive immune systems, cells communicate information about invading organisms by the secretion of chemical mediators. Which are these mediators? Mark all that apply.

a. Virulence factors

b. Chemokines

c. Colony-stimulating factors

d. Coxiella

15. There are many cells that comprise the passive and adaptive immune systems. Which cells are responsible for the specificity and memory of adaptive immunity? Mark all that apply.

a. Phagocytes

b. T lymphocytes

c. Dendritic cells

d. Natural killer cells

e. B lymphocytes

CHAPTER 18

Inflammation, Tissue Repair, and Wound Healing

SECTION I: LEARNING OBJECTIVES

1. State the five cardinal signs of acute inflammation and describe the physiologic mechanisms involved in production of these signs

2. Describe the vascular changes in an acute inflammatory response

3. Characterize the interaction of adhesion molecules, chemokines, and cytokines in leukocyte adhesion, migration, and phagocytosis, which are part of the cellular phase of inflammation

4. List four types of inflammatory mediators and state their function

5. Contrast acute and chronic inflammation

6. Define the systemic manifestations of inflammation, including the characteristics of an acute-phase response

7. Define the terms *parenchymal* and *stromal* as they relate to the tissues of an organ

8. Compare labile, stable, and permanent cell types in terms of their capacity for regeneration

9. Describe healing by primary and secondary intention

10. Explain the effects of soluble mediators and the extracellular matrix on tissue repair and wound healing

11. Trace the wound-healing process through the inflammatory, proliferative, and remodeling phases

12. Explain the effects of malnutrition; ischemia and oxygen deprivation; impaired immune and inflammatory responses; and infection, wound separation, and foreign bodies on wound healing

13. Discuss the effect of age on wound healing

SECTION II: ASSESSING YOUR UNDERSTANDING

Activity A *Fill in the blanks.*

1. _____ is a protective response intended to eliminate the initial cause of cell injury, remove the damaged tissue, and generate new tissue.

2. The cardinal signs of inflammation are _____, _____, _____, and _____.

3. In addition to the cardinal signs that appear at the site of injury, _____ manifestations may occur as chemical mediators produced at the site of inflammation gain entrance to the circulatory system.

4. _____ inflammation is of relatively short duration, lasting for a few minutes, whereas _____ inflammation is of a longer duration, lasting for days to years.

5. Acute inflammation involves two major components: the _____ and _____ stages.

6. Increased circulating white blood cells are a condition known as _____.

7. _____ produce prostaglandins and leukotrienes, platelet activating factor, inflammatory cytokines, and growth factors that promote regeneration of tissues.

8. _____ changes that occur with inflammation involve the arterioles, capillaries, and venules of the microcirculation.

9. The selectins function in adhesion of _____ to endothelial cells.

10. The integrins promote _____ and cell-to-extracellular matrix interactions.

11. Chemotaxis is dynamic and energy-directed process of directed _____.

12. Groups of proteins that direct the trafficking of leukocytes during the early stages of inflammation or injury are known as _____.

13. The _____ pathways generate toxic oxygen and nitrogen products.

14. The plasma-derived mediators of inflammation include the _____ factors and the _____ proteins.

15. Histamine causes _____ of arterioles and increases the _____ of venules.

16. The _____ family of inflammatory mediators consists of prostaglandins, leukotrienes, and related metabolites.

17. The _____ induce inflammation and potentiate the effects of histamine and other inflammatory mediators.

18. Aspirin and the nonsteroidal anti-inflammatory drugs reduce inflammation by inactivating the first enzyme in the _____ pathway for prostaglandin synthesis.

19. Eating oily fish and other foods that are high in _____ results in partial replacement of arachidonic acid in inflammatory cell membranes, which leads to decreased production of arachidonic acid–derived inflammatory mediators.

20. _____ fragments contribute to the inflammatory response by causing vasodilation, increasing vascular permeability; and enhancing the activity of phagocytes.

21. Activation of the _____ system results in release of bradykinin, which increases vascular permeability and causes contraction of _____, dilation of blood vessels, and _____.

22. _____, a cytokine that will induce endothelial cells to express adhesion molecules and release cytokines, chemokines, and reactive oxygen species, is released from mast cells.

23. The _____ radical, _____ radical, and _____ radical are the major free oxygen radicals produced within the cell.

24. At higher levels, free radical mediators can produce _____.

25. The acute inflammatory response involves the production of _____; they can be serous, hemorrhagic, fibrinous, membranous, or purulent.

26. Agents that evoke chronic inflammation typically are low-grade, persistent infections or irritants that are unable to _____ or _____.

27. The function of the acute phase protein _____ is believed to be protective, in that it binds to the surface of invading microorganisms and targets them for destruction by complement and phagocytosis.

28. Body organs and tissues are composed of two types of structures: _____ and _____.

29. _____are those that continue to divide and replicate throughout life, replacing cells that are continually being destroyed.

30. Cells that are capable of undergoing regeneration when confronted with an appropriate stimulus and are thus capable of reconstituting the tissue of origin are termed _____.

31. _____ tissue is a glistening red, moist connective tissue that contains newly formed capillaries, proliferating fibroblasts, and residual inflammatory cells.

32. The elderly have reduced _____ and _____ synthesis, impaired wound contraction, and slower reepithelialization of open wounds.

33. The _____ is often born with immature organ systems and minimal energy stores but high metabolic requirements—a condition that predisposes to impaired wound healing.

Activity B *Consider the following figure.*

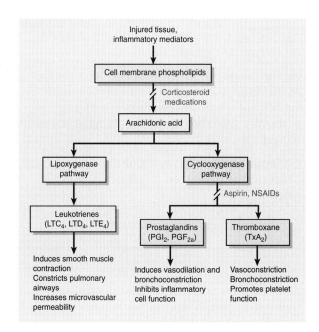

1. What does this figure represent? Explain the process that is depicted.

_____

_____

_____

Activity C *Match the key terms in Column A with their definitions in Column B.*

Column A

____ 1. Endothelial cells

____ 2. Eosinophils

____ 3. Edema

____ 4. Neutrophils

____ 5. Exudate

____ 6. Nitric oxide

____ 7. Margination

____ 8. Thrombocytes

____ 9. Mast cells

____ 10. Basophils

Column B

a. Increase in the blood during allergic reactions

b. Leukocyte accumulation

c. Regulate leukocyte extravasation

d. Stimulate inflammatory reaction in response to injury or infection

e. Circulating cells similar to mast cells

f. Primary phagocyte that arrives early at the site of inflammation

g. Stimulator of vasodilation

h. Activation affects vascular permeability, chemotactic, adhesive, and proteolytic properties

i. Swelling due to movement of fluid from vasculature into tissues

j. Outpouring of a protein-rich fluid into the tissue and extravascular space

Activity D *Put the following events in the proper order:*

a. Chemotaxis
b. Margination and adhesion to endothelium
c. Activation and phagocytosis
d. Transmigration across endothelium

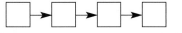

Activity E *Briefly answer the following.*

1. The cardinal signs of inflammation result from the physiologic processes of the inflammatory cells and protein systems. List the signs, and give a brief explanation as to its cause.

   _____

   _____

   _____

2. Describe and differentiate between acute and chronic inflammation.

   _____

   _____

   _____

3. The vascular response of inflammation follows one of three patterns. Describe these patterns, and explain why it is necessary to have multiple responses.

   _____

   _____

   _____

4. Many leukocytes have the ability to phagocytose foreign material and dispose of it. The process involves three steps. List and explain these steps.

   _____

   _____

   _____

5. There are many mediators of the inflammatory system. They may be grouped by function. Describe each group, and give a brief example of each.

   _____

   _____

   _____

6. Explain and describe the two types of chronic inflammation.

   _____

   _____

   _____

7. What is the purpose of the acute phase response of inflammation?

   _____

   _____

   _____

8. Explain the concept of wound healing by first and second intent.

   _____

   _____

   _____

SECTION III: APPLYING YOUR KNOWLEDGE

Activity F *Consider the following scenario and answer the questions.*

You are the nurse caring for a burn victim who has sustained second- and third-degree burns over 50% of his body. The family is asking you questions about the care that is being given to their relative.

1. A family member asks about the drainage she sees on the bandages. What would you tell her?

   _____

   _____

   _____

2. Several days post injury, a family member asks why the client is not eating. What kind of information would you give her?

   _____

   _____

   _____

SECTION IV: PRACTICING FOR NCLEX

Activity G *Answer the following questions.*

1. The cardinal signs of inflammation include swelling, pain, redness, and heat. What is the fifth cardinal sign of inflammation?
   a. Loss of function
   b. Altered level of consciousness
   c. Sepsis
   d. Fever

2. The cells that are associated with allergic disorders and the inflammation associated with immediate hypersensitive reactions are known as what? Mark all that apply.
   a. Macrophages
   b. Eosinophils
   c. Mast cells
   d. Neutrophils
   e. Basophils

3. Inflammation can be either acute or chronic. The immune system is believed to play a role in chronic inflammation and may be one of the reasons chronic inflammation may persist for days to months to years. Why is the risk of scarring and deformity greater in chronic inflammation than it is in acute inflammation?
   a. Chronic inflammation is the persistent destruction of healthy tissue.
   b. Fibroblasts instead of exudates proliferate in chronic inflammation.
   c. Typically, agents that evoke chronic inflammation are infections or irritants that penetrate deeply and spread rapidly.
   d. Chronic inflammation is often the result of allergic reactions.

4. A class of student nurses is hearing a lecture on wound healing. The professor explains about primary and secondary healing. The professor continues to talk about the phases of wound healing and states that in both primary and secondary healing the phases of wound healing occur at different rates. What are the phases of wound healing? Mark all that apply.
   a. Activation phase
   b. Proliferative phase
   c. Nutritional phase
   d. Inflammatory phase
   e. Maturational phase

5. Hyperbaric treatment for wound healing is used for wounds that have problems in healing due to hypoxia or infection. It works by raising the partial pressure of oxygen in plasma. How does hyperbaric oxygen treatment enhance wound healing?
   a. Destruction of anaerobic bacteria
   b. Increased action of eosinophils
   c. Promotion of angiogenesis
   d. Decrease in fibroblast activity

6. As a nurse in the emergency department, you would know that research has shown that the possibility of infection in a bite wound is tied to what caused the bite, the location of the bite, and the type of injury inflicted by the bite. Which bite would have the highest possibility of infection?
   a. Bite inflicted by a child
   b. Wound caused by a cat bite
   c. Bite inflicted by an adult
   d. Wound caused by a dog bite

7. Wound healing is more difficult for persons at both ends of the age spectrum, although the reasons differ. In the elderly, wound healing is impaired or delayed because of structural and functional changes in the skin that occur with aging and the chronicity of wounds in the elderly. Why do neonates and small children have problems with wound healing?
   a. Their bodies are not yet capable of an inflammatory response.
   b. Their skin is fragile.
   c. They do not have the reserves needed.
   d. Their immune systems are hypersensitive to infectious agents.

8. All wounds are considered contaminated at the time they occur. Usually, the natural defenses in our bodies can deal with the invading microorganisms; however, there are times when a wound is badly contaminated and host defenses are overwhelmed. What happens to the healing process when host defenses are overwhelmed by infectious agents?

   a. The inflammatory response is shortened and does not complete destruction of the invading organisms.

   b. Fibroblast production becomes malignant due to hypersensitization by invading organisms.

   c. The formation of granulation tissue is impaired.

   d. Collagen fibers cannot draw tissues together.

9. During the acute inflammatory response, there is a period called the transient phase where there is increased vascular permeability. What is considered the principal mediator of the immediate transient phase?

   a. Histamine

   b. Arachidonic acid

   c. Fibroblasts

   d. Cytokines

10. Inflammation can be either local or systemic. What are the most prominent systemic manifestations of inflammation?

    a. Fever, leukocytosis or leukopenia, and the acute phase response

    b. Fever, leukocytosis or leukopenia, and the transition phase response

    c. Widening pulse pressure, thrombocytopenia, and the recovery phase response

    d. Widening pulse pressure, thrombocytopenia, and the latent phase response

CHAPTER 19

Disorders of the Immune Response

SECTION I: LEARNING OBJECTIVES

1. State the difference in causes of primary and secondary immunodeficiency disorders

2. Compare and contrast pathology and manifestations of humoral (B-cell), cellular (T-cell), and combined T- and B-cell immunodeficiency disorders

3. State the function of the complement system and relate it to the manifestations of complement deficiencies and hereditary angioneurotic edema

4. State the proposed mechanisms of dysfunction and manifestations of phagocytosis disorders

5. Differentiate between adaptive immune responses that protect against microbial agents and hypersensitivity responses

6. Describe the immune mechanisms involved in a type I, type II, type III, and type IV hypersensitivity reaction

7. Describe the pathogenesis of allergic rhinitis, food allergy, serum sickness, Arthus reaction, contact dermatitis, and hypersensitivity pneumonitis

8. Characterize the differences in latex allergy caused by a type I, IgE-mediated hypersensitivity response and that caused by a type IV, cell-mediated response

9. Discuss the rationale for matching of human leukocyte antigen or major histocompatibility complex types in organ transplantation

10. Compare the immune mechanisms involved in allogeneic transplant rejection

11. Describe the mechanisms and manifestations of graft-versus-host disease

12. Relate the mechanisms of self-tolerance to the possible explanations for development of autoimmune disease

13. Name four or more diseases attributed to autoimmunity

14. Describe three or more postulated mechanisms underlying autoimmune disease

15. State the criteria for establishing an autoimmune basis for a disease

SECTION II: ASSESSING YOUR UNDERSTANDING

Activity A *Fill in the blanks.*

1. Under normal conditions, the _____ response deters or prevents disease.

2. _____ can be defined as an abnormality in the immune system that renders a person susceptible to diseases normally prevented by an intact immune system.

3. The _____ immune system is comprised of the phagocytic leukocytes, natural killer cells, and complement proteins.

4. The _____ immune response is composed mainly of T and B cells and responds to infections more slowly, but more specifically than the innate immune system.

5. The adaptive immune system is further divided into the _____ and _____ immune systems.

6. A large number of primary immunodeficiency diseases have been mapped to the _____ chromosome.

7. Defects in humoral immunity increase the risk of recurrent _____ infections.

8. During the first few months of life, infants are protected from infection by IgG antibodies that originate in _____ circulation during fetal life.

9. Of all the primary immunodeficiency diseases, those affecting _____ production are the most frequent.

10. Abnormal immunoglobulin loss can occur with chronic _____ disease; due to abnormal glomerular filtration, patients lose serum IgA and IgG in their urine.

11. Secondary humoral immunodeficiency's can also result from a number of _____, including chronic lymphocytic leukemia, lymphoma, and multiple myeloma that interfere with normal immunoglobulin production.

12. T cells can be functionally divided into two subtypes: _____ and _____ T cells.

13. Collectively, _____ protect against fungal, protozoan, viral, and intracellular bacterial infections; control malignant cell proliferation; and are responsible for coordinating the overall immune response.

14. Disorders that affect both B and T lymphocytes, with resultant defects in both humoral and cell-mediated immunity, fall under the broad classification of _____ syndrome.

15. In _____, genetic mutations lead to absence of all T- and B-cell function and, in some cases, a lack of natural killer cells.

16. Severe combined immunodeficiency disease is more commonly found in _____ because it is X linked.

17. Hereditary angioneurotic edema is a form of _____ deficiency.

18. Chronic cirrhosis of the liver would reduce the production of complement proteins; this type of deficiency would be classified as _____.

19. Chédiak-Higashi syndrome is an abnormality of _____ of phagocytes.

20. Chronic granulomatous disease is a group of inherited disorders that greatly reduce or inactivate the ability of phagocytic cells to produce the _____.

21. _____ disorders refer to excessive or inappropriate activation of the immune system.

22. Type I hypersensitivity reactions to antigens are referred to as _____.

23. _____ is a systemic life-threatening hypersensitivity reaction characterized by widespread edema, vascular shock secondary to vasodilation, and difficulty breathing.

24. Persons with _____ allergic conditions tend to have high serum levels of IgE and increased numbers of basophils and mast cells.

25. Allergic _____ is characterized by symptoms of sneezing, itching, and watery discharge from the nose and eyes.

26. There are three different types of antibody-mediated mechanisms involved in _____ reactions: opsonization and complement- and antibody receptor–mediated phagocytosis, complement- and antibody receptor–mediated inflammation, and antibody-mediated cellular dysfunction.

27. With _____ destruction, cells that are coated with low levels of IgG antibody are killed by a variety of effector cells, which bind to their target by their receptors for IgG, and cell lysis occur without phagocytosis.

28. _____ hypersensitivity reactions are responsible for the vasculitis seen in certain autoimmune diseases such as systemic lupus erythematous or the kidney damage seen with acute glomerulonephritis.

29. _____ sickness is a systemic immune complex disorder that is triggered by the deposition of insoluble antigen-antibody complexes in blood vessels, joints, heart, and kidney tissue.

30. A term used by pathologists and immunologists to describe localized tissue necrosis caused by immune complexes is the _____.

31. Hypersensitivity reactions that are mediated by specifically sensitized T lymphocytes are divided into two basic types—direct cell-mediated cytotoxicity and delayed-type hypersensitivity—and generally classified as _____.

32. Allergic _____ denotes an inflammatory response confined to the skin that is initiated by reexposure to an allergen to which a person had previously become sensitized.

33. A major barrier to _____ is the process of rejection in which the recipient's immune system recognizes the graft as foreign and attacks it.

34. Transplanted tissue can be categorized as an _____ graft if donor and recipient are the same person, _____ graft if the donor and recipient are identical twins, and _____ if the donor and recipient are related or unrelated but share similar human leukocyte antigen types.

35. _____ occurs when immunologically competent cells or precursors are transplanted into recipients who are immunologically compromised.

36. _____ diseases represent a group of disorders that are caused by a breakdown in the ability of the immune system to differentiate between self- and nonself-antigens.

37. The ability of the immune system to differentiate self from nonself is called _____.

38. Loss of self-tolerance with development of _____ is characteristic of a number of autoimmune disorders.

Activity B *Consider the following figure.*

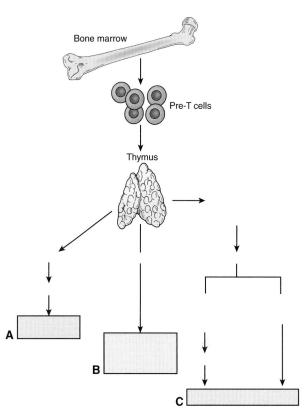

In this figure, label and diagram the process of T cell selection. Be sure to include the end result of each pathway.

Activity C *Match the key terms in Column A with their definitions in Column B.*

Column A

____ 1. DiGeorge syndrome

____ 2. Secondary immunodeficiency

____ 3. Hyper-IgM syndrome

____ 4. X-linked agammaglobulinemia

____ 5. Selective IgA deficiency

Column B

a. Essentially undetectable levels of all serum immunoglobulins

b. Complement-mediated immune disorders

c. Decreases in one or more IgG subgroups

d. Repeated bouts of upper respiratory and middle ear infections

_____ **6.** Adenosine deaminase deficiencies and T-cell cytokine receptor mutations

_____ **7.** Transient hypogamma-globulinemia of infancy

_____ **8.** Ataxia-telangiectasia

_____ **9.** Common variable immuno-deficiency

_____ **10.** Immuno-globulin G subclass deficiency

_____ **11.** Wiskott-Aldrich syndrome

_____ **12.** Type I hypersensitivity reaction

_____ **13.** Type II hypersensitivity reaction

_____ **14.** Type III hypersensitivity reaction

_____ **15.** Type IV hypersensitivity reaction

e. Partial or complete failure of develop-ment of the thymus and parathyroid glands

f. In levels of serum and secretory IgA

g. Antibody-mediated disorders

h. Acquired later in life

i. Terminal differenti-ation of mature B cells to plasma cells is blocked

j. Ig-E–mediated dis-orders

k. Lymphopenia and a decrease in the ratio of CD4$^+$ helper T cells to CD8$^+$ sup-pressor T cells

l. Low IgG and IgA levels, high IgM concentrations

m. Cause of severe combined immun-odeficiency disease

n. Susceptible to infec-tions caused by encapsulated microorganisms

o. T-cell–mediated disorders

Activity D *Put the normal sequence of actions of a polymorphonuclear phagocyte in order in the following boxes.*

1. Phagocytosis

2. Kill the ingested pathogens

3. Chemotaxis

4. Generate microbicidal substances

5. Adherence

Activity E *Briefly answer the following.*

1. What is the difference between a primary and a secondary immunodeficiency?

_____

_____

_____

2. Why does it take up to 6 months for the symp-toms of a primary immunodeficiency to ap-pear?

_____

_____

_____

3. Explain how a patient can become sensitized to an allergen (antigen) in a type I hypersensi-tivity reaction.

_____

_____

_____

4. Compare the direct cell-mediated cytotoxicity of type IV hypersensitivity reactions with the delayed-type hypersensitivity reactions.

_____

_____

_____

5. What is severe combined immunodeficiency disease?

_____

_____

_____

SECTION III: APPLYING YOUR KNOWLEDGE

Activity F *Consider the following scenario and answer the questions.*

A 30-year-old woman has just been diagnosed with systemic lupus erythematosus. She presents with arthritis, a "butterfly rash," weight loss, weakness, and fatigue. She is distraught and states, "How can the doctor be sure that I have this disease?"

1. The correct response to this patient about the diagnosis would include information about which test?

_____

_____

_____

2. When planning patient education for this woman, what medications would the nurse tell the patient about?

_____

_____

_____

SECTION IV: PRACTICING FOR NCLEX

Activity G *Answer the following questions.*

1. Infants are born with a passive immunity that occurs when immunoglobulin antibodies cross the placenta from the maternal circulation prior to birth. Which immunoglobulin is capable of crossing the placenta?

a. IgM
b. IgD
c. IgG
d. IgE

2. Drug-induced secondary hypogammaglobulinemia are reversible. Which drugs produce hypogammaglobulinemia? Mark all that apply.

a. Phenytoin
b. Corticosteroids
c. Carbamazepine
d. Disease-modifying antirheumatic drugs
e. Interferon-beta 1a drugs

3. Primary cell-mediated disorders of the immune system cause severe problems with infections. Children with these disorders rarely survive beyond childhood without a bone marrow transplant. Which of the following is a disease that involves primary cell-mediated disorders of the immune system?

a. DiGeorge syndrome
b. Y-linked hyper-IgM syndrome
c. X-linked agammaglobulinemia
d. Y-linked agammaglobulinemia

4. Combined immunodeficiency syndrome is a disorder in which both B and T lymphocytes are affected. This results in defects in both humoral and cell-mediated immunity. What could be the cause of this disorder?

a. Multiple misplaced genes that influence lymphocyte development and response
b. A single mutation in any gene that influences major histocompatibility antigens
c. A single misplaced gene that influences major histocompatibility
d. Multiple mutations in genes that influence lymphocyte development and response

5. Combined immunodeficiency syndrome (CIDS) is distinguished by low, not absent, T-cell function. These diseases are usually associated with other disorders and arise from diverse genetic causes. Which of the following diseases is considered a CIDS?

a. Pierre-Robin syndrome
b. Angelman syndrome
c. Ataxia-telangiectasia
d. Adair-Dighton syndrome

6. The immune system typically responds to invaders of all types in our bodies. However, it can also cause tissue injury and disease. What is this effect called?

a. Hypersensitivity action
b. Antigen reaction
c. Mediator response action
d. Allergen stimulating reaction

7. Some people are so sensitive to certain antigens that they react within minutes by developing itching, hives, and skin erythema, followed shortly thereafter by bronchospasm and respiratory distress. What is this commonly known as?

a. Antigen reaction
b. Anaphylactic reaction
c. Hyposensitive reaction
d. Arthus reaction

8. A systemic immune complex disorder that is caused by insoluble antigen-antibody complexes being deposited in blood vessels, the joints, the heart, or kidney tissue is called what?

    a. Anti-immune disease

    b. Systemic lupus erythematosus

    c. Serum sickness

    d. Antigen-antibody sickness

9. The incidence of latex allergy is skyrocketing because of diseases such as HIV. It is known that the use of latex examining gloves has played a major role in the increasing incidence of latex allergy. What plays a significant role in the allergic response to latex gloves?

    a. Baking powder used inside the gloves

    b. Airborne pieces of latex

    c. Latex proteins that attach to clothing

    d. Cornstarch powder used inside the gloves

10. A transplant reaction that occurs immediately after transplantation is caused by _____ antibodies.

11. It has been postulated that an autoimmune disease needs a "trigger event" for it to clinically manifest itself in the body. What are these "trigger events" believed to be? Mark all that apply.

    a. A. microorganism or virus

    b. A self-antigen from a previously sequestered body tissue

    c. A breakdown in the antigen-antibody response

    d. A chemical substance

    e. A systemic ability for self-tolerance

CHAPTER 20

Acquired Immunodeficiency Syndrome

SECTION I: LEARNING OBJECTIVES

1. Briefly trace the history of the AIDS epidemic

2. State the virus responsible for AIDS and explain how it differs from most other viruses

3. Describe the mechanisms of HIV transmission and relate them to the need for public awareness and concern regarding the spread of AIDS

4. Describe the structure of HIV and trace its entry and steps in replication within the $CD4^+$ T lymphocyte

5. Describe the alterations in immune function that occur in persons with AIDS

6. Describe the CDC HIV/AIDS classification system

7. Relate the altered immune function in persons with HIV infection and AIDS to the development of opportunistic infections, malignant tumors, nervous system manifestations, the wasting syndrome, and metabolic disorders

8. Discuss the transmission of HIV

9. Describe preventive strategies to decrease the transmission of HIV

10. Explain the possible significance of a positive antibody test for HIV infection

11. Differentiate between the enzyme immunoassay (enzyme-linked immunosorbent assay) and Western blot antibody detection tests for HIV infection

12. Describe the methods used in the early management of HIV infection

13. Compare the actions of the reverse transcriptase inhibitors (e.g., nucleoside reverse transcriptase inhibitors, nucleotide analog reverse transcriptase inhibitors), non-nucleoside reverse transcriptase inhibitors, protease inhibitors, and fusion inhibitors in terms of controlling HIV replication

14. Enumerate some of the psychosocial issues associated with HIV/AIDS

15. Discuss the vertical transmission of HIV from mother to child and recommended prevention measures

16. Cite problems with the diagnosis of HIV infection in the infant

17. Compare the progress of HIV infection in infants and children with HIV infection in adults

SECTION II: ASSESSING YOUR UNDERSTANDING

Activity A *Fill in the blanks.*

1. AIDS is a disease caused by infection with _____ and is characterized by profound _____ with associated _____ infections, malignancies, wasting, and central nervous system degeneration.

2. HIV is a _____ that selectively attacks the _____ T lymphocytes, the immune cells responsible for orchestrating and coordinating the immune response to infection.

3. HIV is transmitted from one person to another through _____ contact, _____ contact, or _____.

4. _____ contact is the most frequent way that HIV is transmitted.

5. Because HIV is found in _____, the use of needles, syringes, and other drug injection paraphernalia is a direct route for transmission.

6. Occupational risk of infection for health care workers is most often associated with _____ or _____ of blood from a patient with HIV.

7. HIV infects a limited number of cell types in the body, including a subset of lymphocytes called _____, _____, and _____ cells.

8. $CD4^+$ T cell recognizes foreign antigens and helps activate _____ and _____ immunity.

9. Treatment of HIV/AIDS relies on the use of agents that _____ steps of the HIV replication process.

10. HIV replication involves the killing of the _____ cell and the release of copies of HIV into the bloodstream.

11. _____ infections begin to occur as the immune system becomes severely compromised.

12. The most common causes of respiratory disease in persons with HIV infection are _____, Pneumocystis carinii pneumonia, and pulmonary _____.

13. _____ syndrome is common in persons with HIV infection or AIDS.

14. The term _____ is frequently used to describe the body composition changes with or without the other metabolic derangements.

15. The development of _____ or _____ behaviors will prevent HIV transmission.

16. The most accurate and inexpensive method for identifying HIV is the _____ test.

17. The _____ test is more specific than the HIV antibody test.

18. Polymerase chain reaction is a technique for detecting HIV _____.

19. The medications that are currently available to treat HIV _____ the amount of virus in the body, but they do not _____ HIV.

20. Many people with HIV have preexisting mental health conditions like _____ or _____ disorders as well as alcohol and other drug problems.

21. _____ for HIV DNA is used most often to diagnose HIV in infants younger than 18 months.

Activity B *Match the key terms in Column A with their definitions in Column B.*

Column A

_____ 1. HIV-associated neurocognitive disorders

_____ 2. *Mycobacterium tuberculosis*

_____ 3. Human papillomavirus

_____ 4. *Pneumocystis carinii*

_____ 5. Progressive multifocal leukoencephalopathy

_____ 6. *Toxoplasma gondii*

_____ 7. Kaposi sarcoma

_____ 8. HIV-associated dementia

_____ 9. *Streptococcus pneumoniae*

Column B

a. Demyelinating disease of the central nervous system

b. Malignancy of the endothelial cells that line small blood vessels

c. Organism common in the environment that causes pneumonia in AIDS patients

d. Usually a late complication of HIV manifested via decrease in neural speed

e. Most common cause of death for people with HIV

f. Brain parasite

g. Causes bacterial pneumonia in AIDS patients

h. Syndrome of cognitive impairment with motor dysfunction

i. Causes cervical and anal carcinoma

Activity C *Put the following steps of viral replication in the correct order.*

Cleavage of protein product into separate proteins for new viruses; transcription of viral DNA into mRNA; binding of the virus to the CD4$^+$ T cell; DNA synthesis via reverse transcriptase; attachment and uncoating of the virus, allowing the genetic material to enter the host cell; translation of mRNA into a protein; assemblage of new HIV; integration into the host DNA.

Activity D *Briefly answer the following.*

1. How does HIV make a patient immunodeficient?

_____

_____

_____

2. What is the typical course of HIV?

_____

_____

_____

3. What is the goal of highly active antiretroviral therapy (HAART)?

_____

_____

_____

4. What are the primary classes of medication used in HAART, and what is the goal of each?

_____

_____

_____

5. What is the most common route of HIV infection for children?

_____

_____

_____

SECTION III: APPLYING YOUR KNOWLEDGE

Activity E *Consider the following scenario and answer the questions.*

A 15-year-old boy is coming to the clinic with his parents after being diagnosed with HIV/AIDS. The client and his family want to learn about the treatment plan that is being recommended.

1. As the nurse, you are preparing the educational plan for the family. What essential elements will you include in the education of the client and family?

_____

_____

_____

2. At this clinic visit, you know that a baseline evaluation will be performed. What will this evaluation include?

_____

_____

_____

SECTION IV: PRACTICING FOR NCLEX

Activity F *Answer the following questions.*

1. You are a school nurse teaching a health class to a group of high school students. You are preparing a lecture on HIV/AIDS. You would know to include what information about the transmission of AIDS in your lecture? Mark all that apply.

a. AIDS is transmitted through the bite of an insect.

b. AIDS is transmitted through sexual contact.

c. AIDS is transmitted through blood-to-blood contact.

d. AIDS is transmitted from the mother to her unborn baby.

e. AIDS is transmitted through nonsexual household contact.

2. The HIV virus, once inside the body, replicates through an eight-step process. Take the eight steps that are listed and put them in the correct order.

a. DNA synthesis

b. Binding of virus to $CD4^+$ T cell

c. Cleavage

d. Assembly and release from $CD4^+$ T cell

e. Integration

f. Transcription

g. Translation

h. Internalization

3. A new patient presents at the clinic with the following history: a $CD4^+$ cell count of 400 cells/μL, generalized lymphadenopathy, and a positive HIV test 8 years ago. Based on this information, you would know that the patient is in what phase of the HIV infection?

a. Latent phase

b. Overt AIDS phase

c. Primary infection phase

d. Conversion phase

4. A 21-year-old woman diagnosed with HIV/AIDS 4 years ago now presents with cytomegalovirus. The nurse explains to the woman that this infection is caused by a common organism that normally does not cause infection in someone with a healthy immune system. This type of infection is called what?

a. HIV infection

b. Opportunistic infection

c. Autoimmune infection

d. Suppression infection

5. In the United States, the most common opportunistic infection in people with HIV/AIDS infections is respiratory infection. When the $CD4^+$ level drops below 200 cells/μL, it is time to start prophylaxis. What is the drug of choice for prophylaxis?

a. Trimethobenzamide

b. Triamterene

c. Trimethoprim-sulfate

d. Trimipramine

6. Kaposi sarcoma is an opportunistic malignancy that is found on the skin, in the oral cavity, in the gastrointestinal tract, and in the lungs of immunocompromised people. Many people with skin lesions caused by Kaposi sarcoma also have gastrointestinal involvement. What are the presenting symptoms of Kaposi sarcoma in the gastrointestinal tract? Mark all that apply.
   a. Bleeding
   b. Rectal burning
   c. Pain
   d. Diarrhea
   e. Obstruction

7. While doing patient education at a public health clinic, a nurse teaches about sexually transmitted disease prevention. In the education is a segment on HIV/AIDS. Which of the following statements from a client would indicate that more teaching is needed?
   a. "Latex condoms provide protection from HIV/AIDS."
   b. "There is no cure for HIV/AIDS."
   c. "Natural or lambskin condoms are as protective as latex condoms."
   d. "Adopting risk-free or low-risk behavior is the best protection against HIV/AIDS."

8. A 20-year-old male presents at the clinic complaining of severe fatigue, night sweats, and fever. While taking the client's history, he reports having multiple sexual partners and unprotected sex. HIV/AIDS is suspected. What diagnostic test would be ordered to confirm the diagnosis?
   a. Complete metabolic panel
   b. Western blot assay
   c. ALEA
   d. Eastern blot assay

9. The treatment of HIV/AIDS is complicated because different drugs act on different stages of the replication cycle of the virus. Therefore, treatment includes combinations of two, three, or more drugs. What is this treatment called?
   a. DHHS treatment
   b. Anti-AIDS treatment
   c. HAART treatment
   d. HEELP treatment

10. A client presents at the clinic complaining of unplanned weight loss of up to 10% of her body weight. She states that she has had diarrhea, more than twice a day. She goes on to say the she has fever and weakness that "just won't go away." After a complete history and physical, an enzyme-linked immunoabsorbent assay test is ordered. This order is based on what suspected diagnosis?
    a. Wasting syndrome
    b. AIDS syndrome
    c. Beal syndrome
    d. WAGAR syndrome

11. Psychosocial issues are faced by every patient diagnosed with HIV/AIDS and their families. These issues include which of the following? Mark all that apply.
    a. Condemnation of risk behaviors
    b. Helplessness
    c. Lack of control
    d. Decreased strain on relationships with support persons
    e. Acceptance of lifestyle

12. Perinatal transmission of HIV/AIDS from the mother to the baby have dropped drastically with the advent of new treatment methods and drug therapies. What increases the risk of perinatal transmission of the virus?
    a. Low viral load
    b. High CD4+ counts
    c. Breast-feeding
    d. Mother in primary phase of disease

Structure and Function of the Cardiovascular System

SECTION I: LEARNING OBJECTIVES

1. Compare the function and distribution of blood flow and blood pressure in the systemic and pulmonary circulations

2. State the relation between blood volume and blood pressure in arteries, veins, and capillaries of the circulatory system

3. Define the term *hemodynamics* and describe the effects of blood pressure, vessel radius, vessel length, vessel cross-sectional area, and blood viscosity on blood flow

4. Use the law of Laplace to explain the effect of radius size on the pressure and wall tension in a vessel.

5. Use the term *compliance* to describe the characteristics of arterial and venous blood vessels

6. Describe the structural components and function of the pericardium, myocardium, endocardium, and the heart valves and fibrous skeleton

7. Draw a figure of the cardiac cycle, incorporating the volume, pressure, phonocardiographic, and electrocardiographic changes that occur during atrial and ventricular systole and diastole

8. Define the terms *preload* and *afterload*

9. State the formula for calculating the cardiac output and explain the effects that venous return, cardiac contractility, and heart rate have on cardiac output

10. Describe the cardiac reserve and relate it to the Frank-Starling mechanism

11. Compare the structure and function of arteries and veins

12. Describe the structure and function of vascular smooth muscle

13. Use the equation blood pressure = cardiac output $\times$ peripheral vascular resistance to explain the regulation of arterial blood pressure

14. Define autoregulation and characterize mechanisms responsible for short-term and long-term regulation of blood flow

15. Describe mechanisms involved in the humoral control of blood flow

16. Define the term *microcirculation*

17. Describe the structure and function of the capillaries

18. Explain the forces that control the fluid exchange between the capillaries and the interstitial spaces

19. Describe the structures of the lymphatic system and relate them to the role of the lymphatics in controlling interstitial fluid volume

20. Describe the roles of the medullary vasomotor and cardioinhibitory centers in controlling the function of the heart and blood vessels

21. Relate the performance of baroreceptors and chemoreceptors in the control of cardiovascular function

22. Describe the distribution of sympathetic and parasympathetic nervous system in the innervation of the circulatory system and their effects on heart rate and cardiac contractility

23. Relate the role of the central nervous system in terms of regulating circulatory function

SECTION II: ASSESSING YOUR UNDERSTANDING

Activity A *Fill in the blanks.*

1. The circulatory system delivers _____ and nutrients needed for metabolic processes to the tissues, carries _____ products from the tissues to the kidneys and other excretory organs for elimination, and circulates electrolytes and _____ needed to regulate body function.

2. The circulatory system can be divided into two parts: the _____ circulation and the _____ circulation.

3. The _____ circulation consists of the right heart, the pulmonary artery, the pulmonary capillaries, and the pulmonary veins.

4. The _____ circulation consists of the left heart, the aorta and its branches, the capillaries that supply the brain and peripheral tissues, and the systemic venous system and the vena cava.

5. The _____ pressure of the pulmonary circulation allows blood to move through the lungs more slowly, which is important for gas exchange.

6. The _____ function as collection chambers for blood, and the _____ are the main pumping chambers of the heart.

7. Because it is a closed system, the effective function of the circulatory system requires that the outputs of both sides of the heart pump the _____ amount of blood over time.

8. Blood flow in the circulatory system depends on a blood _____ that is sufficient to fill the blood vessels and a _____ difference across the system that provides the force to move blood forward.

9. The term _____ refers to the principles that govern blood flow in the circulatory system.

10. Because flow is directly related to the radius, small changes in vessel radius can produce _____ changes in flow to an organ or tissue.

11. _____ is the resistance to flow caused by the friction of molecules in a fluid.

12. _____ blood flow may predispose to clot formation as platelets and other coagulation factors are exposed to the endothelial lining of the vessel.

13. Wall tension is inversely related to wall thickness, such that the _____ the vessel wall, the lower the tension.

14. The total quantity of blood that can be stored in a given portion of the circulation for each millimeter rise in pressure is termed compliance and reflects the _____ of the blood vessel.

15. The _____ and _____ valves control the movement of blood out of the ventricles.

16. The electrical activity, recorded on the ECG, _____ the mechanical events of the cardiac cycle.

17. The aorta is highly _____ and, as such, stretches during systole to accommodate the blood that is being ejected from the left heart during systole.

18. _____ is marked by ventricular relaxation and filling.

19. The difference between the end diastolic and end systolic volumes (approximately 70 mL) is called the _____.

20. The stroke volume divided by the end diastolic volume is the _____ fraction.

21. The efficiency of the heart as a pump is often measured in terms of the _____ or the amount of blood the heart pumps each minute.

22. The _____ refers to the maximum percentage of increase in cardiac output that can be achieved above the normal resting level.

23. The _____ mechanism allows the heart to adjust its pumping ability to accommodate various levels of venous return.

24. The _____ determines the frequency with which blood is ejected from the heart.

25. The outermost layer of a vessel, the _____, is composed primarily of loosely woven collagen fibers. The middle layer, the _____, is largely a smooth muscle layer. The innermost layer, the _____, consists of a single layer of flattened endothelial cells.

26. The _____ represents the energy that is transmitted from molecule to molecule along the length of the vessel.

27. With peripheral arterial disease, there is a delay in the transmission of the reflected wave so that the pulse _____ in amplitude.

28. Pressure in the right atrium is called the _____.

29. _____ in the veins of extremities prevent retrograde flow with the help of skeletal muscles that surround and intermittently compress the leg veins to move blood forward to the heart.

30. _____ of blood flow is mediated by changes in blood vessel tone due to changes in flow through the vessel or by local tissue factors.

31. An increase in local blood flow is called _____.

32. In the heart and other vital structures, _____ channels exist between some of the smaller arteries.

33. The term _____ refers to the functions of the smallest blood vessels, the capillaries, and the neighboring lymphatic vessels.

34. Water-filled junctions, called the _____, join the capillary endothelial cells and provide a pathway for passage of substances through the capillary wall.

35. The key factor that restrains fluid loss from the capillaries is the _____ pressure generated by the plasma proteins.

36. The neural control centers for the integration and modulation of cardiac function and blood pressure are located bilaterally in the _____.

37. The neural control of the circulatory system occurs primarily through the _____ and _____ divisions of the autonomic nervous system.

38. When the intracranial pressure rises to levels that equal intraarterial pressure, blood vessels to the vasomotor center become compressed, initiating the central nervous system ischemic response. This is known as the _____.

Activity B   *Consider the following figures.*

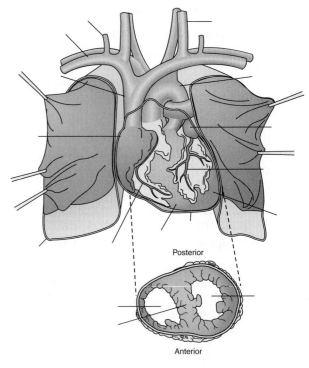

Posterior

Anterior

1. Label the following structures.

- Pericardium
- Pleura
- Right ventricle

- Right coronary artery
- Right atrium
- Subclavian vein
- External jugular vein
- Internal jugular vein
- Intraventricular septum
- Aortic arch
- Left atrium
- Left coronary artery
- Left ventricle
- Superior vena cava

2. Label the following structures.
   - Chordae tendineae
   - Tricuspid valve
   - Superior vena cava
   - Inferior vena cava
   - Pulmonic valve
   - Papillary muscle
   - Left pulmonary artery
   - Right pulmonary artery
   - Pulmonary veins
   - Aortic valve
   - Mitral valve
   - Left atrium
   - Right atrium
   - Left ventricle
   - Right ventricle
   - Descending aorta
   - Papillary muscles

Activity C *Match the key terms in Column A with their definitions in Column B.*

Column A

____ 1. Diastole

____ 2. Pericardium

____ 3. End diastolic volume

____ 4. Preload

____ 5. Myocardium

____ 6. Cardiac output

____ 7. Heart valves

____ 8. End systolic volume

____ 9. Systole

____ 10. Afterload

Column B

a. Contractile phase of cardiac cycle

b. Sac that covers the heart

c. Ventricular filling

d. Resting phase of cardiac cycle

e. Semilunar and atrioventricular

f. Residual blood volume following contraction

g. Resistance to ejection of blood from heart

h. Heart rate × stroke volume

i. Muscular wall of heart

j. Volume in heart following passive filling phase

Activity D *Briefly answer the following.*

1. What are the factors involved in regulating the flow of blood, and how are they related?

   _____

   _____

   _____

2. The velocity of blood in the circulatory system varies considerably between large vessels and capillaries. Normally, when fluid flows from a large vessel to a smaller vessel, the velocity increases, but this does not occur in the circulatory system. Why, and for what purpose?

   _____

   _____

   _____

3. What is the importance of the Frank-Starling mechanism?

_____

_____

_____

4. How is blood vessel diameter controlled?

_____

_____

_____

5. What are the factors that travel in the blood-stream that will regulate blood flow? Indicate whether it is a dilator or a vasoconstrictor.

_____

_____

_____

SECTION III: APPLYING YOUR KNOWLEDGE

Activity E   _Consider the following scenario and answer the question._

As a nurse on the telemetry floor, you are caring for a 77-year-old man who was admitted with a cardiac dysrhythmia. He has spent the day having diagnostic tests performed and complains of being very tired and feeling weak. He states, "I feel like I am suffocating; I think I am going to die." You note that his telemetry is showing ST segment elevations. You have read his chart and know that he has a history of variant angina.

1. You know that variant angina is caused by severe spasms of the coronary artery. What medications would you expect to give this client to reverse the spasm of the artery?

_____

_____

_____

SECTION IV: PRACTICING FOR NCLEX

Activity F   _Answer the following questions._

1. Blood volume is dictated by age and body weight. Neonates have a higher blood volume per kilogram than does an adult. What is the blood volume range per kilogram in an adult?

   a. 70 to 75 mL/kg

   b. 85 to 90 mL/kg

   c. 60 to 65 mL/kg

   d. 90 to 100 mL/kg

2. Resistance to flow is determined by the blood vessels and the blood vessel itself. An equation has been developed for understanding the relationship between the diameter of the blood vessel, the viscosity of the blood, and resistance. What is the equation called?

   a. Laplace law

   b. Poiseuille law

   c. Laminar law

   d. Pierre law

3. The distensibility of the blood vessel is the major factor in which of the vessels characteristics?

   a. Wall tension

   b. Compliance

   c. Laminar blood flow

   d. Resistance

4. When intracranial pressure (ICP) equals intraarterial pressure, the central nervous system ischemic response is initiated. This response is directed at raising arterial pressure above ICP, thereby reestablishing blood flow to the vasomotor center of the brain. What is this response called?

   a. Cushing law

   b. Cushing response

   c. Cushing reflex

   d. Cushing syndrome

5. The troponin complex is one of a number of important proteins that regulate actin-myosin binding. Troponin works in striated muscle to help regulate calcium-mediated contraction of the muscle. Which of the troponin complexes are diagnostic of a myocardial infarction?

a. Troponin C and Troponin T
b. Troponin A and Troponin I
c. Troponin T and Troponin I
d. Troponin A and Troponin C

6. The stroke volume is the amount of blood ejected with every contraction of the ventricle. It is broken down into quarters. What is the approximate amount of the stroke volume per quarter?

a. 25%, 25%, 25%, and 25%
b. 50%, 30%, 20%, and little blood
c. 40%, 40%, 10%, and 10%
d. 60%, 20%, 20%, and little blood

7. Downstream peripheral pulses have a higher pulse pressure because the pressure wave travels faster than the blood itself. What occurs in peripheral arterial disease?

a. The pulse decreases rather than increases in amplitude.
b. The reflected wave is transmitted more rapidly through the aorta.
c. Downstream peripheral pulses are increased even more than normal.
d. Downstream peripheral pulses are greater than upstream pulses.

8. Cardiac output (CO) is used to measure the efficiency of the heart as a pump. What is the equation used to express CO?

a. $CO = HR \times AV$
b. $CO = SV \times HR$
c. $CO = AV \times SV$
d. $CO = HR \times EF$

9. As the needs of the body change, the heart's ability to increase output necessarily needs to change. This ability in the heart depends on what factors? Mark all that apply.

a. Cardiac reserve
b. Cardiac contractility
c. Heart rate
d. Preload
e. Afterload

10. Nitroglycerin is the drug of choice in treating angina. What does nitroglycerin release into the vascular smooth muscle of the target tissues?

a. Antithrombin factor
b. Platelet aggregating factor
c. Calcium channel blocker
d. Nitric oxide

11. Colloidal osmotic pressure acts differently than the osmotic effects of the plasma proteins. What is its action?

a. Pulls fluid back into the capillary
b. Pushes fluid into the extracellular spaces
c. Controls the direction of the fluid flow in the large arteries
d. Pulls fluid into the interstitial spaces

12. The lymph system correlates with the vascular system without actually being part of the vascular system. Among other things, the lymph system is the main route for the absorption of fats from the gastrointestinal system. The lymph system empties into the right and left thoracic ducts, which are the points of juncture with the vascular system. What are these points of juncture?

a. Bifurcation of the common carotid arteries
b. Internal and external jugular veins
c. Junctions of the subclavian and internal jugular veins
d. Junctions of the subclavian and pulmonary veins

13. The heart and blood vessels receive both sympathetic and parasympathetic innervation from neural control. What controls the parasympathetic-mediated slowing of the heart rate?

a. Vasomotor center
b. Cardioinhibitory center
c. Medullary center
d. Innervation center

22

Disorders of Blood Flow in the Systemic Circulation

SECTION I: LEARNING OBJECTIVES

1. Describe the functions of the endothelial cells and define the term *endothelial dysfunction*

2. Describe the function of vascular smooth muscle and its role in vascular repair

3. List the five types of lipoproteins and state their function in terms of lipid transport and development of atherosclerosis

4. Describe the role of lipoprotein receptors in removal of cholesterol from the blood

5. Cite the criteria for diagnosis of hypercholesterolemia

6. Describe possible mechanisms involved in the development of atherosclerosis

7. List risk factors in atherosclerosis

8. List the vessels most commonly affected by atherosclerosis and describe the vessel changes that occur

9. State the signs and symptoms of acute arterial occlusion

10. Describe the pathology associated with the vasculitides and relate it to four disease conditions associated with vasculitis

11. Compare the mechanisms and manifestations of ischemia associated with atherosclerotic peripheral vascular disease, Raynaud phenomenon, and thromboangiitis obliterans (*i.e.,* Buerger disease)

12. Distinguish between the pathology and manifestations of aortic aneurysms and dissection of the aorta

13. Describe venous return of blood from the lower extremities, including the function of the muscle pumps and the effects of gravity, and relate to the development of varicose veins

14. Differentiate primary from secondary varicose veins

15. Characterize the pathology of venous insufficiency and relate to the development of stasis dermatitis and venous ulcers

16. List the four most common causes of lower leg ulcer

17. Cite risk factors associated with venous thrombosis and describe the manifestation of the disorder and its treatment

SECTION II: ASSESSING YOUR UNDERSTANDING

Activity A *Fill in the blanks.*

1. Although the heart is the center of the cardio-vascular system, _____ transport blood throughout the body.

2. Endothelial cells form a continuous lining for the entire vascular system called the _____.

3. Vascular smooth muscle cells, which form the predominant cellular layer in the tunica media, produce _____ or _____ of blood vessels.

4. The term _____ denotes a reduction in arterial flow to a level that is insufficient to meet the oxygen demands of the tissues.

5. _____ refers to an area of ischemic necrosis in an organ produced by occlusion of its arterial blood supply or its venous drainage.

6. Elevated levels of blood _____ are implicated in the development of atherosclerosis with its attendant risk of heart attack and stroke.

7. Because _____ and _____ are insoluble in plasma, they are encapsulated by a stabilizing coat of water-soluble lipoproteins.

8. The _____ transport cholesterol and triglyceride to various tissues for energy utilization, lipid deposition, steroid hormone production, and bile acid formation.

9. Some of the apoproteins activate the _____ enzymes that facilitate the removal of lipids from the lipoproteins.

10. There are two sites of lipoprotein synthesis: the _____ and the _____.

11. _____ transfer their triglycerides to the cells of adipose and skeletal muscle tissue.

12. Low-density lipoprotein, sometimes called the _____, is the main carrier of cholesterol.

13. Low-density lipoprotein is removed from the circulation either by _____ or by _____ cells.

14. The uptake of low-density lipoprotein by macrophages in the arterial wall can result in the accumulation of insoluble cholesterol esters, the formation of foam cells, and the development of _____.

15. High-density lipoprotein is synthesized in the liver and is often referred to as the _____.

16. Lipoprotein measurements are particularly important in persons at high risk for development of _____.

17. Many types of primary hypercholesterolemia have a _____ basis.

18. Causes of _____ hyperlipoproteinemia include obesity with high-calorie intake and diabetes mellitus.

19. Excess calories consistently _____ high-density lipoprotein and less consistently _____ low-density lipoprotein.

20. _____ is a type of arteriosclerosis or hardening of the arteries.

21. The major risk factor for atherosclerosis is _____.

22. _____ is closely linked with coronary heart disease and sudden death.

23. Considerable interest in the role of _____ in the etiology of atherosclerosis has emerged over the last few years.

24. _____ is a serum marker for systemic inflammation.

25. _____ inhibits elements of the anticoagulant cascade and is associated with endothelial damage, which is believed to be an important first step in the development of atherosclerosis.

26. Activated macrophages release _____ that oxidize low-density lipoprotein.

27. Small vessel _____ are sometimes associated with antineutrophil cytoplasmic antibodies.

28. An _____ is a freely moving particle such as a blood clot that breaks loose and travels in the larger vessels of the circulation until lodging in a smaller vessel and occluding blood flow.

29. _____ is an inflammatory arterial disorder that causes thrombus formation.

30. _____ is a functional disorder caused by intense vasospasm of the arteries and arterioles in the fingers and, less often, the toes.

31. An _____ is an abnormal localized dilatation of a blood vessel.

32. An aneurysm may also be _____, with the first evidence of its presence being associated with vessel _____.

33. Aortic dissection involves _____ into the vessel wall with longitudinal tearing of the vessel wall to form a blood-filled channel.

34. Venous _____ prevent the retrograde flow of blood.

35. The most common cause of secondary varicose veins is _____.

36. _____ leads to tissue congestion, edema, and eventual impairment of tissue nutrition.

37. Virchow described the triad that has come to be associated with venous thrombosis: _____, _____, and _____.

Activity B *Consider the following figure.*

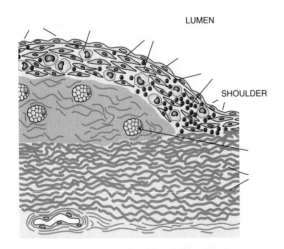

LUMEN

SHOULDER

In this figure, label the following: media, lymphocytes, endothelial cells, smooth muscle cells, macrophages, CAP region, and necrotic core.

Activity C *Match the key terms in Column A with their definitions in Column B.*

Column A

_____ 1. Chylomicrons

_____ 2. C-reactive protein

_____ 3. Familial hypercholesterolemia

_____ 4. Xanthomas

_____ 5. Hypercholesterolemia

_____ 6. Vasculitis

_____ 7. Very low-density lipoprotein

_____ 8. Homocysteine

_____ 9. Atherosclerosis

_____ 10. Low-density lipoprotein (LDL)

Column B

a. Necrosis of the blood vessel wall

b. Main carrier of cholesterol

c. Derived from the metabolism of dietary methionine

d. Elevated levels of blood cholesterol

e. LDL-related arteriosclerosis

f. Carries large amounts of triglycerides

g. Caused by LDL receptor deficiency, which prevents uptake of LDL

h. Transfer triglycerides to skeletal muscle, smaller than very low-density lipoproteins

i. Elevated levels associated with arterial disease

j. Cholesterol deposits

Activity D *Put the following sequence of events of atherosclerotic pathogenesis in chronologic order:*

formation of fibrofatty plaque, foam cell formation, endothelial injury, complicated lesion, development of fatty streak.

Activity E *Briefly answer the following.*

1. Describe the role of the endothelium.

_____

_____

_____

2. Describe the causation of secondary hyper-lipoproteinemia.

_____

_____

_____

3. Describe the general mechanisms of drug therapy to lower serum low-density lipoprotein levels.

_____

_____

_____

4. What are the seven signs and symptoms of acute arterial occlusion?

_____

_____

_____

5. What are the physical effects of Raynaud phenomenon?

_____

_____

_____

6. How do skeletal muscles of the leg contribute to returning blood to the heart?

_____

_____

_____

SECTION III: APPLYING YOUR KNOWLEDGE

Activity F _Consider the following scenario and answer the questions._

A 72-year-old man is brought to the emergency department (ED) by his wife. She says that her husband "just started moaning and complaining of pain in his back." She goes on to say that "she has never seen him in this much pain." In the triage area of the ED, the client's blood pressure was mildly elevated. He complained of syncope that became worse over time. On admission to the ED, the patient's blood pressure and pulse were unobtainable in his left arm, and his pain and syncope were worse. The nurse suspects a diagnosis of a dissecting aneurysm of the descending aorta.

1. What orders would the nurse expect to receive from the physician to confirm a diagnosis of a dissecting aneurysm?

_____

_____

_____

2. Once the diagnosis of dissecting aneurysm is confirmed, what would be the priority nursing action for this patient?

_____

_____

_____

_____

SECTION IV: PRACTICING FOR NCLEX

Activity G _Answer the following questions._

1. A variety of etiologies are responsible for altering the blood flow in the systemic circulation. Match the disturbance of blood flow with the cause.

Disturbance in Blood Flow	Cause
____ **1.** Abnormal vessel dilation	**a.** Atherosclerosis (arterial)
____ **2.** Pathologic changes in vessel wall	**b.** Raynaud phenomenon (vasospasm)
____ **3.** Acute vessel obstruction	**c.** Venous thrombosis (venous)
____ **4.** Pathologic changesin vessel wall	**d.** Varicose veins (venous)
____ **5.** Abnormal vessel dilation	**e.** Vasculitis (arterial)
____ **6.** Acute vessel obstruction	**f.** Arterial aneurysms (arterial)

2. Where in the body is lipoprotein is synthesized? Mark all that apply.
   a. Small intestine
   b. Large intestine
   c. Pancreas
   d. Liver

3. A 35-year-old man presents to the emergency department complaining of chest pain for the past 2 hours. He describes the pain as crushing, like a huge weight is on his chest. He also states that the pain goes up into his neck and down his left arm. An acute myocardial infarction (MI) is diagnosed. When taking his history, the following things are noted:

   • Hyperlipoproteinemia for past 7 years
   • Family history of early MI
   • Cholesterol deposits along the tendons (diagnosed 1 year ago)
   • Atherosclerosis (diagnosed 6 months ago)
   • Diabetes mellitus (type 1) (diagnosed at age 16 years)

   The nurse suspects which of the following diagnosis will be made?
   a. Familial hypercholesterolemia (type 2A)
   b. Homozygotic cutaneous xanthoma
   c. Adult onset hypercholesterolemia (type 1A)
   d. Secondary hyperlipoproteinemia

4. Atherosclerosis begins in an insidious manner with symptoms becoming apparent as long as 20 to 40 years after the onset of the disease. Although an exact etiology of the disease has not been identified, epidemiologic studies have shown that there are predisposing risk factors to this disease. What is the major risk factor for developing atherosclerosis?
   a. Male sex
   b. Hypercholesterolemia
   c. Familial history of premature coronary heart disease
   d. Increasing age

5. A group of vascular disorders called vasculitides cause inflammatory injury and necrosis of the blood vessel wall (i.e., vasculitis). These disorders are common pathways for tissue and organ involvement in many different disease conditions. What is the most common of the vasculitides?
   a. Polyarteritis nodosa
   b. Raynaud disease
   c. Temporal arteritis
   d. Varicose veins

6. A 69-year-old man is admitted to the floor following a popliteal embolectomy. He asks the nurse why he had to have surgery on his leg. What is the best response by the nurse?
   a. "The doctor wanted to look into your artery to make sure everything was okay."
   b. "Didn't the doctor explain everything to you before your surgery?"
   c. "The artery that runs behind your knee was blocked by a blood clot, and the doctor removed it."
   d. "Your upper leg wasn't getting enough blood, so the doctor had to fix it."

7. A 45-year-old woman with a diagnosis of multiple sclerosis comes to the clinic complaining of coldness and pain in her fingers. She says that her fingers turn blue and then red, and they throb and tingle. The nurse would expect what diagnosis and treatment for this patient? Mark all that apply.
   a. Raynaud disease; protecting the digits from cold
   b. Arterial thrombosis; streptokinase
   c. Peripheral artery disease; aspirin
   d. Raynaud phenomenon; stop smoking

8. Aortic aneurysms take varied forms and can occur anywhere along the aorta. What are the types of aneurysm termed abdominal aortic aneurysms? Mark all that apply.
   a. Berry aneurysms
   b. Dissecting aneurysms
   c. Saccular aneurysms
   d. Fusiform aneurysms
   e. Bifurcating aneurysms

9. A 56-year-old woman presents at the clinic complaining of the unsightliness of her varicose veins and wants to know what can be done about them. The nurse explains that the treatment for varicose veins includes which of the following interventions?

   a. Surgical or fibrotherapy
   b. Sclerotherapy or surgery
   c. Trendelenburg therapy or sclerotherapy
   d. Surgery or Trendelenburg therapy

10. Venous thrombosis most commonly occurs in the lower extremities. Risk factors for venous thrombosis include which of the following?

   a. Stasis of blood, hypercoagulability, inflammation
   b. Hypocoagulability, vessel wall injury, increased pressure on deep veins
   c. Vessel wall injury, hypocoagulability, decreased venous blood flow
   d. Stasis of blood, hypercoagulability, vessel wall injury

23

Disorders of Blood Pressure Regulation

SECTION I: LEARNING OBJECTIVES

1. Define the terms *systolic blood pressure, diastolic blood pressure, pulse pressure*, and *mean arterial blood pressure*

2. Explain how cardiac output and peripheral vascular resistance interact in determining systolic and diastolic blood pressure

3. Describe the mechanisms for short-term and long-term regulation of blood pressure

4. Describe the requirements for accurate and reliable blood pressure measurement in terms of cuff size, determining the maximum inflation pressure, and deflation rate

5. Cite the definition of hypertension put forth by the seventh report of the Joint National Committee on Detection, Evaluation, and Treatment of Hypertension

6. Differentiate essential, systolic, secondary, and malignant forms of hypertension

7. Describe the possible influence of genetics, age, race, obesity, diet and sodium intake, and alcohol consumption on the development of essential hypertension

8. Cite the risks of hypertension in terms of target-organ damage

9. Describe behavior modification strategies used in the prevention and treatment of hypertension

10. List the different categories of drugs used to treat hypertension and state their mechanisms of action in the treatment of high blood pressure

11. Explain the changes in blood pressure that accompany normal pregnancy and describe the four types of hypertension that can occur during pregnancy

12. Cite the criteria for the diagnosis of high blood pressure in children

13. Define systolic hypertension and relate the circulatory changes that occur with aging that predispose to the development of systolic hypertension

14. Define the term *orthostatic hypotension*

15. Describe the cardiovascular, neurohumoral, and muscular responses that serve to maintain blood pressure when moving from the supine to standing position

16. Explain how fluid deficit, medications, aging, disorders of the ANS, and bed rest contribute to the development of orthostatic hypotension

SECTION II: ASSESSING YOUR UNDERSTANDING

Activity A *Fill in the blanks.*

1. _____ blood pressure reflects the rhythmic ejection of blood from the left ventricle into the aorta.

2. The pressure at the height of the pressure pulse is _____ pressure, and the lowest pressure is the _____ pressure.

3. The difference between the systolic and diastolic pressure (approximately 40 mm Hg) is called the _____.

4. The _____ represents the average pressure in the arterial system during ventricular contraction and relaxation.

5. The mean arterial blood pressure is determined mainly by the _____ and the _____.

6. The renin-angiotensin-aldosterone system plays a central role in blood pressure by increasing _____ and _____.

7. The extracellular fluid volume and arterial blood pressure are regulated around an _____ point, which represents the normal pressure for a given individual.

8. The role that the _____ play in blood pressure regulation is emphasized by the fact that many hypertension medications produce their blood pressure lowering effects by increasing _____ and _____ elimination.

9. _____ hypertension is the term applied to 95% of cases in which no cause for hypertension can be identified. In _____ hypertension, the elevation of blood pressure results from some other disorder.

10. A diagnosis of hypertension is made if the systolic blood pressure is _____ or higher and the diastolic blood pressure is _____ or higher.

11. The _____ risk factors include a family history of hypertension, race, and age-related increases in blood pressure.

12. An elevation in blood pressure increases the workload of the _____ by increasing the pressure against which the heart must pump as it ejects blood into the systemic circulation.

13. Chronic hypertension leads to _____, a common cause of chronic kidney disease.

14. Hypertension is a major risk factor for _____ stroke and intracerebral _____.

15. The main objective for treatment of essential hypertension is to achieve and maintain arterial blood pressure below _____.

16. _____ lower blood pressure initially by decreasing vascular volume and cardiac output.

17. The _____ blockers are effective in treating hypertension because they are cardioselective and thus decrease heart rate and cardiac output.

18. The _____ drugs inhibit the movement of calcium into cardiac and vascular smooth muscle.

19. Elevated pressures during _____ favor the development of left ventricular hypertrophy, increased myocardial oxygen demands, and eventual left heart failure.

20. Many of the conditions causing _____ hypertension can be corrected or cured by surgery or specific medical treatment.

21. The use of _____ pills is probably the most common cause of secondary hypertension in young women.

22. _____ hypertension is characterized by sudden marked elevations in blood pressure, with diastolic values above 120 mm Hg complicated by evidence of acute or rapidly progressive life-threatening organ dysfunction.

23. _____ is defined as an elevation in blood pressure and proteinuria developing after 20 weeks of gestation.

24. Any disease condition that reduces blood volume, impairs mobility, results in prolonged inactivity, or impairs autonomic nerve system function may also predispose to _____.

25. _____ drugs and _____ drugs are the most common cause of chronic orthostatic hypotension.

Activity B *Consider the following figures.*

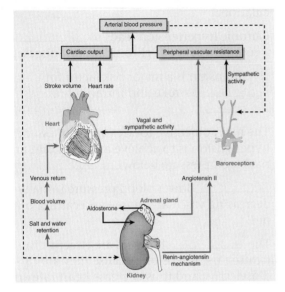

1. What does this figure depict? What do the solid lines and the dashed lines represent?

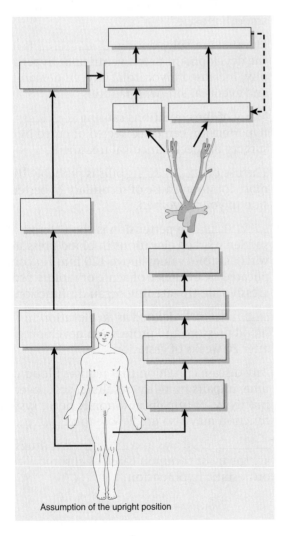

Assumption of the upright position

2. In this figure, fill in the following terms that apply to maintaining blood pressure on standing:

- Action of skeletal muscle pumps
- Compression of veins
- Increased venous return
- Pooling of blood in lower body
- Decreased venous return to the heart
- Decreased cardiac output
- Drop in blood pressure
- Increased heart rate
- Increased cardiac output
- Vasoconstriction
- Blood pressure returns to normal

Activity C *Match the key terms in Column A with their definitions in Column B.*

Column A

_____ 1. Dippers

_____ 2. Systolic hypertension

_____ 3. Vasopressin

_____ 4. Angiotensin-converting enzyme inhibitors

_____ 5. Postural hypotension

_____ 6. Indirect auscultatory method

_____ 7. Diastolic hypertension

_____ 8. Coarctation of the aorta

_____ 9. Angiotensin II

_____ 10. Nondippers

Column B

a. Abnormal drop in blood pressure on assumption of the standing position

b. Noninvasive blood pressure measurement

c. Persons with flat blood pressure profile

d. Increases renal water retention

e. Diastolic pressure over 90 mm Hg

f. Strong vasoconstrictor, reduces sodium excretion

g. Narrowing of the aorta

h. Systolic pressure over 140 mm Hg

i. Persons whose blood pressure follows circadian rhythms

j. Block formation of angiotensin II

Activity D

1. Put the sequence and actions of the RAAS system in chronological order.

   a. Water retention

   b. Stimulation of juxtaglomerular apparatus

   c. Conversion of angiotensinogen to angiotensin I

   d. Conversion of angiotensin I to angiotensin II by angiotensin-converting enzyme

   e. Increased vascular resistance, release of aldosterone

   f. Release of renin

   g. Decrease in blood pressure

   h. Na^+ retention, stimulation of ADH release

Activity E *Briefly answer the following.*

1. Explain the short-term regulation of blood pressure.

   _____

   _____

   _____

2. Why does the kidney play a major role in the development of secondary hypertension?

   _____

   _____

   _____

3. How does the RAAS system influence blood pressure?

   _____

   _____

   _____

4. Why are the elderly predisposed to hypertension?

   _____

   _____

   _____

SECTION III: APPLYING YOUR KNOWLEDGE

Activity F *Consider the following scenario and answer the questions.*

An 87-year-old African American male is brought to the clinic by his son for a routine physical exam. His son states, "Dad has been complaining of feeling dizzy, and he is afraid he is going to fall." When taking the patient's vital signs, the nurse notes that the his blood pressure has reached orthostatic levels and needs further evaluation.

1. What assessments need to be made in further evaluating this patient?

   _____

   _____

   _____

2. The son asks what his father's treatment will be to correct this condition. What is the nurse's best response?

   _____

   _____

   _____

3. The son asks what else can be done to help his father if it is not possible to correct the cause of the orthostatic hypertension. What is the nurse's best response?

   _____

   _____

   _____

SECTION IV: PRACTICING FOR NCLEX

Activity G *Answer the following questions.*

1. For people who suffer from hypertension and other diseases that affect blood pressure, important information about the status of their disease is gathered from measurements including systolic and diastolic pressures, pulse pressure, and mean arterial pressure.

What is the mean arterial pressure estimated to be when the blood pressure is 130/85 mm Hg?

a. 90

b. 95

c. 100

d. 105

2. Although the etiology of essential hypertension is mainly unknown, several risk factors have been identified. These risk factors fall under the categories of constitutional risk factors and lifestyle factors. What are the primary risk factors for essential hypertension? Mark all that apply.

a. Race and excessive sodium chloride intake

b. Type 2 diabetes and obesity

c. Age and high intake of potassium

d. Race and smoking

e. Family history and excessive alcohol consumption

3. A 37-year-old woman is admitted to your unit with a differential diagnosis of rule out pheochromocytoma. What are the most common symptoms you would expect this patient to exhibit?

a. Nervousness and periodic severe headache

b. Variability in blood pressure and weight loss

c. Excessive sweating and pallor

d. Periodic severe headache and marked variability in blood pressure

4. The extended, severe exposure of the walls of the blood vessels to the exaggerated pressures that occur in malignant hypertension cause injuries to the walls of the arterioles. Blood vessels in the renal system are particularly vulnerable to this type of damage. Because hypertension is a chronic disease, and it is associated with autoregulatory changes in the blood flow to major organs, what would be the initial treatment goal for malignant hypertension?

a. Partial reduction in blood pressure to less critical values

b. Reduction to normotensive levels of blood pressure

c. Rapid decrease in blood pressure to less critical levels

d. Slow, gradual decrease in blood pressure to normotensive blood pressures

5. A client with malignant hypertension is at risk for a hypertensive crisis, including the cerebral vascular system often causing cerebral edema. As the nurse caring for this patient, what are the signs and symptoms you would assess for?

a. Papilledema and lethargy

b. Headache and confusion

c. Restlessness and nervousness

d. Stupor and hyperreflexia

6. Pregnancy-induced hypertension is a serious condition affecting between 5% and 10% of pregnant women. The most serious classification of hypertension in pregnancy is preeclampsia-eclampsia. It is a pregnancy-specific syndrome that can have both maternal and fetal manifestations. What is a life-threatening manifestation of the preeclampsia-eclampsia classification of pregnancy-induced hypertension?

a. Hepatocellular necrosis

b. Thrombocytopenia

c. HELLP syndrome

d. Decreased renal filtration rate

7. In infants and children, secondary hypertension is the most common form of hypertension. What is the most common cause of hypertension in an infant?

a. Cerebral vascular bleed

b. Coarctation of the aorta

c. Pheochromocytoma

d. Renal artery thrombosis

8. Hypertension in the elderly is a common finding. This is due to the age-related rise in systolic blood pressure. Among the aging processes, what is a contributor to hypertension?

a. Baroreceptor sensitivity

b. Aortic softening

c. Decreased peripheral vascular resistance

d. Increased renal blood flow

9. A 75-year-old male presents at the clinic for a routine physical check-up. He is found to be hypertensive. While taking his blood pressure in the sitting, standing, and lying positions, the nurse notes that the brachial artery is pulseless at a high cuff pressure, but she can still feel it. What condition would the nurse suspect?

   a. Essential hypertension

   b. Pseudohypertension

   c. Orthostatic hypertension

   d. Secondary hypertension

10. The rennin-angiotensin-aldosterone system is a negative feedback system that plays a central role in blood pressure regulation. How does the end result of this feedback loop regulate blood pressure in the body?

   a. Vasodilates blood vessels to decrease blood pressure

   b. Vasoconstricts blood vessels to increase blood pressure

   c. Increases salt and water retention by the kidney

   d. Decreases salt and water retention by the kidney

Disorders of Cardiac Function

SECTION I: LEARNING OBJECTIVES

1. Characterize the function of the pericardium

2. Compare the clinical manifestations of acute pericarditis and chronic pericarditis

3. Describe the physiologic impact of pleural effusion on cardiac function and relate it to the life-threatening nature of cardiac tamponade

4. Relate the pathophysiology of constrictive pericarditis to its clinical manifestations

5. Describe blood flow in the coronary circulation and relate it to the determinants of myocardial oxygen supply and demand

6. Define the term *acute coronary syndrome* and distinguish among chronic stable angina, unstable angina, non–ST-segment elevation myocardial infarction, and ST-segment elevation infarction in terms of pathology, symptomatology, ECG changes, and serum cardiac markers

7. Compare the treatment goals for stable angina and the acute coronary syndromes

8. Define the term *cardiomyopathy* as it relates to both the mechanical and electrical function of the myocardium

9. Describe the role of genetics in the etiology of the primary cardiomyopathies

10. Differentiate among the pathophysiologic changes that occur with hypertrophic cardiomyopathy, arrhythmogenic right ventricular cardiomyopathy, dilated cardiomyopathies, and myocarditis

11. List four causes of secondary cardiomyopathy

12. Describe the treatment strategies of both primary and secondary cardiomyopathy

13. Distinguish between the roles of infectious organisms and the immune system in infective endocarditis and rheumatic fever

14. Describe the relation between the infective vegetations associated with infective endocarditis and the extracardiac manifestations of the disease

15. Describe the long-term effects of rheumatic fever and primary and secondary prevention strategies for rheumatic fever and rheumatic heart disease

16. State the function of the heart valves and relate alterations in hemodynamic function of the heart that occur with valvular disease

17. Compare the effects of stenotic and regurgitant mitral and aortic valvular heart disease on cardiovascular function

18. Compare the methods of and diagnostic information obtained from cardiac auscultation and echocardiography as they relate to valvular heart disease

19. Trace the flow of blood in the fetal circulation, state the function of the foramen ovale and ductus arteriosus, and describe the changes in circulatory function that occur at birth

20. Compare the effects of left-to-right and right-to-left shunts on the pulmonary circulation and production of cyanosis

21. Describe the anatomic defects and altered patterns of blood flow in children with atrial septal defects, ventricular septal defects, endocardial cushion defects, pulmonary stenosis, tetralogy of Fallot, patent ductus arteriosus, transposition of the great vessels, coarctation of the aorta, and single-ventricle anatomy

22. Describe the prevalence of the condition and issues of concern for adults with congenital heart disease.

23. Describe the manifestations related to the acute, subacute, and convalescent phases of Kawasaki disease

SECTION II: ASSESSING YOUR UNDERSTANDING

Activity A *Fill in the blanks.*

1. The _____ is a double-layered serous membrane that isolates the heart from other thoracic structures, maintains its position in the thorax, prevents it from overfilling, and serves as a barrier to infection.

2. Pericardial fluid acts as a lubricant that prevents _____ forces from developing as the heart contracts and relaxes.

3. The manifestations of acute _____ include a triad of chest pain, pericardial friction rub, and ECG changes.

4. Pericardial _____ refers to the accumulation of fluid in the pericardial cavity, usually because of an inflammatory and/or infectious process.

5. Pericardial effusion can lead to cardiac _____, in which there is compression of the heart due to the accumulation of fluid, pus, or blood in the pericardial sac.

6. In _____ pericarditis, fibrous, calcified scar tissue develops between the visceral and parietal layers of the serous pericardium.

7. In most cases, coronary artery disease is caused by _____.

8. Myocardial blood flow, in turn, is largely regulated by the _____ of the myocardium and _____ mechanisms that control vessel dilation.

9. There is little oxygen reserve in the blood; therefore, coronary arteries must increase their flow to meet the metabolic needs of the myocardium during periods of _____.

10. The _____ is the most frequently used cardiovascular diagnostic procedure.

11. _____ uses ultrasound signals that are inaudible to the human ear.

12. _____ is by far the most common cause of coronary artery disease.

13. There are two types of atherosclerotic lesions: the _____ plaque, which obstructs blood flow, and the _____ plaque, which can rupture and cause platelet adhesion and thrombus formation.

14. Coronary artery disease is commonly divided into two types of disorders: _____ and _____.

15. The classic ECG changes that occur with acute coronary syndrome involve _____, _____, and _____.

16. Acute severe ischemia reduces the _____ and shortens the duration of the action potential in the ischemic area.

17. The _____ have high specificity for myocardial tissue and have become the primary biomarker for the diagnosis of myocardial infarction.

18. _____ myocardial infarction is characterized by the ischemic death of myocardial tissue associated with atherosclerotic disease of the coronary arteries.

19. Irreversible myocardial cell death occurs after _____ minutes of severe ischemia.

20. Infarcted and noninfarcted areas of the heart muscle in patients with ST-segment elevation myocardial infarction can change size, shape, and thickness, a term referred to as _____.

21. The gastrointestinal symptoms of ST-segment elevation myocardial infarction are believed to be related to the severity of the pain and _____ stimulation.

22. The medication used to alleviate angina, _____, is given because of its vasodilating effect.

23. _____ is a mechanical technique to remove atherosclerotic tissue during angioplasty.

24. Partial or complete rupture of a _____ is a rare but often fatal complication of transmural myocardial infarction.

25. _____ is the initial manifestation of ischemic heart disease in approximately half of persons with coronary artery disease.

26. Typically, chronic stable angina is provoked by _____ or _____ stress and relieved within minutes by rest or the use of nitroglycerin.

27. The _____ cardiomyopathies include hypertrophic cardiomyopathy, arrhythmogenic right ventricular cardiomyopathy, left ventricular noncompaction cardiomyopathy, inherited conduction system disorders, and ion channelopathies.

28. The _____ cardiomyopathies, which include dilated cardiomyopathy, are of both genetic and nongenetic origin.

29. The physiologic abnormality in _____ is reduced left ventricular chamber size, poor compliance with reduced stroke volume that results from impaired diastolic filling, and dynamic obstruction of left ventricular outflow.

30. _____ cardiomyopathies are characterized by atrophic and hypertrophic myocardial fibers and interstitial fibrosis.

31. _____ is the most common and, frequently, the first manifestation of rheumatic fever.

32. The _____ manifestation of rheumatic fever is Sydenham chorea, where the child often is fidgety, cries easily, begins to walk clumsily, and drops things.

33. The function of the heart _____ is to promote directional flow of blood through the chambers of the heart.

34. Mitral valve_____ represents the incomplete opening of the mitral valve during diastole with left atrial distention and impaired filling of the left ventricle.

35. Mitral valve_____ is characterized by incomplete closure of the mitral valve, with the left ventricular stroke volume being divided between the forward stroke volume that moves into the aorta and the regurgitant stroke volume that moves back into the left atrium during systole.

36. Most persons with mitral valve _____ are asymptomatic, and the disorder is discovered during a routine physical examination.

37. Increased resistance to ejection of blood from the left ventricle into the aorta characterizes aortic valve _____.

38. Aortic _____ is the result of an incompetent aortic valve that allows blood to flow back to the left ventricle during diastole.

39. The major development of the _____ occurs between the fourth and seventh weeks of gestation, and most congenital heart defects arise during this time.

40. Congenital heart defects produce their effects mainly through abnormal shunting of _____, production of _____, and disruption of _____ blood flow.

41. Congenital heart defects that result in a left-to-right shunt are usually categorized as _____ disorders because they do not compromise oxygenation of blood in the pulmonary circulation.

42. A _____ defect is an opening in the ventricular septum that results from an incomplete separation of the ventricles during early fetal development.

43. _____ disease, also known as mucocutaneous lymph node syndrome, is an acute febrile disease of young children.

Activity B *Consider the following figure.*

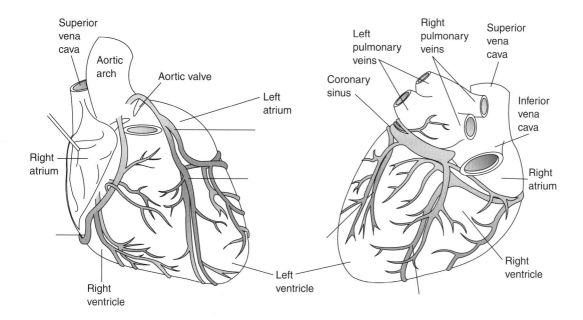

In this figure, label the coronary arteries.

Activity C *Match the key terms in Column A with their definitions in Column B.*

1.

Column A	Column B
____ **1.** Unstable angina	**a.** Chest pain due to a coronary artery spasm
____ **2.** Effusive-constrictive pericarditis	**b.** ST-segment elevation myocardial infarction
____ **3.** Ischemia	**c.** Decreased blood flow to tissue
____ **4.** Pericardial effusion	**d.** Accumulation of fluid in the pericardial cavity
____ **5.** Prinzmetal angina	**e.** Invasion of the heart valves and the mural endocardium by a microbial agent
____ **6.** Cardiac tamponade	**f.** Mechanical compression of the heart
____ **7.** Silent myocardial ischemia	**g.** Occurs in the absence of anginal pain
____ **8.** Heart attack	**h.** Combination of effusion-tamponade and constriction
____ **9.** Infective endocarditis	**i.** Chest pain occurring while at rest
____ **10.** Pulsus paradoxus	**j.** Exaggeration of the normal variation in the pulse during the inspiratory phase of respiration

2.

Column A	Column B
____ **1.** Restrictive cardiomyopathy	**a.** Ventricular enlargement, a reduction in ventricular wall thickness, and impaired systolic function
____ **2.** Ion channelopathies	
____ **3.** Myocarditis	**b.** An inflammation of the heart
____ **4.** Arrhythmogenic right ventricular cardiomyopathy	**c.** Disproportionate thickening of the ventricular septum and left ventricle
____ **5.** Dilated cardiomyopathy	
____ **6.** Stress cardiomyopathy	**d.** Occurs during the last trimester of pregnancy or the first 6 months after delivery
____ **7.** Hypertrophic cardiomyopathy	
____ **8.** Left ventricular noncompaction	

_____ **9.** Secondary cardiomyopathy

_____ **10.** Peripartum cardiomyopathy

e. Conduction disorders in the heart resulting from abnormal membrane potentials (long QT/short QT syndromes)

f. Left ventricular dysfunction in response to profound psychological or emotional stress

g. Ventricular filling restricted because of excessive rigidity of the ventricular walls

h. Heart muscle disease that affects primarily the right ventricle

i. Heart muscle disease in the presence of a multisystem disorder

j. Failure of trabecular compaction in the developing myocardium

Activity D

1. Construct a flowchart using the following conditions and manifestations of coronary heart disease:

- Chronic ischemic heart disease
- Acute coronary syndrome
- Stable angina
- Unstable angina
- Variant angina
- Non-ST-segment elevation
- Silent myocardial ischemia
- ST-segment elevation
- Q-wave AMI
- No ST-elevation

Activity E   *Briefly answer the following.*

1. Why does pericardial effusion demonstrate signs of right-sided heart failure?

_____

_____

_____

2. What factors determine myocardial oxygen supply and demand?

_____

_____

_____

3. How does an atherosclerotic plaque stimulate thrombosis?

_____

_____

_____

4. What changes are seen in the blood (serum) during acute coronary syndromes?

_____

_____

_____

5. Describe the pathologic process that is seen in unstable angina/non–ST-segment elevation myocardial infarction.

_____

_____

_____

6. What is the damage that results from an acute myocardial infarction, and what are the factors that determine severity?

_____

_____

_____

7. What is meant by "reperfusion therapy," and what is its goal?

_____

_____

_____

8. What is the definition of a cardiomyopathy (according to the American Heart Association)?

_____

_____

_____

_____

9. What is the relationship between strep throat and heart valve disorders?

_____

_____

_____

10. Describe the clinical manifestation of patent ductus arteriosus.

_____

_____

_____

11. Describe the tetralogy of Fallot.

_____

_____

_____

SECTION III: APPLYING YOUR KNOWLEDGE

Activity F *Consider the following scenario and answer the questions.*

A 55-year-old woman is brought to the emergency department by ambulance complaining of severe, acute chest pain. The patient states, "It just came on all of a sudden. Like someone sitting on my chest crushing me." An ECG shows ST segment elevation, and the presumptive diagnosis is acute ST-segment elevation myocardial infarction (STEMI).

1. While taking a history on this patient, what symptoms should the nurse pay particular attention to because they are further indications of a STEMI?

_____

_____

_____

2. What are the emergency department goals of management for a patient with a STEMI?

_____

_____

_____

SECTION IV: PRACTICING FOR NCLEX

Activity G *Answer the following questions.*

1. Nearly everyone with pericarditis has chest pain. With acute pericarditis, the pain is abrupt in onset and sharp, and radiates to the neck, back, abdomen, or sides. What can be done to ease the pain of acute pericarditis?
   a. Have patient sit up and lean forward
   b. Have patient change positions to unaffected side
   c. Have patient breath deeply
   d. Have patient swallow slowly and frequently

2. Cardiac tamponade is a serious life-threatening condition that can arise from a number of other conditions. What is a key diagnostic finding in cardiac tamponade?
   a. Increase in stroke volume
   b. Pulsus paradoxus
   c. Narrowed pulse pressure
   d. Rise in systolic blood pressure

3. The scar tissue that occurs between the layers of the pericardium becomes rigid and constrictive from scar tissue in constrictive pericarditis. What is a physiologic sign of constrictive pericarditis?
   a. Kussmaul breathing
   b. Pulsus paradoxus
   c. Kussmaul sign
   d. Widening pulse pressure

4. Unstable plaque, a condition of atherosclerotic heart disease, occurs in unstable angina and myocardial infarction. Unstable plaque can rupture, causing platelet aggregation and thrombus formation. What are the major determinants of the vulnerability of plaque to rupture? Mark all that apply.
   a. Size of lipid-rich core
   b. Preponderance of smooth muscle cells
   c. Presence of inflammation
   d. Decrease in blood pressure and coronary blood flow
   e. Thickness of fibrous cap

5. A patient with a suspected myocardial infarction (MI) is brought to the emergency department by ambulance. As the nurse caring for this patient, what lab work would you expect to receive an order for to confirm a diagnosis of MI?

   a. Creatine kinase marker
   b. Complete blood components
   c. Calcium level
   d. Troponin level

6. Unstable angina/non–ST-segment elevation myocardial infarction is a clinical syndrome that ranges in severity between stable angina to myocardial infarction (MI). It is classified according to its risk of causing an acute MI and is diagnosed based on what? Mark all that apply.

   a. Severity of pain and abruptness of onset
   b. Serum biomarkers
   c. Coexisting chronic conditions
   d. ECG pattern
   e. Blood flow angiography

7. When an acute myocardial infarction (MI) occurs, many physiologic changes occur very rapidly. What causes the loss of contractile function of the heart within seconds of the onset of an MI?

   a. Conversion from aerobic to anaerobic metabolism
   b. Overproduction of energy capable of sustaining normal myocardial function
   c. Conversion from anaerobic to aerobic metabolism
   d. Inadequate production of glycogen with mitochondrial shrinkage

8. ST-elevated myocardial infarction (STEMI) is accompanied by severe, crushing pain. Morphine is the drug of choice used to treat the pain of STEMI when the pain cannot be relieved with oxygen and nitrates. Why is morphine considered the drug of choice in STEMI?

   a. Action increases autonomic nervous system activity
   b. Action decreases metabolic demands of the heart
   c. Action increases anxiety, thus increasing metabolic demands of heart
   d. Action relieves pain and gives sense of depression

9. During an acute myocardial infarction (MI), there is ischemic damage to the heart muscle. The location and extent of the ischemic damage is the major predictor of complications, ranging from cardiac insufficiency to death, following an MI. What is the "window of opportunity" in restoring blood flow to the affected area so as to diminish the ischemic damage to the heart and maintain the viability of the cells?

   a. 10 to 20 minutes
   b. 30 to 40 minutes
   c. 20 to 40 minutes
   d. 10 to 30 minutes

10. Angina pectoris is a chronic ischemic coronary artery disease that is characterized by a symptomatic paroxysmal chest pain or pressure sensation associated with transient myocardial ischemia. What precipitates an attack of angina pectoris?

    a. Exposure to heat
    b. Sedentary lifestyle
    c. Abrupt change in position
    d. Emotional stress

11. The diagnosis of chronic stable angina is based on a detailed pain history, the presence of risk factors, invasive and noninvasive studies, and laboratory studies. What test is not used in the diagnosis of angina?

    a. Serum biochemical markers
    b. Cardiac catheterization
    c. Echocardiogram
    d. Nuclear imaging studies

12. Cardiomyopathies are classified as either primary or secondary. The primary cardiomyopathies are further classified as genetic, mixed, or acquired. Identify the following conditions as *genetic, acquired,* or *mixed.*

    Hypertrophic cardiomyopathy

    Left ventricular noncompaction

    Myocarditis

    Dilated cardiomyopathy

    Peripartum cardiomyopathy

13. It is known that more than 100 distinct myocardial diseases can demonstrate clinical features associated with dilated cardiomyopathy (DCM). What is the most common identifiable cause of DCM in the United States?

a. Hepatic cardiomyopathy

b. Alcoholic cardiomyopathy

c. Cardiotoxic cardiomyopathy

d. Exercise-induced cardiomyopathy

14. In infective endocarditis, vegetative lesions grow on the valves of the heart. These vegetative lesions consist of a collection of infectious organisms and cellular debris enmeshed in the fibrin strands of clotted blood. What are the possible systemic effects of these vegetative lesions?

a. They can block the heart valves from closing completely.

b. They can keep the heart valves from opening.

c. They can fragment and cause cerebral emboli.

d. They can fragment and make the lesions larger.

15. Antibodies directed against the M protein of certain strains of streptococcal bacteria seem to cross-react with glycoprotein antigens in the heart, joint, and other tissues to produce an autoimmune response resulting in rheumatic fever and rheumatic heart disease. This occurs through what phenomenon?

a. Aschoff reaction

b. Sydenham reaction

c. C-reactive mimicry

d. Molecular mimicry

16. Mitral valve prolapse occurs frequently in the population at large. Its treatment is aimed at relieving symptoms and preventing complications of the disorder. Which drug is used in the treatment of mitral valve prolapse to relieve symptoms and aid in preventing complications?

a. β-adrenergic blocking drugs

b. Calcium channel blocking drugs

c. Antianxiety drugs

d. Broad-spectrum antibiotic drugs

17. Heart failure in an infant usually manifests itself as tachypnea or dyspnea, both at rest and on exertion. When does this most commonly occur with an infant?

a. During bathing

b. During feeding

c. During burping

d. During sleep

18. Tetralogy of Fallot is a congenital condition of the heart that manifests in four distinct anomalies of the infant heart. It is considered a cyanotic heart defect due to the right-to-left shunting of the blood through the ventricular septal defect. A hallmark of this condition is the "tet spells" that occur in these children. What is a tet spell?

a. A stressful period right after birth that occurs without evidence of cyanosis

b. A hyperoxygenated period when the infant is at rest

c. A hypercyanotic attack brought on by periods of stress

d. A hyperpneic attack in which the infant loses consciousness

CHAPTER 25

Disorders of Cardiac Conduction and Rhythm

SECTION I: LEARNING OBJECTIVES

1. Describe the cardiac conduction system and relate it to the mechanical functioning of the heart

2. Characterize the four phases of a cardiac action potential and differentiate between the fast and slow responses

3. Draw an ECG tracing and state the origin of the component parts of the tracing

4. Provide a rationale for the importance of careful lead placement and monitoring of ischemic events

5. Describe the possible mechanisms for arrhythmia generation

6. Compare sinus arrhythmias with atrial arrhythmias

7. Characterize the effects of atrial flutter and atrial fibrillation on heart rhythm

8. Describe the significance of long QT syndrome

9. Describe the characteristics of first-, second-, and third-degree heart block

10. Compare the effects of premature ventricular contractions, ventricular tachycardia, and ventricular fibrillation on cardiac function

11. Cite the types of cardiac conditions that can be diagnosed using the ECG

12. Describe the methods used in diagnosis of cardiac arrhythmias

13. Explain the mechanisms, criteria for use, and benefits of antiarrhythmic drugs, internal cardioverter-defibrillator therapy, ablation therapy, and surgical procedures in the treatment of persons with recurrent, symptomatic arrhythmias

SECTION II: ASSESSING YOUR UNDERSTANDING

Activity A *Fill in the blanks.*

1. Specialized _____ cells generate impulses at a faster rate than other types of heart tissue, and the conduction tissue transmits these impulses at a more rapid rate than other cardiac cell types.

2. Coronary heart disease that _____ blood flow through the vessels supplying tissues of the conduction system can induce serious and sometimes fatal disturbances in cardiac rhythm.

3. Blood supply to the sinoatrial node is provided by means of the _____ artery.

4. The _____, which supplies the ventricles, has large fibers that allow for rapid conduction and almost simultaneous excitation.

5. _____ represents the period during which the negative potential inside the cell reverses and becomes positive.

_____ involves reestablishment of the
ng membrane potential.

longer length of the _____ of car-
muscle is important in maintaining the
rnating contraction and relaxation that is
ntial to the pumping action of the heart
for the prevention of fatal arrhythmias.

_____ records the potential differ-
e in charge between two electrodes as de-
rization and repolarization waves move
ugh the heart and are conducted to the
surface.

six limb leads view the electrical forces as
pass through the heart on the
_____ plane, and the six chest leads
ide a view of the electrical forces as they
through the heart on the _____
e.

y forms of cardiac diagnostic criteria are
_____.

e are two types of disorders of the cardiac
duction system: disorders of _____
disorders of _____.

e sinoatrial (SA) node fires more slowly or
ode conduction is blocked, then another
that is capable of _____ takes over
acemaker.

ost all tachyarrhythmias are the result of
enomenon known as _____.

ythmias that arise because of anatomic
try are _____.

ormal _____, a P wave precedes
QRS complex, and the RR intervals re-
relatively constant over time.

_____ are contractions that originate
e atrial conduction pathways or atrial
cle cells and occur before the next ex-
ed sinoatrial node impulse.

xysmal supraventricular tachycardias
nate above the bifurcation of the
_____ and have a sudden onset and
ination.

pical atrial flutter, the ECG reveals a de-
_____ pattern in leads aVF, V1,
V5.

_____ is characterized by chaotic im-
es propagating in different directions and
ing disorganized atrial depolarization
out effective atrial contraction.

20. The long QT syndrome may result in
_____ and sudden cardiac death.

21. A _____ is caused by a ventricular ectopic pacemaker and leaves the ventricle unable to repolarize sufficiently to respond to
the next impulse that arises in the sinoatrial
node.

22. _____ is dangerous because it elimi-
nates atrial kick and can cause a reduction in
diastolic filling time to the point where cardiac
output is severely diminished or nonexistent.

23. In ventricular fibrillation, the ventricle
_____ but does not contract.

24. _____ refers to abnormalities of impulse conduction.

25. _____-degree block may be the result
of disease in the atrioventricular node, such
as ischemia or infarction, or of infections,
such as rheumatic fever or myocarditis.

26. _____ heart disease is the primary
cause for the development of ventricular
fibrillation.

27. _____ tachycardia is characterized by
ventricular tachycardia, syncope, and sudden
death occurring in familial or sporadic cases
in the absence of cardiac disease or ECG abnormalities.

28. The correction of conduction defects, brady-
cardias, and tachycardias can involve the use
of an electronic _____, _____,
or _____.

Activity B   *Consider the following figure.*

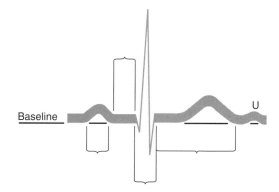

Baseline

U

In this figure, label the following:
- P wave
- QRS complex

- T wave
- Delay in atrioventricular node
- Atrial depolarization
- Ventricular depolarization
- Ventricular repolarization

Activity C *Match the key terms in Column A with their definitions in Column B.*

Column A

_____ 1. Automaticity

_____ 2. Sinus bradycardia

_____ 3. ECG

_____ 4. Sinus arrest

_____ 5. Bradyarrhythmias

_____ 6. Sick sinus syndrome

_____ 7. Ectopic pacemaker

_____ 8. Arrhythmia

_____ 9. Sinus tachycardia

_____ 10. Tachyarrhythmias

_____ 11. First-degree atrioventricular block

_____ 12. Second-degree atrioventricular block

_____ 13. Third-degree atrioventricular block

Column B

a. Failure of the sinoatrial node to discharge

b. Conduction link between the atria and ventricles is lost

c. Disorders of cardiac rhythm

d. Prolonged PR interval

e. Ability of certain cells to spontaneously initiate an action potential

f. Intermittent failure of conduction of one or more P waves

g. Decreased systemic perfusion

h. Heart rate >100 beats/minute

i. Graphic recording of the electrical activity of the heart

j. Excitable focus outside the normally functioning sinoatrial node

k. Bradycardia-tachycardia syndrome

l. Heart rate <60 beats/minute

m. Reduce the diastolic filling time

Activity D *Put the events of cardiac conduction in the order in which the structures are depolarized.*

_____ Atrioventricular node depolarization

_____ Bundle branches

_____ Sinoatrial node depolarization

_____ Bundle of His

_____ Purkinje fibers

Activity E *Briefly answer the following.*

1. Describe the phases of the cardiac action potential and relate each phase to the ECG.

_____

_____

_____

2. What is believed to be the cause(s) of many arrhythmias?

_____

_____

_____

3. Describe the treatment options for atrial fibrillation.

_____

_____

_____

4. Explain the effects on the cardiac cell membrane that result in long QT syndrome.

_____

_____

_____

5. What is an exercise stress test, and what is its purpose?

_____

_____

_____

6. What is the physiologic aim of pharmacologic treatment of arrhythmia?

_____

_____

_____

SECTION III: APPLYING YOUR KNOWLEDGE

Activity F *Consider the following scenario and answer the questions.*

A 75-year-old woman is brought to the emergency department by ambulance. She has a 6-month history of atrial fibrillation. She is complaining of palpitations and extreme fatigue. The paramedic reports that she has a wet sounding, nonproductive cough. Her respiratory rate is 35 breaths/minute; her heart rate is variable with a ventricular rate ranging from 80 to 160 beats/minute. Her ECG confirms atrial fibrillation.

1. What medications would the nurse expect this patient to be taking?

   _____

   _____

   _____

2. What treatment is used to convert atrial fibrillation to sinus rhythm, and what are the complications of this treatment?

   _____

   _____

   _____

SECTION IV: PRACTICING FOR NCLEX

Activity G *Answer the following questions.*

1. ECG monitoring has been found to be more sensitive than a patient's report of symptoms when identifying transient ongoing myocardial ischemia. Why is this?
   a. Most ECG-detected ischemic events are clinically silent.
   b. The ECG can look at ischemic events from different directions.
   c. ECG monitoring is reliable only when the patient remains still.
   d. Most ECG-detected ischemic events cause a great deal of pain.

2. Respiratory sinus arrhythmia is considered a more optimal rhythm than a rhythm where all RR intervals are equal. In respiratory sinus arrhythmia, what is the variation in cardiac cycles related to?
   a. Intraabdominal pressure changes that occur with respiration
   b. Intrathoracic pressure changes that occur with respiration
   c. Intraabdominal pressure changes due to vagal nerve stimulus
   d. Intrathoracic pressure changes due to inadequate oxygenation

3. In children, what is sick sinus syndrome most commonly associated with?
   a. Congenital heart defects prior to corrective cardiac surgery
   b. Destruction of the sinoatrial node
   c. Congenital heart defects following corrective cardiac surgery
   d. Destruction of the atrioventricular node

4. Atrial fibrillation is the most common chronic arrhythmia whose incidence increases with age. Atrial fibrillation may present as asymptomatic to severe symptomatology. What is the treatment of atrial fibrillation dependent on? Mark all that apply.
   a. Recency of onset
   b. Etiology
   c. Persistence of arrhythmia
   d. Size of pulse deficit
   e. Atrial rate

5. Torsade de pointes is a specific type of polymorphic ventricular tachycardia in which the polarity of the QRS complex swings between positive and negative, often on a beat-to-beat basis. It is the result of the long QT syndrome and can cause sudden cardiac death. Which medication is not linked to torsade de pointes as a causative agent?
   a. Verapamil
   b. Procainamide
   c. Digitalis
   d. Tetracycline

6. In second-degree atrioventricular block, there is a relationship between the P waves and the QRS complex resulting in recurring PR intervals. What does this mean?

  a. The association of P waves and QRS complexes is not random.

  b. The relationship between the P waves and the QRS complexes is a widening PR interval.

  c. The association of P waves and QRS complexes is random.

  d. The relationship between the P waves and the QRS complexes is a narrowing PR interval.

7. Brugada syndrome, an autosomal dominant disorder, manifests in adulthood as ST segment elevation, right bundle branch block, and susceptibility to ventricular tachycardia. In Brugada syndrome, the timing of cardiac events is significant. When do these cardiac events typically occur?

  a. During exercise

  b. When first arising in the morning

  c. Just before bedtime at night

  d. During sleep or rest

8. A Holter monitor is a small ECG recording device used for long-term monitoring of cardiac activity, usually for up to 48 hours. These devices are used in correlation with event markers (on the device itself) and activity logs, or diaries of the person's activities. What cardiac problems is a Holter monitor useful in documenting? Mark all that apply.

  a. Conduction abnormalities

  b. Acquired cardiac deficiencies

  c. Congenital cardiac problems

  d. ST segment changes

  e. PR interval changes

9. An exercise stress test challenges the heart to respond to the increased demands of exercise in a controlled and monitored environment. Not only do exercise stress tests show changes in heart rate, blood pressure, and perceived level of exercise, but they have also been found useful in determining what?

  a. ECG ischemic-type ST segment changes

  b. ECG ischemic-type QRS changes

  c. ECG documented conduction abnormalities

  d. ECG documented hemodynamic hyperreactions

10. Antiarrhythmic drugs are classified into four major groups. The drugs in one may act similarly on cardiac conduction their hemodynamic action may vary significantly. Match the name of the drug to its classification and use in the following chart:

Uses: supraventricular arrhythmias and tachyarrhythmias; slowing the sinoatrial node pacemaker and inhibiting conduction in the atrioventricular node; supraventricular and ventricular arrhythmias; treating ventricular arrhythmias only; treatment of serious ventricular arrhythmias

Classifications: Class IA, Class IB, Class II, Class III, Class IV

Drug	Use	Class
Procainamide		
Atenolol		
Amiodarone		
Diltiazem		
Lidocaine		

11. When a patient has a recurrent, life-threatening arrhythmia originating either supraventricularly or ventricularly, ablation therapy is an option for treatment. What does ablation therapy do?

  a. Removes hyperexcitable cardiac tissue through open heart surgery

  b. Isolates and destroys arrhythmogenic cardiac tissue

  c. Identifies and excises ischemic cardiac tissue

  d. Uses a catheter technique to reestablish conductivity to mild infarcts

CHAPTER 26

Heart Failure and Circulatory Shock

SECTION I: LEARNING OBJECTIVES

1. Define heart failure

2. Describe the contractile properties of the myocardium

3. Explain how the Frank-Starling mechanism, sympathetic nervous system, renin-angiotensin-aldosterone mechanism, natriuretic peptides, endothelins, and myocardial hypertrophy and remodeling function as adaptive and maladaptive mechanisms in heart failure

4. Differentiate high-output versus low-output heart failure, systolic versus diastolic heart failure, and right-sided versus left-sided heart failure in terms of causes, impact on cardiac function, and major manifestations

5. Differentiate chronic heart failure from acute heart failure syndromes

6. Describe the manifestations of heart failure and relate to the function of the heart

7. Describe the methods used in diagnosis and assessment of cardiac function in persons with heart failure

8. Relate the pharmacologic actions of angiotensin-converting enzyme inhibitors and receptor blockers, β-adrenergic–blockers, diuretics, digoxin, and vasodilatory agents to the treatment of heart failure

9. Relate the use of cardiac resynchronization, implantable cardioverter-debrillators, left ventricular assist devices, heart transplantation, and other surgical alternatives to the treatment of selected types of heart failure

10. State a clinical definition of shock

11. Compare the causes, pathophysiology, and chief characteristics of cardiogenic, hypovolemic, obstructive, and distributive shock

12. Describe the complications of shock as they relate to the lungs, kidneys, gastrointestinal tract, and blood clotting

13. State the rationale for treatment measures to correct and reverse shock

14. Define multiple organ dysfunction syndrome and cite its significance in shock

15. Describe the causes of heart failure in infants and children

16. Cite how the aging process affects cardiac function and predisposes to ventricular dysfunction

17. State how the signs and symptoms of heart failure may differ between younger and older adults

SECTION II: ASSESSING YOUR UNDERSTANDING

Activity A *Fill in the blanks.*

1. _____ has been defined as a complex syndrome that results from any functional or

structural disorder of the heart that causes decreased pumping.

2. Among the most common causes of heart failure are _____, _____, dilated cardiomyopathy, and _____ heart disease.

3. Endurance athletes have _____ cardiac reserves.

4. _____ can be expressed as the product of the heart rate and stroke volume.

5. The heart rate is regulated by a balance between the activity of the _____ nervous system, which produces an increase in heart rate, and the _____ nervous system, which slows it down.

6. The _____ is a function of preload, afterload, and myocardial contractility.

7. _____ is the percentage of blood pumped out of the ventricles with each contraction.

8. In systolic ventricular dysfunction, myocardial contractility is impaired, leading to a _____ in the ejection fraction and cardiac output.

9. Diastolic ventricular dysfunction is characterized by a _____ ejection fraction but impaired diastolic ventricular relaxation, leading to a decrease in ventricular filling that ultimately causes a decrease in preload, stroke volume, and cardiac output.

10. With both systolic and diastolic ventricular dysfunction, _____ are usually able to maintain adequate resting cardiac function until the later stages of heart failure.

11. The rise in preload seen in systolic dysfunction is believed to be a compensatory mechanism to help maintain stroke volume via the _____ mechanism despite a drop in ejection fraction.

12. Systolic dysfunction commonly results from conditions that impair the _____ performance of the heart (e.g., ischemic heart disease, cardiomyopathy), produce a _____ (e.g., valvular insufficiency, anemia), or generate a _____ (e.g., hypertension, valvular stenosis) on the heart.

13. In _____ dysfunction, cardiac output is compromised by the abnormal filling of the ventricle.

14. Among the conditions that cause diastolic dysfunction are those that _____ the ventricle (e.g., pericardial effusion, constrictive pericarditis), those that _____ wall thickness and reduce chamber size (e.g., myocardial hypertrophy, hypertrophic cardiomyopathy), and those that _____ diastolic relaxation (e.g., aging, ischemic heart disease).

15. Diastolic dysfunction can be aggravated by _____ and can be improved by a reduction in heart rate.

16. Heart failure can be classified according to the _____ of the heart that is primarily affected.

17. A major effect of right-sided heart failure is the development of _____.

18. As venous distention progresses in right-sided heart failure, blood backs up in the _____ veins that drain into the inferior vena cava, and the liver becomes engorged.

19. _____ is the most common cause of right ventricular failure.

20. The most common causes of _____ ventricular dysfunction are acute myocardial infarction and cardiomyopathy.

21. _____ is an uncommon type of heart failure that is caused by an excessive need for cardiac output.

22. _____ is caused by disorders that impair the pumping ability of the heart, such as ischemic heart disease and cardiomyopathy.

23. Elevated _____ levels have been shown to be predictive of the development of heart failure.

24. The development of _____ constitutes one of the principal mechanisms by which the heart compensates for an increase in workload.

25. A gradual or rapid change in heart failure signs and symptoms resulting in a need for urgent therapy is defined as _____ syndrome.

26. _____ dyspnea is a sudden attack of dyspnea that occurs during sleep.

27. _____ is the most dramatic symptom of acute heart failure syndromes.

28. In acute or severe left-sided failure, cardiac output may fall to levels that are insufficient for providing the _____ with adequate oxygen.

29. Ascites is a common manifestation associated with _____ ventricular failure and long-standing elevation of systemic venous pressures.

30. Central cyanosis is caused by conditions that impair _____ of the arterial blood.

31. In persons with ventricular dysfunction, sudden death is caused most commonly by _____ tachycardia or fibrillation.

32. Measurements of _____ are recommended to confirm the diagnosis of heart failure, to evaluate the severity of left ventricular compromise and estimate the prognosis and predict future cardiac events such as sudden death, and to evaluate the effectiveness of treatment.

33. β-Adrenergic receptor blocking drugs are used to decrease _____ dysfunction associated with activation of the sympathetic nervous system.

34. _____ can be described as an acute failure of the circulatory system to supply the peripheral tissues and organs of the body with an adequate blood supply, resulting in cellular hypoxia.

35. The most common cause of cardiogenic shock is _____.

36. _____ shock is characterized by diminished blood volume such that there is inadequate filling of the vascular compartment.

37. _____ shock is characterized by loss of blood vessel tone, enlargement of the vascular compartment, and displacement of the vascular volume away from the heart and central circulation.

38. A defect in the vasomotor center in the brain stem or the sympathetic outflow to the blood vessels is known as _____.

39. Anaphylactic shock results from an _____-mediated reaction in which vasodilator substances such as histamine are released into the blood.

40. _____ heart defects are the most common cause of heart failure in children.

41. _____ is associated with impaired left ventricular filling that is due to changes in myocardial relaxation and compliance.

Activity B *Match the key terms in Column A with their definitions in Column B.*

1.

Column A	Column B
___ 1. Inotropy	a. Volume or loading conditions of the ventricle at the end of diastole
___ 2. Cardiac output	
___ 3. Afterload	b. Right heart failure occurs in response to chronic pulmonary disease
___ 4. Pulmonary congestion	
___ 5. Cardiac reserve	c. Ability to increase cardiac output during increased activity
___ 6. Cor pulmonale	d. Force that the contracting heart muscle must generate to eject blood from the filled heart
___ 7. High-output failure	
___ 8. Preload	e. Failure that is caused by an excessive need for cardiac output
___ 9. Systolic dysfunction	f. Amount of blood the ventricles eject each minute
___ 10. Endothelin	g. Ejection fraction less than 40%
	h. Potent vasoconstrictors
	i. Common sign of left ventricular failure
	j. Contractile performance of the heart

2.

Column A	Column B
___ 1. Hydrothorax	a. Periodic breathing characterized by gradual increase in depth, followed by a decrease resulting in apnea
___ 2. Cyanosis	
___ 3. Cheyne-Stokes respiration	
___ 4. Dyspnea	b. Bronchospasm due to congestion of the bronchial mucosa

_____ 5. Cardiac asthma

_____ 6. Circulatory failure

_____ 7. Orthopnea

_____ 8. Ascites

c. Bluish discoloration of the skin

d. Labored breathing

e. Transudation of fluid into the peritoneal cavity

f. Hypoperfusion of organs and tissues

g. Transudation of fluid into the pleural cavity

h. Shortness of breath when supine

3.

Column A	Column B
_____ 1. Cardiogenic shock	a. Acute failure of the circulatory system to supply the peripheral tissues and organs of the body with an adequate blood supply
_____ 2. Obstructive shock	
_____ 3. Distributive shock	b. Caused by excessive vasodilation with maldistribution of blood flow
_____ 4. Hypovolemic shock	c. Caused by alteration in cardiac function
_____ 5. Circulatory shock	d. Caused by a decrease in blood volume
	e. Caused by obstruction of blood flow through the circulatory system

Activity C

1. The pathophysiology of right- and left-sided heart failure has distinct features. Construct a flowchart of the following symptoms and their causes:
   - Right heart failure
   - Left heart failure
   - Orthopnea
   - Cyanosis
   - Activity intolerance
   - Anorexia
   - Weight loss
   - Impaired liver function
   - Gastrointestinal tract congestion
   - Impaired gas exchange
   - Pulmonary edema
   - Dependent edema and ascites
   - Congestion of peripheral tissues
   - Decreased cardiac output
   - Pulmonary congestion

Activity D *Briefly answer the following.*

1. How is cardiac contractility regulated?

   _____

   _____

   _____

2. Why is it advisable to test cardiac function during exercise (stress) rather than at rest?

   _____

   _____

   _____

3. How does diastolic dysfunction produce the typical signs and symptoms that characterize the condition?

   _____

   _____

   _____

4. Often, the early signs of heart failure are silent. This is due to the many compensatory mechanisms of the cardiovascular system. Explain, briefly, how these mechanisms work and why, in the end, they only serve to make the heart failure worse.

   _____

   _____

   _____

5. What are the common manifestations of heart failure? Why?

   _____

   _____

   _____

6. What effect does diuretic therapy have on heart failure?

   _____

   _____

   _____

7. What are the cellular consequences of shock?

   _____

   _____

   _____

8. What are the five major complications of severe shock?

_____

_____

_____

SECTION III: APPLYING YOUR KNOWLEDGE

Activity E *Consider the following scenario and answer the questions.*

The parents of a 1-month-old boy born with tetralogy of Fallot are in the emergency department with their child, who is exhibiting a respiratory rate of 65 breaths/minute, heart rate of 160 beats/minute, and urine output of <1 cc/kg/hour. The child is diaphoretic, his extremities are cool, and he is lethargic and will not eat. The suspected diagnosis is heart failure.

1. What diagnostic tests would the nurse expect to be ordered for this child?

_____

_____

_____

2. What drugs are used in the treatment of heart failure in infants and children, and what are the dosages based on?

_____

_____

_____

SECTION IV: PRACTICING FOR NCLEX

Activity F *Answer the following questions.*

1. Match the following conditions with the type of heart failure they cause.

Condition

____ 1. Valvular insufficiency

____ 2. Ischemic heart disease

____ 3. Aortic or mitral stenosis

Type of Heart Failure

a. Diastolic dysfunction

b. Left ventricular dysfunction

____ 4. Acute myocardial infarction

____ 5. Paget disease

____ 6. Cardiomyopathy

c. Right ventricular dysfunction

d. Low-output failure

e. High-output failure

f. Systolic dysfunction

2. What are the signs and symptoms of heart failure? Mark all that apply.
   a. Fluid retention
   b. Ruddy complexion
   c. Fatigue
   d. Bradycardia
   e. Chronic productive cough

3. When an acute event occurs and the circulatory system can no longer provide the body with adequate perfusion of its tissues and organs, cellular hypoxia occurs, and the body goes into shock. What are the causes of shock in the human body? Mark all that apply.
   a. Maldistribution of blood flow
   b. Hypovolemia
   c. Excessive vasoconstriction
   d. Obstruction of blood flow
   e. Hypervolemia

4. What are the physiologic signs and symptoms of cardiogenic shock? Mark all that apply.
   a. Decreased mean arterial blood pressures
   b. Increased urine output related to increased renal perfusion
   c. Increased central venous pressure
   d. Hypercapnic lips and nail beds
   e. Increased extraction of O_2 from hemoglobin

5. In hypovolemic shock, the main purpose of treatment is correcting or controlling the underlying cause of the hypovolemia and improving the perfusion of the tissues and organs of the body. Which of the following treatments is *not* a primary form of therapy for hypovolemic shock?
   a. Surgery
   b. Administration of IV fluids and blood
   c. Vasoconstrictive drugs
   d. Infusion of blood and blood products

6. Neurogenic shock, or spinal shock, is a phenomenon caused by the inability of the vasomotor center in the brain stem to control blood vessel tone through the sympathetic outflow to the blood vessels. In neurogenic shock, what happens to the heart rate and the skin?

    a. Heart rate slower than normal; skin warm and dry

    b. Heart rate faster than normal; skin cool and moist

    c. Heart rate slower than normal; skin cool and moist

    d. Heart rate slower than normal; skin warm and dry

7. Anaphylactic shock is the most severe form of systemic allergic reaction. Immunologically medicated substances are released into the blood, causing vasodilation and an increase in capillary permeability. What physiologic response often accompanies the vascular response in anaphylaxis?

    a. Uterine smooth muscle relaxation

    b. Laryngeal edema

    c. Bronchodilation

    d. Gastrointestinal relaxation

8. Sepsis is a growing incidence in the United States. Its pathogenesis includes neutrophil activation that kills microorganisms. Neutrophils also injure the endothelium, releasing mediators that increase vascular permeability. What else do neutrophils do in sepsis?

    a. Release nitric oxide

    b. Vasoconstrict the capillary bed

    c. Cause bradycardia

    d. Activate erythropoiesis

9. What is the primary physiologic result of obstructive shock?

    a. Left ventricular hypertrophy

    b. Elevated right heart pressure

    c. Right atrial hypertrophy

    d. Decreased right heart pressure

10. An important factor in the mortality of severe shock is acute renal failure. What is the degree of renal damage related to in shock?

    a. Loss of perfusion and duration of shock

    b. Loss of perfusion and degree of immune-mediated response

    c. Severity and duration of shock

    d. Severity of shock and degree of immune-mediated response

11. The pathogenesis of multiorgan dysfunction syndrome (MODS) is not clearly understood at this time. Supportive management is currently the focus of treatment in this disorder. What is not a major risk factor in MODS?

    a. Advanced age

    b. Alcohol abuse

    c. Respiratory dysfunction

    d. Infarcted bowel

12. What is the primary cause of heart failure in infants and children?

    a. Idiopathic heart disease

    b. Structural heart defects

    c. Hyperkalemia

    d. Reaction to medications

CHAPTER 27

Structure and Function of the Respiratory System

SECTION I: LEARNING OBJECTIVES

1. State the difference between the conducting and the respiratory airways

2. Trace the movement of air through the airways, beginning in the nose and oropharynx and moving into the respiratory tissues of the lung

3. Describe the function of the mucociliary blanket

4. Compare the supporting structures of the large and small airways in terms of cartilaginous and smooth muscle support

5. State the function of the two types of alveolar cells

6. Differentiate the function of the bronchial and pulmonary circulations that supply the lungs

7. Describe the basic properties of gases in relation to their partial pressures and their pressures in relation to volume and temperature

8. State the definition of intrathoracic, intrapleural, and intra-alveolar pressures, and state how each of these pressures changes in relation to atmospheric pressure during inspiration and expiration

9. Use the law of Laplace to explain the need for surfactant in maintaining the inflation of small alveoli

10. Differentiate between the determinants of airway resistance and lung compliance and their effect on the work of breathing

11. Define inspiratory reserve, expiratory reserve, vital capacity, residual lung volume, and $FEV_{1.0}$

12. Trace the exchange of gases between the air in the alveoli and the blood in the pulmonary capillaries

13. Differentiate between pulmonary and alveolar ventilation

14. Explain why ventilation and perfusion must be matched

15. Cite the difference between dead air space and shunt

16. List four factors that affect the diffusion of gases in the alveoli

17. Explain the difference between PO_2 and hemoglobin-bound oxygen and O_2 saturation, and oxygen content

18. Explain the significance of a shift to the right and a shift to the left in the oxygen–hemoglobin dissociation curve

19. Compare the neural control of the respiratory muscles, which control breathing, with that of cardiac muscle, which controls the pumping action of the heart

20. Describe the function of the chemoreceptors and lung receptors in the regulation of ventilation

21. Trace the integration of the cough reflex from stimulus to explosive expulsion of air that constitutes the cough

22. Describe the type of periodic breathing known as Cheyne-Stokes breathing

23. Define dyspnea and list three types of conditions in which dyspnea occurs

SECTION II: ASSESSING YOUR UNDERSTANDING

Activity A *Fill in the blanks.*

1. The primary function of the respiratory system is _____.

2. Functionally, the respiratory system can be divided into two parts: the _____ airways, through which air moves as it passes between the atmosphere and the lungs, and the _____ tissues of the lungs, where gas exchange takes place.

3. The _____ airways consist of the nasal passages, mouth and pharynx, larynx, trachea, bronchi, and bronchioles.

4. The air we breathe is _____, _____, and _____ as it moves through the conducting airways.

5. The _____ produced by the epithelial cells in the conducting airways forms a layer that protects the respiratory system by entrapping dust, bacteria, and other foreign particles that enter the airways.

6. The vocal folds and the elongated opening between them are called the _____.

7. The walls of the trachea are supported by horseshoe- or C-shaped rings of _____ cartilage, which prevent it from collapsing when the pressure in the thorax becomes negative.

8. Each primary bronchus, accompanied by the pulmonary arteries, veins, and lymph vessels, enters the lung through a slit called the _____.

9. Each _____ is supplied by a branch of a terminal bronchiole, an arteriole, the pulmonary capillaries, and a venule.

10. The _____ are the terminal air spaces of the respiratory tract and the actual sites of gas exchange between the air and the blood.

11. The pulmonary circulation arises from the _____ artery and provides for the gas exchange function of the lungs.

12. Particulate matter entering the lung is partly removed by _____ vessels, as are the plasma proteins that have escaped from the pulmonary capillaries.

13. It is _____ stimulation, through the vagus nerve, that is responsible for the slightly constricted smooth muscle tone in the normal resting lung.

14. Stimulation of the _____ nervous system causes airway relaxation, blood vessel constriction, and inhibition of glandular secretion.

15. The pressure exerted by a single gas in a mixture is called the _____.

16. Air moves between the atmosphere and the lungs because of a _____.

17. The pressure in the pleural cavity is called the _____ pressure.

18. The _____ maneuver is used to study the cardiovascular effects of increased intrathoracic pressure on peripheral venous pressures, cardiac filling, and cardiac output, as well as poststrain heart rate and blood pressure responses.

19. Lung _____ refers to the ease with which the lungs can be inflated.

20. The _____ is the volume of air inspired (or exhaled) with each breath.

21. The maximum amount of air that can be inspired in excess of the normal tidal volume (TV) is called the _____, and the maximum amount that can be exhaled in excess of the normal TV is the _____.

22. The _____ is the amount of air a person can breathe in beginning at the normal expiratory level and distending the lungs to the maximal amount.

23. The _____ equals the inspiratory reserve volume plus the tidal volume plus the expiratory reserve volume and is the amount of air that can be exhaled from the point of maximal inspiration.

24. The _____ is the amount of air that is exchanged in 1 minute.

25. _____ ventilation refers to the total exchange of gases between the atmosphere and the lungs; _____ ventilation is the exchange of gases within the gas exchange portion of the lungs.

26. Even at low lung volumes, some air remains in the alveoli of the lower portion of the lungs, preventing their _____.

27. _____ refers to the air that is moved with each breath but does not participate in gas exchange.

28. Both dead air space and shunt produce a _____ of ventilation and perfusion.

29. Although the lungs are responsible for the exchange of gases with the external environment, the _____ transports gases between the lungs and body tissues.

30. _____ carries about 98% to 99% of oxygen in the blood and is the main transporter of oxygen.

31. Oxygen binds _____ with the heme groups on the hemoglobin molecule.

32. Hemoglobin's affinity for oxygen is influenced by _____, _____ concentration, and body _____.

33. Carbon dioxide is transported in the blood in three forms as _____ (10%), attached to _____ (30%), and as _____ (60%).

34. The pacemaker properties of the respiratory center result from the cycling of the two groups of respiratory neurons: the _____ center in the upper pons and the _____ center in the lower pons.

35. The automatic regulation of ventilation is controlled by input from two types of sensors or receptors: _____ and _____ receptors.

36. The _____ content in the blood regulates ventilation through its effect on the pH of the extracellular fluid of the brain.

37. _____ is a subjective sensation or a person's perception of difficulty in breathing that includes the perception of labored breathing and the reaction to that sensation.

Activity B *Consider the following figure.*

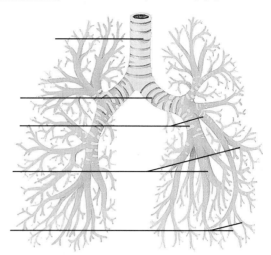

In this figure of the respiratory system, label the following structures:

- Secondary bronchi
- Tracheal cartilage
- Left primary bronchus
- Terminal bronchioles
- Segmental bronchi

Activity C *Match the key terms in Column A with their definitions in Column B.*

Column A	Column B
____ 1. Mediastinum	a. Mucus lining of the conducting airways
____ 2. Elastic recoil	b. Form part of respiratory membrane
____ 3. Epiglottis	
____ 4. Type I pneumocytes	c. Pressure inside the airways and alveoli
____ 5. Angiogenesis	d. Trachea, bronchi, and bronchioles
____ 6. Mucociliary blanket	e. Synthesize pulmonary surfactant
____ 7. Alveolar pressure	f. Space between lungs that contains heart, blood vessels, lymph nodes, nerves, and esophagus
____ 8. Brush cells	
____ 9. Tracheobronchial	
____ 10. Type II pneumocytes	

(continues)

g. Ability of the elastic components of the lung to recoil to their original position

h. Routes liquids and foods into the esophagus

i. Formation of new blood vessels

j. Act as receptors that monitor the air quality of the lungs

Activity D *Put these respiratory structures in anatomic order:*

a. Nasopharynx

b. Trachea

c. Epiglottis

d. Alveoli

e. Respiratory bronchiole

f. Intrapulmonary bronchus

g. Extrapulmonary bronchus

Activity E *Briefly answer the following.*

1. Describe the pleura and explain its function.

_____

_____

_____

2. Describe the events of the respiratory cycle.

_____

_____

_____

3. What is the function of pulmonary surfactant?

_____

_____

_____

4. What is the mathematical formula used to describe the diffusion of gas across the respiratory membrane?

_____

_____

_____

5. In the clinic, what type of blood is used for blood gas measurements, and why?

_____

_____

_____

6. What causes us to cough?

_____

_____

_____

SECTION III: APPLYING YOUR KNOWLEDGE

Activity F *Consider the following scenario and answer the questions.*

Seventy-nine-year-old Mr. Borden is brought to the clinic by his daughter, who says, "I am worried about him. He is so stubborn, he just won't complain. When he walks, he gets so short of breath. I don't think he is getting enough oxygen!" Mr. Borden's O_2 level is 87%, and his nail beds are dusky with a delayed capillary refill time. There is no clubbing to Mr. Borden's fingertips.

1. How would the nurse explain generalized hypoxia to Mr. Borden's daughter?

_____

_____

_____

2. What diagnostic tests would the doctor order to confirm a diagnosis of generalized hypoxia?

_____

_____

_____

SECTION IV: PRACTICING FOR NCLEX

Activity G *Answer the following questions.*

1. The lungs are the working structures of the respiratory system, and they have several

functions. What are the functions of the lungs? Mark all that apply.

a. To produce heparin

b. To activate vasoactive substances

c. To convert angiotensin I to angiotensin II

d. To activate bradykinin

e. To convert glucose to glycogen

2. Bronchial blood vessels have several functions. They warm and humidify incoming air as well as distribute blood to the conducting airways and the supporting structures of the lung. What is it that makes bronchial blood vessels unique in the body?

a. They can undergo angiogenesis.

b. They drain blood into the bronchiole arteries.

c. They participate in gas exchange.

d. They carry oxygenated blood to the lung tissues.

3. Match the respiratory pressures with their definitions.

Pressure	Definition
___ 1. Alveolar pressure	a. Pressure in the thoracic cavity
___ 2. Intrapleural pressure	b. Pressure inside the airways and alveoli of the lungs
___ 3. Transpulmonary pressure	c. Difference between the intra-alveoli and intrapleural pressures
___ 4. Intrathoracic pressure	d. Pressure in the pleural cavity

4. What does the equation $C = \Delta V / \Delta P$ stand for?

a. Surface tension inside the lungs

b. Lung compliance

c. Airway resistance

d. Change in peak expiratory flow

5. An 82-year-old man with chronic obstructive pulmonary disease is at the clinic for a regular check-up. Because of his diagnosis, the nurse would expect his respiratory rate under normal circumstances to be what?

a. Tachypneic

b. ≥18–20 beats/minute

c. ≤18–20 beats/minute

d. Hyperpneic

6. Our ability to oxygenate the tissues and organs of our bodies depends on our ability to ventilate, or exchange gases in our respiratory system. The resultant distribution of ventilation of the areas of the body open to the exchange of gases in our respiratory system depends on what?

a. Effects of gravity intrathoracic pressure

b. Body position and alveolar pressure

c. Effects of gravity and body position

d. Intrathoracic pressure and alveolar pressure

7. Alveolar oxygen levels directly impact the blood vessels in the pulmonary circulation. In a person with lung disease, there is vasoconstriction throughout the lung, causing a generalized hypoxia. What can prolonged hypoxia lead to?

a. Hypertension and increased workload on the left heart

b. Pulmonary hypertension and left ventricular hypertrophy

c. Hypertension and increased workload on the right heart

d. Pulmonary hypertension and increased workload on the right heart

8. When there is a mismatch of ventilation and perfusion within the lung itself, insufficient ventilation occurs. There is a lack of enough oxygen to adequately oxygenate the blood flowing through the alveolar capillaries, thus creating a physiologic shunt. What causes a physiologic right-to-left shunting of blood in the respiratory system?

a. Destructive lung disease or heart failure

b. Obstructive lung disease or heart failure

c. Heart failure or pulmonary hypertension

d. Heart failure or regional hypoxia

9. Blood transports both oxygen and carbon dioxide in a physically dissolved form to the tissues and organs of the body. It is the measurements of the components of the gases in the blood that are used as indicators of the body's status by health care workers. Why is it commonly the blood in the arteries that is measured for its components rather than the blood in the veins?

a. Arterial blood most adequately measures the metabolic demands of the tissues along with the gas exchange function of the lungs.

b. Venous blood measures the metabolic demands of the tissues rather than the gas exchange function of the lungs.

c. Arterial blood only measures the gas exchange function of the lung after it has met the metabolic demands of the tissues.

d. Venous blood only measures the hypoxic reflex of the body, not the gas exchange function of the lungs.

10. Respiration has both automatic and voluntary components that are sent to the respiratory center of the brain from a number of sources. What physiologic forces can exert their influence on respiration through the lower brain centers? Mark all that apply.

a. Fever

b. Cold

c. Pain

d. Endorphins

e. Emotion

11. There are several actions the body makes to initiate a cough. Put these actions into the correct order.

a. Elevation of intrathoracic pressures

b. Rapid opening of glottis

c. Closure of glottis

d. Rapid inspiration of large volume of air

e. Forceful contraction of abdominal and expiratory muscles

12. Dyspnea is defined as an uncomfortable sensation or difficulty in breathing that is subjectively defined by the client. Which of the following disease states is *not* characterized by dyspnea?

a. Pneumonia

b. Emphysema

c. Myasthenia gravis

d. Multiple sclerosis

CHAPTER 28

Respiratory Tract Infections, Neoplasms, and Childhood Disorders

SECTION I: LEARNING OBJECTIVES

1. Describe the transmission of the common cold from one person to another

2. Describe the causes, manifestations, and treatment of acute and chronic sinusitis

3. Relate the characteristics of the influenza virus to its contagious properties and the need for a yearly "flu shot"

4. Characterize community-acquired pneumonia, hospital-acquired pneumonia, and pneumonia in immunocompromised persons in terms of pathogens, manifestations, and prognosis

5. Describe the properties of the immunologic properties of the tubercle bacillus, and differentiate between primary tuberculosis and reactivated tuberculosis on the basis of their pathophysiology

6. State the mechanism for the transmission of fungal infections of the lung

7. Cite risk factors associated with lung cancer

8. Compare small cell lung cancer and non–small cell lung cancer in terms of histopathology, prognosis, and treatment methods

9. Describe the manifestations of lung cancer and list two symptoms of lung cancer that are related to the invasion of the mediastinum

10. Define the term *paraneoplastic* and cite three paraneoplastic manifestations of lung cancer

11. Characterize the effect of age on treatment of lung cancer

12. Trace the development of the respiratory tract through the five stages of embryonic and fetal development

13. Cite the function of surfactant in lung function in the neonate

14. Cite the possible cause and manifestations of respiratory distress syndrome and bronchopulmonary dysplasia

15. Describe the physiologic basis for sternal and chest wall retractions and grunting, stridor, and wheezing as signs of respiratory distress in infants and small children

16. Compare croup, epiglottitis, and bronchiolitis in terms of incidence by age, site of infection, and signs and symptoms

17. List the signs of impending respiratory failure in small children

SECTION II: ASSESSING YOUR UNDERSTANDING

Activity A *Fill in the blanks.*

1. _____ are the most frequent cause of respiratory tract infections.

2. Viral infections can damage _____ epithelium, _____ airways, and lead to secondary _____ infections.

3. The common cold is a viral infection of the _____ respiratory tract.

4. Outbreaks of colds due to _____ are most common in early fall and late spring.

5. _____ are popular over-the-counter treatments for colds because of their action in drying nasal secretions.

6. _____ refers to inflammation of the nasal passages and sinusitis as inflammation of the _____ sinuses.

7. The lower _____ content in the sinuses facilitates the growth of organisms, impairs local defenses, and alters the function of immune cells.

8. Host antibodies to _____ and _____ prevent or ameliorate infection by the influenza virus.

9. The influenza viruses can cause three types of infections: an uncomplicated _____ respiratory infection, _____ pneumonia, and a respiratory viral infection followed by a _____ infection.

10. Because influenza is so highly contagious, prevention relies primarily on _____.

11. Avian strains of the influenza virus do not usually cause outbreaks of disease in humans unless a _____ of the virus genome has occurred within an intermediate mammalian host such as a pig.

12. The term _____ describes inflammation of parenchymal structures of the lung, such as the alveoli and the bronchioles.

13. _____ refers to consolidation of a part or all of a lung lobe, and _____ signifies a patchy consolidation involving more than one lobe.

14. Hospital-acquired, or _____, pneumonia is defined as a lower respiratory tract infection that was not present or incubating on admission to the hospital.

15. The term _____ host is usually applied to persons with a variety of underlying defects in host defenses.

16. _____ disease is a form of bronchopneumonia, an infection that normally occurs by acquiring the organism from the environment.

17. The primary atypical pneumonias are caused by a variety of agents, the most common being _____ pneumonia.

18. _____ is the world's foremost cause of death from a single infectious agent.

19. Mycobacteria are similar to other bacterial organisms except for an outer _____ coating that makes them more resistant to destruction.

20. _____ tuberculosis is a form of the disease that develops in previously unexposed, and therefore, unsensitized persons.

21. The most frequently used screening methods for pulmonary tuberculosis are the _____ tests and chest _____.

22. _____ is caused by the dimorphic fungus *Histoplasma capsulatum* and is one of the most common fungal infections in the United States.

23. _____ respiratory infections produce pulmonary manifestations that resemble tuberculosis.

24. The number of Americans who develop lung cancer is decreasing, primarily due to a decrease in _____.

25. Cigarette smoking causes more than _____ of the cases of lung cancer.

26. _____ are aggressive, locally invasive, and widely metastatic tumors that arise from the epithelial lining of major bronchi.

27. The _____ are small round to oval cells that are approximately the size of a lymphocyte and grow in clusters that exhibit neither glandular nor squamous organization.

28. The _____ include squamous cell carcinomas, adenocarcinomas, and large cell carcinomas.

29. _____ is characterized by inspiratory stridor, hoarseness, and a barking cough.

30. By the _____ weeks of gestation, sufficient terminal air sacs are present to permit survival of the premature infant.

Activity B *Consider the following figures.*

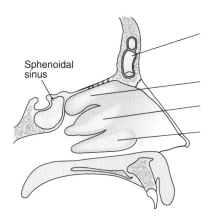

Sphenoidal sinus

In these figures, label the following structures:

- Frontal sinus
- Ethmoid sinuses
- Maxillary sinus
- Superior turbinate
- Middle turbinate
- Inferior turbinate

Activity C *Match the key terms in Column A with their definitions in Column B.*

Column A

_____ **1.** Small cell lung cancers

_____ **2.** Typical pneumonias

_____ **3.** Stridor

_____ **4.** Anergy

_____ **5.** Hemagglutinin

_____ **6.** Squamous cell

_____ **7.** Paraneoplastic syndrome

_____ **8.** Atypical pneumonias

_____ **9.** Neuraminidase

_____ **10.** Reye syndrome

Column B

a. Audible crowing sound during inspiration

b. False-negative tuberculin skin tests

c. Result from infection by bacteria

d. Attachment protein that allows the influenza virus to enter epithelial cells in the respiratory tract

e. Symptoms that develop when substances released by some cancer cells disrupt the normal function

f. Viral and mycoplasma infection

g. Facilitates influenza viral replication and release from the cell

h. Fatty liver with encephalitis

i. Highly aggressive lung cancer

j. Carcinoma associated with the paraneoplastic syndromes that produce hypercalcemia

Activity D

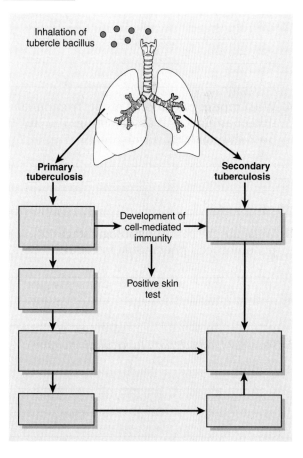

Inhalation of tubercle bacillus

Primary tuberculosis

Secondary tuberculosis

Development of cell-mediated immunity

Positive skin test

Use the following terms to complete the flow-chart:

- Reinfection
- Ghon complex
- Granulomatous inflammatory response
- Healed dormant lesion
- Cell-mediated hypersensitivity response
- Reactivated tuberculosis
- Progressive or disseminated tuberculosis

Activity E *Briefly answer the following.*

1. How is the cold virus spread?

_____

_____

_____

2. How does the influenza virus reinfect someone? How is it so contagious?

_____

_____

_____

3. What is a common complication of influenza (usually of the elderly or those with cardiopulmonary disease)?

_____

_____

_____

4. What type of pneumonia results from inhalation or aspiration of nasopharyngeal secretions during sleep?

_____

_____

_____

5. What are the pathophysiologic stages of pneumococcal pneumonia infection?

_____

_____

_____

6. How is *Mycobacterium tuberculosis hominis* spread?

_____

_____

_____

7. Describe the pathogenic mechanisms of *Mycobacterium tuberculosis hominis*.

_____

_____

_____

8. How is lung cancer categorized?

_____

_____

_____

9. What causes the varied manifestations of lung cancer?

_____

_____

_____

10. What is the result of the absence of surfactant in premature infants?

_____

_____

_____

SECTION III: APPLYING YOUR KNOWLEDGE

Activity F *Consider the following scenario and answer the questions.*

Mr. Jones, a 68-year-old man, presents to the clinic with lack of appetite and weight loss of 30 pounds over the past 6 months. He has a history of a chronic, nonproductive cough; shortness of breath, which is worse on exertion; and wheezing. He tells the nurse that he is now coughing up "bloody stuff," and he wants to know what is wrong with him. When asked about pain he says, "I get heartburn once in awhile, but the pain is dull instead of burning." Routine laboratory work is ordered, and the only abnormal finding is hypercalcemia. The suspected diagnosis is squamous cell cancer of the lung.

1. What diagnostic tests would the nurse expect to be ordered?

_____

_____

_____

2. Mr. Jones wants to know how his cancer will be treated. The nurse knows that treatments are available. Which treatments are used for squamous cell cancer (non–small cell lung cancer) of the lung?

_____

_____

_____

SECTION IV: PRACTICING FOR NCLEX

Activity G *Answer the following questions.*

1. A 23-year-old woman goes to the drugstore to buy a medication to ease the symptoms of her cold. Her friends have told her to buy a medication with an antihistamine in it to help dry up her runny nose and make it easier to breath. The woman talks with the pharmacist, who has known her for many years. The pharmacist recommends that she does not buy a cold medication with a decongestant in it. Why would he do that?

   a. Client has history of hypothyroidism
   b. Client has history of hypotension
   c. Client has history of type 1 diabetes mellitus
   d. Client has history of juvenile rheumatoid arthritis

2. The early stages of influenza pass by as if the infection were any other viral infection. What is the distinguishing feature of an influenza viral infection that makes it different from other viral infections?

   a. Slow onset of upper respiratory symptoms
   b. Rapid onset of profound malaise
   c. Slow onset of fever and chills
   d. Rapid onset of productive cough

3. Influenza A subtype H5N1 has been documented in poultry in both East and Southeast Asian countries. This form of avian flu (bird flu) is highly contagious from bird to bird, but is rarely passed from human to human. There is a large amount of concern that the H5N1 strain might mutate, making it easier to be passed from human to human, carrying with it a high mortality rate. What is the main concern if the H5N1 strain does mutate?

   a. Epidemic in Southeast Asia
   b. Inability to develop a vaccine for the newly infected poultry
   c. Initiation of a pandemic
   d. Several small pockets of infection so widespread that they will be hard to control

4. Community-acquired pneumonia can be categorized according to several indexes. What are these indexes? Mark all that apply.

   a. Radiologic findings
   b. Serologic findings
   c. Age
   d. Presence of coexisting disease
   e. Need for hospitalization in long-term care facility

5. An immunocompromised host is open to pneumonia from all types of organisms. There is, however, a correlation between specific types of immunologic deficits and specific invading organisms. What organism is most likely to cause pneumonia in an immunocompromised host with neutropenia and impaired granulocyte function?

   a. β-Hemolytic *Streptococcus* gram-positive bacilli
   b. Eosinophilic *Bacillus subtilis*
   c. *Haemophilus* influenza
   d. *Staphylococcus aureus*

6. Elderly people are susceptible to pneumonia in all its varieties. The symptoms the elderly exhibit can be different than those of other age groups who have pneumonia. What signs and symptoms are elderly people with pneumonia less likely to experience than people with pneumonia in other age groups?

   a. Marked elevation in temperature
   b. Loss of appetite
   c. Deterioration in mental status
   d. Pleuritic pain

7. Tuberculosis is a highly destructive disease because the tubercle bacillus activates a tissue hypersensitivity to the tubercular antigens. What does the destructive nature of tuberculosis cause in a previously unexposed immunocompetent person?

   a. Cavitation and rapidly progressing pulmonary lesions
   b. Caseating necrosis and cavitation

   c. Rapidly progressing lesions and purulent necrosis

   d. Caseating necrosis and purulent pulmonary lesions

8. Coccidioidomycosis is a pulmonary fungal infection resembling tuberculosis. Less severe forms of the infection are treated with oral antifungal medications. For persons with progressive disease, what is the drug of choice?

   a. IV fluconazole

   b. IV bacillus Calmette-Guérin

   c. IV amphotericin B

   d. IV rifampin

9. Non-small cell lung cancers mimic small cell lung cancers through their abilities to do what?

   a. Synthesize bioactive products and produce panneoplastic syndromes

   b. Neutralize bioactive products that produce paraneoplastic syndromes

   c. Produce paraneoplastic syndromes and synthesize adrenocorticotropic hormone

   d. Synthesize bioactive products and produce paraneoplastic syndromes

10. Premature infants who are treated with mechanical ventilation, mostly for respiratory distress syndrome, are at risk for developing bronchopulmonary dysplasia (BPD), a chronic lung disease. What are the signs and symptoms of BPD?

   a. Rapid, shallow breathing and chest retractions

   b. Weight loss and barrel chest

   c. Tachycardia and slow, shallow breathing

   d. Barrel chest and rapid weight gain

11. For each of the following conditions, identify where it occurs in the respiratory tract of children (upper airway or lower airway.)

Epiglottitis

Acute bronchiolitis

Asthma

Spasmodic croup

Laryngotracheobronchitis

12. What is the underlying cause of respiratory failure in a child with bronchiolitis?

   a. Obstructive process

   b. Impaired gas exchange

   c. Hypoxemia and hypercapnia

   d. Metabolic acidosis

CHAPTER 29

Disorders of Ventilation and Gas Exchange

SECTION I: LEARNING OBJECTIVES

1. Define the terms *hypoxemia* and *hypercapnia*

2. Characterize the mechanisms whereby disorders of ventilation and diffusion cause hypoxemia and hypercapnia

3. Compare the manifestations of hypoxemia and hypercapnia

4. Characterize the pathogenesis and manifestations of transudative and exudative pleural effusion, chylothorax, and hemothorax

5. Differentiate among the causes and manifestations of spontaneous pneumothorax, secondary pneumothorax, and tension pneumothorax

6. Describe the causes of pleurisy and differentiate the characteristics of pleural pain from other types of chest pain

7. Describe the causes and manifestations of atelectasis

8. Describe the physiology of bronchial smooth muscle as it relates to airway disease

9. Describe the interaction between heredity, alterations in the immune response, and environmental agents in the pathogenesis of bronchial asthma

10. Characterize the acute- or early-phase and late-phase responses in the pathogenesis of bronchial asthma and relate them to current methods for treatment of the disorder

11. Explain the changes in pulmonary function studies that occur with chronic airway disease

12. Explain the distinction between chronic bronchitis and emphysema in terms of pathology and clinical manifestations

13. State the chief manifestations of bronchiectasis

14. Describe the genetic abnormality responsible for cystic fibrosis and relate it to the manifestations of the disorder

15. State the difference between chronic obstructive pulmonary diseases and chronic restrictive lung diseases in terms of their pathology and manifestations

16. Cite the characteristics of occupational dusts that determine their pathogenicity in terms of the production of pneumoconiosis

17. Describe the causes of hypersensitivity pneumonitis

18. Characterize the organ involvement in sarcoidosis

19. State the most common cause of pulmonary embolism and the clinical manifestations of the disorder

20. Describe the pathophysiology of pulmonary arterial hypertension and state three causes of secondary pulmonary hypertension

21. Describe the alterations in cardiovascular function that are characteristic of cor pulmonale

22. Describe the pathologic lung changes that occur in acute respiratory distress syndrome and relate them to the clinical manifestations of a general definition of respiratory failure

23. Differentiate between the causes and manifestations of hypoxemic and hypercapnic/hypoxemic respiratory failure

24. Describe the treatment of respiratory failure

SECTION II: ASSESSING YOUR UNDERSTANDING

Activity A *Fill in the blanks.*

1. The primary function of the respiratory system is to remove appropriate amounts of _____ from the blood entering the pulmonary circulation and to add adequate amounts of _____ to the blood leaving the pulmonary circulation.

2. _____ involves the movement of fresh atmospheric air to the alveoli for delivery provision of O_2 and removal of CO_2.

3. As a general rule, _____ of the blood primarily depends on factors that promote diffusion of O_2 from the alveoli into the pulmonary capillaries, whereas _____ primarily depends on the minute ventilation and elimination of CO_2 from the alveoli.

4. _____ refers to a reduction in blood O_2 levels.

5. Hypoxemia produces its effects through tissue _____ and the compensatory mechanisms that the body uses to adapt to the lowered oxygen level.

6. The body compensates for chronic hypoxemia by increased _____, pulmonary _____, and increased production of _____ cells.

7. _____ can occur in a number of disorders that cause hypoventilation or mismatching of ventilation and perfusion resulting in increased arterial CO_2.

8. Elevated levels of PCO_2 produce a decrease in _____ and respiratory _____.

9. _____ refers to an abnormal collection of fluid in the pleural cavity.

10. _____ is a specific type of pleural effusion in which there is blood in the pleural cavity.

11. Primary atelectasis of the newborn implies that the lung has never been _____.

12. Obstructive airway disorders are caused by disorders that limit _____ airflow.

13. Bronchial _____ is a chronic disorder of the airways that causes episodes of airway obstruction, bronchial hyperresponsiveness, and airway inflammation that are usually reversible.

14. Recent research has focused on the role of _____ in the pathogenesis of bronchial asthma.

15. _____ pulmonary disease is characterized by chronic and recurrent obstruction of airflow in the pulmonary airways.

16. In chronic obstructive pulmonary disease, _____ and _____ of the bronchial wall, along with excess mucus secretion, obstruct airflow and cause mismatching of ventilation and perfusion.

17. _____ is believed to result from the breakdown of elastin and other alveolar wall components by enzymes called _____ that digest proteins.

18. A hereditary deficiency in _____ accounts for approximately 1% of all cases of chronic obstructive pulmonary disease and is more common in young persons with emphysema.

19. The earliest feature of chronic bronchitis is _____ in the large airways, associated with hypertrophy of the submucosal glands in the trachea and bronchi.

20. Persons with predominant emphysema are classically referred to as "_____," a reference to the lack of cyanosis, the use of accessory muscles, and pursed-lip breathing.

21. Persons with a clinical syndrome of chronic bronchitis are classically labeled "_____," a reference to cyanosis and fluid retention associated with right-sided heart failure.

22. _____ is a permanent dilation of the bronchi and bronchioles caused by destruction of the muscle and elastic supporting tissue, resulting from a vicious cycle of infection and inflammation.

23. _____ is an autosomal recessive disorder involving fluid secretion in the exocrine glands in the epithelial lining of the respiratory, gastrointestinal, and reproductive tracts.

24. The diffuse _____ diseases are a diverse group of lung disorders that produce similar inflammatory and fibrotic changes in the interalveolar septa of the lung.

25. The interstitial lung disorders exert their effects on the _____ and _____ connective tissue found between the delicate interstitium of the alveolar walls.

26. Pulmonary _____ develops when a blood-borne substance lodges in a branch of the pulmonary artery and obstructs the flow, almost all of which are thrombi that arise from deep vein thrombosis.

27. Chest pain, dyspnea, and increased respiratory rate are the most frequent signs and symptoms of _____.

28. _____ is a disorder characterized by an elevation of pressure within the pulmonary circulation, namely, the pulmonary arterial system.

29. Continued exposure of the pulmonary vessels to _____ is a common cause of pulmonary hypertension.

30. _____ can be viewed as a failure in the gas exchange due to pump failure, lung failure, or both.

Activity B *Consider the following figure.*

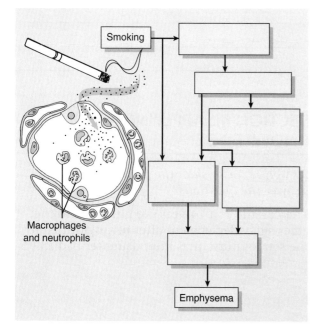

Complete the flowchart using the following items:
- Destruction of elastic fibers in lung
- Decreased α_1-antitrypsin activity
- Action inhibited by α_1-antitrypsin
- Inherited α_1-antitrypsin deficiency
- Release of elastase
- Attraction of inflammatory cells

Activity C *Match the key terms in Column A with their definitions in Column B.*

1.

Column A	Column B
____ 1. Ventilation	a. Ratio of carbon dioxide production to oxygen consumption
____ 2. PF ratio	b. Difference between arterial PO_2 and the fraction of inspired oxygen
____ 3. Cyanosis	
____ 4. Respiratory quotient	
____ 5. Empyema	c. Infection of the pleura
____ 6. Hypercapnia	d. Movement of gas into or out of lungs
____ 7. Venous oxygen saturation	e. Increase in the carbon dioxide content of the arterial blood
____ 8. Pneumothorax	f. Reflects the body's extraction and utilization of O_2 at the tissue levels
____ 9. Hypoxemia	
____ 10. Pleuritis	g. Air in pleural space
	h. Decreased oxygenation
	i. Results from an excessive concentration of reduced hemoglobin
	j. Infection in the pleural cavity

2.

Column A	Column B
____ 1. Cor pulmonale	a. Lung tissue destruction resulting from a vicious cycle of infection and inflammation
____ 2. Pneumoconioses	
____ 3. CFTR	
____ 4. ARDS	b. Caused by the inhalation of inorganic dusts and particulate matter
____ 5. Atelectasis	

___ **6.** Mismatching of ventilation and perfusion

___ **7.** Bronchiectasis

___ **8.** Emphysema

___ **9.** Sarcoidosis

___ **10.** Chronic bronchitis

c. Symptoms are increased mucus production, obstruction of small airways, and a chronic productive cough

d. Incomplete expansion of a lung or portion of a lung

e. Right heart failure resulting from primary lung disease

f. Granulomas found in the lung and lymphatic system

g. Cystic fibrosis transmembrane regulator

h. Enlargement of air spaces and destruction of lung tissue

i. Acute respiratory distress syndrome

j. When areas of the lung are ventilated but not perfused, or when areas are perfused but not ventilated

Activity D *Put the events of IgE-mediated asthma reaction in order in the following boxes:*

a. Infiltration of inflammatory cells

b. Mast cell activation

c. Bronchospasm

d. Increased airway responsiveness

e. Exposure to allergen

f. Airway inflammation

Activity E *Briefly answer the following.*

1. What are the mechanisms of hypoxemia?

_____

_____

_____

2. What are the clinical features of atelectasis?

_____

_____

_____

3. Explain what is meant by the acute response and the late phase reactions of asthma.

_____

_____

_____

4. What factors are causative to the development of bronchiectasis?

_____

_____

_____

5. Describe the pathogenic mechanism of cystic fibrosis.

_____

_____

_____

6. What are the effects of a pulmonary embolism on lung tissue?

_____

_____

_____

7. Describe the disease-producing changes of acute respiratory distress syndrome.

_____

_____

_____

SECTION III: APPLYING YOUR KNOWLEDGE

Activity F *Consider the following scenario and answer the questions.*

The parents of a 14-year-old girl come to the emergency department after being notified by the school nurse that their daughter had a "spell" at school and was taken to the hospital by ambulance. When they arrive, their daughter is sitting up on the stretcher, has oxygen on at 1 L/min, and is answering questions asked by the nurse.

1. The doctor talks to the family and tells them that he suspects their daughter has asthma. What diagnostic tests would the nurse expect to be ordered to confirm the diagnosis of asthma?

_____

_____

_____

2. The parents mention to the nurse that their daughter values her independence. They want to know how her treatment plan will impact it. How would the nurse correctly respond?

_____

_____

_____

SECTION IV: PRACTICING FOR NCLEX

Activity G *Answer the following questions.*

1. There can be many reasons for a patient to present with hypoxemia. For a patient's PO_2 to fall, a respiratory disease is usually involved. Often, patients have involvement from more than one mechanism. Match the mechanism involved with the end result (hypoxemia or decreased levels of PO_2).

Mechanism	Outcome
Decreased oxygen in air	
Inadequate circulation through pulmonary capillaries	
Hypoventilation	
Disease in respiratory system	
Mismatched ventilation and perfusion	
Dysfunction of neurologic system	

2. When CO_2 levels in the blood rise, a state of hypercapnia occurs in the body. What factors contribute to hypercapnia? Mark all that apply.
   a. Alteration in CO_2 production
   b. Abnormalities in respiratory function
   c. Disturbance in gas exchange function
   d. Decrease in CO_2 production
   e. Changes in neural control of respiration

3. The complications of a hemothorax can affect the total body. Left untreated, what can a moderate or large hemothorax cause?
   a. Calcification of the lung tissue
   b. Fibrothorax
   c. Pleuritis
   d. Atelectasis

4. Talc lung can occur from injected or inhaled talc powder that has been mixed with heroin, methamphetamine, or codeine as filler. What are people with talc lung very susceptible to?
   a. Hemothorax
   b. Chylothorax
   c. Fibrothorax
   d. Pneumothorax

5. Pleuritis, an inflammatory process of the pleura, is common in infectious processes that spread to the pleura. Which are the drugs that may be used for treating pleural pain? Mark all that apply.
   a. Indomethacin
   b. Aspirin
   c. Acetaminophen
   d. Inderal

6. Atelectasis is the term used to designate an incomplete expansion of a portion of the lung. Depending on the size of the collapsed area and the type of atelectasis occurring, you may see a shift of the mediastinum and trachea. Which way does the mediastinum and trachea shift in compression atelectasis?
   a. Toward the affected lung
   b. Toward the mediastinum
   c. Away from the affected lung
   d. Away from the trachea

7. Like adults, infants and small children have asthma and need to be medicated. There are special systems manufactured for the delivery of inhaled medications to children. At what age is it recommended that children begin using a metered-dose inhaler with a spacer?

   a. 3–5 years

   b. 4–6 years

   c. 2–4 years

   d. 5–7 years

8. Chronic obstructive pulmonary disease (COPD) is a combination of disease processes. What disease processes have been identified as being part of COPD?

   a. Emphysema and asthma

   b. Chronic obstructive bronchitis and emphysema

   c. Chronic obstructive bronchitis and asthma

   d. Chronic bronchitis and emphysema

9. Bronchiectasis is considered a secondary chronic obstructive pulmonary disease and, with the advent of antibiotics, it is not a common disease entity. In the past, bronchiectasis often followed specific diseases. Which disease did it not follow?

   a. Necrotizing bacterial pneumonia

   b. Complicated measles

   c. Chickenpox

   d. Influenza

10. Cystic fibrosis (CF) is an autosomal recessive disorder involving the secretion of fluids in specific exocrine glands. The genetic defect in CF inclines a person to chronic respiratory infections from a small group of organisms. Which organisms create chronic infection in a child with cystic fibrosis?

    a. *Pseudomonas aeruginosa* and *Escherichia coli*

    b. *Staphylococcus aureus* and hepatitis C

    c. *Haemophilus influenzae* and influenza A

    d. *Pseudomonas aeruginosa* and *Staphylococcus aureus*

11. What etiologic determinants are important in the development of the pneumoconioses? Mark all that apply.

    a. Chemical nature of the dust particle

    b. Size of dust particle

    c. Density of dust particle

    d. Biologic nature of the dust particle

    e. Ability of particle to incite lung destruction

12. There are cytotoxic drugs used in the treatment of cancer that cause pulmonary damage because of their direct toxicity and because they stimulate an influx of inflammatory cells into the alveoli. Which cardiac drug is known for its toxic effect in the lungs?

    a. Amiodarone

    b. Inderal

    c. Methotrexate

    d. Busulfan

13. A pulmonary embolism occurs when there is an obstruction in the pulmonary artery blood flow. Classic signs and symptoms of a pulmonary embolism include dyspnea, chest pain, and increased respiratory rate. What is a classic sign of pulmonary infarction?

    a. Mediastinal shift to the left

    b. Pleuritic pain

    c. Tracheal shift to the right

    d. Pericardial pain

14. Pulmonary hypertension is usually caused by long-term exposure to hypoxemia. When pulmonary vessels are exposed to hypoxemia, what is their response?

    a. Pulmonary vessels dilate

    b. Pulmonary vessels constrict

    c. Pulmonary vessels spasm

    d. Pulmonary vessels infarct

15. The management of cor pulmonale is directed at the underlying lung disease and heart failure. Why is low-flow oxygen therapy part of the management of cor pulmonale?

    a. It stimulates the body to breathe on its own.

    b. It inhibits the respiratory center of the brain from initiating tachypnea.

    c. It reduces pulmonary hypertension and polycythemia associated with chronic lung disease.

    d. It reduces pulmonary hypertension and formation of pulmonary embolism.

16. Acute lung injury and acute respiratory distress syndrome (ARDS) are distinguishable from each other by the extent of hypoxemia involved. What is the clinical presentation of ARDS? Mark all that apply.
    a. Diffuse bilateral infiltrates of lung tissue without cardiac dysfunction
    b. Rapid onset
    c. Signs of respiratory distress
    d. Increase in respiratory rate
    e. Hypoxemia refractory to treatment

17. Acute respiratory failure is commonly signaled by varying degrees of hypoxemia and hypercapnia. Respiratory acidosis develops manifested by what?
    a. Decrease in cerebral blood flow
    b. Arterial vasoconstriction
    c. Increase in cardiac contractility
    d. Increase in cerebral spinal fluid pressure

Structure and Function of the Kidney

SECTION I: LEARNING OBJECTIVES

1. Describe the location and gross structure of the kidney

2. Explain why the kidney receives such a large percentage of the cardiac output and describe the mechanisms for regulating renal blood flow

3. Describe the structure and function of the glomerulus and tubular components of the nephron in terms of regulating the composition of the extracellular fluid compartment

4. Explain the function of sodium in terms of tubular transport mechanisms

5. Describe how the kidney produces concentrated or diluted urine

6. Characterize the function of the juxtaglomerular complex

7. Relate the function of the kidney to drug elimination

8. Explain the endocrine functions of the kidney

9. Relate the sodium reabsorption function of the kidney to action of diuretics

10. Describe the characteristics of normal urine

11. Explain the significance of casts in the urine

12. Explain the value of urine specific gravity in evaluating renal function

13. Explain the concept of the glomerular filtration rate

14. Explain the value of serum creatinine levels in evaluating renal function

15. Describe the methods used in cystoscopic examination of the urinary tract, ultrasonographic studies of the urinary tract, computed tomographic scans, magnetic resonance imaging studies, excretory urography, and renal angiography

SECTION II: ASSESSING YOUR UNDERSTANDING

Activity A *Fill in the blanks.*

1. The _____ are paired, bean-shaped organs that lie outside the peritoneal cavity in the back of the upper abdomen.

2. The _____ is the place where blood vessels and nerves enter and leave the kidney.

3. _____ are the functional units of the kidney.

4. The _____ contains the glomeruli and convoluted tubules of the nephron and blood vessels.

5. The medulla consists of the _____, that are divided by the columns of the cortex.

6. Each kidney is supplied by a single renal artery that arises on either side of the

_____.

7. The afferent arterioles that supply the _____ arise from the intralobular arteries.

8. The _____ is a unique, high-pressure capillary filtration system.

9. _____ are low-pressure vessels that are adapted for reabsorption rather than filtration.

10. The _____ passes through each of these segments before reaching the pelvis of the kidney.

11. The _____ is regulated by the constriction and relaxation of the afferent and efferent arterioles.

12. Substances move from the tubular filtrate into the tubular cell along a _____ gradient, but they require facilitated transport or carrier systems to move across the _____ membrane into the interstitial fluid, where they are absorbed into the peritubular capillaries.

13. _____ uses a carrier system in which the downhill movement of one substance such as sodium is coupled to the uphill movement of another substance such as glucose or an amino acid.

14. In the _____ tubule, there is almost complete reabsorption of nutritionally important substances from the filtrate.

15. The plasma level at which the substance appears in the urine is called the _____.

16. The _____ establishes a high concentration of osmotically active particles in the interstitium surrounding the medullary collecting tubules where the antidiuretic hormone exerts its effects.

17. The thick portion of the loop of Henle contains a _____ cotransport system.

18. The _____ tubule is relatively impermeable to water, and reabsorption of sodium chloride from this segment further dilutes the tubular fluid.

19. The _____ assists in maintenance of the extracellular fluid volume by controlling the permeability of the medullary collecting tubules.

20. Increased _____ activity causes constriction of the afferent and efferent arterioles, and thus a decrease in renal blood flow.

21. Renal _____ is the volume of plasma that is completely cleared each minute of any substance that finds its way into the urine.

22. _____ functions in the regulation of sodium and potassium elimination.

23. Atrial natriuretic peptide contributes to the regulation of _____ elimination.

24. The kidneys regulate body pH by conserving base _____ and eliminating _____ ions.

25. _____ is an end product of protein metabolism.

26. The synthesis of _____ is stimulated by tissue hypoxia, which may be brought about by anemia, residence at high altitudes, or impaired oxygenation of tissues due to cardiac or pulmonary disease.

27. _____ represents excessive protein excretion in the urine.

28. Urine-_____ provides a valuable index of the hydration status and functional ability of the kidneys.

29. _____ levels in the blood and urine can be used to measure glomerular filtration rate.

30. _____, therefore, is not only related to the glomerular filtration rate, but, unlike creatinine, is also influenced by protein intake, gastrointestinal bleeding, and hydration status.

Activity B *Match the key terms in Column A with their definitions in Column B.*

Column A

____ 1. Countertransport

____ 2. Glomerular filtration rate

____ 3. Vasopressin

____ 4. Cortical nephrons

____ 5. Vitamin D

____ 6. Principal cells

Column B

a. Originate in the superficial part of the cortex

b. Originate deeper in the cortex

c. Contribute to regulation of glomerular blood flow

d. Milliliters of filtrate formed per minute

_____ **7.** Juxtamedullary nephrons

_____ **8.** Counter-current

_____ **9.** Transport maximum

_____ **10.** Mesangial cells

e. Movement of one substance enables the movement of a second substance in the opposite direction

f. Maximum amount of substance that can be reabsorbed per unit of time

g. Site of aldosterone action

h. Flow of fluids in opposite directions

i. Stimulate expression of aquaporin-2 channels

j. Converted to active form in kidney

3. How does the juxtaglomerular apparatus regulate glomerular filtration rate?

_____

_____

_____

4. What are the actions of atrial natriuretic peptide?

_____

_____

_____

5. What are the endocrine functions of the kidney?

_____

_____

_____

6. How do Na^+ blockers function as a diuretic?

_____

_____

_____

Activity C

1. Put the components of the renin-angiotensin-aldosterone system in order from stimulation to end hormone action:

- Conversion of angiotensin I to angiotensin II by angiotensin-converting enzyme
- Decreased glomerular filtration rate
- Sodium and water retention
- Angiotensin II stimulates release of antidiuretic hormone and aldosterone
- Juxtaglomerular release of renin
- Conversion of angiotensinogen to angiotensin I by renin

Activity D   *Briefly answer the following.*

1. Describe the three layers of the glomerular membrane.

_____

_____

_____

2. Describe the various methods of transport across the epithelial layer of the renal tubule.

_____

_____

_____

SECTION III: APPLYING YOUR KNOWLEDGE

Activity E   *Consider the following scenario and answer the questions.*

An 18-year-old woman is brought to the emergency department by her friends. Her blood pressure is 115/85 mm Hg, pulse is 99, and respiratory rate in 35 breaths/minute. The girl is doubled over, and she is holding her abdomen saying, "I hurt so bad; I hurt so bad." Her friends deny the girl has been using recreational drugs. They tell the triage nurse that the girl started complaining that her side hurt about 3 hours prior to the trip to the emergency department. Asked if the girl's parents had been notified, the friends tell the triage nurse that they have been unable to reach the girl's parents. On examination, a suspected diagnosis of kidney impairment is arrived at.

1. What tests would the nurse expect to be ordered to either confirm or deny the diagnosis?

   _____

   _____

   _____

2. The girl says, "My father just had a kidney stone removed. Is that what I have?" What noninvasive test should the nurse order to rule out a kidney stone?

   _____

   _____

   _____

SECTION IV: PRACTICING FOR NCLEX

Activity F *Answer the following questions.*

1. Many substances are filtered out of the blood and then reabsorbed into the blood in the kidneys. What is the plasma level at which a specific substance can be found in the urine?

   a. Renal threshold

   b. Renal clearance

   c. Renal filtration rate

   d. Renal transport level

2. You are admitting a 45-year-old female with a presumptive diagnosis of diabetes mellitus to the floor. While taking her history, she mentions that she has been eating a lot of sweets lately. How would you expect this diet to affect her renal system?

   a. Decrease tubular reabsorption

   b. Increase renal blood flow

   c. Decrease renal blood flow

   d. Increase sodium excretion

3. The renal clearance of a substance is measured independently. What are the factors that determine renal clearance of a substance? Mark all that apply.

   a. Ability of the substance to be filtered in the glomeruli

   b. Capacity of the renal tubules to reabsorb or secrete the substance

   c. Normal electrolyte and pH composition of the blood

   d. Rate of renal blood flow

   e. Rate at which sodium is excreted from the body

4. It is known that high levels of uric acid in the blood can cause gout, whereas high levels in the urine can cause kidney stones. What medication competes with uric acid for secretion into the tubular fluid, thereby reducing uric acid secretion?

   a. Ibuprofen

   b. Acetaminophen

   c. Aspirin

   d. Advil

5. Many drugs are eliminated in the urine. These drugs cannot be bound to plasma proteins if the glomerulus is going to filter them out of the blood. In what situation would it be necessary to create either an alkaline or an acid diuresis in a patient?

   a. When there are nontherapeutic drug levels in the patient's blood

   b. If the patient is noncompliant with the medication regimen

   c. In the event that a loading dose of a specific drug must be used and kept in the patient's system for a long time

   d. In the case of a drug overdose

6. The anemia that occurs with end-stage kidney disease is often caused by the kidneys themselves. What inability of the kidneys causes anemia in end-stage kidney disease?

   a. Inability to produce erythropoietin

   b. Inability to produce rennin

   c. Inability to produce angiotensin

   d. Inability to inactivate vitamin D

7. Diuretics can either block the reabsorption of components of the urine, or they can block the reabsorption of water back into the body. What does the increase in urine flow from the body depend on with a patient on diuretics?

   a. Amount of water reabsorption back into the body

   b. Amount of sodium and chloride reabsorption that it blocks

   c. Amount of sodium and chloride that it excretes through the kidney

   d. Amount of water excreted by the body

8. Urine-specific gravity is normally 1.010 to 1.025 with adequate hydration. When there is loss of renal concentrating ability due to impaired renal function, low concentration levels are exhibited. When would the nurse consider low levels of concentration to be significant?

    a. At noon

    b. First void in morning

    c. Last void at night

    d. After a nap

9. An elderly man is brought into the clinic by his daughter who states, "My father hasn't been himself lately. Now I think he looks a little yellow." What test would the nurse expect to have ordered to check this man's creatinine level?

    a. Blood urea nitrogen level

    b. 24-Hour urine test

    c. Urine test—first void in AM

    d. Serum creatinine

10. When the urologist wants to directly visualize the bladder, urethra, and ureteral orifices, what diagnostic test would he use?

    a. Cystoscopy

    b. Ultrasonography

    c. Echocardiogram

    d. Laparoscopy

CHAPTER 31

Disorders of Fluid and Electrolyte Balance

SECTION I: LEARNING OBJECTIVES

1. Define the terms *electrolyte*, *ion*, and *nonelectrolytes*

2. Differentiate the intracellular from the extracellular fluid compartments in terms of distribution and composition of water, electrolytes, and other osmotically active solutes

3. Cite the rationale for the use of concentration rather than absolute values in describing electrolyte content of body fluids

4. Relate the concept of a concentration gradient to the processes of diffusion and osmosis

5. Describe the control of cell volume and the effect of isotonic, hypotonic, and hypertonic solutions on cell size

6. Describe factors that control fluid exchange between the vascular and interstitial fluid compartments and relate them to the development of edema and third spacing of extracellular fluids

7. Describe the manifestations and treatment of edema

8. State the functions and physiologic mechanisms controlling body water levels and sodium concentration, including the effective circulating volume, sympathetic nervous system, renin-angiotensin-aldosterone system, and antidiuretic hormone

9. Describe measures that can be used in assessing body fluid levels and sodium concentration

10. Describe the causes, manifestations, and treatment of psychogenic polydipsia

11. Describe the relationship between antidiuretic hormone and aquaporin-2 channels in reabsorption of water by the kidney

12. Compare the pathology, manifestations, and treatment of diabetes insipidus and the syndrome of inappropriate antidiuretic hormone

13. Compare and contrast the causes, manifestations, and treatment of isotonic fluid volume deficit, isotonic fluid volume excess, hyponatremia with water excess, and hypernatremia with water deficit

14. Characterize the distribution of potassium in the body and explain how extracellular potassium levels are regulated in relation to body gains and losses

15. State the causes of hypokalemia and hyperkalemia in terms of altered intake, output, and transcellular shifts

16. Relate the functions of potassium to the manifestations of hypokalemia and hyperkalemia

17. Describe methods used in diagnosis and treatment of hypokalemia and hyperkalemia

18. Describe the associations among intestinal absorption, renal elimination, bone stores, and the functions of vitamin D and parathyroid hormone in regulating calcium, phosphorus, and magnesium levels

19. State the difference between ionized and bound or chelated forms of calcium in terms of physiologic function

20. Describe the mechanisms of calcium gain and loss and relate them to the causes of hypocalcemia and hypercalcemia

21. Relate the functions of calcium to the manifestations of hypocalcemia and hypercalcemia

22. Describe the mechanisms of phosphorus gain and loss and relate them to causes of hypophosphatemia and hyperphosphatemia

23. Relate the functions of phosphorus to the manifestations of hypophosphatemia and hyperphosphatemia

24. Describe the mechanisms of magnesium gain and loss and relate them to the causes of hypomagnesemia and hypermagnesemia

25. Relate the functions of magnesium to the manifestations of hypomagnesemia and hypermagnesemia

SECTION II: ASSESSING YOUR UNDERSTANDING

Activity A *Fill in the blanks.*

1. The _____ consists of fluid contained within the billions of cells in the body.

2. The _____ contains all fluids outside the cells, including those in the interstitial or tissue spaces and blood vessels.

3. _____ are substances that dissociate in solution to form ions.

4. Particles that do not dissociate into ions such as glucose and urea are called _____.

5. _____ is the movement of charged or uncharged particles along a concentration gradient.

6. _____ is the movement of water across a semipermeable membrane.

7. _____ refers to the osmolar concentration in 1 L of solution and _____ to the osmolar concentration in 1 kg of water.

8. The predominant osmotically active particles in the extracellular fluid are _____ and its associated anions (Cl^- and HCO_3^-).

9. The difference between the calculated and measured osmolality is called the _____.

10. _____ proteins and other organic compounds cannot pass through the membrane.

11. The _____ membrane pump continuously removes three Na^+ ions from the cell for every two K^+ ions that are moved back into the cell.

12. _____ refers to the movement of water through capillary pores because of a mechanical, rather than an osmotic, force.

13. The _____ represents an accessory route whereby fluid from the interstitial spaces can return to the circulation.

14. _____ is a palpable swelling produced by expansion of the interstitial fluid volume.

15. Edema due to decreased capillary colloidal osmotic pressure is usually the result of inadequate production or abnormal loss of _____.

16. _____ edema occurs at times when the accumulation of interstitial fluid exceeds the absorptive capacity of the tissue gel.

17. _____ represent an accumulation or trapping of body fluids that contribute to body weight but not to fluid reserve or function.

18. Water losses that occur through the skin and lungs are referred to as _____ because they occur without a person's awareness.

19. Most sodium losses occur through the _____.

20. The major regulator of sodium and water balance is the maintenance of the _____.

21. The renin-angiotensin-aldosterone system exerts its action through _____ and _____.

22. _____ is primarily a regulator of water intake and _____ a regulator of water output.

23. _____ involves compulsive water drinking and is usually seen in persons with psychiatric disorders, most commonly, schizophrenia.

24. _____ is caused by a deficiency of or a decreased response to antidiuretic hormone.

25. Disorders of sodium concentration produce a change in the osmolality of the extracellular fluid (ECF) with movement of water from the ECF compartment into the intracellular fluid (ICF) compartment, known as _____, or from the ICF compartment into the ECF fluid compartment, known as _____.

26. When the effective circulating blood volume is compromised, the condition is often referred to as _____.

27. _____ cause sequestering of extracellular fluid in the serous cavities, extracellular spaces in injured tissues, or lumen of the gut.

28. Fluid volume excess represents an _____ expansion of the extracellular fluid compartment with increases in both interstitial and vascular volumes.

29. _____ represents a plasma sodium concentration of less than 135 mEq/L.

30. _____ hyponatremia represents retention of water with dilution of sodium while maintaining the extracellular fluid volume within a normal range.

31. MDMA (ecstasy) and its metabolites have been shown to produce enhanced release of _____ from the hypothalamus.

32. _____ implies a plasma sodium level of more than 145 mEq/L.

33. Hypernatremia represents a deficit of _____ in relation to the body's sodium stores.

34. The effects of aldosterone on potassium elimination are mediated through a _____ located in the late distal and cortical collecting tubules of the kidney.

35. The _____ is determined by the ratio of intracellular fluid to extracellular fluid potassium concentration.

36. With severe _____, the resting membrane approaches the threshold potential, causing sustained subthreshold depolarization with a resultant inactivation of the sodium channels and a net decrease in excitability.

37. The renal processes that conserve potassium during _____ interfere with the kidney's ability to concentrate urine.

38. Chronic hyperkalemia is usually associated with _____.

39. The signs and symptoms of potassium _____ are closely related to a decrease in neuromuscular excitability.

40. _____ acts to sustain normal plasma levels of calcium and phosphorus by increasing their absorption from the intestine. It is also necessary for normal bone formation.

41. _____ serves as a cofactor in the generation of cellular energy and is important in the function of second messenger systems.

42. The manifestations of acute _____ reflect the increased neuromuscular excitability.

43. The manifestations of _____ result from a decrease in cellular energy stores due to deficiency in ATP and impaired oxygen transport due to a decrease in red blood cell 2,3-diphosphoglycerate.

44. Many of the signs and symptoms of a phosphorus excess are related to a _____ deficit.

45. _____ acts as a cofactor in many intracellular enzyme reactions, including the transfer of high-energy phosphate groups in the generation of ATP from adenosine diphosphate.

Activity B *Consider the following figure.*

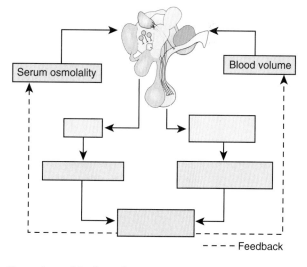

Complete this flowchart using the following terms:

- Extracellular water volume
- Thirst
- Secretion of antidiuretic hormone
- Reabsorption of water by the kidney
- Water ingestion

Activity C *Match the key terms in Column A with their definitions in Column B.*

1.

Column A

_____ **1.** Cations

_____ **2.** Osmotic pressure

_____ **3.** Capillary colloidal osmotic pressure

_____ **4.** Tonicity

_____ **5.** Generalized edema

_____ **6.** Glomerulo-nephritis

_____ **7.** Isotonic solution

_____ **8.** Obligatory urine output

_____ **9.** Anions

_____ **10.** Lymphedema

Column B

a. Effective osmolality same as the intracellular fluid

b. Effect that the osmotic pressure of a solution has on cell size because of water movement across the cell membrane

c. Positively charged ions

d. Negatively charged ions

e. Osmotic pressure generated by the plasma proteins that do not pass through the pores of the capillary wall

f. Increased permeability of glomerulus to proteins

g. Pressure by which water is drawn into a solution through a semipermeable membrane

h. Urine output that is required to eliminate wastes

i. Edema due to impaired lymph drainage

j. Result of increased vascular volume

2.

Column A

_____ **1.** Syndrome of inappropriate antidiuretic hormone

_____ **2.** Aldosterone

_____ **3.** Hypernatremia

_____ **4.** Circulatory overload

_____ **5.** Hyponatremia

_____ **6.** Baroreceptors

_____ **7.** Nephrogenic diabetes insipidus

_____ **8.** Osmoreceptors

_____ **9.** Atrial natriuretic peptide

_____ **10.** Hypodipsia

Column B

a. State of fluid volume excess affecting cardiac function

b. Hypertonic concentration

c. Hypotonic dilution

d. Failure of the negative feedback system that regulates the release and inhibition of antidiuretic hormone

e. Renal insensitivity to antidiuretic hormone

f. Decrease in the ability to sense thirst

g. Respond to changes in extracellular fluid osmolality by swelling or shrinking

h. Acts at the cortical collecting tubules to increase sodium reabsorption

i. Increases sodium excretion by the kidney

j. Respond to pressure-induced stretch of the vessel walls

Activity D

1. Draw a flowchart that puts the following steps of calcium concentration by parathyroid hormone in order. Include the involved organs: parathyroid glands, bone, kidney, and intestine.

- Increased serum calcium
- Increased intestinal calcium absorption
- Activated vitamin D
- Decreased calcium elimination
- Release of calcium from bone
- Decreased serum calcium
- Release of parathyroid hormone

Activity E *Briefly answer the following.*

1. Compare and contrast the intracellular fluid and the extracellular fluid.

_____

_____

_____

2. What are the forces that control the movement of water between the capillary and interstitial spaces?

_____

_____

_____

3. What are the physiologic mechanisms that produce edema?

_____

_____

_____

4. How are sodium and water levels maintained in the body?

_____

_____

_____

5. What are the three types of polydipsia?

_____

_____

_____

6. What are the physical manifestations of an isotonic volume expansion?

_____

_____

_____

7. What are the changes seen in an ECG during hypokalemia, and why are they present?

_____

_____

_____

8. What are the systemic effects of hypercalcemia?

_____

_____

_____

SECTION III: APPLYING YOUR KNOWLEDGE

Activity F *Consider the following scenario and answer the questions.*

The parents of a 10-year-old girl arrive at the burn unit to see their child for the first time since her admission. The client was admitted 8 hours ago with second- and third-degree burns over 60% of her body. She is edematous and in pain.

1. The parents state, "When we left here, just a few hours ago, she wasn't all swollen like that. What causes all that swelling?" What answer would you give?

_____

_____

_____

2. The doctor explains to the parents that because their daughter has a large burned area, she has lost a large amount of fluid. The concern for the client is not only the burn, but also a disorder called fluid volume deficit. After the doctor leaves, the parents ask the nurse whether the doctor is sure their daughter has fluid volume deficit. What should the nurse know about fluid volume deficit?

_____

_____

_____

SECTION IV: PRACTICING FOR NCLEX

Activity G *Answer the following questions.*

1. Edema is an excess in the interstitial fluid volume. What mechanisms play a part in the formation of edema? Mark all that apply.

   a. Mechanisms that increase capillary permeability

   b. Mechanisms that increase capillary filtration pressure

   c. Mechanisms that increase capillary colloidal osmotic pressure

   d. Mechanisms that produce obstruction to the flow of lymph

   e. Mechanisms that decrease capillary colloidal osmotic pressure

2. Match the following elements with their actions in the body.

Element	Action in the body
____ **1.** Sodium	**a.** Increases the absorption of calcium from the intestine
____ **2.** Potassium	**b.** Required for cellular energy metabolism
____ **3.** Calcitriol	**c.** Metabolizes glucose, fat, and protein
____ **4.** Phosphorus	**d.** Regulates the extracellular fluid volume
____ **5.** Magnesium	**e.** Maintains the osmotic integrity of cells

3. The effective circulating volume is the major regulator of water balance in the body. What else does it regulate?

   a. Sodium

   b. Magnesium

   c. Calcium

   d. Potassium

4. Psychogenic polydipsia is most commonly seen in people with schizophrenia. It is a disease that involves compulsive water drinking without thirst and excessive urine output.

   It may be worsened by things that cause by excessive antidiuretic hormone (ADH) secretion. What may be reasons that there is excessive ADH secretion in the body?

   a. Excessive sleeping combined with irregular eating

   b. Antipsychotic medications and smoking

   c. Increased need in the aquaporin channel and coffee drinking

   d. Antipsychotic medications and coffee drinking

5. There are two types of diabetes insipidus (DI), neurogenic and nephrogenic. In nephrogenic DI, there is an inability of the kidney to concentrate urine and to conserve free water. Nephrogenic DI can be either genetic or acquired. What are the causes of nephrogenic DI?

   a. Head injury and cranial surgery

   b. Oral antidiabetic drugs and smoking

   c. Lithium and hypokalemia

   d. Hypocalcemia and hypernatremia

6. In a person with fluid volume deficit, there is a dehydration of brain and nerve cells. What can occur if fluid volume deficit is corrected too rapidly?

   a. Nerve cells absorb too much sodium and cease to function

   b. Brain cells shut down to prevent cerebral edema

   c. Fluid volume increases at a rate the body cannot tolerate

   d. Cerebral edema occurs with potentially severe neurologic impairment

7. Potassium is the major cation in the body. It plays many important roles, including the excitability of nerves and muscles. Where is this action particularly important?

   a. Heart

   b. Brain

   c. Lungs

   d. Liver

8. Vitamin D, although officially classified as a vitamin, functions as a hormone in the body. What other hormone is necessary in the body for vitamin D to work?

   a. Thyroid hormone

   b. Parathyroid hormone

   c. Antidiuretic hormone

   d. Angiotensin II

9. The sodium-phosphate cotransporter (NPT2) creates the action by which phosphate is reabsorbed from the filtrate in the proximal tubule. NPT2 is inhibited by phosphatonin. What condition can cause an overproduction of phosphatonin resulting in hypophosphatemia?

   a. Tumor-induced osteomyelitis

   b. Tumor-induced hypopituitarism

   c. Tumor-induced syndrome of antidiuretic hormone

   d. Tumor-induced osteomalacia

10. Magnesium levels are important indicators to a variety of bodily functions. What is severe hypermagnesemia associated with?

   a. Muscle and respiratory paralysis

   b. Cardiac arrest and pulmonary paralysis

   c. Complete heart block and cardiac arrhythmias

   d. Cardiac arrhythmias and respiratory paralysis

Disorders of Acid-Base Balance

SECTION I: LEARNING OBJECTIVES

1. State the definition of an acid and a base

2. Cite the source of metabolic acids

3. Describe the three forms of carbon dioxide transport and their contribution to acid-base balance

4. Define pH and use the Henderson-Hasselbalch equation to calculate the pH and to compare compensatory mechanisms for regulating pH

5. Describe the intracellular and extracellular mechanisms for buffering changes in body pH

6. Compare the role of the kidneys and respiratory system in regulation of acid-base balance

7. Explain how interactions between potassium and hydrogen cations and between bicarbonate and chloride anions contribute to the regulation of pH

8. Differentiate the terms *acidemia*, *alkalemia*, *acidosis*, and *alkalosis*

9. Describe a clinical situation involving an acid-base disorder in which both primary and compensatory mechanisms are present

10. Define metabolic acidosis, metabolic alkalosis, respiratory acidosis, and respiratory alkalosis

11. Explain the use of the plasma anion gap in differentiating types of metabolic acidosis

12. List common causes of metabolic and respiratory acidosis and metabolic and respiratory alkalosis

13. Contrast and compare the clinical manifestations and treatment of metabolic and respiratory acidosis and of metabolic and respiratory alkalosis

SECTION II: ASSESSING YOUR UNDERSTANDING

Activity A *Fill in the blanks.*

1. Normally, the concentration of body acids and bases is regulated so that the pH of extracellular body fluids is maintained within a very narrow range of _____ to _____.

2. The H^+ concentration is commonly expressed in terms of the _____.

3. Acids are continuously generated as byproducts of _____ processes.

4. Physiologically, these acids fall into two groups: the _____ acid H_2CO_3 and all other _____ acids.

5. The _____ content of the blood can be calculated by multiplying the partial pressure of CO_2 (PCO_2) by its solubility coefficient.

6. The metabolism of _____ and other substances results in the generation of fixed or nonvolatile acids and bases.

7. The plasma pH can be calculated using an equation called the _____.

8. A _____ consists of a weak base and its conjugate acid pair.

9. It has been estimated that as much as 40% of buffering of an acute acid load takes place in _____.

10. The _____ buffer system is the principle extracellular fluid buffer.

11. _____ and _____ are the major protein buffers in the vascular compartment.

12. The kidney regulates pH by excreting excess _____ and reabsorbing _____.

13. There are two important intratubular buffer systems: the phosphate and _____ buffer systems.

14. _____ is a potent stimulus for H^+ secretion and HCO_3^- reabsorption.

15. _____ acts in the collecting duct to stimulate H^+ secretion, while increasing Na^+ reabsorption and K^+ secretion.

16. Arterial blood gases are used for blood gas measurements due to venous blood gas _____, depending on metabolic demands.

17. The _____ describes the difference between the plasma concentration of the major measured cation (Na^+) and the sum of the measured anions (Cl^- and HCO_3^-).

18. The terms _____ and _____ describe the clinical conditions that arise because of changes in dissolved CO_2 and HCO_3^- concentrations.

19. _____ provide a means to control pH when correction is impossible or cannot be immediately achieved.

20. _____ involves a decreased plasma HCO_3^- concentration, along with a decrease in pH.

21. Most cases of _____ acidosis are caused by inadequate oxygen delivery, as in shock or cardiac arrest.

22. An overproduction of _____ occurs when carbohydrate stores are inadequate or when the body cannot use available carbohydrates as a fuel.

23. The _____ cross the blood-brain barrier and directly stimulate the respiratory center, causing hyperventilation and respiratory alkalosis.

24. The enzyme _____ metabolizes methanol and ethylene glycol into their toxic metabolites.

25. _____ disease is the most common cause of chronic metabolic acidosis.

26. Excessive loss of _____ occurs with severe diarrhea; small bowel, pancreatic, or biliary fistula drainage; ileostomy drainage; and intestinal suction.

27. _____ is a systemic disorder caused by an increase in plasma pH due to a primary excess in HCO_3^-.

28. Metabolic alkalosis also leads to a compensatory _____ with development of various degrees of _____ and respiratory acidosis.

29. Respiratory _____ occurs in acute or chronic conditions that impair effective alveolar ventilation and cause an accumulation of PCO_2.

30. Elevated levels of CO_2 produce _____ of cerebral blood vessels, causing headache, blurred vision, irritability, muscle twitching, and psychological disturbances.

31. Respiratory _____ is caused by hyperventilation or a respiratory rate in excess of that needed to maintain normal plasma PCO_2.

Activity B *Consider the following figure.*

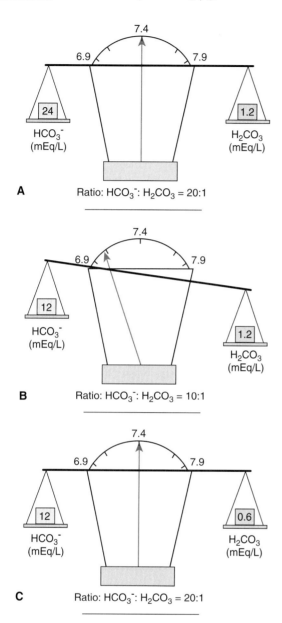

A   Ratio: HCO_3^- : H_2CO_3 = 20:1

_____

$$pH = 6.1 + \log_{10} (\text{ratio } HCO_3^- : H_2CO_3)$$

B   Ratio: HCO_3^- : H_2CO_3 = 10:1

_____

D   Ratio: HCO_3^- : H_2CO_3 = 40:1

_____

C   Ratio: HCO_3^- : H_2CO_3 = 20:1

_____

E   Ratio: HCO_3^- : H_2CO_3 = 20:1

_____

In this diagram, label each scale to reflect the acid-base state and whether there is any compensation present.

- Normal, pH 7.4
- Metabolic acidosis
- Metabolic acidosis with respiratory compensation
- Respiratory alkalosis
- Respiratory alkalosis with renal compensation

Activity C *Match the key terms in Column A with their definitions in Column B.*

Column A

_____ **1.** Amphoteric

_____ **2.** Acid

_____ **3.** Whole blood buffer base

_____ **4.** Delta gap

_____ **5.** MELAS (myopathy,

Column B

a. Molecule that can release H^+

b. Acute increases in HCO_3^-

c. Genetic mitochondrial disorder

d. Ion or molecule that can accept H^+

encephalopathy, lactic acidosis, and strokelike episodes)

_____ **6.** Excess base loading

_____ **7.** Base

_____ **8.** Carbonic anhydrase

_____ **9.** Hypercapnia

_____ **10.** Dissociation constant

e. Can function as acid or base

f. Increase in plasma PCO_2

g. Degree to which an acid or base in a buffer system dissociates

h. Anion gap of urine

i. Measures the level of all buffer systems of the blood

j. Catalyzes bicarbonate reaction

Activity D   *Briefly answer the following.*

1. List the three ways carbon dioxide is transported in the body.

_____

_____

_____

2. Why does someone with kidney disease need to worry about the integrity of his or her skeletal system?

_____

_____

_____

3. How are pH and K^+ related? How do they serve as a buffer?

_____

_____

_____

4. How do the kidneys regulate acid-base balance?

_____

_____

_____

5. What are the two types of acid-base disorders?

_____

_____

_____

6. What are symptoms of metabolic acidosis?

_____

_____

_____

7. Describe the manifestations of respiratory alkalosis.

_____

_____

_____

SECTION III: APPLYING YOUR KNOWLEDGE

Activity E   *Consider the following scenario and answer the questions.*

A female college student is brought to the emergency department by her friend. It is reported by the young woman's friend that they found her wandering around outside the dorm, and she did not know where she was or why she was there. The friend stated that the young woman had complained of being "very tired" lately and that she had lost weight because she was not eating or drinking. Vital signs are blood pressure 118/78 mm Hg, respiratory rate 30 beats/minute, and pulse 66. An arterial blood gas is ordered and results are PO_2 of 95, PCO_2 35, HCO_3^- of 20, and a pH of 7.1.

1. What do this patient's laboratory values indicate?

_____

_____

_____

2. The physician orders a blood glucose level to be drawn. Why would a blood glucose level be important for this patient?

_____

_____

_____

SECTION IV: PRACTICING FOR NCLEX

Activity F   *Answer the following questions.*

1. To calculate the H_2CO_3 content of the blood, you need to measure the PCO_2 (partial pressure of CO_2) by its solubility coefficient. What is the solubility coefficient of CO_2?

a. 0.03
b. 0.3
c. 0.04
d. 0.4

2. The body regulates the pH of its fluids by what mechanism? Mark all that apply.
   a. Chemical buffer systems of the body fluids
   b. Liver
   c. Lungs
   d. Cardiovascular system
   e. Kidneys

3. By reabsorbing HCO_3 from the glomerular filtrate and excreting H^+ from the fixed acids that result from lipid and protein metabolism, the kidneys work to return or maintain the pH of the blood to normal or near-normal values. How long can this mechanism function when there is a change in the pH of body fluids?
   a. Minutes
   b. Hours
   c. Days
   d. Weeks

4. Laboratory tests give us valuable information about what is happening in the body. What laboratory test is a good indicator of the how the buffer systems in the body are working?
   a. Acid-base test
   b. Urine acidity test
   c. H^+ level test
   d. Base excess or deficit test

5. There are both metabolic and respiratory effects on the acid-base balance in the body. How do metabolic disorders change the pH of the body?
   a. Alter the plasma HCO_3
   b. Alter urine H^+ content
   c. Alter CO_2 levels in the lungs
   d. Alter O_2 levels in the major organ systems

6. The body has built-in compensatory mechanisms that take over when correction of pH is not possible or cannot be immediately achieved. What are these compensatory mechanisms considered?

a. Long-term measures that backup first-line correction mechanisms
b. Interim measures that permit survival
c. Short-term measures that depend on first-line correction mechanisms
d. Ways to correct the primary disorder

7. Metabolic acidosis has four main causes. Which laboratory test is used to determine the cause of metabolic acidosis?
   a. Acid-base deficit
   b. Arterial blood gas
   c. Anion gap
   d. Serum bicarbonate

8. A change in the pH of the body affects all organ systems. When the pH falls to less than 7.0, what can occur in the cardiovascular system? Mark all that apply.
   a. Vascular bed can vasodilate, causing the client to go into shock
   b. Vascular bed can vasoconstrict to preserve the primary organs
   c. Cardiac contractility can increase, causing cardiac dysrhythmias
   d. Cardiac contractility can decrease, causing cardiac dysrhythmias

9. Respiratory acidosis occurs when the plasma pH falls below 7.35 and arterial PCO_2 rises above 50 mm Hg. Because CO_2 easily crosses the blood-brain barrier, what signs and symptoms of respiratory acidosis might you see? Mark all that apply.
   a. Irritability
   b. Muscle twitching
   c. Psychological disturbances
   d. Seizures
   e. Psychotic breaks

10. Respiratory alkalosis is caused by hyperventilation, which is recognized as a respiratory rate in excess of that which maintains normal plasma PCO_2 levels. What is a common cause of respiratory alkalosis?
    a. Hyperventilation syndrome
    b. Hypoventilation syndrome
    c. Cluster breathing
    d. Kussmaul breathing

Disorders of Renal Function

SECTION I: LEARNING OBJECTIVES

1. Define the terms *agenesis, hypoplasia,* and *dysgenesis*, and discuss them as they refer to the development of the kidney

2. Cite the effect of urinary obstruction in the fetus

3. Describe the inheritance, pathology, and manifestations of the different types of polycystic kidney disease

4. List four common causes of urinary tract obstruction

5. Define the term *hydronephrosis* and relate it to the destructive effects of urinary tract obstructions

6. Describe the role of urine supersaturation, nucleation, and inhibitors of stone formation in the development of kidney stones

7. Explain the mechanisms of pain and infection that occur with kidney stones

8. Describe methods used in the diagnosis and treatment of kidney stones

9. Cite the organisms most responsible for UTIs and state why urinary catheters, obstruction, and reflux predispose to infections

10. List three physiologic mechanisms that protect against UTIs

11. Describe the signs and symptoms of UTIs

12. Describe factors that predispose to UTIs in children, sexually active women, pregnant women, and older adults

13. Compare the manifestations of UTIs in different age groups, including infants, toddlers, adolescents, adults, and older adults

14. Cite measures used in the diagnosis and treatment of UTIs

15. Describe the two types of immune mechanisms involved in glomerular disorders

16. Use the terms *proliferation, sclerosis, membranous, diffuse, focal, segmental,* and *mesangial* to explain changes in glomerular structure that occur with glomerulonephritis

17. Relate the proteinuria, hematuria, pyuria, oliguria, edema, hypertension, and azotemia that occur with glomerulonephritis to changes in glomerular structure

18. Briefly describe the difference among the nephritic syndromes, rapidly progressive glomerulonephritis, nephrotic syndrome, asymptomatic glomerular disorders, and chronic glomerulonephritis

19. Cite a definition of tubulointerstitial kidney disease

20. Differentiate between the defects in tubular function that occur in proximal and distal tubular acidosis

21. Explain the pathogenesis of kidney damage in acute and chronic pyelonephritis

22. Explain the vulnerability of the kidneys to injury caused by drugs and toxins

23. Characterize Wilms tumor in terms of age of onset, possible oncogenic origin, manifestations, and treatment

24. Cite the risk factors for renal cell carcinoma, describe its manifestations, and explain why the 5-year survival rate has been so low

SECTION II: ASSESSING YOUR UNDERSTANDING

Activity A *Fill in the blanks.*

1. Anomalies in _____ and _____ of the kidneys are the most common form of congenital renal disorder.

2. Dysgenesis refers to a failure of an organ to develop normally and _____ to complete failure of an organ to develop.

3. Newborns with renal agenesis often have characteristic facial features, termed _____, resulting from the effects of oligohydramnios.

4. In renal _____, the kidneys do not develop to normal size.

5. Renal _____ is due to an abnormality in the differentiation of kidney structures during embryonic development.

6. Unilateral _____ renal dysplasia is the most common cause of an abdominal mass in newborns.

7. _____ kidney diseases are a group of kidney disorders characterized by fluid-filled sacs or segments that have their origin in the tubular structures of kidney.

8. In the _____ form of polycystic kidney disease, thousands of large cysts are derived from every segment of the nephron.

9. The _____ effects of urinary obstruction on kidney structures are determined by the degree and duration of the obstruction.

10. _____ of urine predisposes to infection, which may spread throughout the urinary tract.

11. _____ refers to urine-filled dilatation of the renal pelvis and calyces associated with

progressive atrophy of the kidney due to obstruction of urine outflow.

12. Obstruction of the urinary tract may provoke pain due to _____ of the collecting system and renal capsule.

13. The most common cause of upper urinary tract obstruction is urinary _____.

14. In addition to a supersaturated urine, kidney stone formation requires a _____ that facilitates crystal aggregation.

15. Most kidney stones are _____ stones.

16. The major manifestation of kidney stones is _____.

17. Urinary tract infections are the _____ most common type of bacterial infection seen by health care providers.

18. Most uncomplicated lower urinary tract infections are caused by _____.

19. Most urinary tract infections are caused by bacteria that enter through the _____.

20. Urinary tract infections are _____ common in women than men.

21. In urinary tract infections associated with stasis of urine flow, the obstruction may be _____ or _____.

22. _____-associated bacteriuria remains the most frequent cause of gram-negative septicemia in hospitalized patients.

23. An acute episode of _____ is characterized by frequency of urination, lower abdominal or back discomfort, and burning and pain on urination.

24. _____ is the second leading cause of kidney failure worldwide, and it ranks third, after diabetes and hypertension, as a cause of chronic kidney disease in the United States.

25. The _____ syndromes produce a proliferative inflammatory response, whereas the _____ syndrome produces increased permeability of the glomerulus.

26. _____ syndrome is characterized by sudden onset of hematuria, variable degrees of proteinuria, diminished glomerular filtration rate, oliguria, and signs impaired renal function.

27. Acute postinfectious glomerulonephritis usually occurs after infection with certain strains

of group A β-hemolytic streptococci and is caused by _____ of immune complexes.

28. The _____ of postinfectious glomerulonephritis is caused by infiltration of leukocytes, both neutrophils and monocytes; proliferation of endothelial and mesangial cells; and, in severe cases, formation of crescents.

29. _____ syndrome is an uncommon and aggressive form of glomerulonephritis that is caused by antibodies to the glomerular basement membrane.

30. _____ syndrome is characterized by massive proteinuria and lipiduria, along with an associated hypoalbuminemia, generalized edema, and hyperlipidemia.

31. _____ glomerulonephritis is caused by diffuse thickening of the glomerular basement membrane due to deposition of immune complexes.

32. _____ disease is a primary glomerulonephritis characterized by the presence of glomerular IgA immune complex deposits.

33. Alport syndrome represents a hereditary defect of the glomerular _____ that results in hematuria and may progress to chronic renal failure.

34. _____ refers to a group of tubular defects in reabsorption of bicarbonate ions or excretion of hydrogen ions (H^+) that result in metabolic acidosis and its subsequent complications, including metabolic bone disease, kidney stones, and growth failure in children.

35. Proximal renal tubular acidosis involves a defect in proximal tubular reabsorption of _____.

36. _____ represents an infection of the upper urinary tract, specifically the renal parenchyma and renal pelvis.

37. _____ is one of the most common primary neoplasms of young children.

38. Kidney cancer is suspected when there are findings of _____ and a renal _____.

Activity B *Consider the following figure.*

In this figure, identify the common locations and causes of urinary tract obstructions:

- Pregnancy or tumor
- Ureterovesical junction stricture
- Kidney stone
- Scar tissue
- Neurogenic bladder
- Bladder outflow obstruction

Activity C *Match the key terms in Column A with their definitions in Column B.*

Column A

_____ 1. Urease

_____ 2. Hypogenesis

_____ 3. Oliguria

_____ 4. Polycystic kidney disease 1 and 2

_____ 5. Hydronephrosis

_____ 6. Proteinuria

_____ 7. Renal dysplasia

_____ 8. Nephrolithiasis

_____ 9. Hematuria

_____ 10. Oligohydramnios

Column B

a. Low renal mass in infant

b. Blood cells in urine

c. Urea-splitting bacterial enzyme

d. Change in renal structure

e. Dilatation of the renal pelvis and calyces associated with progressive atrophy

f. Very low urine production

g. Genes responsible for autosomal

dominant polycystic kidney disease

h. Kidney stone formation

i. Protein loss in urine

j. Low amniotic fluid levels

Activity D

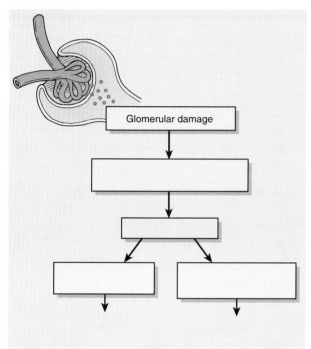

Glomerular damage

Complete this flowchart using the following items:

- Edema
- Hyperlipidemia
- Increased permeability to proteins
- Decreased plasma oncotic pressure
- Hypoproteinemia
- Compensatory synthesis of proteins by liver

Activity E *Briefly answer the following.*

1. What is the mechanism of tissue damage in urinary tract obstructions?

_____

_____

_____

2. What are the factors involved in kidney stone formation?

_____

_____

_____

3. Who are the risk factors for urinary tract infection higher for?

_____

_____

_____

4. What are the host defense mechanisms against the development of a urinary tract infection?

_____

_____

_____

5. What are the cellular changes associated with glomerular disease?

_____

_____

_____

6. Describe the disease progress and the production of symptoms in poststreptococcal glomerulonephritis.

_____

_____

_____

7. Describe the mechanisms of a diabetic nephropathy.

_____

_____

_____

8. How do medications and toxins from the environment damage renal structures?

_____

_____

_____

SECTION III: APPLYING YOUR KNOWLEDGE

Activity F *Consider the following scenario and answer the questions.*

An elderly woman, hospitalized with a broken hip, has an indwelling catheter in place. On the third day of hospitalization, the woman's urine becomes cloudy and foul smelling. The nurse knows that catheters have a high incidence of causing urinary tract infections in hospitalized patients.

1. What orders would the nurse expect to receive for this patient?

_____

_____

_____

2. What actions would the nurse take to prevent further contamination by the indwelling catheter?

_____

_____

_____

SECTION IV: PRACTICING FOR NCLEX

Activity G *Answer the following questions.*

1. Congenital disorders of the kidneys are fairly common, occurring in approximately 1:1000 live births. What is the result to the newborn when bilateral renal dysplasia occurs? Mark all that apply.
   a. Potter facies
   b. Oligohydramnios
   c. Pulmonary hypoplasia
   d. Multicystic kidneys
   e. Renal failure

2. Match the type of polycystic kidney disorder with the characteristic cysts.

   Type of polycystic kidney disorder

   Characteristic cysts

   ____ 1. Autosomal dominant polycystic kidney disease

   ____ 2. Autosomal recessive polycystic kidney disease

   ____ 3. Acquired cysts

   ____ 4. Nephronoph-thisis-medullary cystic kidney disease

   a. Small elongated cysts that form in the collecting ducts and maintain contact with the nephron of origin

   b. Tubule wall, which is lined by a single layer of tubular cells, expands and then rapidly closes the cyst off from the tubule of origin

   c. Cysts that are restricted to the corticomedullary border

   d. Cysts that develop in the kidney as a consequence of aging, dialysis, or other conditions that affect tubular function

3. A young woman presents with signs and symptoms of a urinary tract infection (UTI). The nurse notes that this is the fifth UTI in as many months. What would this information lead the nurse to believe?
   a. There is possible obstruction in the urinary tract.
   b. The woman has multiple sexual partners.
   c. The woman takes too many bubble baths.
   d. The woman does not clean herself properly.

4. Staghorn kidney stones, or struvite stones, are usually located in the renal pelvis. These stones are made from what?
   a. Calcium oxalate
   b. Magnesium ammonium phosphate
   c. Cystine
   d. Uric acid

5. What is the most common cause of a lower urinary tract infection?
   a. *Staphylococcus saprophyticus*
   b. *Pseudomonas aeruginosa*
   c. *Escherichia coli*
   d. *Staphylococcus aureus*

6. Urinary tract infections (UTIs) in children do not generally present as they do in adults. What are the signs and symptoms of a UTI in a toddler? Mark all that apply.
   a. Frequency
   b. Diarrhea
   c. Abdominal pain
   d. Poor growth
   e. Burning

7. Acute postinfectious glomerulonephritis, as its name implies, follows an acute infection somewhere else in the body. What is the most common cause of acute postinfectious glomerulonephritis?
   a. *Escherichia coli*
   b. *Staphylococcus aureus*

c. *Pseudomonas aeruginosa*

d. Group A β-hemolytic streptococci

8. Both type 1 and type 2 diabetes mellitus can cause damage to the glomeruli of the kidneys. What renal disease is diabetic nephropathy associated with?

a. Nephrotic syndrome

b. Acute glomerulonephritis

c. Nephritic syndrome

d. Acute glomerulonephritis

9. Acute pyelonephritis is an infection of the renal parenchyma and renal pelvis. What is the most common cause of acute pyelonephritis?

a. Group A β-hemolytic streptococci

b. *Pseudomonas aeruginosa*

c. *Haemophilus influenza*

d. *Candida albicans*

10. Drug-related nephropathies occur all too often. They involve functional and/or structural changes to the kidney after exposure to a drug. What does the tolerance to drugs depend on?

a. Vesicoureteral reflux

b. Glomerular filtration rate

c. State of hydration

d. Proteinuria

11. Wilms tumor is a tumor of childhood. It is usually an encapsulated mass occurring in any part of the kidney. What are the common presenting signs of a Wilms tumor?

a. Hypotension and a large abdominal mass

b. Vomiting and oliguria

c. Abdominal pain and diarrhea

d. Large asymptomatic abdominal mass and hypertension

34

Acute Renal Failure and Chronic Kidney Disease

SECTION I: LEARNING OBJECTIVES

1. Describe acute renal failure in terms of its causes, treatment, and outcome

2. Differentiate the prerenal, intrinsic, and postrenal forms of acute renal failure in terms of the mechanisms of development and manifestations

3. Cite the two most common causes of acute tubular necrosis and describe the course of the disease in terms of the initiation, maintenance, and recovery phases

4. State the most common causes of chronic kidney disease

5. Describe the five stages of chronic kidney disease

6. Describe the methods used to arrive at an accurate estimation of the GFR and explain the rationale for its use in defining the stages of chronic kidney disease

7. Explain the physiologic mechanisms underlying the common problems associated with chronic kidney disease, including alterations in fluid and electrolyte balance and disorders of skeletal, hematologic, cardiovascular, immune system, neurologic, skin, and sexual function

8. State the basis for adverse drug reactions in patients with chronic kidney disease

9. Describe the scientific principles underlying dialysis treatment, and compare hemodialysis with peritoneal dialysis

10. Cite the possible complications of kidney transplantation

11. State the goals for dietary management of persons with chronic kidney disease

12. List the causes of CKD in children and describe the special problems of children with kidney failure

13. State why CKD is more common in the elderly and describe measures to prevent or delay the onset of kidney failure in this population

14. Describe the treatment of CKD in children and the elderly

SECTION II: ASSESSING YOUR UNDERSTANDING

Activity A *Fill in the blanks.*

1. _____ represents a rapid decline in kidney function sufficient to increase blood levels of nitrogenous wastes and impair fluid and electrolyte balance.

2. The causes of acute renal failure are commonly categorized as _____, _____, or _____.

3. _____ failure, the most common form of acute renal failure, is characterized by a marked decrease in renal blood flow.

4. Because of their high metabolic rate, the _____ cells are most vulnerable to ischemic injury.

5. Prerenal failure is manifested by a sharp decrease in urine output and a disproportionate elevation of _____ in relation to serum creatinine levels.

6. _____ failure results from obstruction of urine outflow from the kidneys.

7. A major concern in the treatment of acute renal failure is identifying and correcting the _____.

8. Regardless of cause, _____ represents a loss of functioning kidney nephrons with progressive deterioration of glomerular filtration, tubular reabsorptive capacity, and endocrine functions of the kidneys.

9. The normal glomerular filtration rate, which varies with age, gender, and body size, is approximately _____ mL/min (1.73 mL/min/m²) for normal young healthy adults.

10. In clinical practice, glomerular filtration rate is usually estimated using the serum _____ concentration.

11. Increased excretion of low-molecular-weight globulins is a marker of _____ disease, and excretion of _____, a marker of chronic kidney disease.

12. The _____ state includes signs and symptoms of altered fluid, electrolyte, and acid-base balance and alterations in regulatory functions.

13. Chronic renal failure can produce _____ or fluid _____, depending on the pathology of the kidney disease.

14. In chronic renal failure, the kidneys lose the ability to regulate _____ excretion.

15. The acidosis that occurs in persons with kidney failure seems to stabilize as the disease progresses, probably because of the tremendous buffering capacity of _____.

16. The term renal _____ is used to describe the skeletal complications of chronic kidney disease.

17. _____ is commonly an early manifestation of chronic renal failure.

18. Anorexia, nausea, and vomiting are common in patients with _____, along with a metallic taste in the mouth.

19. Neuropathy is caused by _____ and _____ of nerve fibers, possibly caused by uremic toxins.

20. Normal aging is associated with a decline in the _____ and, subsequently, with reduced homeostatic regulation under stressful conditions.

Activity B *Consider the following figure.*

In this figure, label the sites of prerenal, intrarenal, and postrenal causes of renal failure.

Activity C *Match the key terms in Column A with their definitions in Column B.*

Column A

_____ 1. Isosthenuria

_____ 2. Azotemia

_____ 3. Creatinine

_____ 4. Salt wasting

_____ 5. Oliguria

_____ 6. Uremic encephalopathy

_____ 7. Prostatic hyperplasia

_____ 8. Hemodialysis

_____ 9. Uremia

_____ 10. Osteitis fibrosa

Column B

a. Decreased urine production

b. Polyuria with urine that is almost isotonic with plasma

c. Increased bone resorption and formation

d. Byproduct of muscle metabolism

e. Decreased central nervous system activity

f. Presence of excessive amounts of urea in the blood

g. Impaired tubular reabsorption of sodium

h. Most common cause of postrenal failure

i. Use of artificial kidney to filter blood

j. Accumulation of nitrogenous wastes in the blood

Activity D *Briefly answer the following.*

1. Name the most common intrarenal cause of renal failure and describe its different forms.

_____

_____

_____

2. Describe the progression of acute tubular necrosis.

_____

_____

_____

3. How is chronic kidney disease classified?

_____

_____

_____

4. Why is chronic kidney disease considered to have an insidious progression?

_____

_____

_____

5. What are the clinical manifestations of chronic kidney disease?

_____

_____

_____

6. How is anemia related to chronic kidney disease?

_____

_____

_____

7. How does renal disease cause cardiovascular disease?

_____

_____

_____

SECTION III: APPLYING YOUR KNOWLEDGE

Activity E *Consider the following scenario and answer the questions.*

The parents of a hospitalized 4-year-old boy have just been told that their son has a chronic renal disease. The nurse is planning discharge teaching for this family.

1. What would the nurse know to include in the discharge teaching for this child and his family?

_____

_____

_____

2. The parents inquire about treatment for their son and the option of kidney transplantation. What would be the nurse's best response?

_____

_____

_____

_____

SECTION IV: PRACTICING FOR NCLEX

Activity F *Answer the following questions.*

1. Acute renal failure occurs at a high rate in seriously ill people who are in intensive care units. What is the most common indicator of acute renal failure?

   a. Azotemia and a decrease in the glomerular filtration rate

   b. Proteinuria and a decrease in the glomerular filtration rate

   c. Azotemia and an increase in the glomerular filtration rate

   d. Proteinuria and an increase in the glomerular filtration rate

2. Acute tubular necrosis (ATN) is the most common cause of intrinsic renal failure. One of the causes of ATN is ischemia. What are the most common causes of ischemic ATN? Mark all that apply.
   a. Severe hypovolemia
   b. Severe hypertension
   c. Burns
   d. Overwhelming sepsis
   e. Severe hypervolemia

3. The glomerular filtration rate (GFR) is considered the best measure of renal function. What is used to estimate the GFR?
   a. Blood urea nitrogen
   b. Serum creatinine
   c. Albumin level
   d. Serum protein

4. Chronic kidney disease (CKD) affects many systems in the body. What is the number one hematologic disorder caused by CKD?
   a. Polycythemia
   b. Erythrocythemia
   c. Anemia
   d. Leukocytosis

5. Uremic pericarditis is a disorder that accompanies chronic kidney disease. What are its presenting signs and symptoms? Mark all that apply.
   a. Pericardial friction rub
   b. Chest pain with respiratory accentuation
   c. Fever without infection
   d. Shortness of breath
   e. Thromboangiitis

6. Neuromuscular disorders can be triggered by chronic kidney disease. For those clients on dialysis, approximately two-thirds suffer from what peripheral neuropathy?
   a. Raynaud syndrome
   b. Burning hands and feet
   c. Tingling and loss of sensation in lower limbs
   d. Restless leg syndrome

7. People with chronic kidney disease have impaired immune responses to infection due to high levels of urea and metabolic wastes in the blood. What is one thing that is missing in an immune response in people with chronic kidney disease?
   a. Failure to mount a fever with infection
   b. Failure of a phagocytic response with infection
   c. Decrease in granulocyte count
   d. Impaired humoral immunity response with infection

8. Sexual dysfunction in people with chronic kidney disease (CKD) is believed to be multifactorial. What are believed to be causes of sexual dysfunction in people with CKD? Mark all that apply.
   a. Antihypertensive drugs
   b. Psychological factors
   c. Uremic toxins
   d. Inability to vasodilate veins
   e. High incidence of sexually transmitted diseases

9. In hemodialysis, access to the vascular system is most commonly through what?
   a. External arteriovenous shunt
   b. Internal arteriovenous fistula
   c. Internal arteriovenous shunt
   d. External arteriovenous fistula

10. Dietary restrictions placed on people with chronic kidney disease (CKD) include limiting protein in their diet. The recommended sources of protein for people with CKD include what source of protein?
    a. Red meat
    b. Fowl
    c. Milk
    d. Fish

35

Disorders of the Bladder and Lower Urinary Tract

SECTION I: LEARNING OBJECTIVES

1. Trace the ascending sensory and descending motor impulses between the detrusor muscle and external urinary sphincter and the spinal cord, pontine micturition center, and cerebral cortex

2. Explain the mechanism of low-pressure urine storage in the bladder

3. List at least three classes of autonomic drugs and explain their potential effect on bladder function

4. Describe at least three urodynamic studies that can be used to assess bladder function

5. Describe the causes of and compensatory changes that occur with urinary tract obstruction

6. Differentiate lesions that produce storage dysfunction associated with spastic bladder from those that produce emptying dysfunction associated with flaccid bladder in terms of the level of the lesions and their effects on bladder function

7. Describe methods used in treatment of neurogenic bladder

8. Define *incontinence* and differentiate between stress incontinence, overactive bladder/urge incontinence, and overflow incontinence.

9. Describe behavioral, pharmacologic, and surgical methods used in treatment of the different types of incontinence

10. List the treatable causes of incontinence in the elderly

11. Discuss the difference between superficial and invasive bladder cancer in terms of bladder involvement, extension of the disease, and prognosis

12. State the most common sign of bladder cancer

SECTION II: ASSESSING YOUR UNDERSTANDING

Activity A *Fill in the blanks.*

1. The _____ stores urine and controls its elimination from the body.

2. The bladder is a freely movable organ located _____ on the pelvic floor, just posterior to the pubic _____.

3. In the male, the _____ gland surrounds the neck of the bladder where it empties into the urethra.

4. Urine passes from the kidneys to the bladder through the _____.

5. The tonicity and composition of the urine is often quite different from that of the blood, and the _____ of the bladder acts as an effective barrier to prevent the passage of

water and other urine elements between the bladder and the blood.

6. The _____ operates as a reserve mechanism to stop micturition when it is occurring and to maintain continence in the face of unusually high bladder pressure.

7. The motor component of the neural reflex that causes bladder emptying is controlled by the _____ nervous system, whereas the relaxation and storage function of the bladder is controlled by the _____ nervous system.

8. The parasympathetic lower motor neurons for the detrusor muscle of the bladder are located in the _____ segments of the spinal cord; their axons travel to the bladder by way of the _____.

9. The immediate coordination of the normal micturition reflex occurs in the micturition center in the _____, facilitated by descending input from the forebrain and ascending input from the reflex centers in the spinal cord.

10. _____ brain centers enable inhibition of the micturition center in the pons and conscious control of urination.

11. The _____ receptors are found in the detrusor muscle; they produce relaxation of the detrusor muscle, increasing the bladder volume at which the micturition reflex is triggered.

12. The activation of _____ produces contraction of the intramural ureteral musculature, bladder neck, and internal sphincter.

13. Alterations in bladder function include urinary _____ with retention or stasis of urine and urinary _____ with involuntary loss of urine.

14. The most important cause of urinary obstruction in males is external compression of the urethra caused by enlargement of the _____.

15. Neurogenic disorders of bladder function are commonly manifested in one of two ways: failure to _____ urine or failure to _____.

16. Spastic bladder is caused by conditions that produce partial or extensive neural damage above the _____ center in the sacral cord.

17. A mild form of reflex neurogenic bladder can develop after a _____.

18. _____ of the detrusor muscle and loss of the perception of bladder fullness permit the overstretching of the detrusor muscle that contributes to weak and ineffective bladder contractions seen in detrusor muscle areflexia.

19. _____ is the involuntary loss of urine during coughing, laughing, sneezing, or lifting that increases intra-abdominal pressure.

20. Two mechanisms are believed to contribute to its symptomatology of overactive bladder: central nervous system and neural control of bladder sensation and emptying, _____, and those involving the smooth muscle of the bladder itself, _____.

21. Approximately 90% of bladder cancers are derived from the _____ epithelial cells that line the bladder.

22. The most common sign of bladder cancer is painless _____.

Activity B *Consider the following figure.*

1. In this diagram of the bladder, please locate and label the following:

- Detrusor muscle
- Ureters
- Trigone
- Internal sphincter
- External sphincter

Activity C *Match the key terms in Column A with their definitions in Column B.*

Column A

___ **1.** Incontinence

___ **2.** Micturition

___ **3.** Kegel exercises

___ **4.** Muscarinic

___ **5.** Nocturia

___ **6.** Antimus-carinic drugs

___ **7.** Detrusor-sphincter dyssynergia

___ **8.** May cause urinary retention

___ **9.** Nicotinic

___ **10.** Tricyclic anti-depressants

Column B

a. Muscle-tensing exercises of the pelvic muscles

b. Uninhibited spinal reflex–controlled contraction of the bladder without relaxation of the external sphincter

c. Decrease bladder contractility and increase outlet resistance

d. Cholinergic receptor found on external sphincter muscle

e. Antihistamine

f. Passage of urine

g. Decrease detrusor muscle tone and increase bladder capacity

h. Cholinergic receptor found on striated muscle fibers of bladder

i. Involuntary loss or leakage of urine

j. Excessive urination at night

Activity D *Briefly answer the following.*

1. Describe the structural layers of the bladder.

2. List the name and function of the major nerves that regulate bladder function.

3. Describe the activities of the pontine micturition center and cortical brain centers.

4. Describe the actions that take place in the bladder during micturition.

5. What are the necessary factors that every child must possess in order to attain conscious control of bladder function?

6. Describe the effects of prolonged urinary tract obstruction disorders on the bladder.

7. Why do many women develop incontinence following childbirth?

8. Describe how chronic neurologic disorders can contribute to overactive bladder.

9. What are the factors associated with age that contribute to incontinence in the elderly?

SECTION III: APPLYING YOUR KNOWLEDGE

Activity E *Consider the following scenario and answer the questions.*

A 53-year-old woman with multiple sclerosis presents at the clinic with urinary frequency and bladder spasms. A urinalysis is negative for infection. A complete history is taken, and a physical is performed by the primary care physician. The woman asks the nurse why she is having bladder spasms and urinary frequency if she does not have a bladder infection.

1. What would the nurse respond?

_____

_____

_____

2. What would the nurse expect the doctor to do for this woman?

_____

_____

_____

SECTION IV: PRACTICING FOR NCLEX

Activity F *Answer the following questions.*

1. You are caring for a 16-year-old boy, newly diagnosed with a spinal cord injury. He asks you why he can no longer control his bladder. What would you explain to him? Mark all that apply.

  a. "Your spinal cord injury has disrupted the control your brain has over your bladder."

  b. "You will always have to wear an internal catheter."

  c. "You will have to learn how to in-and-out catheterize yourself."

  d. "You have a condition known as a relaxed bladder."

  e. "You have a condition known as detrusor-sphincter dyssynergia."

2. Children usually achieve bladder control by age 5 years. Girls generally achieve bladder control before boys do. What is the general rule for bladder capacity in a child?

  a. Up to the age of 12 to 14 years, the capacity of the bladder is the child's age in years plus 2.

  b. Up to the age of 5 years, the capacity of the bladder is the child's age in years plus 3.

  c. The capacity of the bladder is equal to the child's age in years.

  d. Age has nothing to do with bladder capacity; it has adult capacity from toddlerhood.

3. One of the many tests done during urodynamic studies is the sphincter electromyelogram. What does this test study?

  a. Ability of the bladder to store urine

  b. Activity of the voluntary muscles of the perineal area

  c. Pressure of the bladder during filling and emptying

  d. Flow rate during urination

4. Urinary obstruction in the lower urinary tract triggers changes to the urinary system to compensate for the obstruction. What is an early change the system makes in its effort to cope with an obstruction?

  a. Ability to suppress urination is increased

  b. Stretch receptors in the bladder wall become hypersensitive

  c. Bladder begins to shrink

  d. Bladder contraction weakens

5. What is a common cause of spastic bladder dysfunction?

  a. Central nervous system lesions

  b. Constriction of the internal sphincter muscles

  c. External sphincter spasticity

  d. Vesicoureteral reflux

6. Acute overdistention of the bladder can occur in anyone with a neurogenic bladder that does not empty. How much urine would the nurse empty out of the bladder at one time?

  a. Everything in the bladder, no matter how full it is

  b. No more than 600 cc of urine at one time

  c. No more than 500 cc of urine at one time

  d. No more than 1000 cc of urine at one time.

7. In women, stress incontinence is a common problem. The loss of the angle between the urethrovesical junction and the bladder contributes to stress incontinence. What is the normal angle between the bladder and the urethrovesical junction?

a. 90 to 100 degrees

b. 100 to 110 degrees

c. 80 to 90 degrees

d. 95 to 105 degrees

8. Incontinence can be transient. What are the causes of transient urinary incontinence? Mark all that apply.

a. Spinal cord injury

b. Confusional states

c. Stool impaction

d. Diarrhea

e. Recurrent urinary tract infections

9. Urinary incontinence can be a problem with the elderly. One method of treatment is habit training, or bladder training. When using this treatment with an elderly person, how frequently should they be voiding?

a. Every 1 to 3 hours

b. Every 2 to 4 hours

c. Every 3 to 5 hours

d. Every 4 to 6 hours

10. One of the treatments for bladder cancer in situ is the intervesicular administration of what drug?

a. Adriamycin

b. Mitomycin C

c. Bacillus Calmette-Guérin vaccine

d. Thiotepa

CHAPTER 36

Structure and Function of the Gastrointestinal System

SECTION I: LEARNING OBJECTIVES

1. Describe the anatomic structures of the upper, middle, and lower gastrointestinal tract

2. List the five layers of the gastrointestinal tract wall and describe their function

3. Characterize the structure and function of the peritoneum and describe its attachment to the abdominal wall

4. Characterize the properties of the interstitial smooth muscle cells that act as pacemakers for the GI tract

5. Compare the actions of the enteric and autonomic nervous systems as they relate to motility of the GI tract

6. Trace a bolus of food through the stages of swallowing

7. Differentiate tonic and peristaltic movements in the GI tract

8. Describe the action of the internal and external sphincters in the control of defecation

9. State the source and function of water and electrolytes that are secreted in digestive secretions

10. Explain the protective function of saliva

11. Describe the function of the gastric secretions in the process of digestion

12. List three major GI hormones and cite their function

13. Describe the site of gastric acid and pepsin production and secretion in the stomach

14. Describe the function of the gastric mucosal barrier

15. Describe the functions of the secretions of the small and the large intestine

16. Discuss the function of gut flora in terms of metabolic activities, trophic effects, and protection against invasion by pathogenic microorganisms

17. Differentiate digestion from absorption

18. Relate the characteristics of the small intestine to its absorptive function

19. Explain the function of intestinal brush border enzymes

20. Compare the digestion and absorption of carbohydrates, fats, and proteins

21. Characterize the relationship among anorexia, nausea, retching, and vomiting

22. Describe the neural structures involved in vomiting and their mediators

SECTION II: ASSESSING YOUR UNDERSTANDING

Activity A *Fill in the blanks.*

1. The major physiologic function of the _____ is to digest food and absorb nutrients into the bloodstream.

2. The upper esophageal sphincter, the _____ sphincter, consists of a circular layer of striated muscle.

3. The lower esophageal sphincter, the _____ sphincter, lies just above the area where the esophagus joins the stomach.

4. The _____ lies in the left side of the abdomen and serves as a food storage reservoir during the early stages of digestion.

5. The small intestine, which forms the middle portion of the digestive tract, consists of three subdivisions: the _____, _____, and _____.

6. Bile and pancreatic juices enter the intestine through openings for the common bile duct and the main pancreatic duct in the _____.

7. The _____ cells carry out the secretory and absorptive functions of the gastrointestinal tract, and they produce the _____ that lubricates and protects the inner surface of the alimentary canal.

8. _____ fluid forms a moist and slippery surface that prevents friction between the continuously moving abdominal structures.

9. The _____ contains the blood vessels, nerves, and lymphatic vessels that supply the intestinal wall.

10. Like the self-excitable cardiac muscle cells in the heart, some smooth muscle cells of the gastrointestinal tract function as _____ cells.

11. The _____ nervous system consists of the myenteric and submucosal plexuses in the wall of the gastrointestinal tract.

12. _____ monitor the stretch and distention of the gastrointestinal tract wall, and _____ monitor the chemical composition of its contents.

13. Numerous _____ reflexes influence motility and secretions of the digestive tract.

14. Swallowing consists of three phases: an _____ phase, a _____ phase, and an _____ phase.

15. The _____ is the major site for the digestion and absorption of food.

16. _____ is normally initiated by the mass movements of the large intestine.

17. The tract produces _____ that act locally, pass into the general circulation for distribution to more distant sites, and interact with the central nervous system by way of the enteric and autonomic nervous systems.

18. The primary function of _____ is the stimulation of gastric acid secretion.

19. _____ has potent growth hormone–releasing activity and has a stimulatory effect on food intake and digestive function, while reducing energy expenditure.

20. _____ potentiates the action of secretin, increasing the pancreatic bicarbonate response to low circulating levels of secretin; stimulates biliary secretion of fluid and bicarbonate; and regulates gallbladder contraction and gastric emptying.

21. The _____ cells secrete hydrochloric acid and intrinsic factor, which is necessary for the absorption of _____.

22. The chief cells secrete _____, an enzyme that initiates proteolysis or breakdown of proteins.

23. G cells secrete _____.

24. _____ secrete large amounts of alkaline mucus that protect the duodenum from the acid content in the gastric chyme and from the action of the digestive enzymes.

25. The stomach and small intestine contain only a few species of _____, probably due to the composition of luminal contents.

26. The major metabolic function of colonic microflora is the fermentation of _____ and endogenous mucus produced by the epithelial cells.

27. _____ is the process of dismantling foods into their constituent parts.

28. _____ is the process of moving nutrients and other materials from the external environment of the gastrointestinal tract to the internal environment.

29. Each villus is covered with cells called _____ that contribute to the absorptive and digestive functions of the small bowel and goblet cells that provide mucus.

30. The enterocytes secrete _____ that adhere to the border of the villus structures.

31. Triglycerides are broken down by pancreatic _____.

32. _____ represents a loss of appetite.

33. _____ is the conscious sensation resulting from stimulation of the medullary vomiting center that often precedes or accompanies vomiting.

34. _____ is the sudden and forceful oral expulsion of the contents of the stomach.

Activity B *Consider the following figures.*

1. In the transfers section of the digestive tract, locate and label the following layers/structures:

- Mesentery
- Muscularis mucosae
- Serosa (mesothelium)
- Longitudinal muscle
- Circular muscle
- Submucosa
- Mucosa
- Serosa (connective tissue)
- Muscularis externis

2.

1.

2. In the transfers section of the digestive tract, locate and label the following layers/structures:

   • Extruded enterocyte
   • Enterocyte
   • Vein
   • Lacteal
   • Artery
   • Crypt of Lieberkühn

Activity C *Match the key terms in Column A with their definitions in Column B.*

Column A

_____ 1. Amylase

_____ 2. Mastication

_____ 3. Mesentery

_____ 4. Interstitial cells of Cajal

_____ 5. Peritoneum

_____ 6. Submucosal plexus

_____ 7. Haustrations

_____ 8. Chyme

_____ 9. Myenteric plexus

_____ 10. Secretin

Column B

a. Responsible for motility along the length of the gut

b. Blood vessels, nerves, and lymphatic vessels that supply the intestinal wall

c. Breaks down starch

d. Result of chemical breakdown of proteins in stomach

e. Chewing of food

f. Generate slow waves of electrical activity

g. Largest serous membrane in the body

h. Segmental mixing movements of the large intestine

i. Controls function of each segment of intestinal tract

j. Inhibits gastric acid secretion

Activity D *Briefly answer the following.*

1. Describe the functional divisions of the gastrointestinal tract.

   _____

   _____

   _____

2. What factors are involved in stimulating the emptying of the stomach?

   _____

   _____

   _____

3. Describe the two types of contractions seen in the small intestine.

   _____

   _____

   _____

4. Describe the incretin effect.

   _____

   _____

   _____

5. What are the three functions of saliva?

   _____

   _____

   _____

6. What is the mechanism of acid secretion by the parietal cells of the stomach?

   _____

   _____

   _____

7. How are carbohydrates broken down to absorbable units?

   _____

   _____

   _____

8. Describe protein digestion and absorption.

   _____

   _____

   _____

SECTION III: APPLYING YOUR KNOWLEDGE

Activity E *Consider the following scenario and answer the question.*

The nurse is preparing an educational event for a group of children in elementary school who are studying the gastrointestinal tract.

1. What facts would the nurse know to include for these children?

   _____

   _____

   _____

SECTION IV: PRACTICING FOR NCLEX

Activity F *Answer the following questions.*

1. The circular layer of smooth muscle that lies between the stomach and the small intestine is called what?
   a. Pyloric sphincter
   b. Cardiac sphincter
   c. Antrum
   d. Cardiac orifice

2. Where in the gastrointestinal tract is food digested and absorbed?
   a. Colon and ileum
   b. Jejunum and ileum
   c. Stomach and jejunum
   d. Jejunum and colon

3. Some smooth muscle cells in the gastrointestinal tract serve as pacemakers. They display rhythmic spontaneous oscillations in membrane potentials. What are these called?
   a. Peristalsis
   b. Intestinal spasms
   c. Slow waves
   d. Rapid contractility

4. Defecation is controlled by both an internal and an external sphincter. What nerve controls the external sphincter?
   a. Vagus nerve
   b. Femoral nerve
   c. Phrenic nerve
   d. Pudendal nerve

5. The stomach secretes two important hormones in the gastrointestinal tract. One is gastrin. What is the second hormone secreted by the stomach?
   a. Ghrelin
   b. Secretin
   c. Incretin
   d. Cholecystokinin

6. Saliva has more than one function. What are the functions of saliva? Mark all that apply.
   a. Protection
   b. Lubrication
   c. Antibacterial
   d. Initiate digestion of starches
   e. Initiate digestion of protein

7. The colon is home to between 300 and 500 different species of bacteria. What is their main metabolic function?
   a. Digestion of insoluble fiber
   b. Fermentation of undigestible dietary residue
   c. Compaction of metabolic waste prior to leaving the body
   d. Absorption of calcium

8. Absorption is a major function of the gastrointestinal (GI) tract. How is absorption accomplished in the GI tract?
   a. Osmosis and diffusion
   b. Active transport and osmosis
   c. Active transport and diffusion
   d. Diffusion and inactive transport

9. Nausea and vomiting can be side effects of many drugs as well as physiologic disturbances within the body. What is a common cause of nausea?
   a. Distention of the stomach
   b. Distention of the cecum
   c. Distention of the jejunum
   d. Distention of the duodenum

10. Several neurotransmitters have been identified with nausea and vomiting. In this capacity, they act as neuromediators. What neuromediator is believed to be involved in the nausea and vomiting that accompanies chemotherapy?
    a. Serotonin
    b. Dopamine
    c. Acetylcholine receptors
    d. Opioid receptors

Disorders of Gastrointestinal Function

SECTION I: LEARNING OBJECTIVES

1. Define and cite the causes of dysphagia, odynophagia, and achalasia

2. Relate the pathophysiology of gastroesophageal reflux to measures used in the diagnosis and treatment of the disorder in adults and children

3. State the reason for the poor prognosis associated with esophageal cancer

4. Describe the anatomic and physiologic factors that contribute to the gastric mucosal barrier

5. Differentiate between the causes and manifestations of acute and chronic gastritis

6. Characterize the proposed role of *Helicobacter pylori* in the development of chronic gastritis and peptic ulcer and cite methods for diagnosis and treatment of the infection

7. Describe the predisposing factors in development of peptic ulcer and cite the three complications of peptic ulcer

8. Describe the goals for pharmacologic treatment of peptic ulcer disease

9. Cite the etiologic factors in ulcer formation related to Zollinger-Ellison syndrome and stress ulcer

10. List risk factors associated with gastric cancer

11. State the diagnostic criteria for irritable bowel syndrome

12. Compare the characteristics of Crohn disease and ulcerative colitis

13. Relate the use of a high-fiber diet in the treatment of diverticular disease to the etiologic factors for the condition

14. Describe the pathogenesis of the symptoms associated with appendicitis.

15. Compare the causes and manifestations of small-volume diarrhea and large-volume diarrhea

16. Explain why a failure to respond to the defecation urge may result in constipation

17. List five causes of fecal impaction

18. Differentiate between mechanical and paralytic intestinal obstruction in terms of cause and manifestations

19. Describe the characteristics of the peritoneum that increase its vulnerability to and protect it against the effects of peritonitis

20. List three causes of intestinal malabsorption and describe their manifestations

21. List the risk factors associated with colorectal cancer and cite the screening methods for detection

SECTION II: ASSESSING YOUR UNDERSTANDING

Activity A *Fill in the blanks.*

1. The _____ functions primarily as a conduit for passage of food and liquid from the pharynx to the stomach.

2. _____ anomalies of the esophagus require early detection and correction because they are incompatible with life.

3. _____ can result from disorders that produce narrowing of the esophagus, lack of salivary secretion, weakness of the muscular structures that propel the food bolus, or neural networks coordinating the swallowing mechanism.

4. _____ is characterized by a protrusion of the stomach through the esophageal hiatus of the diaphragm.

5. The most frequent symptom of _____ is heartburn.

6. There is considerable evidence linking gastroesophageal reflux with _____.

7. _____ involves mucosal injury to the esophagus, hyperemia, and inflammation.

8. Symptoms of reflux esophagitis in an _____ include evidence of pain when swallowing, hematemesis and anemia due to esophageal bleeding, heartburn, irritability, and sudden or inconsolable crying.

9. Most squamous cell esophageal carcinomas are attributable to _____ and _____ use.

10. The stomach lining is usually _____ to the acid it secretes, a property that allows the stomach to contain acid and pepsin without having its wall digested.

11. The _____ are believed to exert their effect through improved mucosal blood flow, decreased acid secretion, increased bicarbonate ion secretion, and enhanced mucus production.

12. _____ refers to inflammation of the gastric mucosa.

13. _____ is most commonly associated with local irritants such as aspirin or other nonsteroidal antiinflammatory agents, alcohol, or bacterial toxins.

14. _____ is denoted by the absence of grossly visible erosions and the presence of chronic inflammatory changes leading eventually to atrophy of the glandular epithelium of the stomach.

15. Autoimmune gastritis results from the presence of _____ to components of gastric gland parietal cells and intrinsic factor.

16. _____ is a term used to describe a group of ulcerative disorders that occur in areas of the upper gastrointestinal tract that are exposed to acid-pepsin secretions.

17. The most common complications of peptic ulcer are _____, perforation and penetration, and gastric outlet _____.

18. Laboratory findings of hypochromic anemia and occult blood in the stools indicate _____.

19. _____ is the major physiologic mediator for hydrochloric acid secretion.

20. Persons at high risk for development of _____ include those with large surface area burns, trauma, sepsis, acute respiratory distress syndrome, severe liver failure, and major surgical procedures.

21. Gastric _____ is the second most common tumor in the world.

22. _____ is a functional gastrointestinal disorder characterized by a variable combination of chronic and recurrent intestinal symptoms not explained by structural or biochemical abnormalities.

23. The term *inflammatory bowel disease* is used to designate two related inflammatory intestinal disorders: _____ disease and _____.

24. _____ disease is a recurrent, granulomatous type of inflammatory response that can affect any area of the gastrointestinal tract.

25. Ulcerative colitis is confined to the _____ and the _____.

26. _____ deficiencies are common in Crohn disease because of diarrhea, steatorrhea, and other malabsorption problems.

27. Characteristics of ulcerative colitis are the lesions that form in the crypts of _____ in the base of the mucosal layer.

28. _____ of the colon is one of the feared complications of ulcerative colitis.

29. The complications of _____ result from massive fluid loss or destruction of intestinal mucosa.

30. _____ is a condition in which the mucosal layer of the colon herniated through the muscularis layer.

31. _____ is a complication of diverticulosis in which there is inflammation and gross or microscopic perforation of the diverticulum.

32. The pain associated with _____ is caused by stretching of the appendix during the early inflammatory process.

33. The usual definition of _____ is excessively frequent passage of stools.

34. Toxin-producing bacteria or other agents that disrupt the normal absorption or secretory process in the small bowel commonly cause _____.

35. _____ diarrhea is often associated with conditions such as inflammatory bowel disease, irritable bowel syndrome, malabsorption syndrome, endocrine disorders, or radiation colitis.

36. _____ is commonly associated with acute or chronic inflammation or intrinsic disease of the colon, such as ulcerative colitis or Crohn disease.

37. _____ can be defined as the infrequent and/or difficult passage of stools.

38. _____ is the retention of hardened or puttylike stool in the rectum and colon, which interferes with normal passage of feces.

39. Intestinal obstruction designates an impairment of movement of intestinal contents in a _____ direction.

40. _____ obstruction results from neurogenic or muscular impairment of peristalsis.

41. Peritonitis is an inflammatory response of the _____ that lines the abdominal cavity and covers the visceral organs.

42. Celiac disease is an immune-mediated disorder triggered by ingestion of _____ containing grains.

43. _____ provides a means for direct visualization of the rectum and colon.

Activity B *Match the key terms in Column A with their definitions in Column B.*

1.

Column A	Column B
____ 1. Achalasia	a. Swallowing is painful
____ 2. Esophageal atresia	b. Most common cause of chronic gastritis in the United States
____ 3. Odynophagia	c. Ulcer erodes through all layers of the stomach
____ 4. Gastroesophageal reflux	d. Esophagus is connected to the trachea
____ 5. Dysphagia	e. Backward movement of gastric contents into the esophagus
____ 6. Barrett esophagus	f. Upper esophagus ends in a blind pouch
____ 7. Tracheoesophageal fistulae	g. Difficulty passing food into the stomach
____ 8. Mallory-Weiss syndrome	h. Squamous mucosa that lines the esophagus gradually is replaced by columnar epithelium
____ 9. Perforation	i. Tears in the esophagus at the esophagogastric junction
____ 10. *Helicobacter pylori*	j. Difficulty in swallowing

2.

Column A	Column B
____ 1. Fistulas	a. Infection by *Entamoeba histolytica*
____ 2. Zollinger-Ellison syndrome	b. Water is pulled into the bowel by the hyperosmotic nature of its contents
____ 3. Amebiasis	c. Tubelike passages that form connec-
____ 4. Osmotic diarrhea	

_____ 5. Hypergastri-
nemia

_____ 6. Steatorrheic

_____ 7. Cobblestone
appearance

_____ 8. Penetration

_____ 9. Adenomatous
polyps

_____ 10. Rotavirus

tions between dif-
ferent sites in the
gastrointestinal tract

d. Hallmark symptom
of Crohn disease

e. Presence of an ex-
cess of gastrin in
the blood

f. Ulcer crater erodes
into adjacent organs

g. Gastrin-secreting
tumor

h. Causes diarrhea in
children

i. Benign neoplasms
that arise from the
mucosal epithelium
of the intestine

j. Stools contain ex-
cess fat

Activity C *Briefly answer the following.*

1. What is gastroesophageal reflux disease? What
is the mechanism of damage?

_____

_____

_____

2. Describe how the gastric mucosal barrier functions to protect the stomach from its own secretions.

_____

_____

_____

3. Describe the progression and remission of peptic
ulcers.

_____

_____

_____

4. What is the relationship between *Helicobacter
pylori* infection and the development of stomach cancer?

_____

_____

_____

5. What are the typical characteristics of irritable
bowel syndrome?

_____

_____

_____

6. What is hypothesized to be a cause of inflammatory bowel disease (ulcerative colitis and
Crohn disease)?

_____

_____

_____

7. What is the mechanism of diverticulosis formation?

_____

_____

_____

8. What is the pathophysiology of constipation?

_____

_____

_____

9. How does diet expose a patient to colon cancer?

_____

_____

_____

SECTION III: APPLYING YOUR KNOWLEDGE

Activity D *Consider the following scenario
and answer the questions.*

A 67-year-old black man presents at the clinic with
complaints of difficulty swallowing foods of any
kind. He states, "It always feels like I have something caught in my throat." His medical history is
significant for Barrett esophagus, unintentional
weight loss of 15 pounds over the past 4 months,
and some pain when swallowing. The patient is
scheduled for an esophagoscopy, and a diagnosis
of esophageal cancer is subsequently confirmed.
The physician explains that, depending on the
stage of the tumor, there are options for treatment.
The physician recommends chemotherapy
followed by surgical resection of the tumor.

1. The patient arrives for his first treatment of chemotherapy and asks the nurse why he has to have chemotherapy before having the surgery to remove the tumor. The nurse correctly responds by stating what?

   _____

   _____

   _____

2. Subsequent studies show that this patient's tumor has already metastasized. The physician recommends that surgery be done right away, but emphasizes to the patient that there is no cure for his cancer. The patient arrives for surgery and asks the preop nurse why he needs the surgery if it will not cure his cancer. What would be the correct response by the nurse?

   _____

   _____

   _____

SECTION IV: PRACTICING FOR NCLEX

Activity E *Answer the following questions.*

1. Esophageal atresia (EA) is the most common congenital anomaly of the esophagus and is incompatible with life. The majority of children born with EA also have tracheoesophageal fistulae. What are the signs and symptoms of EA in a newborn?

   a. Cyanosis and respiratory distress

   b. Poor feeding and tire easily

   c. Episodes of choking and coughing

   d. Poor feeding and low blood sugar

2. Hiatal hernias can cause severe pain if the hernia is large. Gastroesophageal reflux is a common comorbidity of hiatal hernia, and when this occurs, what might the hernia do?

   a. Increase esophageal acid clearance

   b. Retard esophageal acid clearance

   c. Decrease esophageal acid clearance

   d. Accelerate esophageal acid clearance

3. Infants and children commonly have gastroesophageal reflux. Often, it is asymptomatic and resolves on its own. What are the signs and symptoms of gastroesophageal reflux in infants with severe disease?

   a. Consolable crying and early satiety

   b. Delayed satiety and sleeping after feeding

   c. Tilting of the head to one side and arching of the back

   d. Inconsolable crying and delayed satiety

4. The stomach secretes acid to begin the digestive process on the food that we eat. The gastric mucosal barrier works to prevent acids secreted by the stomach from actually damaging the wall of the stomach. What are the factors that make up the gastric mucosal barrier? Mark all that apply.

   a. Impermeable epithelial cell surface covering

   b. Mechanisms for selective transport of bicarbonate and potassium ions

   c. Characteristics of gastric mucus

   d. Cell coverings that act as antacids

   e. Mechanisms for selective transport of hydrogen and bicarbonate ions

5. *Helicobacter pylori* gastritis has a prevalence in more than 50% of American adults older than 50 years and is believed to be caused by a previous infection when the patient was younger. What can chronic gastritis caused by *H. pylori* cause?

   a. Decreased risk of gastric adenocarcinoma

   b. Decreased risk of low-grade B-cell gastric lymphoma

   c. Duodenal ulcer

   d. Gastric atrophy

6. A 39-year-old Caucasian woman presents at the clinic with complaints of epigastric pain that is cramplike, rhythmic, and just below the xiphoid. She states that it wakes her up around 1 AM and that she is not sleeping well because of it. She further states that this is her third painful episode in the past year. The nurse suspects the patient has a peptic ulcer and expects to receive what orders from the physician?

   a. Schedule patient for a complete metabolic panel and a complete blood count

   b. Schedule patient for laparoscopic examination

c. Schedule patient for a swallow study

d. Schedule patient for a lower gastrointestinal study

7. A patient in a nursing home complains to her nurse that she is not feeling well. When asked to describe how she feels, the patient states that she really is not hungry anymore and seems to have indigestion a lot. The nurse checks the patient's chart and finds that her vital signs are normal, but that she has lost weight over the past 2 months. She also notes that there is a history of gastric cancer in the patient's family. The nurse notifies the physician and expects to receive what orders? Mark all that apply.

a. Schedule a barium x-ray and an endoscopy

b. Perform a Papanicolaou smear on the patient's gastric secretions

c. Order cytologic studies to be done during the endoscopy

d. Schedule a lower gastrointestinal study

e. Have the tech do an endoscopic ultrasound

8. Irritable bowel syndrome is believed to be present in 10% to 15% of the population in the United States. What is its hallmark symptom?

a. Nausea and abdominal pain unrelieved by defecation

b. Abdominal pain relieved by defecation with a change in consistency or frequency of stools

c. Diarrhea and abdominal pain unrelieved by defection

d. Abdominal pain relieved by defecation and bowel impaction

9. Crohn disease is a recurrent inflammatory disease that can affect any area of the bowel. The characteristic of this disease is granulomatous lesions that are sharply demarcated from the surrounding tissue. As the nurse caring for a patient with newly diagnosed Crohn disease, you would know to include what in your teaching?

a. Definition of Crohn disease that indicates that it is a recurrent disease that affects only the large intestine

b. Information on which nonsteroidal anti-inflammatory drugs to take and how often to take them

c. Information on sulfasalazine, including dosage, route, frequency, and side effects of the drug

d. Information on the chemotherapy that will be ordered to cure the disease

10. Rotavirus is a common infection in children younger than 5 years. Like other diseases, rotavirus is most severe in children younger than 24 months. What is a symptom of rotavirus infection?

a. Mild to moderate fever that gets higher after the second day

b. Vomiting that lasts for the course of the disease

c. Fever that disappears after 7 days

d. Vomiting that disappears around the second day

11. Diverticulitis is the herniation of tissue of the large intestine through the muscularis layer of the colon. It is often asymptomatic and is found in approximately 80% of people older than 85 years. Diverticulitis is often asymptomatic, but when symptoms do occur, what is the patient's most common complaint?

a. Lower left quadrant pain with nausea and vomiting

b. Right lower quadrant pain with nausea and vomiting

c. Midepigastric pain with nausea and vomiting

d. Right lower quadrant pain with rebound tenderness on the left

12. Diarrhea is described as a change in frequency of stool passage to where it is excessively frequent. Diarrhea can be acute or chronic, inflammatory or noninflammatory. What are the symptoms of noninflammatory diarrhea? Mark all that apply.

a. Small-volume watery stools

b. Nonbloody stools

c. Periumbilical cramps

d. Nausea and/or vomiting

e. Large-volume bloody stools

13. Peritonitis is an inflammatory condition of the lining of the abdominal cavity. What is one of the most important signs of peritonitis?

    a. Vomiting of coffee ground–appearing emesis

    b. Translocation of extracellular fluid into the peritoneal cavity

    c. Translocation of intracellular fluid into the peritoneal cavity

    d. Vomiting of bloody emesis

14. Celiac disease commonly presents in infancy as failure to thrive. It is an inappropriate T-cell–mediated immune response, and there is no cure for it. What is the treatment of choice for celiac disease?

    a. Removal of protein from the diet

    b. Removal of fat from the diet

    c. Removal of gluten from the diet

    d. Removal of sugar from the diet

15. One of the accepted methods of screening for colorectal cancer is testing for occult blood in the stool. Because it is possible to get a false-positive result on these tests, you would instruct the patient to do what?

    a. Eat a lot of red meat for 3 or 4 days before the test is done.

    b. Take 1,000 mg of vitamin C in supplement form for 1 week prior to testing.

    c. Eat citrus fruits at least five times a day for 2 days prior to testing.

    d. Avoid nonsteroidal anti-inflammatory drugs for 1 week prior to testing.

Disorders of Hepatobiliary and Exocrine Pancreas Function

SECTION I: LEARNING OBJECTIVES

1. Describe the lobular structures of the liver

2. State the source and trace the movement of blood flow into, through, and out of the liver

3. Describe the function of the liver in terms of carbohydrate, protein, and fat metabolism

4. Characterize the function of the liver in terms of bilirubin elimination and describe the pathogenesis of unconjugated and conjugated hyperbilirubinemia

5. Relate the mechanism of bile formation and elimination to the development of cholestasis

6. List four laboratory tests used to assess liver function and relate them to impaired liver function

7. State the three ways by which drugs and other substances are metabolized or inactivated in the liver and provide examples of liver disease related to the toxic effects of drugs and chemical agents

8. Compare hepatitis A, B, C, D, and E in terms of source of infection, incubation period, acute disease manifestations, development of chronic disease, and the carrier state

9. Define chronic hepatitis and compare the pathogenesis of chronic autoimmune and chronic viral hepatitis

10. Characterize the metabolism of alcohol by the liver and state metabolic mechanisms that can be used to explain liver injury

11. Summarize the three patterns of injury that occur with alcohol-induced liver disease.

12. Describe the pathogenesis of intrahepatic biliary tract disease

13. Characterize the liver changes that occur with cirrhosis

14. Describe the physiologic basis for portal hypertension and relate it to the development of ascites, esophageal varices, and splenomegaly

15. Relate the functions of the liver to the manifestations of liver failure.

16. Characterize etiologies of hepatocellular cancer and state the reason for the poor prognosis in persons with this type of cancer

17. Explain the function of the gallbladder in regulating the flow of bile into the duodenum

and relate to the formation of cholelithiasis (gallstones).

18. Describe the clinical manifestations of acute and chronic cholecystitis

19. Characterize the effects of choledocholithiasis and cholangitis on bile flow and the potential for hepatic and pancreatic complications

20. Cite the possible causes and describe the manifestations and treatment of acute pancreatitis

21. Describe the manifestations of chronic pancreatitis

22. State the reason for the poor prognosis in pancreatic cancer

SECTION II: ASSESSING YOUR UNDERSTANDING

Activity A *Fill in the blanks.*

1. The liver, the gallbladder, and the exocrine pancreas are classified as _____ organs of the gastrointestinal tract.

2. Approximately 300 mL of blood per minute enters the liver through the hepatic _____; another 1,050 mL/minute enters by way of the _____.

3. The venous blood delivered by the _____ comes from the digestive tract and major abdominal organs, including the pancreas and spleen.

4. A major exocrine function of the liver is _____ secretion.

5. The most important of liver's secretory proteins is _____ .

6. Acetyl-coenzyme A units from fat metabolism are also used to synthesize _____ and _____ acids in the liver.

7. Almost all _____ synthesis in the body from carbohydrates and proteins occurs in the liver.

8. Whenever a greater quantity of carbohydrates enters the body than can be immediately used, the excess is converted to _____ in the liver.

9. Bile salts serve an important function in digestion; they aid in _____ dietary fats, and they are necessary for the formation of

the _____ that transport fatty acids and fat-soluble vitamins to the surface of the intestinal mucosa for absorption.

10. _____ represents a decrease in bile flow through the intrahepatic canaliculi and a reduction in secretion of water, bilirubin, and bile acids by the hepatocytes.

11. Common to all types of obstructive and hepatocellular cholestasis is the accumulation of _____ pigment in the liver.

12. _____ jaundice occurs when red blood cells are destroyed at a rate in excess of the liver's ability to remove the bilirubin from the blood.

13. _____ of bilirubin is impaired whenever liver cells are damaged, when transport of bilirubin into liver cells becomes deficient, or when the enzymes needed to conjugate the bile are lacking.

14. _____ result in chemical modification of reactive drug groups by oxidation, reduction, hydroxylation, or other chemical reactions carried out in hepatocytes.

15. Drugs such as alcohol and barbiturates can induce certain members of the _____ family to increase enzyme production, accelerating drug metabolism, and decreasing the pharmacologic action of the drug.

16. _____, which involve the conversion of lipid-soluble derivatives to water-soluble substances, may follow phase 1 reactions or proceed independently.

17. Direct hepatotoxic reactions result from drug metabolism and the generation of _____.

18. _____ drug reactions result in decreased secretion of bile or obstruction of the biliary tree.

19. _____ refers to inflammation of the liver.

20. Currently, recreational _____ use is the most common mode of hepatitis C virus (HCV) transmission in the United States and Canada. The main route of transmission of HCV in the past was through contaminated _____ or blood products and _____.

21. _____ hepatitis is a severe type of chronic hepatitis of unknown origin that is

associated with high levels of serum immunoglobulins, including autoantibodies.

22. _____ biliary diseases disrupt the flow of bile through the liver, causing cholestasis and biliary cirrhosis.

23. _____ biliary cirrhosis results from prolonged obstruction of the extrabiliary tree.

24. Obesity, type 2 diabetes, the metabolic syndrome, and hyperlipidemia are coexisting conditions frequently associated with _____ liver disease.

25. _____ represents the end stage of chronic liver disease in which much of the functional liver tissue has been replaced by fibrous tissue.

26. _____ is characterized by increased resistance to flow in the portal venous system and sustained portal vein pressure above 12 mm Hg.

27. Complications of portal hypertension arise from the _____ pressure and _____ of the venous channels behind the obstruction.

28. _____ occurs when the amount of fluid in the peritoneal cavity is increased.

29. _____ is a complication in persons with both cirrhosis and ascites.

30. The _____ syndrome refers to a functional renal failure sometimes seen during the terminal stages of liver failure with ascites.

31. Hepatic _____ refers to the totality of CNS manifestations of liver failure.

32. Among the factors identified as etiologic agents in _____ are chronic viral hepatitis, cirrhosis, long-term exposure to environmental agents such as aflatoxin, and drinking water contaminated with arsenic.

33. The _____ is a distensible, pear-shaped, muscular sac located on the ventral surface of the liver.

34. _____ provides a strong stimulus for gallbladder contraction and is released when food enters the intestines.

35. Gallstones are caused by precipitation of substances contained in bile, mainly _____ and _____.

36. Acute _____ is a diffuse inflammation of the gallbladder, usually secondary to obstruction of the gallbladder outlet.

37. The _____ pancreas is made up of lobules that consist of acinar cells, which secrete digestive enzymes into a system of microscopic ducts.

38. Acute _____ represents a reversible inflammatory process of the pancreatic acini brought about by premature activation of pancreatic enzymes.

39. _____ is characterized by progressive destruction of the exocrine pancreas, fibrosis, and, in the later stages, destruction of the endocrine pancreas.

40. The most significant and reproducible environmental risk factor of pancreatic cancer is _____.

Activity B *Consider the following figure.*

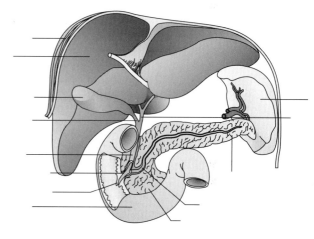

In this figure, label the following structures:

- Liver
- Gallbladder
- Cystic duct
- Common bile duct
- Duodenum
- Tail of pancreas
- Head of pancreas
- Pancreatic duct
- Hepatic duct
- Spleen
- Diaphragm
- Ampulla of Vater
- Sphincter of Oddi

Activity C *Match the key terms in Column A with their definitions in Column B.*

1.

Column A

_____ 1. Kupffer cells

_____ 2. Albumin

_____ 3. Gluconeo-genesis

_____ 4. Oxidative deamination

_____ 5. Beta oxi-dation

_____ 6. Extrahepatic cholestasis

_____ 7. Bilirubin

_____ 8. Jaundice

_____ 9. Steatosis

_____ 10. Cholestatic jaundice

Column B

a. Formed from senescent red blood cells

b. Conversion of amino acids to ketoacids and ammonia

c. Capable of removing and phagocytosing old and defective blood cells

d. Abnormally high accumulation of bilirubin in the blood

e. Splitting of fatty acids into two-carbon acetyl-coenzyme A

f. Transport protein/plasma colloidal osmotic pressure

g. Obstruction of the large bile ducts that reduces bile secretion

h. Amino acids are used for producing glucose

i. Fatty infiltration of the liver

j. Occurs when bile flow is obstructed between the liver and the intestine

2.

Column A

_____ 1. Hepatitis A

_____ 2. Hepatitis B

_____ 3. Hepatitis C

_____ 4. Hepatitis D

_____ 5. Hepatitis E

Column B

a. Infection is linked to hepatitis B

b. Does not cause chronic hepatitis or the carrier state

c. Inoculation with infected blood and/or spread by oral or sexual contact

d. Occurs primarily by the fecal-oral route

e. Most common cause of chronic hepatitis, cirrhosis, and hepatocellular cancer in the world

Activity D

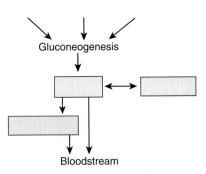

1. Complete the flowchart above for the hepatic pathways for the storage and synthesis of glucose:

- Triglycerides
- Glucose
- Amino acids
- Glycogen
- Glycerol
- Lactic acid

2. Complete the flowchart on the following page using the following terms:

- Increased pressure in peritoneal capillaries
- Portosystemic shunting of blood
- Splenomegaly
- Ascites
- Development of collateral channels
- Shunting of ammonia and toxins into general circulation
- Anemia
- Leukopenia
- Thrombocytopenia
- Hepatic encephalopathy
- Hemorrhoids
- Esophageal varices
- Caput medusae
- Bleeding

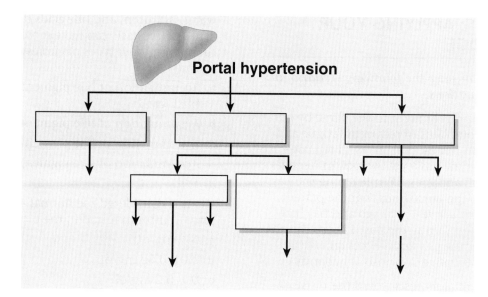

Activity E *Briefly answer the following:*

1. What are the basic functions of the liver?

_____

_____

_____

2. Describe the pathogenesis of cholestasis.

_____

_____

_____

3. List the major causes and categories of jaundice.

_____

_____

_____

4. What is measured in the serum to assess liver dysfunction?

_____

_____

_____

5. Describe the clinical course of viral hepatitis.

_____

_____

_____

6. How does ethanol cause tissue damage?

_____

_____

_____

7. What changes take place in the liver due to the toxic affects of alcohol?

_____

_____

_____

8. What is cirrhosis of the liver?

_____

_____

_____

9. What are the factors that lead to the development of ascites?

_____

_____

_____

10. How does biliary venous obstruction lead to hemorrhoid formation?

_____

_____

_____

SECTION III: APPLYING YOUR KNOWLEDGE

Activity F *Consider the following scenario and answer the questions.*

A 16-year-old girl is brought to the clinic by her mother. She complains of recurrent fatigue and loss of appetite. Her mother states, "I am concerned because she has a yellow look in her eyes. It sort of comes and goes." While taking the patient's history, the nurse finds that the patient became sexually active 1 year ago and has had multiple partners during the past 12 months. On physical exam, the physician notes an enlarged liver. The presumptive diagnosis is hepatitis C.

1. What confirmatory tests would the nurse expect to be ordered?

_____

_____

_____

2. The patient's tests come back positive for hepatitis C. What medications might be ordered for this patient?

_____

_____

_____

SECTION IV: PRACTICING FOR NCLEX

Activity G *Answer the following questions.*

1. The liver has many jobs. One of the most important functions of the liver is to cleanse the portal blood of old and defective blood cells, bacteria in the bloodstream, and any foreign material. Which cells in the liver are capable of removing bacteria and foreign material from the portal blood?
   a. Kupffer cells
   b. Langerhans cells
   c. Epstein cells
   d. Davidoff cells

2. Cholestasis is a condition where there is a decrease in bile flow through the intrahepatic canaliculi and a reduction in secretion of water, bilirubin, and bile acids by the hepatocytes. Cholestasis can have more than one cause, but, in all types of cholestasis, there is what?
   a. Accumulation of bile pigment in the gallbladder
   b. Accumulation of bile pigment in the liver
   c. Accumulation of bile pigment in the blood
   d. Accumulation of bile pigment in the portal vein

3. What is considered the normal amount of serum bilirubin found in the blood?
   a. 1–2 mg/dL
   b. 0.01–0.02 mg/dL
   c. 0.1–0.2 mg/dL
   d. 0.001–0.002 mg/dL

4. Many drugs are metabolized and detoxified in the liver. Most drug metabolizing occurs in the central zones of the liver. What condition is caused by these drug-metabolizing actions?
   a. Central cirrhosis
   b. Lobular cirrhosis
   c. Lobular necrosis
   d. Centrilobular necrosis

5. Primary biliary cirrhosis is an autoimmune disease that destroys the small intrahepatic bile ducts causing cholestasis. It is insidious in onset and is a progressive disease. What are the earliest symptoms of the disease?
   a. Unexplained pruritus
   b. Weight gain
   c. Pale urine
   d. Dark stools

6. One of the jobs the liver performs is to export triglyceride. When the liver's capacity to export triglyceride is maximized, excess fatty acids accumulate in the liver. What is the disease these excess fatty acids contribute to?
   a. Biliary cirrhosis
   b. Nonalcoholic fatty liver disease
   c. Cholelithiasis
   d. Alcoholic fatty liver disease

7. Ascites is an accumulation of fluid in the peritoneal cavity that usually occurs in advanced cirrhosis. What is the treatment of choice for ascites?

a. Paracentesis

b. Thoracentesis

c. Diuretics

d. Desmopressin acetate (DDAVP)

8. A client is suspected of having liver cancer. What diagnostic tests would be ordered to confirm the diagnosis?

a. Serum α-fetoprotein

b. Endoscopy

c. Ultrasound of liver

d. MRI of liver

9. Gallstones are made up mostly of cholesterol. What is believed to be a precursor of gallstones?

a. Gallbladder sludge

b. Thinned mucoprotein

c. Pieces of hard food trapped in the gallbladder

d. Thickened bile

10. What laboratory markers are most commonly used to diagnose acute pancreatitis?

a. Amylase and cholesterol

b. Lipase and amylase

c. Lipase and triglycerides

d. Cholesterol and triglycerides

11. All diseases have risk factors. What is the most significant environmental risk factor for pancreatic cancer?

a. Air pollution

b. Water pollution

c. Cigarette smoking

d. Heavy metal toxicity

Alterations in Nutritional Status

SECTION I: LEARNING OBJECTIVES

1. Define *nutritional status*

2. Define *calorie* and state the number of calories derived from the oxidation of 1 g of protein, fat, or carbohydrate

3. Explain the difference between anabolism and catabolism

4. Relate the processes of glycogenolysis and gluconeogenesis to the regulation of blood glucose by the liver

5. Define *basal metabolic rate* and cite factors that affect it

6. Describe the function of adipose tissue in terms of energy storage and as an endocrine organ

7. State the purpose of the Recommended Dietary Allowance of calories, proteins, fats, carbohydrates, vitamins, and minerals

8. Describe methods used for a nutritional assessment

9. State the factors used in determining body mass index and explain its use in evaluating body weight in terms of undernutrition and overnutrition

10. Define and discuss the causes of obesity and health risks associated with obesity

11. Differentiate upper and lower body obesity and their implications in terms of health risk

12. Discuss the treatment of obesity in terms of diet, behavior modification, exercise, social support, pharmacotherapy, and surgical methods

13. Explain the use of body mass index in evaluating body weight in terms of overnutrition

14. List the major causes of malnutrition and starvation

15. State the difference between protein-calorie starvation (i.e., marasmus) and protein malnutrition (i.e., kwashiorkor)

16. Explain the effect of malnutrition on muscle mass, respiratory function, acid-base balance, wound healing, immune function, bone mineralization, the menstrual cycle, and testicular function

17. State the causes of malnutrition in the severely ill or traumatized patients

18. Compare the eating disorders of anorexia nervosa and bulimia nervosa and the complications associated with each.

SECTION II: ASSESSING YOUR UNDERSTANDING

Activity A *Fill in the blanks.*

1. _____ describes the condition of the body related to the availability and use of nutrients.

2. _____ is the organized process through which nutrients such as carbohydrates, fats, and proteins are broken down, transformed, or otherwise converted into cellular energy.

3. The body transforms carbohydrates, fats, and proteins into the intermediary compound, _____.

4. The _____ refers to the metabolic reactions occurring when the body is at rest.

5. Energy expenditure can be increased by increasing _____ and/or nonexercise activity thermogenesis.

6. More than 90% of body energy is stored in the _____ tissues of the body.

7. _____ acts at the level of the hypothalamus to decrease food intake and increase energy expenditure through an increase in thermogenesis and sympathetic nervous system activity.

8. The _____ defines the intakes that meet the nutrient needs of almost all healthy persons in a specific age and gender group.

9. _____ (% daily vitamins [DV]) tells the consumer what percent of the DV one serving of a food or supplement supplies.

10. _____ are required for growth and maintenance of body tissues, enzymes and antibody formation, fluid and electrolyte balance, and nutrient transport.

11. The rate of protein breakdown can be estimated by measuring the amount of _____ in the urine.

12. The saturated fatty acids _____ blood cholesterol, whereas the monounsaturated and polyunsaturated fats _____ blood cholesterol.

13. Trans-fatty acids _____ low-density lipoprotein cholesterol and _____ high-density lipoprotein cholesterol.

14. There is no specific dietary requirement for _____.

15. _____ are a group of organic compounds that act as catalysts in various chemical reactions.

16. _____ are involved in acid-base balance and in the maintenance of osmotic pressure in body compartments.

17. _____ increases stool bulk and facilitates bowel movements.

18. The _____ contains the feeding center for hunger and satiety.

19. A decrease in blood _____ causes hunger.

20. _____ measurements provide a means for assessing body composition, particularly fat stores and skeletal muscle mass.

21. The _____ uses height and weight to determine healthy weight.

22. Studies have indicated that waist _____ at the abdomen is highly correlated with insulin resistance.

23. _____ is defined as having excess body fat, enlarged fat cells, and even an increased number of fat cells.

24. Research suggests that _____ may be a more important factor for morbidity and mortality than overweight or obesity.

25. _____ has been found to have little or no effect on metabolic variables, central obesity, cardiovascular risk factors, or future amount of weight loss.

26. There is convincing evidence that _____ physical activity decreases the risk of overweight and obesity.

27. _____ does afford significant weight loss, long-term weight loss maintenance, improved quality of life, decreased incidence of associated diseases, and decreased all-cause mortality.

28. Obesity is the most prevalent nutritional disorder affecting the _____ population in the United States.

29. _____ and _____ are conditions in which a person does not receive or is unable to use an adequate amount of nutrients for body function.

30. Protein and energy malnutrition represents a depletion of the body's lean tissues caused by _____ and/or catabolic stress.

31. The child with _____ has a wasted appearance, with loss of muscle mass, stunted growth, and loss of subcutaneous fat.

32. Bulimia nervosa is defined by _____ binge eating and activities such as vomiting;

fasting; excessive exercise; and use of diuretics, laxatives, or enemas to compensate for that behavior.

Activity B *Match the key terms in Column A with their definitions in Column B.*

1.

Column A

____ **1.** Adipocytes

____ **2.** Anabolism

____ **3.** Kwashiorkor

____ **4.** Calorie

____ **5.** Diet-induced thermogenesis

____ **6.** Metabolites

____ **7.** Nitrogen balance

____ **8.** Catabolism

____ **9.** Resting energy equivalent

____ **10.** Kilocalorie

Column B

a. Amount of nitrogen taken in by way of protein is equivalent to the nitrogen excreted

b. Malnutrition caused by inadequate protein intake in the presence of fair to good energy

c. Chemical intermediates of metabolism

d. Storage and synthesis of cell constituents

e. Amount of energy needed to raise the temperature of 1 kg of water by 1°C

f. Fat cells

g. Breakdown of complex molecules

h. Amount of heat or energy required to raise the temperature of 1 g of water by 1°C

i. Energy used by the body for digestion, absorption, and assimilation

j. Used for predicting energy expenditure

2.

Column A

____ **1.** Anorexia nervosa

____ **2.** Ghrelin

Column B

a. Mixture of fatty acids and glycerol

b. Result of a deficiency of linoleic acid

____ **3.** Dermatitis

____ **4.** Triglycerides

____ **5.** Marasmus

____ **6.** Trans-fatty acids

____ **7.** Macro-minerals

c. Hormone that may stimulate hunger

d. Unsaturated oils are partially hydrogenated

e. Minerals present in large amounts in the body

f. Characterized by determined dieting, often accompanied by compulsive exercise

g. Protein and calorie deficiency

Activity C *Briefly answer the following.*

1. What are the two types of adipose tissue? How do they differ?

_____

_____

_____

2. How is bioimpedance performed, and what does it do?

_____

_____

_____

3. What are the nongenetic causes of obesity?

_____

_____

_____

4. What are the causes of anorexia?

_____

_____

_____

5. What are the criteria for the diagnosis of bulimia nervosa?

_____

_____

_____

6. Describe the criteria for a diagnosis of binge-eating disorder.

_____

_____

_____

SECTION III: APPLYING YOUR KNOWLEDGE

Activity D *Consider the following scenario and answer the questions.*

A 14-year-old girl is brought to the clinic by her mother for a sports physical. The young lady is 5'4" tall, weighs 95 pounds, and has a small frame. The nurse notes the client's weight and suspects an eating disorder.

1. What questions would be appropriate in the nursing history to assess for an eating disorder?

_____

_____

_____

2. The nurse knows that the *DSM-IV-TR* diagnostic criteria for anorexia nervosa include what?

_____

_____

_____

SECTION IV: PRACTICING FOR NCLEX

Activity E *Answer the following questions.*

1. Match the term with its action.

Term	Action
____ **1.** Anabolism	**a.** Transform fuel substrates into cellular energy
____ **2.** Catabolism	
____ **3.** Substrate	**b.** Substance on which an enzyme acts
____ **4.** Metabolite	
____ **5.** Enzyme systems	**c.** Breakdown of complex molecules into substances that can be

used in the production of energy

d. Chemical intermediates for anabolism and catabolism

e. Phase of metabolic storage and synthesis of cell constituents

2. Adipose tissue is known to be both an endocrine and a paracrine organ because of the factors it secretes. What are these factors? Mark all that apply.

a. Leptin

b. Growth hormone

c. Adipokine

d. Insulin resistance factor

e. Adiponectin

3. When nutritional requirements are needed for a specific group, what dietary requirements are used?

a. Estimated average requirement

b. Adequate intake

c. Recommended dietary allowance

d. Dietary reference intake

4. Fat is a necessary part of the diet. The Food and Nutrition Board has set what percent of fat as necessary in our diet?

a. 10%

b. 20%

c. 30%

d. 40%

5. It is the hypothalamus that tells us when we are hungry or full. Its message is mediated by input from the gastrointestinal tract. There are also centers in the hypothalamus that regulate energy balance and metabolism based on the secretion of what hormones?

a. Cholecystokinin and glucagonlike peptide-1

b. Ghrelin and thyroid

c. Thyroid and adrenocortical hormones

d. Adrenocortical hormones and cholecystokinin

6. Body mass index (BMI) is the measurement used to determine a person's healthy weight. A BMI between 18.5 and 24.9 is considered the lowest health risk in relation to the weight of a person. How is the BMI calculated?

   a. BMI = weight[lb]/height[ft^2]

   b. BMI = weight[kg]/height[ft^2]

   c. BMI = weight[lb]/height[m^2]

   d. BMI = weight[kg]/height[m^2]

7. Two types of obesity are recognized: upper body obesity and lower body obesity. How is the type of obesity determined?

   a. Waist/hip circumference

   b. Chest circumference/weight

   c. Chest/hip circumference

   d. Waist circumference/weight

8. Anorexia nervosa, bulimia nervosa, and binge-eating disorder are becoming increasingly common, with assessments for these disorders being made in children as young as 9 years. In the adult population, what means of controlling binge eating is most prevalent in men?

   a. Self-induced vomiting

   b. Compulsive exercise

   c. Laxative use

   d. Compulsive working

9. Childhood obesity is recognized as a major problem in the pediatric population. What diseases are pediatricians now seeing in their clients as a direct result of childhood obesity?

   a. Type 1 diabetes

   b. Dyslipidemia

   c. Hypotension

   d. Psychosocial acceptance

10. Malnutrition is not common in the general population in the United States. However, certain populations are more prone to malnutrition than others are. One of these populations is hospitalized patients. Why is this true?

    a. Appetites are increased by fever and pain.

    b. Special diets can increase appetite.

    c. Pain and medications can decrease appetite.

    d. Only healthy diets are served in hospitals.

CHAPTER 40

Mechanisms of Endocrine Controls

SECTION I: LEARNING OBJECTIVES

1. Characterize a hormone

2. Differentiate vesicle-mediated and non–vesicle-mediated mechanisms of hormone synthesis in terms of their stimuli for hormone synthesis and release

3. Describe mechanisms of hormone transport and inactivation

4. State the function of a hormone receptor and the difference between cell surface hormone receptors and intracellular hormone receptors

5. Describe the role of the hypothalamus in regulating pituitary control of endocrine function

6. State the major difference between positive and negative feedback control mechanisms

7. Describe methods used in diagnosis of endocrine disorders

SECTION II: ASSESSING YOUR UNDERSTANDING

Activity A *Fill in the blanks.*

1. The endocrine system uses chemical substances called _____ as a means of regulating and integrating body functions.

2. The functions of the endocrine system are closely linked with those of the _____ system and the _____ system.

3. When hormones act locally on cells other than those that produced the hormone, the action is called _____.

4. Hormones can also exert an _____ action on the cells from which they were produced.

5. Hormones that are released into the bloodstream circulate either as _____ molecules or as hormones _____ to transport carriers.

6. Hormones produce their effects through interaction with _____, which in turn are linked to one or more effector systems within the cell.

7. The structure of hormone _____ varies in a manner that allows target cells to respond to one hormone and not to others.

8. _____ hormones attach to intracellular receptors and form a hormone-receptor complex that travels to the cell nucleus.

9. The synthesis and release of anterior pituitary hormones is regulated by the action of releasing or inhibiting hormones from the _____, which is the coordinating center of the brain for endocrine, behavioral, and autonomic nervous system function.

10. The pituitary gland has been called the _____ because its hormones control the functions of many target glands and cells.

11. The easiest way to measure hormone levels during a specific period are by either blood samples or urine tests to measure _____ or _____.

Activity B *Match the key terms in Column A with their definitions in Column B.*

Column A

____ **1.** Autocrine

____ **2.** Half-life of a hormone

____ **3.** Hormones

____ **4.** Hypophysis

____ **5.** Paracrine

____ **6.** Second messenger

____ **7.** Hormone response element

Column B

a. Time it takes for the body to reduce the concentration of the hormone by one-half

b. Hormone acts on cell that produced it

c. Hormone affecting neighboring cells

d. The hypothalamus and the pituitary

e. Highly specialized organic molecules produced by endocrine organs that exert their action on specific target cells

f. Intracellular signal

g. Activate or suppress intracellular mechanisms such as gene activity

Activity C *Put the steps of hypothalamic-pituitary-target cell feedback mechanism in order. Draw a flowchart using these terms:*

• Effect
• Target
• Peripheral gland
• Tropic hormone
• Central nervous system input
• Hypothalamus
• Pituitary
• Releasing hormone
• Hormone
• Other input

Activity D *Briefly answer the following.*

1. What is a hormone?

_____
_____
_____

2. What is the structure of a hormone?

_____
_____
_____

3. How do tissues regulate a hormone's effect?

_____
_____
_____

4. What are the main types of cell membrane receptors, and how do they exert their effects?

_____
_____
_____

5. Describe the global role of the anterior pituitary hormones.

_____
_____
_____

6. How does negative feedback regulate hormone levels?

_____
_____
_____

SECTION III: APPLYING YOUR KNOWLEDGE

Activity E *Consider the following scenario and answer the questions.*

An 87-year-old woman has come to the clinic for a routine physical exam. She says she has no complaints and is concerned only about a

20-pound weight gain in the past 2 years. She says that she is not as active as she used to be. She also mentions that she has fallen several times and now has a large bruise on her right hip.

1. The nurse knows that this client is at risk for osteoporosis due to her decrease in activity. What test would the nurse expect to be ordered to either confirm or rule out osteoporosis in this patient?

_____

_____

_____

2. With the client's weight gain over the past 2 years and her decrease in activity level, the nurse would expect what test to be ordered to either rule out or confirm type 2 diabetes in this client?

_____

_____

_____

SECTION IV: PRACTICING FOR NCLEX

Activity F *Answer the following questions.*

1. The endocrine system is closely linked with both the immune system and the nervous system. What neurotransmitter can also act as a hormone?
   a. Epinephrine
   b. Norepinephrine
   c. Dopamine
   d. Succinylcholine

2. When hormones act locally rather than being secreted into the bloodstream, their actions are termed what?
   a. Autocratic and paracratic
   b. Autocrine and paracrine
   c. Localized and influential
   d. Preventers and inhibitors

3. Hormones can be synthesized by both vesicle-mediated pathways and nonvesicle-mediated pathways. What hormones are synthesized by nonvesicle-mediated pathways?
   a. Neurotransmitters that are also hormones
   b. Renin and angiotensin
   c. Androgens and estrogens
   d. Pepsin and ghrelin

4. To prevent the accumulation of hormones in our bodies, the hormones are constantly being metabolized and excreted. Where are adrenal and gonadal steroid hormones excreted?
   a. Feces and urine
   b. Bile and lungs
   c. Cell metabolites and lungs
   d. Bile and urine

5. The hypophysis is a unit formed by the pituitary and the hypothalamus. These two glands are connected by the blood flow in what system?
   a. Hypophyseal portal system
   b. Supraoptic portal system
   c. Paraventricular portal system
   d. Hypothalamic portal system

6. The hormone levels in the body need to be kept within an appropriate range. How is this accomplished for many of the hormones in the body?
   a. Positive feedback loop
   b. Negative feedback loop
   c. Regulated feedback loop
   d. Sensory feedback loop

7. Many hormones are measured for diagnostic reasons by using the plasma levels of the hormones. What is used today to measure plasma hormone levels?
   a. Nucleotide assay methods
   b. Selective binding methods
   c. Radioimmunoassay methods
   d. Radiolabeled hormone-antibody methods

8. Sometimes the measurement of hormones is done through a urine sample. What is an advantage of measuring hormone levels through a urine sample rather than a blood sample?
   a. Urine has more accurate measurements of hormones

b. There are more hormone metabolites in urine than in blood

c. Blood sampling has more pure hormone than urine does

d. Urine samples are easily obtained

9. In an adult with acromegaly, a growth hormone-secreting tumor is suspected. What diagnostic test would be used for this client?

a. A growth hormone suppression test

b. A growth hormone stimulation test

c. A growth hormone serum assay test

d. A growth hormone urine assay test

10. Imaging has proven useful in both the diagnosis and follow-up of endocrine disorders. Two types of imaging studies are useful when dealing with endocrine disorders, isotopic imaging and nonisotopic imaging. What is an example of isotopic imaging?

a. MRI

b. Thyroid scan

c. Renal angiography

d. Positron emission topography scan

CHAPTER 41

Disorders of Endocrine Control of Growth and Metabolism

SECTION I: LEARNING OBJECTIVES

1. Describe the mechanisms of endocrine hypofunction and hyperfunction

2. Differentiate primary, secondary, and tertiary endocrine disorders

3. Discuss the classification of pituitary tumors

4. Describe the clinical features and causes of hypopituitarism

5. State the effects of a deficiency in growth hormone

6. Differentiate genetic short stature from constitutional short stature

7. State the mechanisms of short stature in hypothyroidism, poorly controlled diabetes mellitus, chronic treatment with excessive glucocorticoid hormones, malnutrition, and psychosocial dwarfism

8. List three causes of tall stature

9. Relate the functions of growth hormone to the manifestations of acromegaly and adult-onset growth hormone deficiency

10. Explain why children with isosexual precocious puberty are tall-statured children but short-statured adults

11. Characterize the synthesis, transport, and regulation of thyroid hormone

12. Diagram the hypothalamic-pituitary-thyroid feedback system

13. Describe tests in the diagnosis and management of thyroid disorders

14. Relate the functions of thyroid hormone to hypothyroidism and hyperthyroidism

15. Describe the effects of congenital hypothyroidism

16. Characterize the manifestations and treatment of myxedematous coma and thyroid storm

17. Describe the function of the adrenal cortical hormones and their feedback regulation

18. State the underlying cause of congenital adrenal hyperplasia

19. Relate the functions of the adrenal cortical hormones to Addison disease (i.e., adrenal insufficiency) and Cushing syndrome (i.e., glucocorticoid excess)

SECTION II: ASSESSING YOUR UNDERSTANDING

Activity A *Fill in the blanks.*

1. Disturbances of endocrine function can usually be divided into two categories: _____ and _____.

2. _____ defects result in endocrine hypofunction due to the absence or impaired development of the gland or the absence of an enzyme needed for hormone synthesis.

3. Several hormones are essential for normal body _____ and maturation, including growth hormone, insulin, thyroid hormone, and androgens.

4. Growth hormone cannot directly produce bone growth; instead, it acts indirectly by causing the liver to produce _____.

5. _____ secretion is stimulated by hypoglycemia, fasting, starvation, increased blood levels of amino acids, and stress conditions such as trauma, excitement, emotional stress, and heavy exercise.

6. _____ describes children (particularly boys) who have moderately short stature, thin build, delayed skeletal and sexual maturation, and absence of other causes of decreased growth.

7. _____ describes a child who is taller than his or her peers and is growing at a velocity that is within the normal range for bone age.

8. Growth hormone excess occurring before puberty and the fusion of the epiphyses of the long bones results in _____.

9. When growth hormone excess occurs in adulthood or after the epiphyses of the long bones have fused, the condition is referred to as _____.

10. Long-term elevation of growth hormone results in _____ of the beta cells, causing them to literally "burn out."

11. _____ sexual development may be idiopathic or may be caused by gonadal, adrenal, or hypothalamic disease.

12. _____ hormones are bound to thyroxine-binding globulin and other plasma proteins for transport in the blood.

13. Thyroid hormone has two major functions: it increases _____ and _____ synthesis, and it is necessary for growth and development in children.

14. Thyroid hormone increases the _____ of all body tissues except the retina, spleen, testes, and lungs.

15. Measures of T_3, T_4, and thyroid-stimulating hormone have been made available through _____ methods.

16. Congenital hypothyroidism is a common cause of _____.

17. _____ implies the presence of a non-pitting mucus-type edema caused by the accumulation of hydrophobic extracellular matrix substances in the connective tissues of a number of body tissues.

18. _____ is the clinical syndrome that results when tissues are exposed to high levels of circulating thyroid hormone.

19. The most common cause of hyperthyroidism is _____ disease, which is accompanied by ophthalmopathy (or dermopathy) and diffuse goiter.

20. Many of the manifestations of hyperthyroidism are related to the increase in _____ consumption and use of _____ fuels associated with the hypermetabolic state, as well as to the increase in sympathetic nervous system activity that occurs.

21. _____ is manifested by a very high fever, extreme cardiovascular effects, and severe central nervous system effects.

22. The _____ forms the bulk of the gland and is responsible for secreting three types of hormones: the glucocorticoids, the mineralocorticoids, and the adrenal androgens.

23. _____ secretion is regulated by the renin-angiotensin mechanism and by blood levels of potassium.

24. When produced as part of the stress response, _____ hormones aid in regulating the metabolic functions of the body and in controlling the inflammatory response.

25. _____ stimulates glucose production by the liver, promotes protein breakdown, and causes mobilization of fatty acids.

26. Primary adrenal insufficiency, or _____ disease, is caused by destruction of the adrenal gland.

27. _____ refers to the manifestations of hypercortisolism from any cause.

Activity B *Consider the following figure.*

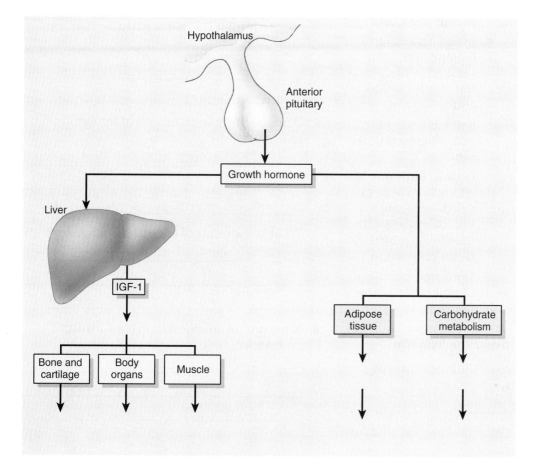

Complete the flowchart with the following terms:

- Antiinsulin effects
- Decreased glucose use
- Decreased adiposity
- Growth-promoting actions
- Increased blood glucose
- Increased lean muscle mass
- Increased linear growth
- Increased lipolysis
- Increased protein synthesis
- Increased size and function

Activity C *Match the key terms in Column A with their definitions in Column B.*

Column A

_____ **1.** Laron-type dwarfism

_____ **2.** Hypopi-tuitarism

_____ **3.** Cretinism

_____ **4.** Hashimoto thyroiditis

Column B

a. Growth hormone-secreting cells

b. Deficiency of all pituitary-derived hormones

c. Dry skin and swelling around lips and nose as well as mental deterioration

_____ **5.** Panhypopi-
tuitarism

_____ **6.** Ophthalmo-
pathy

_____ **7.** Goiter

_____ **8.** Myxedema

_____ **9.** Somatotropes

_____ **10.** Pendred
syndrome

d. Manifestations of
untreated congenital
hypothyroidism

e. Autoimmune disor-
der in which the thy-
roid gland may be
totally destroyed

f. Increase in the size of
the thyroid gland

g. Eyelid retraction,
bulging eyes, light
sensitivity, discom-
fort, double vision,
and vision loss

h. Patients with goiter
and congenital deaf-
ness

i. Growth hormone levels are normal or ele-
vated, but there is a
hereditary defect in
insulinlike growth
factor production

j. Decreased secretion
of pituitary
hormones

Activity D *Briefly answer the following.*

1. Explain the grouping of the root causes of
endocrine disorders.

_____

_____

_____

2. What hormones are directly affected by hypopituitarism? What affect does it have on the
rest of the endocrine system?

_____

_____

_____

3. What are the normal actions of growth
hormone?

_____

_____

_____

4. How is growth hormone release stimulated?
How is it inhibited?

_____

_____

_____

5. Describe the stimulation of the thyroid gland,
and explain the mechanism of negative feedback to inhibit thyroid activity.

_____

_____

_____

6. Describe the manifestations of hypothyroidism.

_____

_____

_____

7. What is the result of adrenal insufficiency?

_____

_____

_____

8. What are the manifestations of Cushing
syndrome?

_____

_____

_____

SECTION III: APPLYING YOUR KNOWLEDGE

Activity E *Consider the following scenario and
answer the questions.*

The parents of a newborn have been notified by
the hospital that they need to bring their newborn back to the hospital for further testing. The
parents are informed that one of the tests done
on the baby when it was first born needs to be repeated. When the parents arrive at the hospital,
they meet with a pediatrician who explains that
their infant's thyroid tests have come back abnormal and need to be repeated. He goes on to
say that it might be a false-negative result on the
original test and not to worry.

1. As the nurse prepares to take the infant's blood, the parents ask what it means if the first test result is not a mistake. The nurse knows the best information to give the parents is what?

_____

_____

_____

2. The parents want to know what will happen to their baby if the thyroid gland is not working correctly. The nurse correctly answers what?

_____

_____

_____

SECTION IV: PRACTICING FOR NCLEX

Activity F *Answer the following questions.*

1. Advances in technology have made it possible to assess hypothalamic-pituitary function by newly developed imaging and radioimmunoassay methods. When baseline tests are not sufficient, what suppression test gives information about combined hypothalamic-pituitary function?
   a. Growth hormone suppression test
   b. ACTH suppression test
   c. Cortisol suppression test
   d. Prolactin suppression test

2. Growth hormone (GH) is secreted by both adults and children. GH deficiency in children is treated by injections of GH on a daily basis. When teaching a family or child to give injections of GH, what is it important to teach them?
   a. Give the injections in the morning so the peak effect is before noon.
   b. Give the injections at bedtime to produce the greatest effect at night.
   c. Give the injections about 3 PM to produce the greatest effect in the evening.
   d. Give the injections in the early afternoon to produce the greatest effect at dinner time.

3. Growth hormone (GH) exerts its effects on the body in many ways. Which of these are effects of GH? Mark all that apply.
   a. Enhances fatty acid mobilization
   b. Increases insulin levels
   c. Facilitates the rate of protein synthesis
   d. Decreases ACTH production
   e. Decreases use of fatty acids for fuel

4. Acromegaly is a disorder that is caused by the production of excessive growth hormone in the adult. Because the person cannot grow taller, the soft tissues continue to grow, presenting a very distinctive appearance. What is it that is distinctive in a person with acromegaly?
   a. Small hands and feet compared to length of arms and legs
   b. Broad, bulbous nose and a protruding lower jaw
   c. Slanting forehead and a receding lower jaw
   d. Protruding lower jaw and forehead

5. Precocious puberty is a disorder that occurs in both boys and girls. What does precocious puberty cause in adults?
   a. Early menopause in females
   b. Early erectile dysfunction problems in males
   c. Short stature in adults
   d. Gigantism in adults

6. When the assessment of thyroid autoantibodies is performed, what is the suspected diagnosis?
   a. Goiter
   b. Thyroid tumor
   c. Congenital hypothyroidism
   d. Hashimoto thyroiditis

7. An elderly woman is brought to the emergency room by her family. They relate to the nurse that the client has had mental status changes and cannot remember her grandchildren's names. They go on to say that she is intolerant of cold and is lethargic. On physical examination, the nurse notes that the client has a husky voice, her face is puffy around the eyes, and her tongue appears enlarged. What diagnosis would the nurse suspect?
   a. Myxedema
   b. Hashimoto thyroiditis
   c. Hyperthyroidism
   d. Congenital hypothyroidism

8. Hyperthyroidism that is inadequately treated can cause a life-threatening condition known as a thyroid storm. What are the manifestations of a thyroid storm? Mark all that apply.

a. Tachycardia

b. Very low fever

c. Delirium

d. Bradycardia

e. Very high fever

9. At times, it is necessary to give medications that suppress the adrenal glands on a long-term basis. When the suppression of the adrenals becomes chronic, the adrenal glands atrophy. What does the abrupt withdrawal of these suppressive drugs cause?

a. Acute adrenal hyperplasia

b. Acute adrenal insufficiency

c. Acute adrenal hypoplasia

d. Acute adrenal cortical hyperplasia

10. Congenital adrenal hyperplasia is a congenital disorder in which a deficiency exists in any of the enzymes necessary for the synthesis of cortisol. Infants of both genders are affected, although boys are not diagnosed at birth unless of enlarged genitalia. Female infants often have ambiguous genitalia because of the oversecretion of adrenal androgens. What are the manifestations of the ambiguous genitalia caused by congenital adrenal hyperplasia?

a. Small clitoris, fused labia, and urogenital sinus

b. Small clitoris, open labia, and urogenital sinus

c. Enlarged clitoris, fused labia, and urogenital sinus

d. Enlarged clitoris, open labia, and urogenital sinus

11. In Addison disease, the majority of the adrenal cortex has been destroyed. This causes a lack of mineralocorticoids and glucocorticoids. Therapy consists of oral replacement with what drug?

a. Cortisol

b. Aldosterone

c. Glucocorticoid

d. Hydrocortisone

12. In an acute adrenal crisis, the onset of symptoms is sudden, and in the case of Addison disease, can be precipitated by exposure to a minor illness or stress. What are the manifestations of acute adrenal crisis? Mark all that apply.

a. Hypertension

b. Muscle weakness

c. Dehydration

d. Altered mental status

e. Vascular collapse

13. The hallmark manifestations of Cushing syndrome are a moon face, a "buffalo hump" between the shoulder blades, and a protruding abdomen. What other manifestations of Cushing syndrome occur?

a. Thin extremities and muscle weakness

b. Muscle wasting and thickened extremities

c. Muscle weakness and thickened extremities

d. Thin extremities and increased strength

CHAPTER 42

Diabetes Mellitus and the Metabolic Syndrome

SECTION I: LEARNING OBJECTIVES

1. State the functions of glucose, fats, and proteins in meeting the energy needs of the body

2. Characterize the actions of insulin with reference to glucose, fat, and protein metabolism

3. Explain what is meant by *counter-regulatory hormones*, and describe the actions of glucagon, epinephrine, growth hormone, and the glucocorticoid hormones in regulation of blood glucose levels

4. Compare the distinguishing features of type 1 and type 2 diabetes mellitus, list causes of other specific types of diabetes, and cite the criteria for gestational diabetes

5. Describe what is meant by the term *prediabetes*

6. Relate the physiologic functions of insulin to the manifestations of diabetes mellitus

7. Define the metabolic syndrome and describe its associations with the development of type 2 diabetes

8. Discuss the role of diet and exercise in the management of diabetes mellitus.

9. Characterize the blood glucose–lowering actions of the hypoglycemic agents used in treatment of type 2 diabetes

10. Name and describe the types (according to duration of action) of insulin

11. Differentiate between the causes and clinical manifestations of diabetic ketoacidosis and the hyperosmolar hyperglycemic state

12. Describe alterations in physiologic function that accompany diabetic peripheral neuropathy, retinopathy, and nephropathy

13. Describe the causes of foot ulcers in people with diabetes mellitus

14. Explain the relation between diabetes mellitus and infection

SECTION II: ASSESSING YOUR UNDERSTANDING

Activity A *Fill in the blanks.*

1. The primary source of energy for the body is _____.

2. Because the _____ can neither synthesize nor store more than a few minutes' supply of glucose, normal cerebral function requires a continuous supply from the circulation.

3. Severe and prolonged _____ can cause brain death.

4. Glucose that is not needed for energy is removed from the blood and stored as _____ or converted to fat.

5. When blood glucose levels fall below normal, as they do between meals, a process called

_____ breaks down glycogen, and glucose is released.

6. In addition to mobilizing its glycogen stores, the liver synthesizes glucose from amino acids, glycerol, and lactic acid in a process called _____.

7. Fat is the most efficient form of fuel storage, providing _____ kcal/g of stored energy, compared with the _____ kcal/g provided by carbohydrates and proteins.

8. _____ are essential for the formation of all body structures, including genes, enzymes, contractile structures in muscle, bone matrix, and hemoglobin of red blood cells.

9. Because _____ cannot be converted to glucose, the body must break down _____ and use the amino acids as a major substrate for gluconeogenesis during periods when metabolic needs exceed food intake.

10. Because cell membranes are impermeable to glucose, they require a special carrier, called a _____, to move glucose from the blood into the cell.

11. _____ is the insulin-dependent glucose transporter for skeletal muscle and adipose tissue.

12. _____ maintains blood glucose between meals and during periods of fasting.

13. The most dramatic effect of glucagon is its ability to initiate _____ and _____.

14. The secretion of growth hormone normally is inhibited by _____ and increased levels of blood glucose.

15. _____ is a disorder of carbohydrate, protein, and fat metabolism resulting from an imbalance between insulin availability and insulin need.

16. A fasting plasma glucose of _____ or a 2-hour oral glucose tolerance test result of _____ is considered normal.

17. _____ diabetes mellitus is characterized by destruction of the pancreatic beta cells.

18. The term _____ type 1B diabetes is used to describe those cases of beta cell destruction in which no evidence of autoimmunity is present.

19. _____ diabetes mellitus is a heterogeneous condition that describes the presence of hyperglycemia in association with relative insulin deficiency.

20. Insulin _____ initially stimulates an increase in insulin secretion, often to a level of modest hyperinsulinemia, as the beta cells attempt to maintain a normal blood glucose level.

21. Although the insulin resistance seen in persons with type 2 diabetes can be caused by a number of factors, it is strongly associated with _____ and _____.

22. A major factor in persons with the metabolic syndrome that leads to type 2 diabetes is _____.

23. _____ diabetes mellitus refers to any degree of glucose intolerance that is first detected during pregnancy.

24. The _____ plasma glucose has been suggested as the preferred diagnostic test because of ease of administration, convenience, patient acceptability, and cost.

25. A _____ plasma glucose concentration that is unequivocally elevated (>_____ mg/dL) in the presence of classic symptoms of diabetes, such as polydipsia, polyphagia, polyuria, and blurred vision, is diagnostic of diabetes mellitus at any age.

26. In uncontrolled diabetes or diabetes with hyperglycemia, there is an increase in the level of _____ in circulation.

27. Type 1 diabetes mellitus always requires treatment with _____, and many people with type 2 diabetes eventually require similar therapy.

28. Diabetic _____ most commonly occurs in a person with type 1 diabetes, in whom the lack of insulin leads to mobilization of fatty acids from adipose tissue because of the unsuppressed adipose cell lipase activity that breaks down triglycerides into fatty acids and glycerol.

29. The _____ is characterized by hyperglycemia (blood glucose >600 mg/dL), hyperosmolarity (plasma osmolarity >310 mOsm/L) and dehydration, the absence of ketoacidosis, and depression of the sensorium.

30. _____ are thought to produce structural defects in the basement membrane of

the microcirculation and to contribute to eye, kidney, and vascular complications.

31. The term _____ is used to describe the combination of lesions that often occur concurrently in the diabetic kidney.

32. _____ is characterized by abnormal retinal vascular permeability, microaneurysm formation, neovascularization and associated hemorrhage, scarring, and retinal detachment.

33. Multiple risk factors for _____, including obesity, hypertension, hyperglycemia, hyperinsulinemia, hyperlipidemia, altered platelet function, endothelial dysfunction, systemic inflammation, and elevated fibrinogen levels, frequently are found in people with diabetes.

Activity B *Match the key terms in Column A with their definitions in Column B.*

Column A

____ **1.** Incretin effect

____ **2.** Somatostatin

____ **3.** Epinephrine

____ **4.** Secretagogues

____ **5.** Adiponectin

____ **6.** Triglyceride

____ **7.** Somogyi effect

____ **8.** PPAR-γ

____ **9.** Amylin

____ **10.** Glucocorticoid

____ **11.** Dawn phenomenon

Column B

a. Three fatty acids linked by a glycerol molecule

b. Produce inhibition of gastric emptying and glucagon secretion

c. Inhibit the release of insulin and glucagon

d. Increase insulin release after an oral nutrient load

e. Agents that cause or stimulate secretion

f. Inhibits insulin release and promotes glycogenolysis

g. Stimulate gluconeogenesis by the liver

h. Increases tissue sensitivity to insulin

i. Nuclear receptor that leads to the regulation of genes controlling free fatty acids (FFA) levels and glucose metabolism

j. Cycle of insulin-induced posthypoglycemic episodes

k. Increased levels of fasting blood glucose without precursor hypoglycemia

Activity C

1. Construct a flowchart, using the terms below, that reflects hormonal and hepatic regulation of blood glucose.

- decreased blood glucose
- removal of glucose from blood
- decreased glucagon
- increased insulin release from beta cells
- deceased hepatic glucose production
- increased blood glucose
- decreased insulin and increased glucagon and gluconeogenesis

Activity D *Briefly answer the following questions.*

1. What are the results/actions of insulin release?

2. How is insulin secretion from beta cells stimulated?

3. Why are patients with type 1 diabetes mellitus especially likely to develop ketoacidosis?

4. What is thought to cause type 1 diabetes mellitus?

5. What are the metabolic changes that precede the development of type 2 diabetes?

6. How does beta cell dysfunction develop in type 2 diabetes?

_____

_____

_____

7. What are the systemic manifestations of metabolic syndrome?

_____

_____

_____

8. What are the effects of insulin resistance and increased glucose production in obese patients with type 2 diabetes?

_____

_____

_____

9. What are the three "polys" and why are they significant?

_____

_____

_____

10. Why do patients with type 1 diabetes lose weight?

_____

_____

_____

11. How does continuous subcutaneous insulin infusion work?

_____

_____

_____

12. What are the three major challenges to normal physiology from diabetic ketoacidosis (DKA)?

_____

_____

_____

13. What are the common complications of chronic diabetes mellitus? How do they develop?

_____

_____

_____

14. What are the pathologic changes observed in peripheral neuropathies that are associated with chronic diabetes mellitus?

_____

_____

_____

15. What are the effects of diabetes mellitus on renal tissue?

_____

_____

_____

SECTION III: APPLYING YOUR KNOWLEDGE

Activity E *Consider the following scenario and answer the questions.*

A 16-year-old boy is admitted to your unit with a new diagnosis of type 1A diabetes mellitus. His blood sugar on admission is 735; he is lethargic; his parents state that he has started eating continuously; and he is urinating much more than he usually does. They say he has lost 10 pounds over the past few months without trying. The patient and his family state that they know nothing about diabetes and ask you for an explanation of the disorder.

1. You would know to include what information in educating the patient and his family about type 1A diabetes mellitus?

_____

_____

2. The patient asks if there is any cure for type 1A diabetes. You would know to respond:

_____

_____

_____

SECTION IV: PRACTICING FOR NCLEX

Activity F *Answer the following questions.*

1. The pancreas is an endocrine organ that is composed of the acini and the islets of Langerhans. The islets of Langerhans have alpha, beta, and delta cells as well as the PP cell. Which cells secrete insulin?
   a. Alpha cells
   b. Beta cells
   c. Delta cells
   d. PP cells

2. Hormones that counteract insulin's storage function when regulating blood glucose during times when glucose intake is limited or glucose stores are depleted are called counter-regulatory hormones. What are the counter regulatory hormones? Mark all that apply.
   a. Glucocorticoids
   b. Growth hormone
   c. Catecholamines
   d. Mineralocorticoids
   e. Glucagon

3. During periods of fasting and starvation, the glucocorticoid and other corticosteroid hormones are critical for survival because of their stimulation of gluconeogenesis by the liver. When the glucocorticoid hormones remain elevated for extended periods of time what can occur?
   a. Hepatomegaly
   b. Portal hypertension
   c. Hyperglycemia
   d. Adrenal hyperplasia

4. Type 1A diabetes is now considered an autoimmune disorder. What factors are considered necessary for type 1A diabetes to occur?
   a. Genetic predisposition, environmental triggering event, and a T lymphocyte-mediated hypersensitivity reaction against some beta cell antigen
   b. Genetic predisposition, physiologic triggering event, allergic reaction to pancreatic alpha cells
   c. Diabetogenic gene from both parents, physiologic triggering event, and an allergic reaction to pancreatic delta cells

   d. Diabetogenic gene from both parents, environmental triggering event, and a B lymphocyte reaction to alpha cell antigens

5. Type 2 diabetes is caused by metabolic abnormalities in the presence of insulin. What are these metabolic abnormalities? Mark all that apply.
   a. Deranged secretion of insulin
   b. Decreased glucose production by the liver
   c. Insulin resistance
   d. Increased glucose production by the liver
   e. Hypersensitivity to insulin

6. Secondary diabetes occurs because of disorders that produce hyperglycemia by stimulating the hepatic production of glucose or decrease the cellular use of glucose. Which disorders can cause secondary diabetes?
   a. Pheochromocytoma and Cushing syndrome
   b. Pancreatic disease and dwarfism
   c. Acromegaly and pancreatic hyperplasia
   d. Hepatomegaly and pheochromocytoma

7. Gestational diabetes mellitus (GDM) is a disorder of glucose intolerance that occurs during pregnancy. It is associated with increased risk for developing type 2 diabetes and with fetal abnormalities. What fetal abnormalities are associated with GDM?
   a. Microsomia and polycythemia
   b. Macrosomia and hypocalcemia
   c. Hypercalcemia and hyperbilirubinemia
   d. Hypoglycemia and hypercalcemia

8. What are the hallmark signs of diabetes mellitus?
   a. Polyuria, polydipsia, and pheochromocytoma
   b. Polyuria, polyphagia, and polycythemia
   c. Polyuria, polydipsia, and polyphagia
   d. Polycythemia, polydipsia, and pheochromocytoma

9. Match the type of oral antidiabetic agent with the name of a drug in its class.

Type of Antidiabetic Agent	**Drug**
___ 1. Insulin secretagogues	a. Exenatide
	b. Rosiglitazone
___ 2. Biguanides	c. Metformin

_____ **3.** α-Glucosidase inhibitors

_____ **4.** Thiazolidinediones

_____ **5.** Dipeptidyl peptidase 4 (DPP-4) enzyme inhibitors

_____ **6.** Glucagonlike poly-peptide 1 agonists

d. Repaglinide

e. Acarbose

f. Alogliptin

10. Diabetic ketoacidosis (DKA) is a condition that mostly occurs in type 1 diabetes. What are the definitive diagnostic criteria for DKA?

a. Blood glucose level >350 mg/dL; bicarbonate <05 mEq/L and pH <7.4

b. Blood glucose level >250 mg/dL; bicarbonate <25 mEq/L and pH <7.3

c. Blood glucose level >350 mg/dL; bicarbonate <05 mEq/L and pH <7.4

d. Blood glucose level >250 mg/dL; bicarbonate <15 mEq/L and pH <7.3

11. A man is brought into the emergency department by paramedics who state that he passed out on the street. The man smells of alcohol and when roused says he has not eaten since yesterday. He is wearing a medic alert bracelet that says he is a diabetic. What diagnosis would you suspect?

a. Hypoglycemia

b. Hyperglycemia

c. Hyponatremia

d. Hypernatremia

12. Hypoglycemia has a sudden onset with a progression of symptoms. What are the signs and symptoms of hypoglycemia?

a. Difficulty problem solving and muscle spasms

b. Altered cerebral function and headache

c. Muscle spasms and headache

d. Altered cerebral function and muscle spasms

13. Research has identified a cycle of insulin-induced posthypoglycemic episodes. What is this phenomenon called?

a. Dawn phenomenon

b. Joslin phenomenon

c. Somogyi effect

d. Sunset effect

14. Peripheral neuropathies occur in people with diabetes mellitus. With the loss of sensation in the lower extremities, diabetics become predisposed to what?

a. Denervation of the large muscles of the foot and bunions

b. Displacement of the submetatarsal fat pad posteriorly and hammer toes

c. Impairment of temperature and touch sensations

d. Clawing of toes and denervation of the small muscles of the foot

15. Diabetics are at higher risk than most of the population for injury to organ systems in the body. Which organs are most at risk?

a. Kidneys and eyes

b. Kidneys and liver

c. Liver and eyes

d. Pancreas and eyes

16. Macrovascular disease includes coronary artery disease, cerebrovascular disease, and peripheral vascular disease. People with both type 1 and type 2 diabetes are at high risk for developing macrovascular disease. What are the risk factors for macrovascular disease in diabetics? Mark all that apply.

a. Elevated fibrinogen levels and hyperinsulinemia

b. Hyperlipidemia and hypotension

c. Hyperglycemia and hypoinsulinemia

d. Decreased fibrinogen levels and systemic inflammation

17. Diabetics are hospitalized for a number of reasons. What is the most common complication of diabetes requiring hospitalization?

a. Diabetic ketoacidosis

b. Foot problems

c. Hypertensive crisis

d. Macrovascular disease

18. Infections are common in people with diabetes. Which infection is thought to be related to a neurogenic bladder?

a. Nephrotic syndrome

b. Urinary retention

c. Pyelonephritis

d. Urinary incontinence

Structure and Function of the Male Genitourinary System

SECTION I: LEARNING OBJECTIVES

1. Characterize the embryonic development of the male reproductive organs and genitalia

2. Describe the structure and function of the testes and scrotum, the genital ducts, accessory organs, and penis

3. Describe the process of spermatogenesis

4. State the functions of testosterone

5. Draw a diagram illustrating the secretion, site of action, and feedback control of gonadotropin-releasing hormone, luteinizing hormone, follicle-stimulating hormone and inhibin

6. Describe the function of follicle-stimulating hormone in terms of spermatogenesis

7. Describe the classification and clinical features of male hypogonadism

8. Describe the autonomic and nonautonomic nervous system's control of erection, emission, and ejaculation

9. Describe changes in the male reproductive system that occur with aging

SECTION II: ASSESSING YOUR UNDERSTANDING

Activity A *Fill in the blanks.*

1. The male _____ system is composed of the paired gonads, or testes, genital ducts, accessory organs, and penis.

2. The testicular cells of a male embryo produce an _____, which prevents development of the uterus and fallopian tubes in the male, and testosterone.

3. _____ stimulates the wolffian ducts to develop into the epididymis, vas deferens, and seminal vesicles.

4. After descent of the testes, the _____ closes almost completely.

5. The male _____ consist of the seminal vesicles, the prostate gland, and the bulbourethral glands.

6. The _____ is a fibromuscular and glandular organ lying just inferior to the bladder.

7. _____ refers to the generation of spermatozoa or sperm.

8. _____ is produced and secreted by the interstitial Leydig's cells in the testes.

9. All or almost all of the actions of testosterone and other androgens result from increased _____ in target tissues.

10. The term _____ has been used to describe an ill-defined collection of symptoms in aging men, typically those older than 50 years, who have a relative or absolute hypogonadism associated with aging.

Activity B *Consider the following figures:*

1. In the figure above, locate and label the following structures:

- ampulla
- urethra
- spongy urethra
- membranous urethra
- prostatic urethra
- seminiferous tubules
- epididymis
- ductus deferens
- ejaculatory duct
- prostate gland
- urinary bladder opening
- urinary bladder surface
- seminal vesicle
- testis

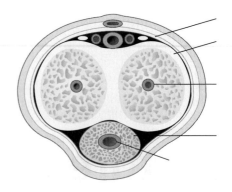

2. In the figure above, locate and label the following structures:

- deep penile fascia
- corpus cavernosum
- central artery
- corpus spongiosum
- urethra

Activity C

Match the key terms in Column A with their definitions in Column B.

Column A

_____ **1.** SRY gene

_____ **2.** Cryptorchidism

_____ **3.** Follicle-stimulating hormone

_____ **4.** Hypogonadism

_____ **5.** Erectile dysfunction

_____ **6.** Ejaculation

_____ **7.** Emission

_____ **8.** Luteinizing hormone

_____ **9.** Corpora cavernosa

_____ **10.** Seminiferous tubules

Column B

a. Expulsion of the sperm from the urethra

b. Sperm move from the epididymis to the urethra

c. Persistent inability to achieve and maintain an erection

d. Androgen deficiency

e. Initiation of spermatogenesis

f. Controls production of testosterone

g. Becomes engorged with blood during erection

h. Site of sperm production

i. Failure of the testes to descend into the scrotum

j. The sex-determining region of the Y chromosome

Activity D *Briefly answer the following:*

1. What are the endocrine changes that occur to stimulate male puberty?

_____

_____

_____

2. Describe the process of spermatogenesis.

_____

_____

_____

3. What are the side effects of excess synthetic androgens?

_____

_____

_____

4. How does the penis become erect?

_____

_____

_____

SECTION III: APPLYING YOUR KNOWLEDGE

Activity E *Consider the following scenario and answer the questions.*

A 35-year-old man comes into the clinic complaining of decreased sexual desire and activity, depression, and fatigue. He states that he and his wife want to conceive, but he has developed erectile dysfunction and, over the last 6 months, he has lost a lot of his body hair. You consider a possible diagnosis of impaired testosterone secretion or hypogonadism.

1. For what tests would you expect to receive an order?

_____

_____

_____

2. The diagnosis of secondary hypogonadism is confirmed. The patient asks what the treatment will be. What would be your correct response?

_____

_____

_____

SECTION IV: PRACTICING FOR NCLEX

Activity F *Answer the following questions.*

1. Sperm production by the testes is optimal at 2°C to 3°C below body temperature. Two systems of the body maintain the temperature of the testes at a level that allows sperm production. What is the system that assists in maintaining the testes at a temperature that allows sperm production?

    a. Pampiniform plexus

    b. Testicular artery

    c. Cremaster veins

    d. Tunica vaginalis

2. Spermatozoa are produced in the seminiferous tubules of the testes and are moved through the genital ducts to be stored in the ampulla of the vas deferens before ejaculation through the penis. Unlike the female egg, which remains briefly fertile, spermatozoa can remain fertile for up to 42 days. Where are the spermatozoa stored so they maintain their fertility?

    a. Vas deferns

    b. Genital ducts

    c. Ampulla

    d. Epididymis

3. The fluid from both the vas deferens and the vagina are acidic. From where do the alkaline secretions that allow mobilization of sperm come?

    a. Vaginal vault

    b. Genital ducts

    c. Prostate

    d. Urethra

4. The penis is a soft, cylindrical shaft that is outside the body. When sexual stimulation occurs the penis becomes firm and elongated due to blood being trapped in what? Mark all that apply.

   a. Corpus spongiosum

   b. Corpora spongiosum

   c. Corpora cavernosa

   d. Corpus cavernosa

   e. Corpus cavernosum

5. Spermatogenesis, or generation of spermatozoa or sperm, begins at approximately 13 years of age and continues as long as a man remains fertile. It is in the seminiferous tubules that spermatogenesis takes place. Of what is the inner lining of the seminiferous tubules composed?

   a. Epididymal cells

   b. Leydig cells

   c. Cowper cells

   d. Sertoli cells

6. The male reproductive system is controlled by the hypothalamus and the anterior pituitary gonadotropic hormones regulated by a negative feedback loop. What gonadotropic hormones regulate control of the male reproductive system?

   a. Follicle-stimulating hormone and luteinizing hormone

   b. Testosterone and antimüllerian hormone

   c. Gonadotropic hormone and follicle-stimulating hormone

   d. Testosterone and luteinizing hormone

7. The practice among some athletes of taking synthetic androgens to improve their performance in their sport can be physiologically harmful. What are the undesired effects of the androgens taken by athletes in supraphysiologic doses? Mark all that apply.

   a. Gynecomastia

   b. Azoospermia

   c. Increased testicular size

   d. Acne

   e. Hypogonadism

8. Sperm begin their life in the Sertoli cells. What factor functions in releasing mature spermatozoa from the Sertoli cells?

   a. Prostate secretions

   b. Plasminogen activator

   c. Testosterone

   d. Androgen-binding protein

9. What can cause erectile dysfunction?

   a. Dysfunction of the pampiniform plexus

   b. Damage to Leydig cells

   c. Dysfunction of pudendal nerves

   d. Damage to the Cowper gland

10. The male reproductive system undergoes changes as aging occurs. What is the term used to describe a relative or absolute hypogonadism associated with aging?

   a. Male menopause

   b. Testosterone deficiency

   c. Atherogenisis

   d. Andropause

CHAPTER 44

Disorders of the Male Genitourinary System

SECTION I: LEARNING OBJECTIVES

1. State the difference between hypospadias and epispadias

2. Cite the significance of phimosis

3. Describe the anatomic changes that occur with Peyronie disease

4. Explain the physiology of penile erection and relate it to erectile dysfunction and priapism

5. Describe the appearance of balanitis xerotica obliterans

6. List the signs of penile cancer

7. State the physical manifestations and potential risks associated with uncorrected cryptorchidism

8. Compare the cause, appearance, and significance of hydrocele, hematocele, spermatocele, and varicocele

9. State the difference between extravaginal and intravaginal testicular torsion

10. Describe the symptoms of epididymitis

11. State the manifestations and possible complications of mumps orchitis

12. Relate environmental factors to development of scrotal cancer

13. State the cell types involved in seminoma, embryonal carcinoma, teratoma, and choriocarcinoma tumors of the testes

14. Compare the pathology and symptoms of acute bacterial prostatitis, chronic bacterial prostatitis, and chronic prostatitis/pelvic pain syndrome

15. Describe the urologic manifestations and treatment of benign prostatic hyperplasia

16. List the methods used in the diagnosis and treatment of prostate cancer

SECTION II: ASSESSING YOUR UNDERSTANDING

Activity A *Fill in the blanks.*

1. _____ and _____ are congenital disorders of the penis resulting from embryologic defects in the development of the urethral groove and penile urethra.

2. _____ involves a localized and progressive fibrosis of unknown origin that affects the tunica albuginea.

3. The manifestations of _____ disease include painful erection, bent erection, and the presence of a hard mass at the site of fibrosis.

4. Erection is under the control of the _____ nervous system, and ejaculation and detumescence (penile relaxation) are under the _____ nervous system control.

5. Parasympathetic stimulation results in release of _____, which causes relaxation of trabecular smooth muscle of the corpora cavernosa, permitting inflow of blood into the sinuses of the cavernosa at pressures approaching those of the _____ system.

6. _____ is commonly classified as psychogenic, organic, or mixed psychogenic and organic.

7. Erectile dysfunction, now recognized as a marker for _____ disease, is now considered a component of the _____ syndrome.

8. _____ is caused by impaired blood flow in the corpora cavernosa of the penis.

9. Several risk factors for _____ have been suggested, including increasing age, poor hygiene, smoking, human papillomavirus infections, ultraviolet radiation exposure, and immunodeficiency states.

10. The consequences of _____ include infertility, malignancy, testicular torsion, and the possible psychological effects of an empty scrotum.

11. Sperm concentration and _____ are decreased in men with varicocele.

12. _____ is an inflammation of the epididymis, the elongated cordlike structure that lies along the posterior border of the testis, whose function is the storage, transport, and maturation of spermatozoa.

13. _____ refers to a variety of inflammatory disorders of the prostate gland, some bacterial and some not.

14. The manifestations of _____ include fever and chills, malaise, myalgia, arthralgia, frequent and urgent urination, dysuria, and urethral discharge.

15. As with other cancers, it appears that the development of _____ cancer is a multi-step process involving genes that control cell differentiation and growth.

16. Men with _____ typically have recurrent urinary tract infections with persistence of the same strain of pathogenic bacteria in prostatic fluid and urine.

17. The cause of noninflammatory prostatitis is unknown, but because of the absence of inflammation, the search for the cause of symptoms has been directed toward _____ sources.

18. The level of _____ correlates with the volume and stage of prostate cancer.

Activity B *Consider the following figure:*

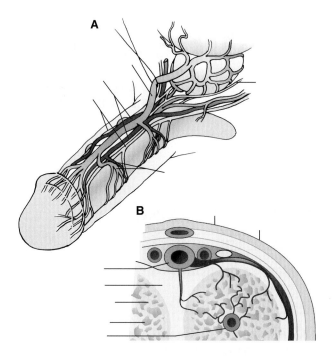

In the figure above, locate and label the structures responsible for penile erection:

- deep dorsal vein
- tunica albuginea
- corpora cavernosa
- cavernous artery
- sinusoidal spaces
- circumflex vein
- circumflex artery
- cavernous nerve
- dorsal nerve
- dorsal artery
- subtunical venular plexus

Activity C *Match the key terms in Column A with their definitions in Column B.*

Column A	Column B
____ **1.** Balanitis	**a.** Inflammation of the glans penis
____ **2.** Smegma	**b.** Undescended testes
____ **3.** Epispadias	**c.** Accumulation under the phimotic foreskin
____ **4.** Hydrocele	

_____ **5.** Cryptorchidism

_____ **6.** Orchitis

_____ **7.** Prostatitis

_____ **8.** Benign prostatic hyperplasia

_____ **9.** Phimosis

_____ **10.** Priapism

d. Excess fluid collects between the layers of the tunica vaginalis

e. Infection of the testes

f. Inflammation of the prostate

g. Tightening of the penile foreskin

h. Opening of the urethra is on the dorsal surface of the penis

i. Involuntary, prolonged, abnormal, and painful erection

j. An age-related, non-malignant enlargement of the prostate gland

Activity D _Briefly answer the following questions._

1. What are some of the known causes of erectile dysfunction?

_____

_____

_____

2. How do drugs like Viagra treat erectile dysfunction?

_____

_____

_____

3. What is testicular torsion? What are the different types?

_____

_____

_____

4. How are testicular cancers staged?

_____

_____

_____

5. How does benign prostatic hyperplasia cause obstruction of the urethra?

_____

_____

_____

6. How is prostate cancer diagnosed?

_____

_____

_____

SECTION III: APPLYING YOUR KNOWLEDGE

Activity E _Consider the following scenario and answer the questions._

A 50-year-old man presents at the clinic complaining of a lump on his penis that has progressed over the past 4 months until he can no longer retract the foreskin over his glans. He states the condition is now painful. He is having difficulty urinating, and a discharge is coming from under his foreskin. He is scheduled for surgery the following day to relieve the phimosis and biopsy the lump. The physician explains the surgery to him and states that, if the lump is malignant, a partial or total penectomy may be necessary.

1. Before the patient leaves, he asks you what causes penile cancer. You correctly respond:

_____

_____

_____

2. The patient is admitted to your unit after having a total penectomy for penile cancer with inguinal lymph node involvement. While caring for him, the client asks you what his prognosis is. What would be your correct response to him?

_____

_____

_____

SECTION IV: PRACTICING FOR NCLEX

Activity F _Answer the following questions._

1. In hypospadias, the treatment of choice is surgery to repair the defect. What influences the timing of the surgical repair? Mark all that apply.

a. Penile size

b. Testicular involvement

c. Psychological effects on a child

d. Presence of an abdominal hernia

e. Anesthetic risk

2. A 75-year-old man presents at the clinic complaining of pain during intercourse and an upward bowing of his penis during erection. His history includes an inflammation of the penis that was treated 3 months ago. The physician's physical examination of him notes beads of scar tissue along the dorsal midline of the penile shaft. What would be the suggested diagnosis for this patient?

a. Peyronie disease

b. Cavernosa disease

c. Balanitic disease

d. Paraphimosic disease

3. Priaprism (a prolonged painful erection not associated with sexual excitement) can occur at any age. In boys, ages 5 to 10 years, what are the most common causes of priapism?

a. Neoplasms or hemophilia

b. Sickle cell disease or neoplasms

c. Hemophilia or sickle cell disease

d. Hypospadias or neoplasms

4. Cryptorchidism, left untreated, is a high risk for testicular cancer and infertility. What are the treatment goals for boys with cryptorchidism?

a. Prevention of testicular cancer

b. Prevention of an associated inguinal hernia

c. Easier cancer detection

d. Decreased fertility

5. The mother of a 5-year-old boy brings him into the clinic because of a firm swelling around one of his testes. What diagnosis is suggested?

a. Peyronie disease

b. Cryptorchidism

c. Priapism

d. Hydrocele

6. In the neonatal and pediatric population, there can be many physiologic problems with the male genitourinary system. What is the most common acute scrotal disorder in the pediatric population?

a. Testicular torsion

b. Hypospadias

c. Balanitis

d. Paraphimosis

7. Epididymitis can be sexually transmitted, or it can be caused by a variety of other reasons, including abnormalities in the genitourinary tract. What are the most common causes of epididymitis in young men without underlying genitourinary disease?

a. *Chlamydia trachomatis* and *Candida albicans*

b. *Chlamydia trachomatis* and *Neisseria gonorrhoeae*

c. *Escherichia coli* and *Neisseria gonorrhoeae*

d. *Candida albicans* and *Escherichia coli*

8. Testicular cancer is highly curable if found and treated early. What are signs of metastatic spread of testicular cancer? Mark all that apply.

a. Hemoptysis

b. Back pain

c. Neck mass

d. Chest mass

e. Hoarse voice

9. A 40-year-old man presents at the clinic complaining of painful urination and rectal pain. His vital signs are as follows: temperature 101.7°F; blood pressure 105/74 mm Hg; pulse 98; respiratory rate 22. While taking a history, you note that the patient has had chills, malaise, and myalgia. What would you suspect as a diagnosis?

a. Benign prostatic hyperplasia

b. Epididymitis

c. Acute bacterial prostatitis

d. Orchitis

10. Although the cause of benign prostatic hyperplasia (BPH) is unknown, its incidence increases with age. In which ethnic group is BPH highest?

a. Japanese

b. Caucasian

c. Native American

d. African American

CHAPTER 45

Structure and Function of the Female Reproductive System

SECTION I: LEARNING OBJECTIVES

1. Describe the anatomic relationship of the structures of the external genitalia

2. Name the three layers of the uterus and describe their function

3. Cite the location of the ovaries in relation to the uterus, fallopian tubes, broad ligaments, and ovarian ligaments

4. Explain the function of the fallopian tubes

5. State the function of endocervical secretions

6. Describe the feedback control of estrogen and progesterone levels by means of gonadotropin-releasing hormone, LH, FSH, and ovarian follicle function

7. List the actions of estrogen and progesterone

8. Describe the four functional compartments of the ovary

9. Relate FSH and LH levels to the stages of follicle development and to estrogen and progesterone production

10. Describe the endometrial changes that occur during the menstrual cycle

11. Describe the composition of normal cervical mucus and the changes that occur during the menstrual cycle

12. Describe the physiology of normal menopause

13. Describe the anatomy of the female breast

14. Describe the influence of hormones on breast development

15. Characterize the changes in breast structure that occur with pregnancy and lactation

SECTION II: ASSESSING YOUR UNDERSTANDING

Activity A *Fill in the blanks.*

1. The _____ is a rounded, skin-covered fat pad located anterior to the symphysis pubis.

2. The _____ are analogous to the male scrotum.

3. The _____ begin anteriorly at the hood of the clitoris and end posteriorly at the base of the vagina.

4. The female _____ is an erectile organ, rich in vascular and nervous supply.

5. The _____ functions as a route for discharge of menses and other secretions.

6. The _____ is a thick-walled muscular organ, located between the bladder and the rectum.

7. The uterus is supported on both sides by four sets of ligaments: the _____ ligaments, which run laterally from the body of the uterus to the pelvic sidewalls; the _____ ligaments, which run from the fundus laterally into each labium majus; the _____ ligaments, which run from the uterocervical junction to the sacrum; and the _____ cervical ligaments.

8. The _____ forms the major portion of the uterine wall.

9. The superficial layer of the _____ is shed during menstruation and regenerated by cells of the basal layer.

10. The end of the _____ nearest the ovary forms a funnel-like opening with fringed, finger-like projections, called fimbriae, which pick up the ovum after its release into the peritoneal cavity after ovulation.

11. The ovaries have a dual function: they store the female germ cells, or ova, and produce the female sex hormones, _____ and _____.

12. Growth, prepubertal maturation, the reproductive cycle, and sex hormone secretion are regulated by _____ and _____ from the anterior pituitary gland.

13. The steroid _____ hormones enter cells by passive diffusion, bind to specific receptor proteins in the cytoplasm, and then move to the nucleus, where they bind to specific sites on the chromosomes.

14. Androgens can be converted to estrogens peripherally, especially in _____.

15. Observational studies indicate a possible preventative role of estrogen in the development of Alzheimer disease through _____ mechanisms to prevent vascular injury, increased cerebral blood flow, and altered brain activation.

16. The corpus luteum of the ovary secretes large amounts of _____ after ovulation.

17. The local effects of progesterone on reproductive organs include the glandular development of the lobular and alveolar tissue of the breasts and the cyclic glandular development of the _____.

18. As estrogen suppresses FSH, the actions of LH predominate, and the mature follicle bursts; the _____, with the corona radiata, is ejected from the follicle.

19. If fertilization does not take place, the corpus luteum atrophies and is replaced by white scar tissue called the _____; the hormonal support of the endometrium is withdrawn and _____ occurs.

20. In the event of fertilization, _____ is produced by the trophoblastic cells in the blastocyst and prevents luteal regression.

21. The functional layer of the _____ arises from the basal layer and undergoes proliferative changes and menstrual sloughing.

22. The absence of _____ of cervical mucus can indicate inadequate estrogen stimulation of the endocervical glands or inhibition of the endocervical glands by increased secretion of progesterone.

23. _____ results from the gradual cessation of ovarian function and the resultant diminished levels of estrogen.

24. Problems that can arise from menopause are a result of _____ and include vaginal dryness, urinary stress incontinence, urgency, nocturia, vaginitis, and urinary tract infection.

25. Consequences of long-term estrogen deprivation include _____ due to an imbalance in bone remodeling, and an increased risk for _____ disease, which is the leading cause of death for women after menopause.

26. The _____ are specialized glandular structures that have an abundant shared nervous, vascular, and lymphatic supply.

27. _____ stimulates increased vascularity of the breasts and the growth and extension of the ductile structures, causing "heaviness" of the breasts.

28. _____ causes marked budding and growth of the alveolar structures.

Activity B *Consider the following figures:*

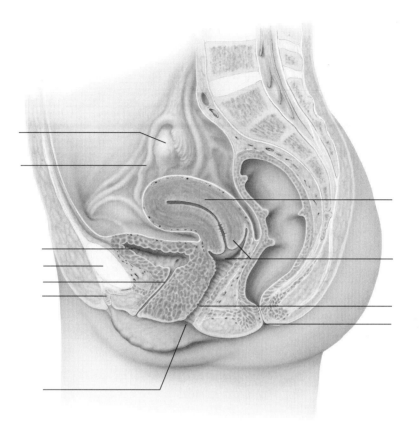

1. In the figure above, locate and label the following structures of the female reproductive system:

- uterus
- cervix
- vagina
- vaginal orifice
- anus

- fallopian tube
- ovary
- urinary bladder
- pubic symphysis
- clitoris
- urethra

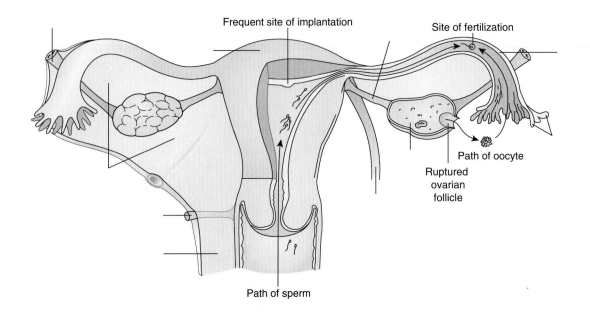

Frequent site of implantation

Site of fertilization

Path of oocyte

Ruptured ovarian follicle

Path of sperm

2. In the figure above, locate and label the following structures of female reproductive organs:

- ovary
- uterine tube
- fimbriae
- ovarian ligament
- fundus
- suspensory ligament of ovary
- broad ligament
- uterosacral ligament
- cardinal ligament
- round ligament of uterus

g. Hormone that stimulates lactation in the postpartum period

h. Tissue located posterior to the vaginal opening and anterior to the anus

i. Glands at urethral opening with lubricating function

j. First menstrual bleeding

Activity C *Match the key terms in Column A with their definitions in Column B.*

Column A

_____ **1.** Oogenesis

_____ **2.** Menarche

_____ **3.** Dyspareunia

_____ **4.** Perineal body

_____ **5.** Spinnbarkeit

_____ **6.** Prolactin

_____ **7.** Skene glands

_____ **8.** Menopause

_____ **9.** Dysmenorrhea

_____ **10.** Montgomery tubercles

Column B

a. Technique to examine properties of cervical mucus

b. Cessation of menstrual cycles

c. Painful intercourse

d. Pain accompanying the contractions associated with menses

e. Sebaceous glands that keep the nipple area soft and elastic

f. Generation of ova by mitotic division

Activity D *Briefly answer the following.*

1. How and why is the vagina kept at an acidic pH?

_____

_____

_____

2. What relationship is there between body composition and a normal menstrual cycle?

_____

_____

_____

3. What is the cardioprotective effect of estrogen?

_____

_____

_____

4. What is the normal role of estrogen in female development?

_____

_____

_____

5. What were the posited benefits of hormone replacement therapy? How has it been shown to be incorrect?

_____

_____

_____

6. How does lactation occur?

_____

_____

_____

SECTION III: APPLYING YOUR KNOWLEDGE

Activity E *Consider the following scenario and answer the questions.*

A 55-year-old woman has just been told by her physician that she is going through menopause. The physician discusses with her the adverse effects menopause can have on a woman's body and explains that most of these effects are caused by a significant decrease in the estrogen level of estrogen in her body. After leaving the clinic, the patient calls back and, speaking with you, asks about hormone replacement therapy.

1. What information about hormone therapy (HT) would you tell her?

_____

_____

_____

2. The patient asks if HT can reverse the symptoms of aging (e.g., decrease in body hair and subcutaneous fat) in her body? You would know that the best response is what?

_____

_____

_____

SECTION IV: PRACTICING FOR NCLEX

Activity F *Answer the following questions.*

1. The female external genitalia are made up of several components. What is in the vestibule of the female external genitalia?

  a. Bartholin glands

  b. Skene glands

  c. Cowper glands

  d. Bulbourethral glands

2. Estrogen stimulates the vaginal wall to thicken and increase the secretion of glycogen. What causes the glycogen in the vagina to ferment to lactic acid?

  a. *Escherichia coli*

  b. Döderlein's bacilli

  c. *Candida albicans*

  d. *Staphylococcus aureus*

3. The perimetrium reflects over the bladder wall and forms what?

  a. Opening to fallopian tubes

  b. The external cervical os

  c. The pouch of Douglas

  d. Bartholin's pouch

4. The fallopian tubes are narrow tubes that attach bilaterally to the uterus. Within the fallopian tube, fertilization of the ovum takes place. The end of the fallopian tube nearest the ovary is funnel-like. What are the fringed, fingerlike projections around the funnel-shaped opening of the fallopian tube called?

  a. Fallopian fingers

  b. Oviducts

  c. Cilia

  d. Fimbriae

5. The ovarian follicle becomes luteinized once ovulation has taken place. As the corpus luteum, the now empty follicle produces what?

   a. Estrogen and progesterone

   b. Follicle-stimulating hormone and luteinizing hormone

   c. Testosterone and estrogen

   d. Glycogen and testosterone

6. The ovaries secrete both estrogen and progesterone. What is one function of progesterone in the body?

   a. Causes moderate retention of sodium and water

   b. Increases body temperature at ovulation

   c. Reduces levels or rennin

   d. Enhances the coagulability of blood

7. Follicle-stimulating hormone (FSH) and luteinizing hormone (LH) produce profound effects on the ovaries. What do high levels of estrogen do to FSH and LH?

   a. ↑FSH and ↓LH

   b. ↑LH and ↓estradiol

   c. ↑ LH and ↓ FSH

   d. ↑ FSH and ↓ renin

8. Menopause signals the end of the menstrual cycle. It is caused by the end of ovarian function and the decreased levels of estrogen this brings to the body. What are problems that can arise from the onset of menopause? Mark all that apply.

   a. Nocturia

   b. Urinary stress incontinence

   c. Upper respiratory infection

   d. Vaginitis

   e. Urinary retention

9. What are the small bumps or projections on the areolar surface called?

   a. Cowper cells

   b. Bartholin gland

   c. Climacteric glands

   d. Montgomery tubercles

10. Lactation occurs under the control of the anterior pituitary hormone prolactin. What causes the ejection of milk from the ductile system in the breast?

    a. Oxytocin

    b. Prolactin

    c. Estrogen

    d. Progesterone

CHAPTER 46

Disorders of the Female Reproductive System

SECTION I: LEARNING OBJECTIVES

1. Compare the abnormalities associated with Bartholin cyst, non-neoplastic epithelial disorders, vulvodynia, and cancer of the vulva

2. State the role of Döderlein bacilli in maintaining the normal ecology of the vagina

3. Describe the conditions that predispose to vaginal infections and the methods used to prevent and treat these infections

4. Describe the importance of the cervical transformation zone in the pathogenesis of cervical cancer

5. Compare the lesions associated with nabothian cysts and cervical polyps

6. List the complications of untreated cervicitis

7. Describe the development of cervical cancer from the appearance of atypical cells to the development of invasive cervical cancer and relate to the importance of the Pap smear in early detection of cervical cancer

8. Cite the rationale for describing cervical cancer as a sexually transmitted infection and the rationale for use of the HPV vaccine in prevention of cervical cancer

9. Compare the pathology and manifestations of endometriosis and adenomyosis

10. Cite the major early symptom of endometrial cancer and describe the relationship between unopposed estrogen stimulation of the endometrium and development of endometrial cancer

11. Compare the location and manifestations of intramural and subserosal leiomyomas

12. List the common causes and symptoms of pelvic inflammatory disease

13. Describe the risk factors and symptoms of ectopic pregnancy

14. State the underlying cause of ovarian cysts

15. Differentiate benign ovarian cyst from polycystic ovary syndrome

16. List the hormones produced by the three types of functioning ovarian tumors

17. State the reason that ovarian cancer may be difficult to detect in an early stage

18. Characterize the function of the supporting ligaments and pelvic floor muscles in maintaining the position of the pelvic organs, including the uterus, bladder, and rectum

19. Describe the manifestations of cystocele, rectocele, and enterocele

20. Explain how uterine anteflexion, retroflexion, and retroversion differ from normal uterine position

21. Describe the cause and manifestations of uterine prolapse

22. Define the terms amenorrhea, hypomenor-
rhea, oligomenorrhea, menorrhagia, metror-
rhagia, and menometrorrhagia

23. Relate the alteration in estrogen and progesterone levels to the development of dysfunctional menstrual cycles

24. Differentiate between primary dysmenorrhea
and secondary dysmenorrhea

25. Characterize the manifestations of the pre-
menstrual syndrome, its possible causes, and
the methods of treatment

26. Describe changes in breast function that
occur with galactorrhea, mastitis, and ductal
ectasia

27. Describe the manifestations of fibrocystic
breast changes

28. Cite the risk factors for breast cancer, the importance of clinical breast examination, and
recommendations for mammography

29. Describe the methods used in the diagnosis
and treatment of breast cancer

30. Provide a definition of infertility

31. List male and female factors that contribute
to infertility

32. Briefly describe methods used in the treatment of infertility

SECTION II: ASSESSING YOUR UNDERSTANDING

Activity A *Fill in the blanks.*

1. Diseases of the external genitalia are similar
to those that affect _____ skin elsewhere in the body.

2. The _____ is particularly susceptible to
skin infections because it is constantly being
exposed to secretions and moisture.

3. A _____ is a fluid-filled sac that results
from occlusion of the duct system in
Bartholin's gland.

4. _____ presents as thickened, gray-
white plaques with an irregular surface.

5. The normal vaginal _____ depends on
the delicate balance of hormones and bacterial flora.

6. _____ represents an inflammation of
the vagina that is characterized by vaginal
discharge and burning, itching, redness, and
swelling of vaginal tissues.

7. The most common symptom of vaginal carcinoma is abnormal _____.

8. During _____, the newly developed
squamous epithelial cells of the cervix are
vulnerable to development of dysplasia
and genetic change if exposed to cancer-
producing agents.

9. _____ cancer is readily detected and, if
detected early, is the most easily cured of all
the cancers of the female reproductive
system.

10. Untreated _____ may extend to include the development of pelvic cellulitis, low
back pain, dyspareunia, cervical stenosis, dysmenorrhea, and ascending infection of the
uterus or fallopian tubes.

11. _____ are the most common lesions of
the cervix.

12. A preponderance of evidence suggests a
causal link between _____ infection
and cervical cancer.

13. _____ is the condition in which functional endometrial tissue is found in ectopic
sites outside the uterus.

14. _____ is the condition in which endometrial glands and stroma are found
within the myometrium, interspersed between the smooth muscle fibers.

15. _____ and _____, which con-
sists of dilating the cervix and scraping the
uterine cavity, is the definitive procedure for
diagnosis of endometrial cancer because it
provides a more thorough evaluation.

16. Uterine _____ are benign neoplasms of
smooth muscle origin.

17. _____ is a polymicrobial infection of
the upper reproductive tract associated with
sexually transmitted and endogenous organisms.

18. _____ occurs when a fertilized ovum
implants outside the uterine cavity, the most
common site being the fallopian tube.

19. Disorders of the ovaries frequently cause
_____ and _____ problems.

20. _____ syndrome is characterized by varying degrees of menstrual irregularity, signs of hyperandrogenism, and infertility.

21. Most women with polycystic ovary syndrome (PCOS) have elevated _____ levels with normal estrogen and follicle-stimulating hormone (FSH) production.

22. _____ tumors are common, most are benign, but malignant tumors are the leading cause of death from reproductive cancers.

23. The most significant risk factor for ovarian cancer appears to be _____ —the length of time during a woman's life when her ovarian cycle is not suppressed by pregnancy, lactation, or oral contraceptive use.

24. The breast cancer susceptibility genes, *BRACA1* and *BRCA2*, which are _____ genes are incriminated in approximately 10% of hereditary ovarian cancers despite being identified as breast cancer genes.

25. _____ is the herniation of the rectum into the vagina.

26. Uterine prolapse is the bulging of the uterus into the vagina that occurs when the _____ ligaments are stretched.

27. Removal of the uterus through the vagina with appropriate repair of the vaginal wall often is done when _____ is accompanied by cystocele or rectocele.

28. Primary _____ is the failure to menstruate by 15 years of age or by 13 years of age if failure to menstruate is accompanied by absence of secondary sex characteristics.

29. _____ is the secretion of breast milk in a nonlactating breast.

30. _____ is inflammation of the breast.

31. _____ are firm, rubbery, sharply defined round masses in breast tissue.

32. _____ changes usually present as nodular granular breast masses that are more prominent and painful during the luteal or progesterone-dominant portion of the menstrual cycle.

33. _____ disease presents as an eczemoid lesion of the nipple and areola.

34. _____ is the inability to conceive a child after 1 year of unprotected intercourse.

Activity B *Consider the following figure:*

In the figure above, locate and label all the common locations of endometriosis within the pelvis and abdomen.

Activity C *Match the key terms in Column A with their definitions in Column B.*

1.

Column A	Column B
____ 1. Papanicolaou smear	a. Insertion of radioactive materials into the body
____ 2. Menorrhagia	b. Commonly called fibroids
____ 3. Vulvodynia	c. Unexplained vulvar pain
____ 4. Leiomyomas	d. Herniation of the bladder into the vagina
____ 5. Cystocele	e. Inflammation of the vagina that occurs after menopause
____ 6. Curettage	f. Surgical procedure used to scrape out the surface of the endometrium
____ 7. Atrophic vaginitis	g. Inflammation of the cervix
____ 8. Lichen sclerosus	h. Excessive menstrual bleeding
____ 9. Brachytherapy	
____ 10. Cervicitis	

i. Vaginal cytology to detect vaginal or cervical cancer

j. Inflammatory disease of the vulva

2.

Column A	Column B
____ **1.** Amenorrhea	**a.** Frequent menstruation
____ **2.** Hypo-menorrhea	**b.** Infrequent menstruation
____ **3.** Oligo-menorrhea	**c.** Bleeding between periods
____ **4.** Poly-menorrhea	**d.** Absence of menstruation
____ **5.** Menorrhagia	**e.** Heavy bleeding during and between menstrual periods
____ **6.** Metrorrhagia	**f.** Scanty menstruation
____ **7.** Meno-metrorrhagia	**g.** Excessive menstruation

Activity D *Briefly answer the following.*

1. What measures should be taken to avoid vaginal infections?

_____

_____

_____

2. What is the only approved vaccine for cervical cancer and how does it work?

_____

_____

_____

3. What is the normal method of detecting/diagnosis cervical cancer?

_____

_____

_____

4. What are the three most prominent theories of the pathogenesis of endometriosis?

_____

_____

_____

5. What is the mechanism of infection in pelvic inflammatory disease?

_____

_____

_____

6. Why should you be concerned about the future of your patient with polycystic ovarian syndrome?

_____

_____

_____

7. Describe the functional anatomy of normal pelvic support.

_____

_____

_____

8. Describe the alterations in a normal period and name the hormone thought to be responsible.

_____

_____

_____

9. What is the genetic component of breast cancer?

_____

_____

_____

SECTION III: APPLYING YOUR KNOWLEDGE

Activity E *Consider the following scenario and answer the questions.*

A 23-year-old woman is being seen in her physician's office as a follow-up to an abnormal Papanicolaou smear. The physician tells the patient that she may have cervical cancer, and he wants to do a colposcopy so he can diagnose and treat any lesions he may find. The patient gives her consent.

1. While preparing the patient for the procedure, she asks you for an explanation of the colposcopy and the reason it is being done. How would you correctly respond?

_____

_____

_____

2. The colposcopy shows dysplastic lesions, and the physician wants to do a large loop electro-surgical excision procedure (LEEP) of the transformation zone. The patient gives her consent, but wants to know what this proce-dure is. How would you explain the procedure to the patient?

_____

_____

_____

SECTION IV: PRACTICING FOR NCLEX

Activity F *Answer the following questions.*

1. Bartholin gland obstruction of the ductal sys-tem will cause a cyst. Sometimes the cyst be-comes infected and an abscess occurs. What is the surgical procedure to remove a Bartholin cyst or abscess when a wedge of vulvar skin is removed along with the cyst wall?

   a. Marsupialization

   b. Vulvectomy

   c. Bartholectomy

   d. Incision and drainage

2. There are two types of vulvar cancer. One type is found in older women, and one type is found in younger women, generally younger than 40 years of age. The type found in younger women thought to be caused by which of the following?

   a. Multiple sexual partners

   b. Human papillomavirus (HPV)

   c. Nonsquamous cell lesions

   d. Lichen sclerotic lesions

3. Vaginal infections can occur in young girls before menarche. These infections generally have nonspecific causes. What are some of the causes of vaginal infections in premenar-chal girls? Mark all that apply.

   a. Presence of foreign bodies

   b. Intestinal parasites

   c. Poor hygiene

   d. Vaginal deodorants

   e. Tampon

4. The endocervix is covered with large-branched mucous secreting glands. During the menstrual cycle, they undergo functional changes, and the amount and properties of the mucus that they secret varies according to the stage of the cycle. When one of these glands gets blocked, what kind of cyst forms within the cervix?

   a. Bartholin cysts

   b. Bulbouretheral cysts

   c. Nabothian cysts

   d. Metaplastic cysts

5. Endometriosis is the condition where en-dometrial tissue is found growing outside of the uterus in the pelvic cavity. What are risk factors for endometriosis?

   a. Late menarche and regular periods with longer cycles than 27 days

   b. Early menarche and lighter flow

   c. Increased menstrual pain and periods of shorter than 7 days

   d. Periods longer than 7 days and increased menstrual pain

6. Leiomyomas, or intrauterine fibroids, are the most common form of pelvic tumor. Approximately half the time leiomyomas are asymptomatic. What are the symptoms of leiomyomas that are not asymptomatic?

   a. Anemia and urinary frequency

   b. Diarrhea and rectal pressure

   c. Menorrhagia and urinary retention

   d. Abdominal distention and diarrhea

7. An 18-year-old woman presents at the clinic complaining new-onset breakthrough bleed-ing, even though she is on contraceptives. What contraceptive use, along with new-onset breakthrough bleeding, has been associ-ated with pelvic inflammatory disease.

   a. Intrauterine device

   b. Depo-Provera

   c. Spermicidal foam

   d. Diaphragm

8. Ectopic pregnancies are true gynecologic emergencies and are considered the leading cause of maternal death in the first trimester.

What diagnostic test would you expect to have ordered for a suspected ectopic pregnancy?

a. Transvaginal ultrasound if pregnancy is <5 weeks' gestation

b. Serial β-human chorionic gonadotropin (hCG) with higher than normal hCG production

c. Ultrasonography followed by serial hCG tests

d. Amniocentesis

9. Polycystic ovary syndrome is an endocrine disorder and a common cause of chronic anovulation. In addition to the clinical manifestations of PCOS, long-term health problems, including cardiovascular disease and diabetes, have been linked to PCOS. What drug has emerged as an important part of PCOS treatment?

a. Dehydroepiandrosterone

b. Methotrexate

c. Mineralocorticoids

d. Metformin

10. Ovarian cancer, once thought to be asymptomatic, has now been shown to produce nonspecific symptoms, which makes the diagnosis of ovarian cancer difficult. What symptoms are believed to have a strong association to ovarian cancer? Mark all that apply.

a. Difficulty eating

b. Increased intestinal gas

c. Bloating

d. Increased appetite

e. Abdominal or pelvic pain

11. Uterine prolapse is a disorder of pelvic support and uterine position. It can range in severity from a slight descent of the uterus into the vagina, all the way to the entire uterus protruding through the vaginal opening. In women who want to have children or in older women who are at significant risk if surgery is performed, what device is inserted to hold the uterus in place?

a. A pessary

b. A Colpexin sphere

c. A vesicourethral suspenser

d. A retroversion inducer

12. In primary dysmenorrheal when contraception is not desired, what is the treatment of choice?

a. Aspirin

b. Ibuprofen

c. Acetaminophen

d. Metformic acid

13. Mastitis is an inflammation of the breast that can occur at any time. What is the treatment for mastitis?

a. Opioid analgesics

b. Nonsteroidal anti-inflammatory drugs

c. Application of heat or cold

d. Tylenol 3

14. Fibrocystic changes in the breast are not uncommon. How is the diagnosis of fibrocystic changes made?

a. Physical examination and client history

b. Galactography and biopsy

c. Mammography and galactography

d. Ultrasonography and mammography

15. Cancer of the breast is the most common cancer in women. Many breast cancers are found by women themselves while doing breast self-examination. When should postmenopausal women perform breast self-examination?

a. Any day of the month

b. 2 days following menses

c. On the first day of every month

d. On the 15th of every month

16. The causes of infertility can be in either the male or the female. Male tests for infertility require a specimen of ejaculate that is collected when?

a. Any time

b. After 3 days of abstinence

c. After 3 consecutive days of intercourse

d. After 3 weeks of abstinence

17. Couples who are being treated for infertility often choose to try in vitro fertilization (IVF). When using this technique, the eggs are inseminated with sperm in a culture dish. After a period of time, the ova are evaluated for signs of fertilization. If signs of fertilization are present, when are the fertilized eggs placed in the woman's uterus?

a. 12 to 24 hours after egg retrieval

b. 36 to 48 hours after egg retrieval

c. 48 to 72 hours after egg retrieval

d. 24 to 36 hours after egg retrieval

CHAPTER 47

Sexually Transmitted Infections

SECTION I: LEARNING OBJECTIVES

1. Define what is meant by a sexually transmitted infection (STI)

2. List common portals of entry for STIs

3. Name the organisms responsible for condylomata acuminata, genital herpes, molluscum contagiosum, chancroid, granuloma inguinale, and lymphogranuloma venereum

4. State the significance of being infected with high-risk strains of the human papillomavirus

5. Explain the pathogenesis of recurrent genital herpes infections

6. State the difference between wet-mount slide and culture methods of diagnosis of STIs

7. Compare the signs and symptoms of infections caused by *Candida albicans*, *Trichomonas vaginalis*, and bacterial vaginosis

8. Compare the signs and symptoms of gonorrhea in the male and female

9. Describe the three stages of syphilis

10. State the genital and nongenital complications that can occur with chlamydial infections, gonorrhea, and syphilis

11. State the treatment for chlamydial urogenital infections, gonorrhea, nonspecific urogenital infections, and syphilis

SECTION II: ASSESSING YOUR UNDERSTANDING

Activity A *Fill in the blanks.*

1. STIs can selectively infect the _____ tissues of the external genitalia, primarily cause vaginitis in women, or they can produce both genitourinary and systemic effects.

2. STIs can be transmitted by an infected mother to a _____, causing congenital defects or death of the child.

3. _____ are caused by the human papillomavirus (HPV).

4. Genital warts typically present as soft, raised, fleshy lesions on the _____, including the penis, vulva, scrotum, perineum, and perianal skin.

5. _____ is one of the most common causes of genital ulcers in patients in the United States.

6. Herpes simplex virus type-1 and herpes simplex virus type-2 are _____ viruses, meaning that they grow in neurons and share the biologic property of latency.

7. Herpes simplex virus _____ is responsible for greater than 90% of recurrent genital herpes infections.

8. The initial symptoms of _____ infections include tingling, itching, and pain in the genital area, followed by eruption of small pustules and vesicles.

9. _____ is a common viral disease of the skin that gives rise to multiple umbilicated papules.

10. *Candida albicans* is the most commonly identified organism in vaginal _____ infections, but other *Candida* species, such as *Candida glabrata* and *Candida tropicalis* may also be present.

11. _____ can reside in the paraurethral glands of both sexes.

12. _____ vaginosis is the most prevalent form of vaginal infection seen by health care professionals.

13. _____ exist in two forms: elementary bodies, which are the infectious particles capable of entering uninfected cells, and the initiator or reticulate bodies, which multiply by binary fission to produce the inclusions identified in stained cells.

14. Untreated chlamydial infection results in _____ damage in female patients.

15. The _____ is a pyogenic (i.e., pus-forming) gram-negative diplococcus that evokes inflammatory reactions characterized by purulent exudates.

16. _____ is spread by direct contact with an infectious moist lesion, usually through sexual intercourse.

Activity B *Match the key terms in Column A with their definitions in Column B.*

Column A

____ 1. *Granuloma inguinale*

____ 2. *Condylomata cuminata*

____ 3. *Trichomonas vaginalis*

____ 4. Chancroid

____ 5. *Treponema pallidum*

____ 6. Candidiasis

____ 7. *Chlamydia trachomatis*

____ 8. *Lymphogranuloma venereum*

____ 9. Donovan bodies

____ 10. Döderlein cytolysis

Column B

a. Anaerobic protozoan that can be transmitted sexually

b. Development of large, tender, and sometimes fluctuant inguinal lymph nodes called buboes

c. Excess of lactobacilli

d. Disease of the external genitalia and lymph nodes

e. Large mononuclear cells filled with intracytoplasmic gram-negative rods

f. Yeast infection

g. Spirochete responsible for syphilitic infection

h. Genital warts

i. Obligate intracellular bacterial pathogen that resembles a virus but, as does bacteria, has RNA and DNA and is susceptible to some antibiotics.

j. In late stages, it is associated with the development of enlarged and elephantoid external genitalia

Activity C *Briefly answer the following.*

1. What are the risk factors for acquiring the human papillomavirus (HPV) and how is it spread?

_____

_____

_____

2. How do herpes simplex virus (HSV)-1 and HSV-2 spread, and where do they reside in the body?

_____

_____

_____

3. What are the risk factors for developing a candidiasis infection?

_____

_____

_____

4. What are the potential complications of trichomoniasis in male and female patients?

_____

_____

_____

5. What are the sex-specific manifestations of gonorrhea?

_____

_____

_____

6. What is the clinical course of syphilis?

_____

_____

_____

SECTION III: APPLYING YOUR KNOWLEDGE

Activity D _Consider the following scenario and answer the questions._

A 35-year-old man presents at the clinic complaining of painful joints of the left leg and pain on urination. Also noted are mucocutaneous lesions on the palms of his hands.

1. What would be important for you to note while taking a nursing history?

_____

_____

_____

2. The patient is diagnosed with a chlamydial infection complicated by Reiter syndrome. What would be the expected treatment for this patient?

_____

_____

_____

SECTION IV: PRACTICING FOR NCLEX

Activity E _Answer the following questions._

1. After inoculation with human papilloma virus (HPV), genital warts may begin to grow. They usually manifest as soft, raised fleshy lesions on the external genitalia of either a male or female patient. What is the incubation period for HPV-induced genital warts?

   a. 6 weeks to 8 months

   b. 6 weeks to 8 weeks

   c. 6 months to 8 months

   d. 6 days to 8 days

2. Primary genital herpes is a sexually transmitted infection (STI) caused by either the herpes simplex virus type 1 (HSV-1) or the herpes simplex virus type 2 (HSV-2). What are the initial symptoms of primary genital herpes infections? Mark all that apply.

   a. Itching

   b. Chancres

   c. Genital pain

   d. Eczemalike lesions

   e. Small pustules

3. There is no known cure for genital herpes and methods of treatment are often symptomatic. Pharmacologic treatment of genital herpes includes which drugs?

   a. Zidovudine

   b. Famciclovir

   c. Nonsteroidal anti-inflammatory drugs

   d. Topical corticosteroid compounds

4. Chancroid or soft chancre is a highly contagious STI usually found in the Southeast Asian and North African populations. What is the recommended treatment for chancroid?

   a. Tetracycline

   b. Sulfamethoxazole

   c. Erythromycin

   d. Acyclovir

5. A male patient presents at the clinic with flu-like symptoms, weight loss of 10 pounds without trying. On physical examination, he is found to have splenomegaly and large, tender, fluctuant inguinal lymph nodes. While taking the nursing history, it is discovered that the patient prefers male sexual partners, and 2 weeks ago he had small, painless papules. What disease would the nurse suspect the client has?

   a. Genital herpes

   b. Chancroid

   c. Syphilis

   d. _Lymphogranuloma venereum_ (LGV)

6. Candidiasis is a leading cause of vaginal infections. Which antifungal agent is not available without prescription to treat candidiasis?

    a. Terconazole

    b. Clotrimazole

    c. Miconazole

    d. Butaconazole

7. Trichomoniasis is an STI that can occur in either sex. Men carry the protozoan in the urethra and prostate and remain asymptomatic. This anerobic protozoan can cause a number of complications. What is a risk factor for trichomoniasis in both men and women?

    a. Atypical pelvic inflammatory disease (PID)

    b. Human immunodeficiency virus (HIV) transmission

    c. Blockage of tubes and ducts

    d. Ovarian and testicular cysts

8. Bacterial vaginosis is the most common vaginal infection seen by health care providers. What is the predominant symptom of bacterial vaginosis?

    a. Thick, cottage cheese-like discharge with a fishy odor

    b. Painless chancres

    c. Grayish white discharge with a fishy odor

    d. Small, painless papules

9. Gonorrhea is an STI that affects both men and women. When diagnosing gonorrhea, specimens should be collected from the appropriate site and inoculated onto the correct medium. From what sites can specimens be collected when diagnosing gonorrhea? Mark all that apply.

    a. Oropharynx

    b. Urethra

    c. Nasal passages

    d. Exocervix

    e. Anal canal

10. Tertiary syphilis is a delayed response of untreated primary syphilis that can occur as long as 20 years after the primary disease. When tertiary syphilis progresses to a symptomatic stage, it can produce localized necrotic lesions. What are these lesions called?

    a. Chancres

    b. Chancroids

    c. Gummies

    d. Gummas

CHAPTER 48

Organization and Control of Neural Function

SECTION I: LEARNING OBJECTIVES

1. Distinguish between the functions of the neurons and supporting cells of the nervous system

2. List the three parts of a neuron and describe their structure and function

3. Name the supporting cells in the central nervous system and peripheral nervous system and state their functions

4. Describe the energy requirements of nervous tissue

5. Describe the three phases of an action potential and relate the functional importance of ion channels to the different phases

6. State the difference between electrical and chemical synapses

7. Describe the interaction of the presynaptic and postsynaptic terminals

8. Characterize the role of excitatory and inhibitory postsynaptic potentials as they relate to spatial and temporal summation of membrane potentials

9. Briefly describe how neurotransmitters are synthesized, stored, released, and inactivated

10. Use the segmental approach to explain the development of the nervous system and the organization of the postembryonic nervous system

11. Define the terms *afferent, efferent, ganglia, association neuron, cell column,* and *tract*

12. State the origin and destination of nerve fibers contained in the dorsal and ventral roots

13. State the structures innervated by general somatic afferent, special visceral afferent, general visceral afferent, special somatic afferent, general visceral efferent, pharyngeal efferent, and general somatic efferent neurons

14. Describe the longitudinal and transverse structures of the spinal cord

15. Trace an afferent and efferent neuron from its site in the periphery through its entrance into or exit from the spinal cord

16. Explain the innervation and function of spinal cord reflexes

17. List the structures of the hindbrain, midbrain, and forebrain and describe their functions

18. Name the cranial nerves and cite their location and function

19. Describe the characteristics of the CSF and trace its passage through the ventricular system

20. Contrast and compare the blood-brain and CSF-brain barriers

21. Compare the sensory and motor components of the autonomic nervous system with those of the CNS

22. Compare the anatomic location and functions of the sympathetic and parasympathetic nervous systems

23. Describe neurotransmitter synthesis, release, and degradation, and receptor function in the sympathetic and parasympathetic nervous systems

SECTION II: ASSESSING YOUR UNDERSTANDING

Activity A *Fill in the blanks.*

1. The _____ are the functional cells of the nervous system.

2. The supporting cells, such as _____ in the PNS and the _____ cells in the CNS, protect the nervous system and provide metabolic support for the neurons.

3. Neurons have three distinct parts: the cell _____, and its cytoplasm-filled processes, the _____ and _____, which form the functional connections, or _____, with other nerve cells, with receptor cells, or with effector cells.

4. _____ are multiple, short-branched extensions of the nerve cell body; they conduct information toward the cell body and are the main source of information for the neuron.

5. A bidirectional axonal transport system exists to carry materials to the nerve terminal (_____ direction) and back to the cell body (_____ direction).

6. Supporting cells of the nervous system, the _____ and _____ cells of the PNS and the several types of neuroglial cells of the CNS, give the neurons protection and metabolic support.

7. _____ cells secrete a basement membrane that protects the cell body from the diffusion of large molecules.

8. In some pathologic conditions, such as multiple sclerosis in the CNS and Guillain-Barré syndrome in the PNS, the _____ may degenerate or be destroyed.

9. The _____ increase nerve conduction by allowing the impulse to jump from node to node through the extracellular fluid in a process called _____.

10. The _____ form the myelin in the CNS.

11. _____ is the major fuel source for the nervous system.

12. Nerve signals are transmitted by _____, which are abrupt, pulsatile changes in the membrane potential.

13. The excitability of neurons can be affected by conditions that alter the _____, moving it either closer to or further from the threshold potential.

14. Neurons communicate with each other through structures known as _____.

15. _____ synapses involve special presynaptic and postsynaptic membrane structures, separated by a synaptic cleft.

16. The secreted neurotransmitters diffuse into the _____ and unite with receptors on the postsynaptic membrane.

17. In excitatory synapses, binding of the neurotransmitter to the receptor produces _____ of the postsynaptic membrane, whereas the binding of the neurotransmitter to the receptor in an inhibitory synapse induces _____ of the postsynaptic membrane by making the membrane more permeable to potassium or chloride.

18. When the combination of a neurotransmitter with a receptor site causes partial depolarization of the postsynaptic membrane, it is called an _____ potential.

19. The process of _____ involves the synthesis, storage, and release of a neurotransmitter; the reaction of the neurotransmitter with a receptor; and termination of the receptor action.

20. _____ molecules react with presynaptic or postsynaptic receptors to alter the release of or response to neurotransmitters.

21. _____ factors are required to maintain the long-term survival of the postsynaptic cell and are secreted by axon terminals independent of action potentials.

22. A functional system called the _____ operates in the lateral portions of the reticular formation of the medulla, pons, and especially the midbrain.

23. The spinal cord and the dorsal and ventral roots are covered by a connective tissue sheath, the _____, which also contains the blood vessels that supply the white and gray matter of the cord.

24. The peripheral nerves that carry information to and from the spinal cord are called _____.

25. Each spinal cord segment communicates with its corresponding body segment through the _____.

26. Spinal nerves do not go directly to skin and muscle fibers; instead, they form complicated nerve networks called _____.

27. A _____ is a highly predictable relationship between a stimulus and an elicited motor response.

28. The _____ reflex is stimulated by a damaging stimulus and quickly moves the body part away from the offending stimulus, usually by flexing a limb part.

29. Based on its embryonic development, the brain is divided into three regions, the _____, the _____, and the _____.

30. Damage to the _____ nerve results in weakness or paralysis of tongue muscles.

31. Sensory and motor components of the _____ nerve innervate the pharynx, the gastrointestinal tract, the heart, the spleen, and the lungs.

32. The sternocleidomastoid, a powerful head-turning muscle, and the trapezius muscle, which elevates the shoulders, are innervated by the _____.

33. The dorsolateral _____ contains the same components as the vagus nerve, but for a more rostral segment of the gastrointestinal tract and the pharynx.

34. The special sensory afferent _____ is attached laterally at the junction of the medulla oblongata and the pons, often called the caudal pons.

35. The _____ innervates the nasopharynx and taste buds of the palate.

36. The _____ nerve abducts the eye.

37. The _____ is the main sensory nerve conveying the modalities of pain, tempera-ture, touch, and proprioception to the super-ficial and deep regions of the face.

38. The _____ makes continuous adjust-ments, resulting in smoothness of movement, particularly during the delicate maneuvers.

39. The _____ plays a role in relaying criti-cal information regarding motor activities to and from selected areas of the motor cortex.

40. A _____ is the ridge between two grooves, and the groove is called a _____.

41. The _____ supply axial and proximal unlearned and learned postures and move-ments, which enhance and add gracefulness to UMN-controlled manipulative movements.

42. The _____ is necessary for somesthetic perception, especially concerning perception of "where" the stimulus is in space and in re-lation to body parts.

43. Inside the skull and vertebral column, the brain and spinal cord are loosely suspended and protected by several connective tissue sheaths called the _____.

44. The _____ provides a supporting and protective fluid in which the brain and spinal cord float.

45. The ability to maintain homeostasis and per-form the activities of daily living in an ever-changing physical environment is largely vested in the _____.

46. The functions of the _____ are con-cerned with conservation of energy, resource replenishment and storage, and maintenance of organ function during periods of minimal activity—the *rest and digest* response.

Activity B *Consider the following figures.*

1.

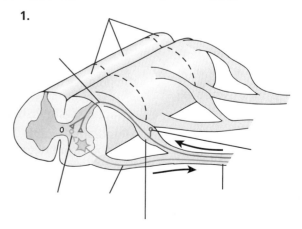

1. In the figure above of the segments of the spinal
   cord, please label the following structures:

   - IA neuron
   - segments
   - ventral root
   - dorsal root ganglion neuron
   - spinal nerve
   - dorsal root ganglion

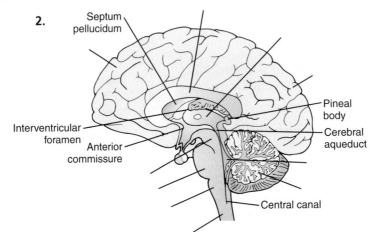

2.

Septum
pellucidum

Interventricular
foramen
Anterior
commissure

Pineal
body

Cerebral
aqueduct

Central canal

2. In the above figure of the brain, please label
   the following structures:

   - spinal cord
   - medulla oblongata
   - pons
   - midbrain
   - frontal lobe
   - corpus callosum
   - occipital lobe
   - third ventricle
   - fourth ventricle
   - cerebellum

_____ 6. Synaptic
   vesicles

_____ 7. Ependymal

_____ 8. Plexus

_____ 9. Threshold
   potential

_____ 10. Oligoden-
   drocytes

e. Chemical transmitter
   molecules

f. Small phagocytic cell
   that is available for
   cleaning up debris
   after cellular damage,
   infection, or cell
   death

g. Membrane potential
   at which neurons or
   other excitable tissues
   are stimulated

h. Flow of electrically
   charged ions toward
   an equilibrium

i. Production of CNS
   myelin

j. Site of intermixing
   nerve branches

Activity C *Match the key terms in Column A
with their definitions in Column B.*

1.

Column A

_____ 1. Microglia

_____ 2. Depolari-
   zation

_____ 3. Neurotrans-
   mitters

_____ 4. Repolari-
   zation

_____ 5. Astrocytes

Column B

a. Forms the lining of
   the neural tube cavity

b. Phase during which
   the polarity of the
   resting membrane po-
   tential is reestablished

c. Membrane-bound
   sacs that store neuro-
   transmitters

d. Form the blood–brain
   barrier

2.

Column A

_____ 1. Afferent

_____ 2. Bell's palsy

_____ 3. Efferent

_____ 4. Proprioception

_____ 5. Ganglia

Column B

a. Neurons that com-
   municate with the
   central nervous
   system and periph-
   eral neural cells

b. Nerves that con-
   duct impulses from

_____ **6.** Association neuron

_____ **7.** Muscle spindles

_____ **8.** Cell column

_____ **9.** Tract

the periphery of the body to the brain or spinal cord.

c. Longitudinal columns of neurons

d. Communication over distances between neighboring and distal segment of neural tube

e. Carrying impulses from the central nervous system to an effector

f. Group of neural cell bodies

g. Sense of body movement and position

h. Stretch receptors distributed throughout the belly of a muscle

i. Unilateral loss of facial nerve function

Activity D *Briefly answer the following.*

1. Describe the formation and attachment of myelin to the axonal membrane.

_____

_____

_____

2. Explain the fragileness of neural cells in regard to metabolic requirements.

_____

_____

_____

3. How do neural cell bodies interpret the numerous incoming signals (action potentials) from other neurons?

_____

_____

_____

4. How are neurotransmitters inactivated in the synaptic space following release?

_____

_____

_____

5. Describe the basic embryological development of the nervous system.

_____

_____

_____

6. How are the cell columns organized in the dorsal and ventral horns of the spinal cord?

_____

_____

_____

7. What is the importance of cerebral spinal fluid?

_____

_____

_____

8. How does the blood–brain barrier affect drug/toxin actions on the brain?

_____

_____

_____

SECTION III: APPLYING YOUR KNOWLEDGE

Activity E *Consider the following scenario and answer the questions.*

A woman in her fourth month of pregnancy comes to the clinic to have an ultrasound done. When the ultrasound is read, the physician tells the woman that her fetus has a neural tube defect, and, when the infant is born, it will have a cystlike pouch on its lower back that contains cerebrospinal fluid, meninges, and spinal nerves.

1. The patient asks if there is a name for the defect her child has. What is your correct response to the patient's question?

_____

_____

_____

2. The patient asks what this defect will mean for her baby. What would be your correct response?

_____

_____

_____

SECTION IV: PRACTICING FOR NCLEX

Activity F *Answer the following questions.*

1. There are two types of nervous tissue cells. One type is neurons, and the other type is the supporting cells. What is the function of the supporting cells?

a. Protect nervous system and provide metabolic support for the neurons

b. Transmit messages between parts of the peripheral nervous system (PNS)

c. Transmit messages between the central nervous system and the PNS

d. Provide metabolic support for the neurons and the PNS

2. Ion channels in nervous system cells generate action potentials in the cells. What are the ion channels guarded by?

a. Schwann cells

b. Voltage-dependent gates

c. Ligand-gates

d. Leyte cells

3. Neurons communicate through the use of synapses. These synapses may link neurons into functional circuits. What is the most common type of synapse?

a. Electrical synapse

b. Excitatory synapse

c. Chemical synapse

d. Inhibitory synapse

4. Neurotransmitters are small molecules that exert their actions through specific proteins, called receptors, embedded in the postsynaptic membrane. Where are neurotransmitters synthesized?

a. In the dendrite terminal

b. In the presynaptic junction

c. In the postsynaptic junction

d. In the axon terminal

5. Neuromodulators can produce slower and longer-lasting changes in membrane excitability by acting on postsynaptic receptors. What do neuromodulators do?

a. Alter the release or response to neurotransmitters

b. Alter the inhibitory response of postsynaptic electrical receptors

c. Alter the metabolic function of Schwann cells

d. Alter the Ligand-gate response to electrical activity

6. The basis for assessing the function of any peripheral nerve lies in what?

a. Peripheral nerves contain only afferent processes from the cell columns

b. Peripheral nerves contain processes of more than one of the four afferent and three efferent cell columns

c. Peripheral nerves contain only efferent processes from the cell columns

d. Peripheral nerves contain no processes from the seven cell columns

7. The spinal cord does not hang freely within the spinal column. What is it supported by?

a. The pia mater and the posterior vertebra

b. The denticulate ligaments and the vertebral blood vessels

c. The pia mater and the denticulate ligaments

d. The vertebral blood vessels and the posterior vertebra

8. One of the spinal motor reflexes is the myotatic reflex. What does this reflex do for the body?

a. Provides information to withdraw the body from noxious stimuli

b. Provides information about nociceptive stimuli

c. Provides information about equilibrium

d. Provides information about proprioception

9. The cerebellum, separated from the cerebral hemispheres by the tentorium cerebelli, lies in the posterior fossa of the cranium. What is one of the functions of the cerebellum?

a. Coordinates smooth and accurate movements of the body

b. Conveys the senses of pain, temperature, touch, and proprioception to the superficial and deep regions of the face

c. Contains the pontine nuclei

d. Contains the main motor pathways between the forebrain and the pons.

10. The basal ganglia, part of the cerebral hemispheres, are damaged by diseases such as Parkinson disease and Huntington chorea. What does this result in?

a. Uncontrollable tremors on movement

b. Abnormal movement patterns

c. Explosive, inappropriate speech

d. Inappropriate emotions

11. The blood–brain barrier excludes most highly water-soluble drugs, but allows lipid-soluble drugs to easily cross. What antibiotic is highly lipid soluble and readily enters the brain?

a. Ceftriaxone

b. Penicillin

c. Chloramphenicol

d. Cefadroxil

12. The sympathetic and the parasympathetic nervous systems are continuously at work in our bodies. This continual action gives a basal activity to all parts of the body. What is this basal activity referred to as?

a. Tension

b. Relaxation

c. Tone

d. Strength

13. Dopamine is an intermediate compound made during the synthesis of norepinephrine. It is the principal inhibitory transmitter of the internuncial neurons in the sympathetic ganglia. What other action does it have?

a. Vasoconstricts renal and coronary blood vessels when given intravenously (IV)

b. Acts as a neuromoderator in the hindbrain

c. Acts as a neuromoderator in the forebrain

d. Vasodilates renal and coronary blood vessels when given IV

Somatosensory Function, Pain, and Headache

SECTION I: LEARNING OBJECTIVES

1. Describe the four major classes of somatosensory modalities

2. Describe the organization of the somatosensory system in terms of first-, second-, and third-order neurons

3. Characterize the structure and function of the dorsal root ganglion neurons in terms of sensory receptors, conduction velocities, and spinal cord projections

4. Compare the discriminative pathway with the anterolateral pathway, and explain the clinical usefulness of this distinction

5. Compare the tactile, thermal, and position sense modalities in terms of receptors, adequate stimuli, ascending pathways, and central integrative mechanisms

6. Describe the role of clinical examination in assessing somatosensory function

7. Differentiate among the specificity, pattern, gate control, and neuromatrix theories of pain

8. Characterize the response of nociceptors to stimuli that produce pain

9. State the difference between the $A\delta$- and C-fiber neurons in the transmission of pain information

10. Trace the transmission of pain signals with reference to the neospinothalamic, paleospinothalamic, and reticulospinal pathways, including the role of chemical mediators and factors that modulate pain transmission

11. Describe the function of endogenous analgesic mechanisms as they relate to transmission of pain information

12. Compare pain threshold and pain tolerance

13. Differentiate acute pain from chronic pain in terms of mechanisms, manifestations, and treatment

14. Describe the mechanisms of referred pain, and list the common sites of referral for cardiac and other types of visceral pain

15. Describe three methods for assessing pain

16. State the proposed mechanisms of pain relief associated with the use of heat, cold, transcutaneous electrical nerve stimulation, and acupuncture and acupressure

17. Cite the mechanisms whereby non-narcotic and narcotic analgesics, tricyclic antidepressants, and antiseizure drugs relieve pain

18. Define allodynia, hypoesthesia, hyperesthesia, paresthesias, hyperpathia, analgesia, and hypoalgesia and hyperalgesia.

19. Describe the cause and characteristics and treatment of neuropathic pain, trigeminal neuralgia, postherpetic neuralgia, and complex regional pain syndrome.

20. Cite possible mechanisms of phantom limb pain

21. State the importance of distinguishing between primary and secondary types of headache

22. Differentiate between the periodicity of occurrence and manifestations of migraine headache, cluster headache, tension-type headache, and headache due to temporomandibular joint syndrome

23. Characterize the nonpharmacologic and pharmacologic methods used in treatment of headache

24. Cite the most common cause of temporomandibular joint pain

25. State how the pain response may differ in children and older adults

26. Explain how pain assessment may differ in children and older adults

27. Explain how pain treatment may differ in children and older adults

SECTION II: ASSESSING YOUR UNDERSTANDING

Activity A *Fill in the blanks.*

1. The _____ system is designed to provide the central nervous system (CNS) with information related to deep and superficial body structures as contrasted to special senses, such sight and hearing.

2. _____ somatic afferent neurons have branches with widespread distribution throughout the body and with many distinct types of receptors that result in sensations such as pain, touch, and temperature.

3. _____ somatic afferent neurons sense position and movement of the body.

4. General _____ afferent neurons have receptors on various visceral structures that sense fullness and discomfort.

5. Somatosensory information from the face and cranial structures is transmitted by the _____ sensory neurons, which function in the same manner as the dorsal root ganglion neurons.

6. The region of the body wall that is supplied by a single pair of dorsal root ganglia is called a _____.

7. The _____ pathway is used for the rapid transmission of sensory information, such as discriminative touch.

8. The _____ pathway provides for transmission of sensory information, such as pain, thermal sensations, crude touch, and pressure that does not require discrete localization of signal source or fine discrimination of intensity.

9. Somatosensory experience can be divided into _____, a term used for qualitative, subjective distinctions between sensations, such as touch, heat, and pain.

10. The receptive endings of different afferent neurons can initiate _____ to many forms of energy at high energy levels, but they usually are highly tuned to be differentially sensitive to low levels of a particular energy type.

11. The ability to discriminate the location of a somesthetic stimulus is called _____ and is based on the sensory field in a dermatome innervated by an afferent neuron.

12. The _____ system, which relays sensory information regarding touch, pressure, and vibration, is considered the basic somatosensory system.

13. _____ sensation is discriminated by three types of receptors: cold receptors, warmth receptors, and pain receptors.

14. Attention, motivation, past experience, and the meaning of the situation can influence the individual's reaction to _____.

15. The experience of pain depends on both _____ stimulation and _____.

16. _____ pain arises from direct injury or dysfunction of the sensory axons of peripheral or central nerves.

17. The _____ theory proposes that the brain contains a widely distributed neural network that contains somatosensory, limbic, and thalamocortical components.

18. _____ stimuli are objectively defined as stimuli of such intensity that they cause or are close to causing tissue damage.

19. Nociceptive stimulation that activates _____ can cause a response known as *neurogenic inflammation* that produces vasodilation and an increased release of chemical mediators to which nociceptors respond.

20. The faster-conducting fibers in the _____ tract are associated mainly with the transmission of sharp-fast pain information to the thalamus.

21. The _____ tract is a slower-conducting, multisynaptic tract concerned with the diffuse, dull, aching, and unpleasant sensations that commonly are associated with chronic and visceral pain.

22. Through research, it was found that electrical stimulation of the midbrain _____ regions produced a state of analgesia that lasted for many hours.

23. Three families of endogenous opioid peptides have been identified: the _____, _____, and _____.

24. Pain _____ and tolerance affect an individual's response to a painful stimulus.

25. _____ pain arises from superficial structures, such as the skin and subcutaneous tissues.

26. _____ pain originates in deep body structures, such as the periosteum, muscles, tendons, joints, and blood vessels.

27. The purpose of acute pain is to serve as a _____ system.

28. An _____ drug is a medication that acts on the nervous system to decrease or eliminate pain without inducing loss of consciousness.

29. Primary _____ describes pain sensitivity that occurs directly in damaged tissues.

30. _____ is the absence of pain on noxious stimulation or the relief of pain without loss of consciousness.

31. _____ is characterized by severe, brief, often repetitive attacks of lightninglike or throbbing pain.

32. _____ headache is a type of primary neurovascular headache that typically includes severe, unrelenting, unilateral pain located, in order of decreasing frequency, in the orbital, retro-orbital, temporal, supraorbital, and infraorbital region.

33. The most common type of headache is _____ headache.

34. A common cause of head pain is _____ syndrome.

Activity B *Consider the following figures.*

1. In the figure above, label the flowing structures:

- receptor
- dorsal root ganglion
- first order neuron
- second order neuron
- thalamus
- somatosensory cortex
- third order neuron

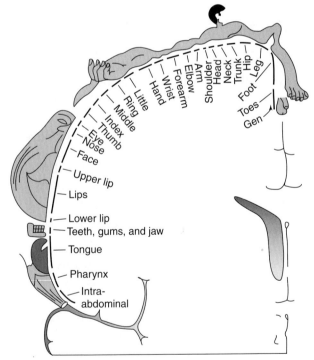

2. Using the figure above, please answer the following questions.

- Which area has the smallest receptor field?
- Which area has the largest receptor field?
- Which area has the highest acuity?

Activity C *Match the key terms in Column A with their definitions in Column B.*

1.

Column A

_____ 1. Perception
_____ 2. Somesthesia
_____ 3. Type A fibers
_____ 4. Polymodal receptors
_____ 5. Type B fibers
_____ 6. Hunting reflex
_____ 7. Primary somato-sensory cortex
_____ 8. Hyperpathia
_____ 9. Type C fibers
_____ 10. Type Aα fibers

Column B

a. The perception of tactual, proprioceptive, or gut sensations

b. Transmit information about muscle length and tendon stretch

c. Sensory threshold is raised

d. Convey cutaneous pressure and touch sensation, cold sensation, mechanical pain, and heat pain

e. Circulation to a cooled area undergoes alternating periods of pallor caused by ischemia and flushing caused by hyperemia

f. Awareness of the stimuli, localization and discrimination of their characteristics, and interpretation of their meaning

g. Receives primary sensory information by way of direct projections from the thalamus

h. Convey warm-hot sensation and mechanical and chemical as well as heat- and cold-induced pain sensation

i. Respond to mechanical, thermal, and chemical stimuli

j. Transmit information from cutaneous and subcutaneous mechanoreceptors

2.

Column A

_____ 1. Free nerve endings
_____ 2. Meissner corpuscles
_____ 3. Merkel disks
_____ 4. Pacinian corpuscles
_____ 5. Hair follicle end-organs
_____ 6. Ruffini end-organs

Column B

a. Stimulated by rapid movements of the tissues and adapts within a few hundredths of a second

b. Unmyelinated fibers entwined around most of the length of the hair follicle that detect movement on the surface of the body

c. Are responsible for giving steady-state signals that allow for continuous determination of touch against the skin

d. Detect touch and pressure

e. Found in joint capsules

f. Elongated, encapsulated nerve ending that is present in non-hairy parts of the skin

Activity D *Briefly answer the following.*

1. How are sensory systems organized?

_____

_____

_____

2. What are the types of sensory information that can be perceived by our sensory receptors?

_____

_____

_____

3. How much information can be obtained from a single pinprick to the bottom of your patient's foot?

_____

_____

_____

4. What is the gate control theory of pain?

_____

_____

_____

5. How can the phenomenon of referred pain be explained?

_____

_____

_____

6. In many sports injuries the athlete may be instructed to place heat on the injured area. What is the effect on pain originating from the injury?

_____

_____

_____

7. What is phantom limb pain and what are some of the theories postulated to explain its presence?

_____

_____

_____

8. What are the differences and similarities between migraine headaches with aura and migraine headaches without aura?

_____

_____

_____

9. What is known about the pathology of pain during a migrainous headache?

_____

_____

_____

SECTION III: APPLYING YOUR KNOWLEDGE

Activity E *Consider the following scenario and answer the questions.*

An 82-year-old woman is brought to the emergency department by ambulance from a local nursing home. The report from the accompanying staff member is that she suffers from a physiologic dementia and that 2 days ago she fell in the bathroom. The patient denies pain, but has been restless and agitated since the fall, and today she will not use her right arm.

1. The caregiver asks the nurse how the healthcare team is going to assess this client's pain since the client cannot give them any accurate information. What is your best response?

_____

_____

_____

2. The patient is diagnosed with a fractured right ulna. She is taken to the OR, where the arm is aligned and cast. When she is ready for release back to the nursing home, the caregiver asks what can be done for her discomfort. What information would you include at discharge?

_____

_____

_____

SECTION IV: PRACTICING FOR NCLEX

Activity F *Answer the following questions.*

1. Match the type of neuron with the information it transmits and where it transmits it.

Type of Neuron	Information Transmitted and Site
____ 1. Special somatic afferent neurons	a. Sensations such as pain, touch, and temperature
____ 2. General somatic afferent neurons	b. Transmit sensory information from the periphery to the CNS
____ 3. General visceral afferent neurons	c. Communicate with various reflex networks and sensory pathways in the spinal cord and travel directly to the thalamus
____ 4. First-order neurons	
____ 5. Second-order neurons	
____ 6. Third-order neurons	

_____ **7.** Dorsal root ganglion neurons

_____ **8.** Trigeminal sensory neurons

d. Transmits all somatosensory information from the limbs and trunk

e. Sense position and movement of the body

f. Somatosensory information from the face and cranial structures

g. Sense fullness and discomfort

h. Relay information from the thalamus to the cerebral cortex

2. Match the term with the definition.

Term

_____ **1.** Discriminative touch

_____ **2.** Sensory unit

_____ **3.** Type A fibers

_____ **4.** Type Aα and Aδ fibers

_____ **5.** Type B fibers

_____ **6.** Dermatome

_____ **7.** Discriminative pathway

_____ **8.** Stereognosis

_____ **9.** Anterolateral pathway

_____ **10.** Free nerve endings

_____ **11.** Nociceptors

Definition

a. The region of the body wall that is supplied by a single pair of dorsal root ganglia

b. Stimulate autonomic nervous system responses, such as a rise in heart rate and blood pressure, dilation of the pupils, and the pale, moist skin that results from constriction of the cutaneous blood vessels and activation of the sweat glands

c. Identifies the size and shape of objects and their movement across the skin, temperature sensation, sense of movement of the limbs and joints of the body, and nociception, or pain

d. Transmit information about muscle length and tendon stretch

e. Sensory receptors that are activated by noxious insults to peripheral tissues

f. Carry the information from the spinal cord to the thalamic level of sensation and relay precise information regarding spatial orientation

g. The cell body of the dorsal root ganglion neuron, its peripheral branch (which innervates a small area of periphery), and its central axon (which projects to the CNS)

h. Transmit information from cutaneous and subcutaneous mechanoreceptors

i. Convey cutaneous pressure and touch sensation, cold sensation, mechanical pain, and heat pain

j. The sense of shape and size of an object in the absence of visualization

k. Detect touch and pressure

3. A neurologic assessment of the somatosensory function of the body is often necessary for diagnostic information. How is this assessment done?

a. Testing the integrity of spinal segmental nerves

b. Testing the integrity of cranial nerves

c. Testing the integrity of peripheral nerves

d. Testing the integrity of the CNS

4. When testing nociceptive stimuli to elicit a withdrawal reflex in the body, what stimuli are commonly used?

a. Weak electrical current

b. Pressure from a sharp object

c. Skin temperature damp cotton ball

d. Water heated to 5°C above skin temperature

5. One of the neurotransmitters between the nociceptive neurons and the dorsal horn neurons is a major excitatory neurotransmitter. What is this neurotransmitter?

a. Norepinephrine

b. Substance P

c. Glutamate

d. Dopamine

6. Which tract in the spinal cord conducts the diffuse, dull, aching sensations that are associated with chronic and visceral pain?

a. Multisynaptic tract

b. Neospinothalamic tract

c. Anterolateral tract

d. Paleospinothalamic tract

7. Match the type of pain with its description

Type of Pain	Description of Pain
____ **1.** Deep somatic pain	a. Extends for long periods of time and generally represents low levels of underlying pathology that does not explain the presence and/or extent of the pain
____ **2.** Cutaneous pain	
____ **3.** Visceral pain	
____ **4.** Referred pain	b. The pain's location, radiation, intensity, and duration, as well as those factors that aggravate or relieve it provide essential diagnostic clues
____ **5.** Guarding	
____ **6.** Acute pain	
____ **7.** Chronic pain	

c. Type of pain experienced from a sprained ankle

d. A sharp pain with a burning quality that may be abrupt or slow in onset.

e. A protective reflex rigidity; its purpose is to protect the affected body parts

f. Diffuse and poorly localized nature with a tendency to be referred to other locations

g. Perceived at a site different from its point of origin, but innervated by the same spinal segment

8. It is often necessary to assess a patient's pain. What factors would you assess when assessing pain? Mark all that apply.

a. Nature and severity of pain

b. Severity and spinal reflex involvement of pain

c. Location and radiation of pain

d. Spinal reflex involvement and nature of pain

e. Spinal tract involvement and radiation of pain

9. When giving medicine for acute pain, health care workers are reluctant to provide much needed opioid pain medicine. What is your major concern when providing opioid pain relief?

a. Fear of addiction

b. Fear of depressed respirations

c. Fear of over-sedation

d. Fear of adverse reactions

10. Chronic pain is difficult to treat. Cancer, a common cause of chronic pain, has been especially addressed by the World Health Organization (WHO). What has WHO created to assist clinicians in choosing appropriate analgesics?

a. An opioid ladder for pain control

b. An analgesic ladder for pain control

c. Stepping stones for pain control

d. A list of nonpharmacologic ways to control pain

11. In describing the ideal analgesic, what factors would be included? Mark all that apply.

a. Inexpensive

b. Have minimal adverse effects

c. Effective

d. Addictive

e. Decrease the level of consciousness

12. Using surgery to relieve severe, intractable pain has been successful to a degree. For what can surgery be used when a person is in pain?

a. Relief of severe peripheral contractures

b. Cure inoperable cancer

c. Block transmission of phantom limb pain

d. Cure severe myalgia

13. When a peripheral nerve is sufficiently irritated, it becomes hypersensitive to the noxious stimuli, which results in increased painfulness or hyperalgesia. Health care professionals recognize both primary and secondary forms of hyperalgesia. What is primary hyperalgesia?

a. Pain that occurs in the tissue surrounding an injury.

b. Pain sensitivity that lasts longer than 1 week

c. Pain sensitivity that occurs in the viscera

d. Pain sensitivity that occurs directly in damaged tissues

14. Match the type of pain with its description.

Type of Pain	Description
___ **1.** Neuropathic pain	a. Manifested by facial tics or spasms and characterized by paroxysmal attacks of stabbing pain that usually are limited to the unilateral sensory distribution of one or more branches of the trigeminal nerve, most often the maxillary or mandibular divisions.
___ **2.** Neuralgia	
___ **3.** Tic douloureux	
___ **4.** Postherpetic neuralgia	b. Characterized by severe, brief, often repetitive attacks of lightninglike or throbbing pain.
	c. Affected sensory ganglia and the peripheral nerve to the skin of the corresponding dermatomes cause a unilateral localized vesicular eruption and hyperpathia (i.e., abnormally exaggerated subjective response to pain).
	d. Widespread pain that is not otherwise explainable, burning pain, and attacks of pain that occur without seeming provocation.

15. Phantom limb pain is a little understood pain that develops after an amputation. Because it is little understood, it is difficult to treat, even though the patient is experiencing severe pain. What are the treatments for phantom limb pain?

a. Sympathetic blocks and hypnosis

b. Relaxation training and transcutaneous electrical nerve stimulation (TENS) on the efferents in the area

c. Narcotic analgesics and relaxation training

d. Biofeedback and nonsteroidal anti-inflammatory drugs (NSAIDs)

16. Migraine headaches affect millions of people worldwide. What are first-line agents for the treatment of migraine headaches?

a. Ondansetron and morphine

b. Naproxen sodium and metoclopramide

c. Sumatriptan and Tramadol

d. Caffeine and syrup of ipecac

17. A severe type of headache that occurs more frequently in men than in women and is described as having unrelenting, unilateral pain located most frequently in the orbit is called what?

a. Migraine headache

b. Tension headache

c. Cluster headache

d. Chronic daily headache

18. When assessing pain in children, it is important to use the correct pain rating scale. What would be the appropriate pain rating scale with children who are 3 to 8 years of age?

a. COMFORT pain scale

b. FLACC pain scale

c. CRIES pain scale

d. FACES pain scale

19. Children feel pain just as much as adults do. What is the major principle in pain management in the pediatric population?

a. Treat on individual basis and match analgesic agent with cause and level of pain

b. Always use nonpharmacologic pain treatment before using pharmacologic pain treatment

c. Base treatment of pain on gender and age group

d. Treat pediatric pain the way the parents wish

50

Disorders of Motor Function

SECTION I: LEARNING OBJECTIVES

1. Relate the functional hierarchy of motor function to the performance of a complicated movement such as writing your name or throwing a ball

2. Define the term *motor unit* and characterize its mechanism of controlling skeletal muscle movement

3. Describe the distribution of upper and lower motor neurons in relation to the central nervous system

4. Differentiate between the functions of the primary, premotor, and supplemental motor cortices

5. Compare the effect of upper and lower motor neuron lesions on the spinal cord stretch reflex function and muscle tone

6. Describe muscle atrophy and differentiate between disuse and degenerative atrophy

7. Relate the molecular changes in muscle structure that occur in Duchenne muscular dystrophy to the clinical manifestations of the disease

8. Describe the actions of *Clostridium botulinum* neurotoxins in terms of their pathologic and therapeutic potential

9. Relate the clinical manifestations of myasthenia gravis to its cause

10. Define the term *peripheral nervous system* and describe the characteristics of peripheral nerves

11. Trace the steps in regeneration of an injured peripheral nerve

12. Compare the cause and manifestations of peripheral mononeuropathies with polyneuropathies

13. Describe the manifestation of peripheral nerve root injury due to a ruptured intervertebral disk

14. Relate the functions of the cerebellum to production of vestibulocerebellar ataxia, decomposition of movement, and cerebellar tremor

15. Describe the functional organization of the basal ganglia and communication pathways with the thalamus and cerebral cortex

16. State the possible mechanisms responsible for the development of Parkinson disease and characterize the manifestations and treatment of the disorder

17. Relate the pathologic UMN and LMN changes that occur in amyotrophic lateral sclerosis to the manifestations of the disease

18. Explain the significance of demyelination and plaque formation in multiple sclerosis

19. Describe the manifestations of multiple sclerosis

20. Relate the structures of the vertebral column to mechanisms of spinal cord injury

21. Explain how loss of UMN function contributes to the muscle spasms that occur after recovery from spinal cord injury

22. State the effects of spinal cord injury on ventilation and communication, the autonomic nervous system, cardiovascular function, sensorimotor function, and bowel, bladder, and sexual function

SECTION II: ASSESSING YOUR UNDERSTANDING

Activity A *Fill in the blanks.*

1. _____, whether it involves walking, running, or precise finger movements, requires movement and maintenance of posture.

2. The _____ contains the neuronal circuits that mediate a variety of reflexes and automatic rhythmic movements.

3. Most reflexes are _____, meaning that they involve one or more interposed interneurons.

4. The medial descending systems of the brain stem contribute to the control of _____ by integrating visual, vestibular, and somatosensory information.

5. The _____ is the highest level of motor function.

6. The primary _____ cortex is located on the rostral surface and adjacent portions of the central sulcus.

7. The _____ and _____ provide feedback circuits that regulate cortical and brain stem motor areas.

8. Cerebellar _____ are involved with the timing and coordination of movements that are in progress and with the learning of motor skills.

9. The _____, which are distributed throughout the belly of a muscle, relay information about muscle length and rate of stretch.

10. _____ are found in muscle tendons and transmit information about muscle tension or force of contraction at the junction of the muscle and the tendon that attaches to bone.

11. Stretch reflexes tend to be hypoactive or absent in cases of _____ nerve damage or ventral horn injury involving the test area.

12. Abnormalities in any part of the _____ pathway can produce muscle weakness.

13. Muscular _____ usually results from lower motor neuron (LMN) lesions as well as diseases of the muscle themselves.

14. Any interruption of the myotatic or stretch reflex circuitry by peripheral nerve injury, pathology of the neuromuscular junction, injury to the spinal cord, or damage to the corticospinal system can results in disturbances of _____.

15. Hyperactive reflexes are suggestive of an _____ disorder.

16. _____ suggests the presence of an LMN lesion.

17. Disorders affecting the nerve cell body are often referred to _____ those affecting the nerve axon as _____ neuropathies, and primary disorders affecting the muscle fibers as _____.

18. Muscular _____ is a term applied to a number of genetic disorders that produce progressive deterioration of skeletal muscles because of mixed muscle cell hypertrophy, atrophy, and necrosis.

19. If the LMN dies or its axon is destroyed, the skeletal muscle cell begins to have temporary spontaneous contractions, called _____.

20. _____ muscular dystrophy is inherited as a recessive single-gene defect on the X chromosome and it is transmitted from the mother to her male offspring.

21. The _____ serves as a synapse between a motor neuron and a skeletal muscle fiber.

22. Neurotoxins from the botulism organism (*Clostridium botulinum*) produce paralysis by blocking _____ release.

23. _____ is a disorder of transmission at the neuromuscular junction that affects communication between the motor neuron and the innervated muscle cell.

24. LMN diseases are progressive neurologic illnesses that selectively affect the anterior horn cells of the _____ and _____ motor neurons.

25. There are two main types of _____ injury based on the target of the insult: segmental demyelination involving the Schwann cell and axonal degeneration involving the neuronal cell body and/or its axon.

26. _____ usually are caused by localized conditions, such as trauma, compression, or infections, that affect a single spinal nerve, plexus, or peripheral nerve trunk.

27. _____ involve demyelination or axonal degeneration of multiple peripheral nerves that leads to symmetric sensory, motor, or mixed sensorimotor deficits.

28. The signs and symptoms of a _____ are localized to the area of the body innervated by the nerve roots and include both motor and sensory manifestations.

29. Loss of _____ function can result in total incoordination of these functions even though its loss does not result in paralysis.

30. The _____ are a group of deep, interrelated subcortical nuclei that play an essential role in control of movement.

31. Disorders of the basal ganglia comprise a complex group of motor disturbances characterized by _____ and other involuntary movements, changes in posture and muscle tone, and poverty and slowness of movement.

32. _____ disease is a degenerative disorder of basal ganglia function that results in variable combinations of tremor, rigidity, and bradykinesia.

33. The cardinal manifestations of Parkinson disease are tremor, rigidity, and _____ or slowness of movement.

34. _____ affects motor neurons in three locations: the anterior horn cells of the spinal cord; the motor nuclei of the brain stem, particularly the hypoglossal nuclei; and the UMNs of the cerebral cortex.

35. _____ is characterized by inflammation and selective destruction of central nervous system myelin.

36. The pathophysiology of multiple sclerosis involves the _____ of nerve fibers in the white matter of the brain, spinal cord, and optic nerve.

37. The most common cause of _____ is motor vehicle accidents, followed by falls, violence (primarily gunshot wounds), and recreational sporting activities.

38. Sudden complete transection of the spinal cord results in complete _____ of motor, sensory, reflex, and autonomic function below the level of injury.

39. _____ is the impairment or loss of motor or sensory function (or both) after damage to neural structures in the cervical segments of the spinal cord.

40. _____ refers to impairment or loss of motor or sensory function (or both) in the thoracic, lumbar, or sacral segments of the spinal cord from damage of neural elements in the spinal canal.

41. Vagal stimulation that causes a marked bradycardia is called the _____ response.

42. _____ hypotension usually occurs in persons with injuries at T4 to T6 and above and is related to the interruption of descending control of sympathetic outflow to blood vessels in the extremities and abdomen.

43. The high risk for _____ in patients with acute SCI is owing to immobility, decreased vasomotor tone below the level of injury, and hypercoagulability and stasis of blood flow.

Activity B *Consider the following figure:*

In the figure above, locate and label the following areas of the brain:

- premotor cortex
- motor cortex
- Broca area
- vestibular cortex
- primary auditory cortex
- primary visual cortex
- somatosensory cortex
- frontal eye fields

Activity C *Match the key terms in Column A with their definitions in Column B.*

1.

Column A	Column B
_____ **1.** Clonus	**a.** Increased muscle resistance that varies and commonly becomes worse at the extremities of the range of motion
_____ **2.** Paralysis	
_____ **3.** Fasciculations	
_____ **4.** Motor homunculus	**b.** Incomplete loss of strength
_____ **5.** Spasticity	**c.** Loss of movement
_____ **6.** Dysdiadochokinesia	**d.** Rhythmic contraction and alternate relaxation of a limb
_____ **7.** Reflex	**e.** Somatotopic array of the body representing motor areas
_____ **8.** Ataxia	
_____ **9.** Proprioception	**f.** The failure to accurately perform rapid alternating movements
_____ **10.** Paresis	**g.** Sense of body movement and position
	h. A wide-based, unsteady gait
	i. Visible squirming and twitching movements of muscle
	j. Involuntary motor responses

2.

Column A	Column B
_____ **1.** Bradykinesia	**a.** Muscle shrinkage owing to loss of neural stimulus
_____ **2.** Dystonia	
_____ **3.** Chorea	**b.** Involuntary jerking movement
_____ **4.** Truncal ataxia	**c.** Slowness of movements
_____ **5.** Myoclonus	

_____ **6.** Parkinsonism	**d.** Rhythmic movements of a particular body part
_____ **7.** Dysmetria	
_____ **8.** Denervation atrophy	**e.** Abnormal simultaneous contractions of agonist and antagonist muscles
_____ **9.** Constant conjugate readjustment of eye position	**f.** Abnormal writhing movements
_____ **10.** Tremor	**g.** Inaccuracies of movements, leading to a failure to reach a specified target
	h. Nystagmus
	i. Unsteadiness of the trunk
	j. Syndrome arising from the degenerative changes in basal ganglia function

Activity D

1. In the boxes below, put the following events regarding synaptic transmission in order:

  1. Inactivation by acetylcholinesterase

  2. Action potential arrives at synaptic terminal

  3. Depolarization of motor-end plate

  4. Release of acetylcholine into synapse

  5. Influx of Ca^{2+}

Activity E *Briefly answer the following.*

1. Describe the basic hierarchy of the organization of motor movement.

_____

_____

_____

2. What is the basic unit of motor control? How does it vary between gross motor movement and fine motor movements?

_____

_____

_____

3. What is a muscle spindle and how does it work?

_____

_____

_____

4. What areas must be integrated for muscle movement to be coordinated?

_____

_____

_____

5. Describe the molecular causation of Duchene muscular dystrophy.

_____

_____

_____

6. Compare segmental demyelination with axonal degeneration in relation to peripheral nerve injuries.

_____

_____

_____

7. What is carpal tunnel syndrome?

_____

_____

_____

8. What are the clinical manifestations of Guillain-Barré syndrome?

_____

_____

_____

9. What is the current theory of the pathogenesis of Parkinson disease?

_____

_____

_____

10. What does amyotrophic lateral sclerosis imply?

_____

_____

_____

11. What are the two pathologic types of spinal chord injury?

_____

_____

_____

SECTION III: APPLYING YOUR KNOWLEDGE

Activity F *Consider the following scenario and answer the questions.*

A 27-year-old man is brought into the emergency department after falling out of a tree stand while deer hunting. He is awake and alert and states that he cannot feel or move his legs. A magnetic resonance image (MRI) indicates a subluxation of the vertebrae with fractures above and below the subluxation.

1. The man's wife arrives at the emergency department. She asks you what medicine is in the intravenous medication and why her husband is receiving it. What would you include in your answer to her?

_____

_____

_____

2. The patient is transferred to a neurosurgic intensive care unit. As the nurse caring for this client, what orders would you expect to receive?

_____

_____

_____

SECTION IV: PRACTICING FOR NCLEX

Activity G *Answer the following questions.*

1. The spinal cord contains the basic factors necessary to coordinate function when a movement is planned. It is the lowest level of function. What is the highest level of function in planning movement?

   a. Frontal cortex

   b. Cerebral cortex

   c. Pons

   d. Cerebellum

2. Match the neurons with their function/description.

Neuron	Function/Description
___ **1.** Motor neurons	**a.** Motor neuron and the group of muscle fibers it innervates in a muscle
___ **2.** Motor unit	**b.** Control motor function
___ **3.** Lower motor neurons (LMNs)	**c.** Project from the motor strip in the cerebral cortex to the ventral horn and are fully contained within the central nervous system
___ **4.** Upper motor neurons (UMNs)	**d.** The motor neurons supplying a motor unit are located in the ventral horn of the spinal cord

3. Reflexes are basically "hard-wired" into the central nervous system. Anatomically, the basis of a reflex is an afferent neuron that synapses directly with an effector neuron that causes muscle movement. Sometimes the afferent neuron synapses with what intermediary between the afferent and effector neurons?

a. Neurotransmitter

b. Interneuron

c. Intersegmental effectors

d. Suprasegmental effectors

4. The signs and symptoms produced by disorders of the motor system are useful in finding the disorder. What signs and symptoms would you assess when looking for a disorder of the motor system? Mark all that apply.

a. Spinal reflex activity

b. Bulk

c. Motor coordination

d. Muscle innervation

e. Tone

5. Duchenne muscular dystrophy usually does not produce any signs or symptoms until between the ages of 2 and 3. What muscles are usually first to be affected in Duchenne muscular dystrophy?

a. Muscles of the upper arms

b. Large muscles of the legs

c. Postural muscles of hip and shoulder

d. Spinal and neck muscles

6. Antibiotics, such as gentamicin, can produce a disturbance in the body that is similar to botulism by preventing the release of acetylcholine from nerve endings. In persons with preexisting neuromuscular transmission disturbances, these drugs can be dangerous. What disease falls into this category?

a. Multiple sclerosis

b. Duchenne muscular dystrophy

c. Becker muscular dystrophy

d. Myasthenia gravis

7. In myasthenia gravis, periods of stress can produce myasthenia crisis. When does myasthenia crisis occur?

a. When muscle weakness becomes sufficiently severe to compromise ventilation

b. When the patient is too weak to hold up his or her head

c. When the patient is so weak he or she cannot lift his or her arms

d. When the patient can no longer walk

8. Peripheral nerve disorders are not uncommon. What is an example of a fairly common mononeuropathy?

a. Guillain-Barré syndrome

b. Carpal tunnel syndrome

c. Myasthenia gravis

d. Phalen syndrome

9. Herniated disks occur when the nucleus pulposus is compressed enough that it protrudes through the annulus fibrosus putting pressure on the nerve root. This type of injury occurs most often in the cervical and lumbar region of the spine. What is an important diagnostic test for a herniated disk in the lumbar region?

a. Hip flexion test

b. Computed tomography (CT) scan

c. Straight-leg test

d. Electromyelography

10. Match the cerebellar pathway with its function.

    **Cerebellar
    Pathway**   **Function**

    ____ **1.** Vestibulocere-   **a.** Maintains equilib-
            bellar pathway   rium and posture

    ____ **2.** Spinocerebellar   **b.** Provides the cir-
            pathway   cuitry for coordi-
                                      nating the
    ____ **3.** Cerebrocere-   movements of the
            bellar   distal portions of
            pathway   the limbs

                                  c. Coordinates se-
                                      quential body and
                                      limb movements

11. The basal ganglia play a role in coordinated movements. Part of the basal ganglia system is the striatum which involves local cholinergic interneurons. What disease is thought to be related to the destruction of the cholinergic interneurons?

    a. Parkinson syndrome

    b. Guillain-Barré syndrome

    c. Myasthenia gravis

    d. Huntington disease

12. What disease results from the degeneration of the dopamine nigrostriatal system of the basal ganglia?

    a. Parkinson disease

    b. Huntington disease

    c. Guillain-Barré syndrome

    d. Myasthenia gravis

13. Amyotrophic lateral sclerosis (ALS) is considered a disease of the upper motor neurons. What is the most common clinical presentation of ALS?

    a. Rapidly progressive weakness and atrophy in distal muscles of both upper extremities

    b. Slowly progressive weakness and atrophy in distal muscles of one upper extremity

    c. Rapidly progressive weakness and atrophy in distal muscles of both lower extremities

    d. Slowly progressive weakness and atrophy in distal muscles of one lower extremity

14. Although no laboratory test is diagnostic for multiple sclerosis (MS), some patients have alterations in their cerebrospinal fluid (CSF) that can be seen when a portion of the CSF is removed during a spinal tap. What finding in CSF is suggestive of MS?

    a. Decreased immunoglobulin G levels

    b. Decreased total protein levels

    c. Oligoclonal patterns

    d. Decreased lymphocytes

15. At what level of the cervical spine would an injury allow finger flexion?

    a. C5

    b. C6

    c. C7

    d. C8

16. A 14-year-old girl has been thrown from the back of a pick-up truck. MRI shows broken vertebrae at the C2 level. What is the main significance of an injury at this level of the spinal column?

    a. Cannot breathe on own, needs ventilator assistance

    b. Partial or full diaphragmatic function, ventilation is diminished because of the loss of intercostal muscle function, resulting in shallow breaths and a weak cough

    c. Intercostal and abdominal musculature is affected, the ability to take a deep breath and cough is less impaired

    d. Needs maintenance therapy to strengthen existing muscles for endurance and mobilization of secretions

17. Approximately 6 months after a spinal cord injury, a 29-year-old man has an episode of autonomic dysreflexia. What are the characteristics of autonomic dysreflexia? Mark all that apply.

    a. Hypertension

    b. Fever

    c. Skin pallor

    d. Vasoconstriction

    e. Piloerector response

18. Bowel dysfunction is one of the most difficult problems to handle after a spinal cord injury. After a spinal cord injury, most people experience constipation. Why does this occur?

    a. Innervation of the bowel is absent

    b. Defecation reflex is lost

    c. Internal anal sphincter will not relax

    d. Peristaltic movements are not sufficiently strong to move stool through the colon

Disorders of Brain Function

SECTION I: LEARNING OBJECTIVES

1. Differentiate cerebral hypoxia from cerebral ischemia and focal from global ischemia

2. Characterize the role of excitatory amino acids as a common pathway for neurologic disorders

3. State the determinants of intracranial pressure and describe compensatory mechanisms used to prevent large changes in intracranial pressure when there are changes in brain, blood, and cerebrospinal fluid volumes

4. Explain the causes of tentorial herniation of the brain and its consequences

5. Compare the causes of communicating and noncommunicating hydrocephalus

6. Compare cytotoxic, vasogenic, and interstitial cerebral edema

7. Differentiate primary and secondary brain injuries due to head trauma

8. Describe the mechanism of brain damage in coup–contrecoup injuries

9. List the constellation of symptoms involved in the postconcussion syndrome

10. Differentiate among the location, manifestations, and morbidity of epidural, subdural, and intracerebral hematoma

11. Define consciousness and trace the rostral-to-caudal progression of consciousness in terms of pupillary changes, respiration, and motor function as the effects of brain dysfunction progress to involve structures in the diencephalon, midbrain, pons, and medulla

12. State two criteria for the diagnosis of brain death

13. List the major vessels in the cerebral circulation and state the contribution of the internal carotid arteries, the vertebral arteries, and the circle of Willis to the cerebral circulation

14. Describe the autoregulation of cerebral blood flow

15. Explain the substitution of "brain attack" for stroke in terms of making a case for early diagnosis and treatment

16. Differentiate the pathologies of ischemic and hemorrhagic stroke

17. Explain the significance of transient ischemic attacks, the ischemic penumbra, and watershed zones of infarction and how these conditions relate to ischemic stroke

18. Cite the most common cause of subarachnoid hemorrhage and state the complications associated with subarachnoid hemorrhage

19. Describe the alterations in cerebral vasculature that occur with arteriovenous malformations

20. Describe the patterns of motor deficits and typical problems with speech and language that occur as a result of stroke

21. List the sequence of events that occur with meningitis

22. Describe the symptoms of encephalitis

23. List the major categories of brain tumors and interpret the meaning of benign and malignant as related to brain tumors

24. Describe the general manifestations of brain tumors

25. List the methods used in diagnosis and treatment of brain tumors

26. Explain the difference between a seizure and epilepsy

27. State four or more causes of seizures other than epilepsy

28. Differentiate between the origin of seizure activity in partial and generalized forms of epilepsy and compare the manifestations of simple partial seizures with those of complex partial seizures and major and minor motor seizures

29. Characterize status epilepticus

SECTION II: ASSESSING YOUR UNDERSTANDING

Activity A *Fill in the blanks.*

1. A number of regulatory mechanisms, including the blood–brain barrier and autoregulatory mechanisms that ensure its blood supply, maintain the _____ electrically active cells.

2. Although the brain makes up only 2% of the body weight, it receives 15% of the resting cardiac output and accounts for _____ % of the oxygen consumption.

3. Because _____ indicates decreased oxygen levels in all brain tissue, it produces a generalized depressant effect on the brain.

4. Cerebral ischemia can be _____, as in stroke, or _____, as in cardiac arrest.

5. Excessive influx of _____ during neural ischemia results in neuronal and interstitial edema.

6. _____ refers to short serpiginous segments of necrosis that occur within and parallel to the cerebral cortex, in areas supplied by the penetrating arteries during an ischemic event.

7. In many neurologic disorders, various mediators, including excitatory _____, catecholamines, nitric oxide, free radicals, inflammatory cells, apoptosis, and intracellular _____ can cause injury to neurons.

8. Increased _____ pressure is a common pathway for brain injury from different types of insults and agents.

9. Brain _____ represents a displacement of brain tissue under the falx cerebri or through the tentorial notch or incisura of the tentorium cerebelli.

10. Cerebral _____ is an increase in tissue volume secondary to abnormal fluid accumulation.

11. The functional manifestations of _____ edema include focal neurologic deficits, disturbances in consciousness, and severe intracranial hypertension.

12. _____ edema involves an increase in intracellular fluid.

13. The effects of traumatic head injuries can be divided into two categories: _____ injuries, in which damage is caused by impact; and secondary injuries, in which damage results from the subsequent brain swelling, infection, or _____.

14. _____ usually are caused by head injury in which the skull is fractured.

15. A subdural hematoma develops in the area between the dura and the arachnoid and usually is the result of a _____ in the small bridging veins that connect veins on the surface of the cortex to dural sinuses.

16. _____ is the state of awareness of self and the environment and of being able to become oriented to new stimuli.

17. Brain death is defined as the irreversible loss of function of the _____, including the brain stem.

18. The _____ state is characterized by loss of all cognitive functions and the unawareness of self and surroundings.

19. Cerebral _____ has been classically defined as the ability of the brain to maintain

constant cerebral blood flow despite changes in systemic arterial pressure.

20. At least three metabolic factors affect cerebral blood flow: _____, _____, and _____ concentration.

21. _____ is the syndrome of acute focal neurologic deficit from a vascular disorder that injures brain tissue.

22. _____ strokes are caused by an interruption of blood flow in a cerebral vessel and _____ strokes are caused by bleeding into brain tissue.

23. Transient ischemic attack (TIA) or "_____" is equivalent to "brain angina" and reflects a temporary disturbance in focal cerebral blood flow, which reverses before infarction occurs, analogous to _____ in relation to heart attack.

24. _____ are the most common cause of ischemic strokes, usually occurring in atherosclerotic blood vessels.

25. _____ infarcts result from occlusion of the smaller penetrating branches of large cerebral arteries, commonly the middle cerebral and posterior cerebral arteries.

26. An _____ stroke is caused by a moving blood clot that travels from its origin to the brain.

27. The most frequently fatal stroke is a spontaneous _____ into the brain.

28. The specific manifestations of stroke or TIA are determined by the _____ that is affected by the area of brain tissue that is supplied by that vessel and by the adequacy of the collateral circulation.

29. Aneurysmal subarachnoid hemorrhage represents bleeding into the subarachnoid space caused by a ruptured _____.

30. _____ malformations are a complex tangle of abnormal arteries and veins linked by one or more fistulas.

31. _____ represents a generalized infection of the parenchyma of the brain or spinal cord.

32. _____ occurs with or without nausea, may be projectile, and is a common symptom of increased intracranial pressure (ICP) and brain stem compression.

33. The use of _____ for brain tumors is somewhat limited by the blood–brain barrier.

34. A _____ represents the abnormal behavior caused by an electrical discharge from neurons in the cerebral cortex.

35. _____ seizures usually involve only one hemisphere and are not accompanied by loss of consciousness or responsiveness.

36. _____ seizures involve impairment of consciousness and often arise from the temporal lobe.

37. Myoclonic seizures involve brief, involuntary _____ induced by stimuli of cerebral origin.

38. _____ seizures usually present with a person having a vague warning and experience a sharp tonic contraction of the muscles with extension of the extremities and immediate loss of consciousness.

39. Seizures that do not stop spontaneously or occur in succession without recovery are called _____.

Activity B *Consider the following figure.*

Anterior

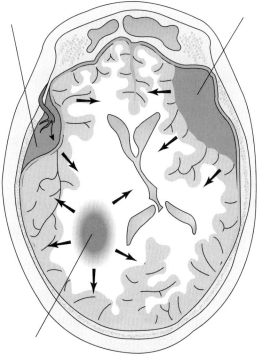

Posterior

In the figure above, identify the subdural hematoma, the epidural hematoma, and the intracerebral hematoma.

Activity C *Match the key terms in Column A with their definitions in Column B.*

Column A

_____ **1.** Vasogenic edema

_____ **2.** Hypoxia

_____ **3.** Tentorium cerebelli

_____ **4.** Hydrocephalus

_____ **5.** Aphasia

_____ **6.** Microneurons

_____ **7.** Ischemia

_____ **8.** Decorticate posturing

_____ **9.** Hemineglect

_____ **10.** Macroneurons

Column B

a. To attend to and react to stimuli coming from the contralateral side

b. Inability to comprehend, integrate, and express language

c. Small cells intimately involved in local circuitry

d. Divides the cranial cavity into anterior and posterior fossae

e. Reduced or interrupted blood flow

f. Occurs when integrity of the blood–brain barrier is disrupted

g. Deprivation of oxygen with maintained blood flow

h. Results from lesions of the cerebral hemisphere

i. Large cells with long axons that leave the local network of intercommunicating neurons to send action potentials to other regions of the nervous system

j. Abnormal increase in cerebrospinal fluid (CSF) volume in any part or all of the ventricular system

Activity D

In the boxes below, put the pathologic process of bacterial meningitis in order:

1. Release endotoxins

2. Development of a cloudy, purulent exudate in CSF

3. Endotoxins initiate inflammatory response

4. Meninges thicken and adhesions form

5. Bacteria replicate and undergo lysis in CSF

6. Vascular congestion and infarction in the surrounding tissues

7. Pathogens, neutrophils, and albumin to move across the capillary wall into the CSF

8. Adhesions may impinge on the cranial nerves or impair the outflow of CSF

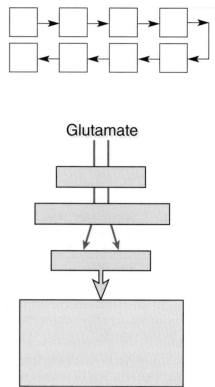

2. Complete the flowchart above using the following terms:

- release of intracellular proteases, free radicals, and fragmentation of nuclei
- calcium cascade
- opening calcium channels
- N-methyl-D-aspartate (NMDA) receptor activation

Activity E *Briefly answer the following.*

1. To what does "global ischemia" refer and what is the result of global ischemia?

_____

_____

_____

2. Explain what watershed infarcts are and why they occur.

_____

_____

_____

3. What is the mechanism of toxicity of excito-toxic amino acids?

4. What is postconcussion syndrome?

5. Compare the general manifestations of global and focal brain injury.

6. What are the two components of consciousness? What are the signs of altered consciousness?

7. How are pupillary reflexes used to evaluate levels of brain function?

8. What is the ischemic penumbra of an ischemic stroke and how does it affect the degree of irreversible damage?

9. Why do arteriovenous malformations predispose a patient to stroke?

10. What are some of the possible causes of a seizure?

SECTION III: APPLYING YOUR KNOWLEDGE

Activity F *Consider the following scenario and answer the questions.*

A 78-year-old African American woman is brought to the emergency department by ambulance. She was found on the floor of her bedroom by her daughter in a confused state, and she could not move her left leg. A diagnosis of stroke is suspected.

1. When taking the nursing history, for what risk factors would you assess?

2. The diagnosis of ischemic stroke is confirmed. What orders would the nurse expect to receive from the physician for acute ischemic stroke?

SECTION IV: PRACTICING FOR NCLEX

Activity G *Answer the following questions.*

1. Match the type of brain insult to its definition.

Type
_____ 1. Hypoxic
_____ 2. Ischemic
_____ 3. Excitotoxic
_____ 4. Increased intercranial volume and pressure
_____ 5. Brain herniation
_____ 6. Cerebral edema
_____ 7. Hydro-cephalus

Definition
a. Excessive activity of the excitatory neurotransmitters and their receptor-mediated effects
b. Displacement of brain tissue under the falx cerebri or through the tentorial notch or incisura of the tentorium cerebelli
c. Interferes with delivery of oxygen and glucose as well as the removal of metabolic wastes

d. An abnormal increase in cerebrospinal fluid volume in any part or all of the ventricular system

e. Swelling of the brain

f. Increase in intercranial tissue causing an increase in intracranial pressure

g. Decreased oxygen levels in all brain tissue

2. Match the type of brain insult to its effect on the brain

Type

_____ 1. Brain herniation

_____ 2. Hypoxic

_____ 3. Ischemic

_____ 4. Increased intercranial volume and pressure

_____ 5. Excitotoxic

_____ 6. Hydrocephalus

_____ 7. Cerebral edema

Effect on Brain

a. Can be focal or global, with only one part of the brain being underperfused or all of the brain being compromised

b. Neuronal cell injury and death

c. Clouding of consciousness, bilaterally small pupils (approximately 2 mm in diameter) with a full range of constriction, and motor responses to pain that are purposeful or semipurposeful (localizing) and often asymmetric

d. Depends on the brain's compensatory mechanisms and the extent of the swelling

e. Generalized depressant effect on the brain

f. Cerebral hemispheres become enlarged, and the ventricular system beyond the point of obstruction is

dilated. The sulci on the surface of the brain become effaced and shallow, and the white matter is reduced in volume.

g. Tissue perfusion becomes inadequate, cellular hypoxia results, and neuronal death can occur.

3. Several types of brain injuries can occur. What are the primary (or direct) brain injuries? Mark all that apply.

a. Focal lesions of laceration

b. Contusion

c. Hypoxic

d. Diffuse axonal

e. Hemorrhage

4. Global and focal brain injuries manifest differently. What is almost always a manifestation of a global brain injury?

a. Altered level of consciousness

b. Change in behavior

c. Respiratory instability

d. Loss of eye movement reflexes

5. You are the nurse caring for a 31-year-old trauma victim admitted to the neurologic intensive care unit (ICU). During your initial assessment, you find that the patient is flexing arms, wrists, and fingers. There is abduction of the upper extremities with internal rotation and plantar flexion of the lower extremities. How would you describe this in your nursing notes?

a. Decerebrate posturing

b. Decorticate posturing

c. Extensor posturing

d. Diencephalon posturing

6. Brain death is the term used when irreversible loss of function of the entire brain occurs. A clinical examination must be done and repeated at least 6 hours later with the same findings for brain death to be declared. What is not assessed in the clinical examination for brain death?

a. Blink reflex

b. Responsiveness

c. Electrocardiographic (ECG) findings

d. Respiratory effort

7. Much as with brain death, there are criteria for the diagnosis of a persistent vegetative state, and the criteria have to have lasted for more than 1 month. What are criteria for the diagnosis of persistent vegetative state? Mark all that apply.
   a. Bowel and bladder incontinence
   b. Ability to open the eyes
   c. Lack of language comprehension
   d. Lack of sufficient hypothalamic function to maintain life
   e. Variable preserved cranial nerve reflexes

8. The regulation of cerebral blood flow is accomplished through both autoregulation and local regulation. This allows for the brain to meet its metabolic needs. What is the low parameter for blood pressure before cerebral blood flow becomes severely compromised?
   a. 30 mm Hg
   b. 40 mm Hg
   c. 50 mm Hg
   d. 60 mm Hg

9. Intracranial aneurysms that rupture cause subarachnoid hemorrhage in the patient. How is the diagnosis of intracranial aneurysms and subarachnoid hemorrhage made?
   a. Lumbar puncture
   b. Magnetic resonance imaging (MRI)
   c. Loss of cranial nerve reflexes
   d. Venography

10. When the suspected diagnosis is bacterial meningitis, what assessment techniques can assist in determining the presence of meningeal irritation?
   a. Kernig sign and Chadwick sign
   b. Brudzinski sign and Kernig sign
   c. Brudzinski sign and Chadwick sign
   d. Chvostek sign and Guedel sign

11. Manifestations of brain tumors are focal disturbances in brain function and increased intracranial pressure (ICP). What causes the focal disturbances manifested by brain tumors?
   a. Tumor infiltration and increased blood pressure
   b. Brain compression and decreased ICP
   c. Brain edema and disturbances in blood flow
   d. Tumor infiltration and decreased ICP

12. Match the type of seizure with its definition.

Type of Seizure
____ 1. Unprovoked
____ 2. Complex partial seizures
____ 3. Generalized-onset
____ 4. Absence seizures
____ 5. Atonic
____ 6. Tonic-clonic

Definition
a. Motion takes the form of automatisms such as lip smacking, mild clonic motion (usually in the eyelids), increased or decreased postural tone, and autonomic phenomena
b. These seizures also are known as drop attacks
c. Most common major motor seizure
d. Clinical signs, symptoms, and supporting electroencephalographic (EEG) changes indicate involvement of both hemispheres at onset
e. Begins in a localized area of the brain but may progress rapidly to involve both hemispheres
f. No identifiable cause can be determined

13. For seizure disorders that do not respond to anticonvulsant medications, an option for surgical treatment exists. What is removed in the most common surgery for seizure disorders?
   a. Temporal neocortex
   b. Hippocampus
   c. Entorhinal cortex
   d. Amygdala

14. Generalized convulsive status epilepticus is a medical emergency caused by a tonic-clonic seizure that does not spontaneously end, or recurs in succession without recovery. What is the first-line drug of choice to treat status epilepticus?
   a. Intravenous (IV) diazepam
   b. Intramuscular (IM) lorazepam
   c. IV cyclobenzaprine
   d. IM cyproheptadine

CHAPTER 52

Sleep and Sleep Disorders

SECTION I: LEARNING OBJECTIVES

1. Cite the major brain structures that are involved in sleep

2. Describe the different stages of sleep in terms of the electroencephalogram (EEG) tracing, eye movements, motor movements, heart rate, blood pressure, and cerebral activity

3. Characterize the circadian rhythm as it relates to sleep and wakefulness

4. Describe the possible role of melatonin in regulation of sleep

5. List the four categories of sleep disorders included in the *International Classification of Sleep Disorders*

6. Describe the methods used in diagnosis of sleep disorders, including the sleep history, sleep diary, polysomnography, and wrist actigraphy

7. Characterize the non–24-hour sleep–wake syndrome experienced by visually impaired individuals, sleep disorders associated with acute shifts in the sleep–wake cycle due to intercontinental travel and shift work, and advanced sleep phase and delayed sleep phase circadian rhythm sleep disorders

8. Describe the causes, manifestations, diagnosis, and treatment of acute and chronic insomnia

9. Differentiate periodic limb movement disorder and restless legs syndrome in terms of manifestations and treatment

10. Explain the physiologic mechanisms, contributing factors, and manifestations of obstructive sleep apnea and describe the methods used in diagnosis and treatment of the disorder

11. Define the term *parasomnias* and relate it to the manifestations of nightmare, sleep terrors, and sleep walking

12. Characterize normal sleep patterns of the infant and small child and relate them to the development of sleep disorders

13. Describe the normal changes in sleep stages that occur with aging and relate them to sleep problems in the elderly

SECTION II: ASSESSING YOUR UNDERSTANDING

Activity A *Fill in the blanks.*

1. _____ is a time of mental activity and energy expenditure; _____ is a period of inactivity and restoration of mental and physical function.

2. Many hormones, such as growth hormone, are produced in a cyclic manner correlating with the sleep–wake cycle, suggesting that _____ and tissue _____ may occur during sleep.

3. The _____ of the midbrain, pons, and brain stem monitors and modulates the activity of various circuits controlling wakefulness.

4. The normal _____ consists of brain waves of various frequencies rather than the combined activity and "cross-talk" among

288

many hundreds of neurons responding to a given stimulus.

5. _____ sleep is a quiet type of sleep characterized by a relatively inactive, yet fully regulating brain, and fully movable body.

6. _____ sleep is associated with rapid eye movements, loss of muscle movements, and vivid dreaming.

7. It has been shown that adequate amounts of _____ sleep are necessary for normal daytime functioning.

8. _____, a hormone produced by the pineal gland, is thought to help regulate the sleep–wake cycle and, possibly, circadian rhythm.

9. A _____ is fundamental to the process of identifying the nature of a sleep disorder.

10. The _____ are disorders that produce either excessive sleepiness or difficulty initiating or maintaining sleep.

11. The non–24-hour sleep–wake syndrome consists of a lack of _____ between the internal sleep–wake rhythm and the external 24-hour day.

12. _____ is caused by the sudden loss of synchrony between a traveler's intrinsic circadian clock and the local time of the flight's destination.

13. People with _____ have trouble staying awake in the evening and have to curtail evening activities to avoid falling asleep.

14. _____ has been defined as three or more of the following: difficulty initiating sleep, difficulty maintaining sleep, waking up too early, or sleep that is chronically non-restorative or poor in quality.

15. Sleep _____ refers to a set of rules and information about personal and environmental activities that affect sleep.

16. _____ is characterized by episodes of repetitive movement of the large toe with flexion of the ankle, knee, and hip during sleep.

17. Apnea is defined as cessation of airflow through the nose and mouth for _____ or longer.

18. _____ are vivid and terrifying nocturnal episodes in which the dreamer is abruptly awakened from sleep.

19. _____ persons have more fragmented sleep and shorter duration of stage 3 and 4 sleep.

Activity B *Consider the following figure.*

In the figure above, label the structures of the mouth and throat; highlight those involved in obstructive sleep apnea.

- uvula
- soft palate
- nasopharynx
- oropharynx
- laryngopharynx
- tongue
- epiglottis

Activity C *Match the key terms in Column A with their definitions in Column B.*

Column A

____ **1.** Thalamo-cortical loop

____ **2.** Narcolepsy

____ **3.** Periodic breathing

Column B

a. A sudden recurrent uncontrollable compulsion to sleep

b. Interrupted sleep caused by disordered breathing

_____ **4.** Confusional arousals

_____ **5.** Alpha rhythm

_____ **6.** Actigraphy

_____ **7.** Dreams

_____ **8.** Sleep apnea

_____ **9.** Entrainment

_____ **10.** Beta rhythm

c. EEG pattern that occurs when a persons eyes are open

d. Measures muscle motion

e. Recollections of mental activity that occurred during sleep

f. Marked confusion, slow and inappropriate responses to questions, and nonpurposeful activities

g. EEG pattern that occurs when a person is awake with eyes closed

h. Daily resetting of the circadian clock

i. Differential patterns of breathing associated with non-REM sleep

j. Pathways between each sensory area of the thalamus and the cortex

Activity D *Briefly answer the following.*

1. What is the sleep–wake cycle? Describe both what it means to sleep and to be awake.

2. What are the four stages of non-REM sleep and what occurs during each stage?

3. What are the physiologic changes that are seen during REM sleep?

4. What are the categories of sleep disorders set by the American Sleep Disorders Association?

5. What are the components of a typical polysomnography?

6. What are some of the common causes of chronic insomnia?

7. How does the National Institute of Health define restless leg syndrome (RLS)?

8. What is the pathologic mechanism of sleep apnea?

SECTION III: APPLYING YOUR KNOWLEDGE

Activity E *Consider the following scenario and answer the questions.*

A 52-year-old man is being admitted for a sleep study. He reports a history of severe snoring, obesity for more than 10 years, falling asleep at work, and waking frequently during the night. His presumptive diagnosis is obstructive sleep apnea.

1. As he is being prepared for the study, the patient asks what obstructive sleep apnea is. Your correct response would be what?

2. The patient asks how many episodes of apnea does it take to be diagnosed with obstructive sleep apnea. Your correction response would be what?

_____

_____

_____

3. The patient asks what his treatment would be if he is diagnosed with severe sleep apnea. You would expect orders for what?

_____

_____

_____

SECTION IV: PRACTICING FOR NCLEX

Activity F *Answer the following questions.*

1. One of the stages of sleep is the rapid eye movement, or REM, stage. What is it that the brain cannot do during REM sleep?

　a. Acquire new sensory information

　b. Regulate blood pressure

　c. Replay previous memories

　d. Arouse auditory and visual systems

2. What hormone does the pineal gland synthesize and release under the direct control of the suprachiasmatic nucleus (SCN)?

　a. Growth hormone

　b. Melatonin

　c. Cortisol

　d. Dehydroepiandrosterone (DHEA)

3. The multiple sleep latency test (MSLT) is a diagnostic sleep study used to evaluate daytime sleepiness. What result of an MSLT would be considered abnormal?

　a. 10 minutes

　b. 12 minutes

　c. 4 minutes

　d. 5 minutes

4. Restless leg syndrome (RLS) is a disorder that has its peak onset in middle age. Diagnosis of RLS is based on a history of what?

　a. Compelling urge to rest legs

　b. Motor relaxation

　c. Symptoms that are worse in the afternoon

　d. Symptoms that become worse at rest

5. Match the type of dyssomnia with their definition.

Type of Dyssomnia	Definition
____ **1.** Jet lag	**a.** A lack of synchronization between the internal sleep–wake rhythm and the external 24-hour day
____ **2.** Change in sleep phase disorder	
	b. Advanced or delayed sleep phase syndrome
____ **3.** Shift work sleep disorder	**c.** Clash between shift demands for wakefulness as part of the work environment and the sleep setting of the worker's intrinsic circadian clock.
____ **4.** Non–24-hour sleep–wake syndrome	
____ **5.** Insomnia	**d.** Sudden loss of synchrony between a traveler's intrinsic circadian clock and the local time of the flight's destination.
____ **6.** Narcolepsy	
	e. A syndrome characterized by abnormal sleep tendencies, including excessive daytime sleepiness, disturbed nocturnal sleep, and manifestations related to REM sleep, such as cataplexy (brief periods of muscle weakness), hypnagogic hallucinations, and sleep paralysis.
	f. Sleep that is chronically nonrestorative or poor in quality

6. Sleepwalking can occur in both adults and children. Typically, what does someone who is sleepwalking do?

　a. Refuse to respond to communication efforts of other people

　b. Go outside

　c. Appear alert

　d. Fix something to eat

7. The onset of sleep terrors is usually between the ages of 2 and 4 years. What are the manifestations of sleep terrors? Mark all that apply.

   a. Dilated pupils

   b. Rapid breathing

   c. Tachycardia

   d. Screams on awakening

   e. Refuses to go to sleep in own bed

8. The prevalence of sleep disorders increases with age. Medication use is one reason for this. What medication can have a stimulating effect that interferes with sleep?

   a. Vasoconstrictors

   b. Antihypertensives

   c. Beta blockers

   d. Vasodilators

9. In what disease is often seen more frequent periods of nighttime awakening and daytime sleeping?

   a. Parkinson disease

   b. Huntington disease

   c. Alzheimer disease

   d. Amyotrophic lateral sclerosis (ALS)

10. Actigraphy can be used to diagnose sleep disturbances. The actigraph is worn on the wrist and is used most commonly with what?

   a. A sleep diary

   b. CPAP

   c. Video tape of sleep

   d. Trial pharmacologic substances

CHAPTER 53

Disorders of Thought, Mood, and Memory

SECTION I: LEARNING OBJECTIVES

1. Define the terms *biologic psychiatry* and *psychosocial psychiatry* and compare them in terms of their definitions of the origins of mental disease

2. Describe the changes in the treatment of mental illness over the past three centuries

3. Explain the role that heredity plays in the epidemiology and development of mental illness

4. Name the cerebral cortical structures and structures from the primitive brain involved in thought and emotion

5. Describe the major functions of each brain structure in terms of thought processes, learning, and emotion

6. Describe the cortical pathways by which learning and the development of memory occur

7. Define the terms *synapse*, *synaptic transmission*, and *neuromediators*

8. Name the major neuromediators in the brain, their major location and source, and possible involvement of each in the manifestations of mental illness

9. Define the term *schizophrenia*

10. Describe the epidemiology of schizophrenia

11. Describe the manifestations of schizophrenia, both positive and negative symptoms, and their underlying neuropathophysiology

12. Cite the diagnostic criteria for schizophrenia according to the *DSM-IV-TR* classification

13. Describe the treatment for the positive and negative manifestations of schizophrenia

14. Define the terms *depression* and *mania*

15. Describe the epidemiology of major depression and bipolar depression

16. Describe the manifestations of major depression and bipolar depression

17. Cite the diagnostic criteria for depression according to the *DSM-IV-TR* classification

18. Describe the treatment modalities for depression

19. Define the terms *panic disorder, generalized anxiety disorder, social phobia,* and *obsessive-compulsive disorder*

20. Describe the epidemiology of panic disorder, generalized anxiety disorder, social phobia, and obsessive-compulsive disorder

21. Describe the manifestations of panic disorder, generalized anxiety disorder, social phobia, and obsessive-compulsive disorder and the underlying neuropathophysiology of each

22. Cite the diagnostic criteria for panic disorder, generalized anxiety disorder, social phobia, and obsessive-compulsive disorder according to the *DSM-IV-TR* classification

23. Describe the treatment for panic disorder, generalized anxiety disorder, social phobia, and obsessive-compulsive disorder

24. Define substance dependence

25. Describe the epidemiology of addiction disorders

26. Describe the neurophysiologic alterations associated with substance dependence

27. Cite the actions of medications used in the treatment of substance dependence

28. State the criteria for a diagnosis of dementia

29. Compare the causes associated with Alzheimer disease, vascular dementia, frontotemporal dementia, Creutzfeldt-Jakob disease, Wernicke-Korsakoff syndrome, and Huntington disease

30. Describe the changes in brain tissue that occur with Alzheimer disease

31. Use the three stages of Alzheimer disease to describe its progress

32. Cite the difference between Wernicke disease and the Korsakoff component of the Wernicke-Korsakoff syndrome

SECTION II: ASSESSING YOUR UNDERSTANDING

Activity A *Fill in the blanks.*

1. One view of psychiatric illness is that mental disorders are due to anatomic, developmental, and functional disorders of the brain, and is called _____ psychiatry. Another view is that mental disorders are due to impaired psychological development, a consequence of poor child rearing or environmental stress, and is called _____ psychiatry.

2. The introduction of _____ as a treatment for schizophrenia revolutionized psychiatry because, although it did not cure psychosis, it did control the symptoms of the disease, increasing the potential for more traditional therapies to work and allowing previously institutionalized individuals to lead much more normal lives.

3. There is scientific evidence that anatomic and biochemical _____ in the brain play a critical role in the behaviors observed in mental illness.

4. The _____ lobe is the largest lobe and is often referred to as the chief administrator of the brain.

5. A large part of the cerebral cortex forms _____ areas that add perception and meaning to incoming sensory information.

6. The _____ association area functions in close connection with the motor cortex to plan and execute complex motor movements.

7. Two disorders of information processing, _____ and _____ thoughts, are common symptoms of many psychiatric disorders.

8. _____ hallucinations occur when a normal sensory input is blocked and, as a replacement, stored images are experienced, whereas _____ hallucinations are produced by abnormal neuronal discharges.

9. _____ are characterized by a false belief and the persistent, unshakable acceptance of the false belief.

10. The treatment of many psychiatric disorders is based on pharmacologic interventions that alter _____ or _____ properties of the brain.

11. _____ alleviate depressive symptoms by increasing the activity of norepinephrine and serotonin at postsynaptic membrane receptors.

12. _____ is a chronic debilitating psychotic disorder that affects thinking, feeling, perceiving, behaving, and experiencing the environment without the normal linkages to that environment.

13. Mood disorders are disorders of _____ rather than disturbances of thought.

14. _____ is characterized by the same symptoms as major depression, but in a milder form.

15. _____ is a hypothesized phenomenon in which a stressor creates an electrophysiologic vulnerability to future stressful events by causing long-lasting changes in neuronal function.

16. Dopamine activity has also been implicated in mood disorders, with _____ dopamine activity found in depression, and _____ dopamine activity in mania.

17. Substance _____ refers to repeated use of alcohol or other drugs resulting in functional problems; substance _____ refers to the behaviors exhibited when an individual is unable to control the use of drugs or alcohol and continues to use them despite negative consequences.

18. _____ problems that are associated with normal aging tend to reflect a generalized decrease in the efficiency by which information is processed and retrieved.

19. The diagnosis of _____ is based on assessment of the presenting problem; history about the person that is provided by an informant; complete physical and neurologic examination; evaluation of cognition, behavioral, and functional status; and laboratory and imaging studies.

20. _____ disease is characterized by cortical atrophy and loss of neurons, particularly in the parietal and temporal lobes.

21. The major microscopic features of Alzheimer disease are the presence of _____, _____, and amyloid angiopathy.

22. A major component of the paired helical filaments is an abnormally hyperphosphorylated form of the protein _____, an axonal microtubule-associated protein that enhances microtubule assembly.

23. Death related to Alzheimer disease can occur because of complications related to _____.

24. The use of _____ have been shown to be effective in slowing the progression of Alzheimer disease by potentiating the action of available acetylcholine.

25. _____ dementia is caused by brain injury resulting from ischemic or hemorrhagic damage.

26. Originally known as Pick disease, _____ now refers to a syndrome that includes primary progressive aphasia, corticobasal degeneration, progressive supranuclear palsy, and semantic dementias.

27. Creutzfeldt-Jakob disease is a rare rapidly degenerative form of dementia believed to be caused by an infective protein agent called a _____.

28. _____ disease is characterized by acute weakness and paralysis of the extraocular muscles, nystagmus, ataxia, and confusion.

29. _____ disease is a hereditary disorder characterized by chronic progressive chorea, psychological changes, and dementia.

30. Postmortem studies have shown a decrease of _____ and _____ in the basal ganglia of persons dying of Huntington disease.

Activity B *Consider the following figures.*

A

B

1. In this figure, locate the following structures of the brain that are linked to behavior:

- Amygdala
- Mammillary body
- Olfactory bulb
- Frontal lobe
- Parietal lobe
- Occipital lobe
- Temporal lobe
- Central fissure

- Transverse fissure
- Parietooccipital fissure
- Cingulate gyrus
- Corpus callosum
- Anterior nucleus of thalamus
- Fornix
- Parahippocampus gyrus
- Hippocampus

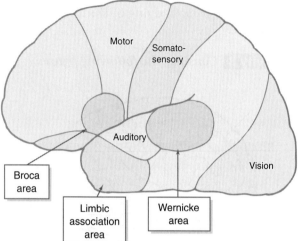

2. In this figure, label the corresponding area of the brain for the following functions:

- Behavior, emotions, motivation
- Word formation
- Planning complex movements and elaboration of thoughts
- Spatial coordinates of body and surroundings
- Language comprehension and intelligence
- Visual processing of words
- Naming of objects

Activity C *Match the key terms in Column A with their definitions in Column B.*

1.

Column A

_____ **1.** Delusions

_____ **2.** Prefrontal lobotomy

_____ **3.** Alogia

_____ **4.** Occipital lobe

_____ **5.** Temporal lobe

_____ **6.** Hallucinations

Column B

a. Using invented words

b. Abnormalities of thought

c. Inability to stick to the original point

d. Tendency to speak very little

e. Integrates and interprets somatic, visual, and auditory information that is critical for recognition of the

_____ **7.** Parietal lobe

_____ **8.** Neologisms

_____ **9.** Wernicke area

_____ **10.** Tangentiality

familiar, as well as appropriate interpretation of and response to social contexts

f. Integration and processing of sensory (visual, tactile, and auditory) input

g. Sensory perceptions with a compelling sense of reality

h. Responsible for language comprehension

i. Receives visual information

j. Severed the connections between the prefrontal areas of the brain and the remainder of the brain

2.

Column A

_____ **1.** Mesolimbic dopamine system

_____ **2.** Disorganized schizophrenia

_____ **3.** Obsessive-compulsive disorder

_____ **4.** Dementia

_____ **5.** Anhedonia

_____ **6.** Dyskinesias

_____ **7.** Mania

_____ **8.** Paranoid schizophrenia

_____ **9.** Amyloid precursor protein

_____ **10.** Anxiety disorder

Column B

a. Cognitive decline caused by any disorder that permanently damages large association areas of the cerebral hemispheres or subcortical areas subserving memory and learning

b. Marked by racing thoughts, high distractibility, and rapid and pressured speech

c. Major component of neuritic plaque

d. Anxiety disorder characterized by recurrent obsessions and compulsions

e. Brain area that adapts to habitual use of drugs

f. Inability to experience pleasure in things that are ordinarily pleasurable

g. Distortion in performing voluntary movements

h. Schizophrenia that manifests with persecutory or grandiose delusions

i. Excessive worry that is not easily controlled

j. Disintegration of the personality and a predominance of negative symptoms

Activity D *Briefly answer the following.*

1. What is known about the genetic potential of mental illness?

2. What is the function of the hippocampus?

3. What can be said about how the brain physiologically perceives thought and memory?

4. Which neurotransmitters have been implicated in metal illness?

5. What are the major types of antidepressants, and how do they work?

6. What are the symptoms of schizophrenia? What is meant by positive and negative?

7. What are the anatomic abnormalities associated with schizophrenia?

8. What is meant by "major depressive disorder?"

9. There are several types of depression. Each is categorized by its manifestations and symptoms. What are the types and their related manifestations?

10. What is the biogenic amine theory of depression?

11. What are the manifestations of a panic attack? Why must it be considered, initially, as a critical health problem?

12. What is believed to be the cause of Alzheimer disease?

SECTION III: APPLYING YOUR KNOWLEDGE

Activity E *Consider the following scenario and answer the question.*

A 65-year-old woman has just been diagnosed with Alzheimer disease. She calls the clinic and asks if she and her family can come in and have someone talk to them about the disease. The nurse sets aside time for this patient and her family.

1. In teaching this family about Alzheimer disease, what are the major points she should convey to them?

   _____

   _____

   _____

SECTION IV: PRACTICING FOR NCLEX

Activity F *Answer the following questions.*

1. In the 1960s, the deinstitutionalization of the mentally ill occurred along with a move to community psychiatry. What was a cause of this movement?
   a. Psychopharmacology
   b. Medicalizing of deviance
   c. Feeling that a calming environment was crucial
   d. Homelessness

2. In the 1990s, studies were conducted on whether mental illness had a genetic basis. What do the results of the studies show?
   a. Mental illness is a Mendelian trait
   b. Mental illness is polygenic
   c. Mental illness is a recessive trait
   d. Mental illness is based solely on environment

3. What are the major neuromediators? Mark all that apply.
   a. Norepinephrine
   b. Gamma-aminobutyric acid
   c. Succinylcholine
   d. Serotonin
   e. Dopamine

4. What is the task of the prefrontal area of the brain?
   a. Control speech
   b. Control hearing
   c. Manage information
   d. Comprehend language

5. Sensory input from the environment is received by what area of the brain?
   a. Hypothalamus
   b. Broca's area
   c. Amygdala
   d. Thalamus

6. Thought and memory pass across synapses in the brain. What are the neural circuits transmitted by new or reactivated pathways called?
   a. Memory traces
   b. Information processing
   c. Information storage
   d. Memory searches

7. Hallucinations can be categorized in several ways. What hallucinations are the products of abnormal neuronal discharges?
   a. Visual
   b. Ictal
   c. Emotional
   d. Release

8. Hallucinations are abnormalities of perception, whereas delusions are abnormalities of thought. What have delusions been associated with?
   a. Sensory overload
   b. Disorders of information management
   c. Sensory deprivation
   d. Disorders of speech

9. The emergence of psychotropic medications gave us the ability to target specific actions in the brain as treatment for mental illness. Which psychotropic medication is a monoamine oxidase inhibitor?
   a. Valium
   b. Halcion
   c. Paxil
   d. Nardil

10. Schizophrenia is a complex disease that strikes men and women equally. What is a common sign or symptom of schizophrenia in its early stages?

    a. Enhancement of senses

    b. Using invented words

    c. Visual hallucinations

    d. Catatonic behavior

11. Match the subclassification of depression or dysthymia with its symptoms.

Subclassification	Symptoms
____ **1.** Catatonic	**a.** Increased emphasis related to the baby
____ **2.** Melancholic	**b.** Low self-esteem, sleep and energy problems
____ **3.** Atypical	
____ **4.** Postpartum	**c.** Hypersomnia
____ **5.** Dysthymia	**d.** Excessive mobility or motoric immobility
	e. Insomnia with early morning awakening

12. Bipolar disorder, also called manic-depressive disorder, has a variety of subclassifications based on the manic episodes of the disorder. What is the severity of manic symptoms called?

    a. Mania

    b. Cyclothymia

    c. Specifier

    d. Kindling

13. Anticonvulsive medications are used in the treatment of bipolar depression. What other drug is used to treat bipolar disorder?

    a. Valium

    b. Flexeril

    c. Lithium

    d. Restoril

14. Panic attacks may result from a "fear network" that has become abnormally sensitive. Where is this "fear network" centered?

    a. Hippocampus

    b. Prefrontal cortex

    c. Thymus

    d. Amygdala

15. Obsessive-compulsive disorder (OCD) is a disorder that remains under investigation as to its actual neurophysiology. What is OCD believed to be a product of?

    a. Dysfunction of the caudate nucleus

    b. Overexcitement of the globus pallidus

    c. Hypersensitive reaction of the frontal cortex

    d. Dysfunction of the amygdala

16. Abuse and addiction are believed to have a neurophysiologic basis. What does habitual use of drugs or alcohol do to the body?

    a. Decrease serotonin reuptake

    b. Increase dopamine transmission

    c. Alter gamma-aminobutyric acid pathways

    d. Reduce the brain's ability to adapt

17. Wernicke-Korsakoff syndrome is a dementia that is associated with chronic alcoholism. It is caused by a deficiency in thiamine (vitamin B_{12}). What is the most distinctive sign or symptom of this syndrome?

    a. Loss of memory

    b. Inability to interact with environment

    c. Confabulation

    d. Isolationism

18. Huntington disease is a genetic disorder that does not usually manifest itself until the patient is in his or her 40s or 50s. What are the most common early psychological changes that occur with Huntington disease? Mark all that apply.

    a. Moodiness

    b. Impulsive behavior

    c. Personality changes

    d. Mania

    e. Heightened sensory awareness

Disorders of Visual Function

SECTION I: LEARNING OBJECTIVES

1. State the cause of eyelid weakness

2. Define the terms *entropion* and *ectropion*

3. Explain the differences between marginal blepharitis, a hordeolum, and a chalazion as to causes and manifestations

4. State the causes and treatment of dry eye

5. Compare symptoms associated with red eye caused by conjunctivitis, corneal irritation, and acute glaucoma

6. Describe the appearance of corneal edema

7. Characterize the manifestations, treatment, and possible complications of bacterial, *Acanthamoeba*, and herpes keratitis

8. Describe the structures of the uveal tract

9. Describe tests used in assessing the pupillary reflex and cite the possible causes of abnormal pupillary reflexes

10. Describe the formation and outflow of aqueous humor from the eye and relate to the development of glaucoma

11. Compare open-angle and angle-closure glaucoma in terms of pathology, symptomatology, and diagnosis and treatment

12. Explain why glaucoma leads to blindness

13. Describe changes in eye structure that occur with near and farsighted vision

14. Describe the changes in lens structure that occur with cataract

15. Cite risk factors and visual changes associated with cataract

16. Describe the treatment of persons with cataracts

17. Relate the phagocytic function of the retinal pigment epithelium to the development of retinitis pigmentosa

18. Cite the manifestations and long-term visual effects of papilledema

19. Describe the pathogenesis of background and proliferative diabetic retinopathies and their mechanisms of visual impairment

20. Relate the role of posterior vitreous detachment to the development of retinal tears and detachment

21. Explain the pathology and visual changes associated with macular degeneration

22. Characterize what is meant by a *visual field defect*

23. Explain the use of perimetry in the diagnosis of a visual field defect

24. Define the terms *hemianopia, quadrantanopia, heteronymous hemianopia,* and *homonymous hemianopia* and relate them to disorders of the optic pathways

25. Describe visual defects associated with disorders of the visual cortex and visual association areas

26. Describe the function and innervation of the extraocular muscles

27. Recognize the use of smooth pursuit, saccadic, and vergence conjugate gaze movements in self or others

28. Explain the difference between paralytic and nonparalytic strabismus

29. Define *amblyopia* and explain its pathogenesis

30. Explain the need for early diagnosis and treatment of eye movement disorders in children

SECTION II: ASSESSING YOUR UNDERSTANDING

Activity A *Fill in the blanks.*

1. The optic globe, commonly called the _____, is a remarkably mobile, nearly spherical structure contained in a pyramid-shaped cavity of the skull called the orbit.

2. The outer layer of the eyeball consists of a tough, opaque, white, fibrous layer called the _____.

3. The upper and lower eyelids, the _____, are modified folds of skin with associated muscle and cartilaginous plates that protect the eyeball.

4. Two striated muscles, the _____ and the _____, provide for movement of the eyelids.

5. _____ is a common bilateral inflammation of the anterior or posterior structures of eyelid margins.

6. _____ blepharitis is usually associated with dandruff of the scalp or brows.

7. The main symptoms of _____ are irritation, burning, redness, and itching of the eyelid margins.

8. _____ blepharitis is inflammation of the eyelids that involves the meibomian glands.

9. Symptoms of _____ are a foreign body sensation, a scratching or burning sensation, itching, and photophobia.

10. _____ conjunctivitis is a severe, sight-threatening ocular infection.

11. The _____ is avascular and obtains its nutrient and oxygen supply by diffusion from blood vessels of the adjacent sclera, from the aqueous humor at its deep surface, and from tears.

12. _____ refers to inflammation of the cornea caused by infections, misuse of contact lenses, hypersensitivity reactions, ischemia, trauma, defects in tearing, and interruption in sensory innervation, as occurs with local anesthesia.

13. Herpes simplex virus _____ with stromal scarring is the most common cause of corneal ulceration and blindness in the Western world.

14. Herpes zoster _____ usually presents with malaise, fever, headache, and burning and itching of the periorbital area.

15. The _____ is an adjustable diaphragm that permits changes in pupil size and in the light entering the eye.

16. Inflammation of the entire uveal tract, which supports the lens and neural components of the eye, is called _____.

17. With diffuse damage to the forebrain involving the thalamus and hypothalamus, the _____ are typically small but respond to light.

18. _____ includes a group of conditions that produce an elevation in intraocular pressure.

19. In persons with glaucoma, temporary or permanent impairment of vision results from _____ changes in the retina and optic nerve and from corneal edema and opacification.

20. _____ glaucoma is caused by a disorder in which the anterior chamber retains its fetal configuration, with aberrant trabecular meshwork extending to the root of the iris, or is covered by a membrane.

21. Nonuniform curvature of the refractive medium comparing the horizontal and vertical planes is called _____.

22. _____ is neurologically associated with convergence of the eyes, pupillary constriction, and results from thickening of the lens through contraction of the ciliary muscle.

23. A _____ is a lens opacity that interferes with the transmission of light to the retina.

24. The function of the _____ is to receive visual images, partially analyze them, and transmit this modified information to the brain.

25. The genetically _____ person has never experienced the full range of normal color vision and is unaware of what he or she is missing.

26. _____ represents a group of hereditary diseases that cause slow degenerative changes in the retinal photoreceptors.

27. _____ degeneration is characterized by degenerative changes in the central portion of the retina that results primarily in loss of central vision.

28. _____ are related inherited or acquired mutations in the retinoblastoma (Rb) tumor suppressor gene, located on the long arm of chromosome 13.

29. The _____ refers to the area that is visible during fixation of vision in one direction.

30. Three pairs of extraocular muscles—the superior and _____, the medial and _____, and the superior and inferior _____—control the movement of each eye.

31. _____ movements are those in which the optical axes of the two eyes are kept parallel, sharing the same visual field.

32. _____ eye movements are sudden, jerky conjugate movements that quickly change the fixation point.

33. _____ refers to any abnormality of eye coordination or alignment that results in loss of binocular vision.

34. _____ describes a decrease in visual acuity resulting from abnormal visual development in infancy or early childhood.

Activity B *Consider the following figures.*

1.

1. In this figure, locate and label the following structures:

- Conjunctiva
- Cornea
- Lens
- Iris
- Meibomian gland
- Orbicularis oculi muscle
- Inferior oblique muscle
- Inferior rectus
- Superior rectus
- Levator palpebrae superioris
- Choroid
- Retina
- Superior tarsal plate
- Ciliary body
- Sclera
- Optic nerve

2.

A

B

C

3.

2. In this figure, which eye represents myopia? Which eye represents hyperopia? Which eye represents normal focal length?

3. In this figure, locate and label the following muscles:
- Medial rectus
- Superior oblique
- Inferior rectus
- Levitator palpebrae
- Lateral rectus
- Temporalis
- Inferior oblique

Activity C *Match the key terms in Column A with their definitions in Column B.*

1.

Column A

_____ **1.** Arcus senilis
_____ **2.** Entropion
_____ **3.** Ophthalmia neonatorum
_____ **4.** Hordeolum
_____ **5.** Pink eye
_____ **6.** Chalazion
_____ **7.** Ptosis
_____ **8.** Dacryo-cystitis
_____ **9.** Ectropion
_____ **10.** Sjögren syndrome

Column B

a. Caused by infection of the sebaceous glands
b. Infection of the lacrimal sac
c. Chronic inflammatory granuloma of a meibomian gland
d. Drooping of the eyelid
e. Extracellular lipid infiltration of the cornea
f. Turning in of the lid margin
g. Conjunctivitis that occurs in newborns and is related to sexually transmitted diseases
h. Diminished salivary and lacrimal secretions, resulting in keratoconjunctivitis sicca and xerostomia
i. Eversion of the lower lid margin
j. Inflammation of the conjunctiva

2.

Column A

_____ **1.** Anopia
_____ **2.** Hyperopia
_____ **3.** Cycloplegia
_____ **4.** Scotoma
_____ **5.** Rhegmato-genous detachment
_____ **6.** Tonometry
_____ **7.** Presbyopia
_____ **8.** Myopia

Column B

a. The vitreous shrinks and partly separates from the retinal surface
b. Hole in the visual field
c. Anterior-posterior dimension of the eyeball is too short
d. Anterior-posterior dimension of the eyeball is too long
e. Measurement of intraocular pressure

_____ **9.** Direct pupillary light reflex
_____ **10.** Papilledema

f. Blindness in one eye
g. Paralysis of the ciliary muscle, with loss of accommodation
h. Leakage of fluid results in edema of the optic papilla
i. Rapid constriction of the pupil exposed to light
j. Decrease in accommodation that occurs because of aging

Activity D *Briefly answer the following.*

1. Where are tears formed, and what purpose(s) do they serve?

_____

_____

_____

2. What is the most common cause of chronic bacterial conjunctivitis, and what are the symptoms?

_____

_____

_____

3. How do the different levels of abrasional trauma (less severe to more severe) affect the cornea, and how fast to the abrasions heal?

_____

_____

_____

4. What is the mechanism of a primary herpes simplex virus optical epithelial infection?

_____

_____

_____

5. What is the cause of acanthamoeba keratitis, and what are the primary symptoms?

_____

_____

_____

6. Explain how the pupil is able to change shape.

7. What is glaucoma? What is primary and secondary glaucoma?

8. What is presbyopia, and how does it affect vision?

9. Retinal hemorrhage can occur at many layers. What are the types of retinal bleeding, and where do they occur?

10. Why is proliferative diabetic retinopathy a major concern for all diabetic patients?

11. What is the relationship between hypertension and the development of a retinopathy?

SECTION III: APPLYING YOUR KNOWLEDGE

Activity E *Consider the following scenario and answer the questions.*

The mother of an 18-month-old girl brings her daughter to the clinic for a well-baby check. During the physical exam, the physician notices that the client has a white reflex in her left eye. He suspects retinoblastoma.

1. What diagnostic measures would the nurse expect the doctor to order?

2. Retinoblastoma is confirmed, and a treatment plan is being made. What are the treatment options for retinoblastoma?

SECTION IV: PRACTICING FOR NCLEX

Activity F *Answer the following questions.*

1. Causes of eyelid weakness include neurologic causes. There can be damage to the cranial nerves that innervate the eyelids, or there can be damage to the central nuclei of the cranial nerves. Where are the central nuclei of cranial nerve (CN) III (oculomotor nerve) and CN VII (facial nerve)?
   a. Midbrain and caudal pons
   b. Faux cerebellum and amygdala
   c. Hypothalamus and pyramid
   d. Medulla oblongata and pineal body

2. Dacryocystitis is an infection in the lacrimal sac. What symptoms indicate dacryocystitis?
   a. Purulent discharge
   b. Swelling
   c. Inflamed conjunctiva
   d. Lack of tears

3. Ophthalmia neonatorum is a conjunctivitis that develops in newborns. It is caused by the agents that cause sexually transmitted diseases. When should ophthalmia neonatorum be suspected?
   a. When a conjunctivitis develops 24 hours after birth
   b. When a conjunctivitis develops 12 hours after birth
   c. When a conjunctivitis develops 48 hours after birth
   d. When a conjunctivitis develops 36 hours after birth

4. Keratitis can be caused by different infectious agents. What is the treatment goal with herpes simplex virus keratitis?

   a. Minimizing pain

   b. Curing the disease

   c. Eliminating viral replication within the cornea

   d. Minimizing spread of virus to other parts of the eye

5. Corneal transplants are performed every day in hospitals around the world. The transplanted corneas come from cadavers. Why do corneal transplants have such a low rejection rate? Mark all that apply.

   a. The cornea is very vascular.

   b. Antigen-presenting cells are not present in great numbers.

   c. The cornea secretes immunosuppressive factors.

   d. The cornea has no lymphatics.

   e. Corneal cells secrete substances that protect against keratitis.

6. Pharmacologic agents can affect dilation of the pupil and the papillary response. What types of drugs produce papillary constriction?

   a. Sympathomimetic agents

   b. Antihistamine agents

   c. Cycloplegic agents

   d. Miotic agents

7. In open-angle glaucoma, there is an increased pressure within the globe of the eye without obstruction at the iridocorneal angle. Usually, this is caused by an abnormality in the trabecular meshwork, which controls the flow or aqueous humor. Where is aqueous humor in a normal eye?

   a. Canal of Schlemm

   b. Ocular canal

   c. Ductus lacrimalis

   d. Behind the pupil

8. Match the terms with their definitions.

Term	Definition
____ 1. Presbyopia	a. Anterior-posterior dimension of the eyeball is too long; the focus point for an infinitely
____ 2. Cycloplegia	
____ 3. Myopia	
____ 4. Hyperopia	distant target is anterior to the retina
____ 5. Astigmatism	b. Paralysis of the ciliary muscle, with loss of accommodation
	c. Anterior-posterior dimension of the eyeball is too short; the image is theoretically focused posterior to (behind) the retina
	d. Range of focus or accommodation is diminished
	e. Asymmetric bowing of the cornea

9. Age-related cataracts are characterized by what?

   a. Everything looking grey

   b. Visual distortion

   c. Narrowing visual field

   d. Blind spots in visual field

10. Vitreous humor occupies the posterior portion of the eyeball. It is an amorphous biologic gel. When liquefaction of the gel occurs, as in aging, what can be seen during head movement?

    a. Blind spots

    b. Meshlike structures

    c. Floaters

    d. Red spots

11. When conditions occur that impair retinal blood flow, such as hyperviscosity of the blood or a sickle cell crisis, what can occur in the eye?

    a. Microaneurysms

    b. Hypertensive retinopathy

    c. Microinfarcts

    d. Neovascularization

12. Age-related macular degeneration that is dry is characterized by what?

    a. Atrophy of the Bruch membrane

    b. Leakage of serous or hemorrhagic fluid

    c. New blood vessels in the eye

    d. Formation of a choroidal neovascular membrane

13. Cortical blindness is the bilateral loss of the primary visual cortex. What is retained in cortical blindness?

a. Red spots seen behind the eyelids

b. Pupillary reflexes

c. Phytosis

d. Myopia

14. Adult strabismus is almost always of the paralytic variety. What is a cause of adult strabismus?

a. Huntington disease

b. Parkinson disease

c. Graves disease

d. Addison disease

15. Amblyopia, or lazy eye, occurs at a time when visual deprivation or abnormal binocular interactions occur in visual infancy. Whether amblyopia is reversible depends on what?

a. Child has to be older than 5 years

b. Maturity of the visual system at time of onset

c. Child has to have bilateral congenital cataracts

d. Child has to be able to wear contact lenses

Disorders of Hearing and Vestibular Function

SECTION I: LEARNING OBJECTIVES

1. List the structures of the external, middle, and inner ear and cite their function

2. Describe two common disorders of the outer ear

3. Relate the functions of the eustachian tube to the development of middle ear problems, including acute otitis media and otitis media with effusion

4. Describe anatomic variations as well as risk factors that make infants and young children more prone to develop acute otitis media

5. List three common symptoms of acute otitis media

6. Describe the disease process associated with otosclerosis and relate it to the progressive conductive hearing loss that occurs

7. Characterize tinnitus

8. Differentiate between conductive, sensorineural, and mixed hearing loss and cite the more common causes of each

9. Describe methods used in the diagnosis and treatment of hearing loss

10. Characterize the causes of hearing loss in infants and children and describe the need for early diagnosis and treatment

11. Explain the function of the vestibular system with respect to postural reflexes and maintaining a stable visual field despite marked changes in head position

12. Relate the function of the vestibular system to nystagmus and vertigo

13. Differentiate the structures of peripheral and central vestibular function

14. Characterize the physiologic cause of motion sickness

15. Compare the manifestations and pathologic processes associated with benign positional vertigo and Ménière disease

16. Differentiate the manifestations of peripheral and central vestibular disorders

SECTION II: ASSESSING YOUR UNDERSTANDING

Activity A *Fill in the blanks.*

1. The external _____ consists of the auricle, which collects sound, and the external

acoustic meatus or ear canal, which conducts sound to the tympanic membrane.

2. Impacted _____ usually produces no symptoms unless it hardens and touches the tympanic membrane or the canal becomes irritated, resulting in symptoms of pain, itching, and a sensation of fullness.

3. _____ is an inflammation of the external ear that can vary in severity from mild allergic dermatitis to severe cellulitis.

4. The tympanic cavity is a small, mucosa-lined cavity within the petrous portion of the _____ bone.

5. The _____ tube, which connects the nasopharynx with the middle ear, is located in a gap in the bone between the anterior and medial walls of the middle ear.

6. The _____ eustachian tube does not close or does not close completely.

7. _____ refers to inflammation of the middle ear without reference to etiology or pathogenesis.

8. _____ is characterized by acute onset of otalgia (or pulling of the ears in an infant), fever, and hearing loss.

9. _____ refers to the formation of new spongy bone around the stapes and oval window, which results in progressive deafness.

10. The spiral canal of the _____, which is shaped like a snail shell, begins at the vestibule and winds around a central core of spongy bone called the modiolus.

11. Persons with damage to _____ of the brain can speak intelligibly and read normally, but are unable to understand the meaning of major aspects of audible speech.

12. _____ hearing loss occurs with disorders that affect the inner ear, auditory nerve, or auditory pathways of the brain.

13. Deafness or some degree of hearing impairment is the most common serious complication of _____ in infants and children.

14. Acoustic neuromas are benign Schwann cell tumors affecting _____.

15. The most common infectious cause of congenital sensorineural hearing loss is _____.

16. The _____ system maintains and assists recovery of stable body and head position through control of postural reflexes, and it maintains a stable visual field despite marked changes in head position.

17. Disorders of vestibular function are characterized by a condition called _____, in which an illusion of motion occurs.

18. _____ is a form of normal physiologic vertigo, caused by repeated rhythmic stimulation of the vestibular system, and encountered in car, air, or boat travel.

19. Benign _____ vertigo is the most common cause of pathologic vertigo.

20. Acute _____ is characterized by an acute onset (usually hours) of vertigo, nausea, and vomiting lasting several days and not associated with auditory or other neurologic manifestations.

21. _____ disease is a disorder of the inner ear due to distention of the endolymphatic compartment of the inner ear, causing a triad of hearing loss, vertigo, and tinnitus.

22. Abnormal nystagmus and vertigo can occur because of central nervous system lesions involving the _____ and lower brain stem.

Activity B *Consider the following figure.*

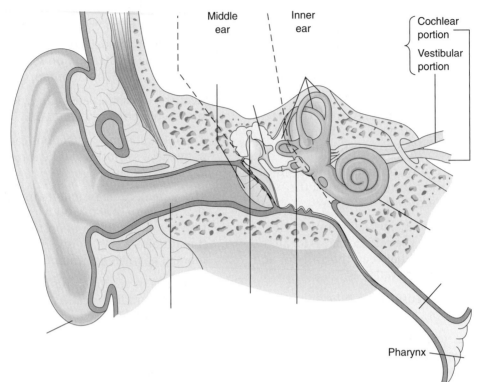

In this figure, locate and label the following structures:

- Auricle
- External acoustic meatus
- Malleus
- Stapes
- Eustachian tube
- Cochlea
- Cranial nerve VIII
- Tympanic membrane
- Incus
- Semicircular canals

Activity C *Match the key terms in Column A with their definitions in Column B.*

Column A

_____ **1.** Otitis media with effusion

_____ **2.** Cerumen

_____ **3.** Tinnitus

_____ **4.** *Streptococcus pneumoniae*

_____ **5.** Electrony-stagmography

Column B

a. Degenerative hearing loss that occurs with advancing age

b. Cystlike lesions of the middle ear

c. Most common cause of bacterial meningitis that results in sensorineural hearing loss after the neonatal period

_____ **6.** Presbycusis

_____ **7.** Nystagmus

_____ **8.** Barotrauma

_____ **9.** Cholestea-tomas

_____ **10.** Frequency

d. Injury resulting from the inability to equalize middle ear with ambient pressures

e. Ringing of the ears, it may also assume a hissing, roaring, buzzing, or humming sound

f. Number of waves per unit time

g. Involuntary rhythmic and oscillatory eye movements that preserve eye fixation on stable objects in the visual field during angular and rotational movements of the head

h. Earwax

i. Examination that records eye movements in response to vestibular, visual, cervical, rotational, and positional stimulation

j. Presence of fluid in the middle ear without signs and symptoms of acute ear infection

Activity D *Briefly answer the following.*

1. What is/are the function(s) of the eustachian tube?

2. What are the complications associated with otitis media?

3. How does otosclerosis lead to progressive deafness?

4. What are the purported causes of subjective tinnitus?

5. What is the cause of hearing loss in conductive hearing loss?

6. How does the vestibular system inform the brain about head and body position?

7. What is the test used to determine vestibular function in an unconscious patient?

SECTION III: APPLYING YOUR KNOWLEDGE

Activity E *Consider the following scenario and answer the question.*

You are the nurse preparing an educational event for the local junior league, which has asked you to speak on hearing loss and deafness. One of the subjects that you will address is ototoxicity.

1. What drugs would you include when talking about ototoxicity?

SECTION IV: PRACTICING FOR NCLEX

Activity F *Answer the following questions.*

1. Otitis externa is an inflammation of the outer ear. What fungi cause otitis externa?
   a. *Aspergillus*
   b. *Pseudomonas aeruginosa*
   c. *Staphylococcus aureus*
   d. *Escherichia coli*

2. The eustachian tube connects the nasopharynx and the middle ear. In infants and children with abnormally patent tubes, what are let into the eustachian tube when the infant or child cries or blows their nose?
   a. Air and cerumen
   b. Air and secretions
   c. Secretions and saliva
   d. Cerumen and saliva

3. Acute otitis media (AOM) is the disorder in children for which antibiotics are most prescribed. What are the risk factors for AOM? Mark all that apply.
   a. Ethnicity
   b. Premature birth
   c. Only child in household
   d. Genetic syndromes
   e. Female gender

4. Otosclerosis is a condition where spongy, pathologic bone grows around the stapes and oval window. It can be treated either medically or surgically. What is the surgical treatment for otosclerosis?
   a. Otosclerotomy
   b. Ovalectomy
   c. Stapedectomy
   d. Amplification surgery

5. What separates the scala vestibule and the scala media?
   a. Corti membrane
   b. Tympani membrane
   c. Modiolus membrane
   d. Reissner membrane

6. Objective tinnitus is tinnitus that someone else can hear. What does the tinnitus that is caused by vascular disorders sound like?
   a. Pulses
   b. Rings
   c. Hums
   d. Roars

7. Conductive hearing loss can occur for a variety of reasons, including foreign bodies in the ear canal, damage to the ear drum, or disease. What disease is associated with conductive hearing loss?
   a. Huntington disease
   b. Paget disease
   c. Alzheimer disease
   d. Parkinson disease

8. Tumors affecting cranial nerve VIII are acoustic neuromas. What are these tumors of?
   a. Inner ear
   b. Organ of Corti
   c. Schwann cells
   d. Labyrinth

9. It is important to differentiate between the kinds of hearing loss so they can be appropriately treated. What is used to test between conductive and sensorineural hearing loss?
   a. AudioScope
   b. Audiometer
   c. Tone analysis
   d. Tuning fork

10. Hearing loss in children can be either conductive or sensorineural, as it is in adults. What is the major cause of sensorineural hearing loss in children?
    a. Genetic causes
    b. Acute otitis media
    c. Paget disease
    d. Ototoxicity

11. Presbycusis is degenerative hearing loss associated with aging. What is the first symptom of this disorder?
    a. Inability to localize sounds
    b. Reduction in ability to understand speech
    c. Inability to detect sound
    d. Reduction in ability to identify sounds

CHAPTER 56

Structure and Function of the Musculoskeletal System

SECTION I: LEARNING OBJECTIVES

1. Describe locations and characteristics of compact and cancellous bone

2. Describe the structure of a long bone

3. Cite the characteristics and name at least one location of elastic cartilage, hyaline cartilage, and fibrocartilage

4. Name and characterize the function of the four types of bone cells

5. State the function of parathyroid hormone, calcitonin, and vitamin D in terms of bone formation and metabolism

6. State the characteristics of tendons and ligaments

7. State the difference between synarthroses and synovial joints

8. Describe the source of blood supply to a synovial joint

9. Explain why pain is often experienced in all the joints of an extremity when only a single joint is affected by a disease process

10. Describe the structure and function of a bursa

11. Explain the pathology associated with a torn meniscus of the knee

SECTION II: ASSESSING YOUR UNDERSTANDING

Activity A *Fill in the blanks.*

1. The bones of the skeletal system serve as a framework for the attachment of _____, _____, and _____.

2. The bones act as a storage reservoir for _____, and the central cavity of some bones contains the hematopoietic connective tissue in which _____ cells are formed.

3. The skeletal system consists of the _____ and _____ skeleton.

4. _____ bone has a densely packed calcified intercellular matrix that makes it more rigid than cancellous bone.

5. _____ are classified by shape as long, short, flat, and irregular.

6. Bones are covered, except at their articular ends, by a membrane called the _____.

7. Bone _____ occupies the medullary cavities of the long bones throughout the skeleton and the cavities of cancellous bone in the vertebrae, ribs, sternum, and flat bones of the pelvis.

8. The _____ enter the bone through a nutrient foramen and supply the marrow space and the internal one-half of the cortex.

9. Bone is _____ tissue in which the intercellular matrix has been impregnated with inorganic _____ salts so that it has great tensile and compressible strength but is light enough to be moved by coordinated muscle contractions.

10. The undifferentiated _____ cells are found in the periosteum, endosteum, and epiphyseal plate of growing bone.

11. _____ are "bone-chewing" cells that function in the resorption of bone, removing the mineral content and the organic matrix.

12. _____ cartilage is found in areas, such as the ear, where some flexibility is important.

13. _____ is found in the intervertebral disks, in areas where tendons are connected to bone, and in the symphysis pubis.

14. _____ cartilage forms the costal cartilages that join the ribs to the sternum and vertebrae, many of the cartilages of the respiratory tract, the articular cartilages, and the epiphyseal plates.

15. _____ inhibits the release of calcium from bone into the extracellular fluid.

16. _____, which attach skeletal muscles to bone, are relatively inextensible because of their richness in collagen fibers.

17. _____ are fibrous thickenings of the articular capsule that join one bone to its articulating mate.

18. _____ are joints that lack a joint cavity and move little or not at all.

19. _____ joints are freely movable joints.

20. The purpose of a _____ sac is to prevent friction on a tendon.

In this figure, locate and label the following structures:

- Proximal epiphysis
- Medullary cavity
- Periosteum
- Nutrient artery
- Compact bone
- Spongy bone
- Yellow marrow
- Diaphysis

Activity C *Match the key terms in Column A with their definitions in Column B.*

Column A	Column B
___ 1. Trabeculae	a. Connect adjacent haversian canals
___ 2. Appendicular skeleton	b. Prebone that will be ossified

_____ **3.** Osteoid

_____ **4.** Lamellar bone

_____ **5.** Haversian canals

_____ **6.** Osteons

_____ **7.** Volkmann canals

_____ **8.** Axial skeleton

_____ **9.** Endosteum

_____ **10.** Chondrocytes

c. Bones of the skull, thorax, and vertebral column

d. Mature bone found in the adult skeleton

e. Contains the blood vessels and nerve supply for the osteon

f. Bones of the upper and lower extremities, including the shoulder and hip

g. Membrane that lines the spaces of spongy bone, the marrow cavities, and the haversian canals

h. Cells that form cartilage

i. Concentric lamellae of bone matrix, surrounding a central canal

j. Lined with osteogenic cells and filled with red or yellow bone marrow

Activity D

1. In this flowchart, put the following in the proper sequence:

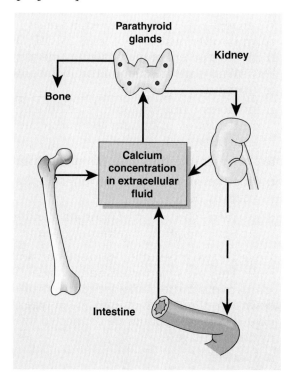

- Reabsorption of calcium via 1,25-dihydroxy-vitamin D_3
- Synthesis of 1,25-dihydroxy-vitamin D_3
- Release of calcium and phosphate
- Reabsorption of calcium
- Urinary excretion of phosphate

Activity E _Briefly answer the following._

1. What is the typical structure of a long bone?

_____

_____

_____

2. What are the two types of bone marrow, and what are their functions?

_____

_____

_____

3. What is the make up of the intercellular matrix of bone tissue?

_____

_____

_____

4. What are the similarities and differences between bone and cartilage?

_____

_____

_____

5. How does parathyroid hormone maintain serum calcium levels?

_____

_____

_____

6. What is the action of vitamin D?

_____

_____

_____

SECTION III: APPLYING YOUR KNOWLEDGE

Activity F *Consider the following scenario and answer the questions.*

A 62-year-old woman with multiple sclerosis (MS) was referred to the orthopedic clinic by her primary care physician due to pain on movement in her upper arms. Because of the MS, the client's legs were extremely weak, and the client had to lift herself out of a chair with her arms. After a physical examination, the orthopedic physician diagnosed her as having bilateral biceps tendonitis.

1. The client asks what causes tendonitis. What would be the correct answer?

   _____

   _____

   _____

2. The client asks if all tendons are like the biceps tendons. What would be the correct answer?

   _____

   _____

   _____

SECTION IV: PRACTICING FOR NCLEX

Activity G *Answer the following questions.*

1. The metaphysis is the part of the bone that fans out toward the epiphysis. What is the metaphysis composed of?
   a. Trabeculae
   b. Cancellous bone
   c. Red bone marrow
   d. Endosteum

2. We have both red and yellow bone marrow in our bodies. What is yellow bone marrow largely composed of?
   a. Hematopoietic cells
   b. Adipose cells
   c. Cancellous cells
   d. Osteogenic cells

3. Lamellar bone is the bone tissue that is found in the adult body. What is lamellar bone largely composed of?
   a. Hematopoietic cells
   b. Spicules
   c. Osteons
   d. Macrocrystalline cells

4. Our bodies contain three types of cartilage: elastic cartilage, hyaline cartilage, and fibrocartilage. Which of these types of cartilage is found in the symphysis pubis?
   a. None
   b. Elastic
   c. Hyaline
   d. Fibrocartilage

5. Parathyroid hormone functions to maintain serum calcium levels. How does it fulfill this function? Mark all that apply.
   a. Initiates calcium release from bone
   b. Enhances intestinal absorption of calcium
   c. Activates conservation of calcium by the kidney
   d. Decreases intestinal absorption of calcium
   e. Inhibits conservation of calcium by the kidney

6. When vitamin D is metabolized, it breaks down into various metabolites. $1,25(OH)_2D_3$ is the most potent of the vitamin D metabolites. What is the function of this metabolite of vitamin D?
   a. Promotes actions of parathyroid hormone on resorption of calcium and phosphate from bone
   b. Decreases intestinal absorption of calcium
   c. Promotes absorption of calcium and phosphate by bone
   d. Decreases absorption of phosphate and increases absorption of calcium by bone

7. There are two types of joints in the human body. They are synarthroses and synovial joints. Synarthroses joints are further broken down into three types of joint. What type of joint occurs when bones are connected by hyaline cartilage?
   a. Synovial
   b. Synchondroses
   c. Syndesmoses
   d. Diarthrodial

8. Rheumatic disorders attack the joints of the body. Which joints are most frequently attacked by rheumatic disorders?
   a. Synchondroses
   b. Articular
   c. Diarthrodial
   d. Synarthroses

9. Each joint capsule has tendons and ligaments? What are the tendons and ligaments of the joint capsule sensitive to?
   a. Position and elevating
   b. Position and lowering
   c. Position and turning
   d. Position and movement

10. Synovial membranes can form sacs called bursae. What is the function of bursae?
    a. Prevent friction on a tendon
    b. Prevent injury to a joint
    c. Prevent friction on a ligament
    d. Cushion the joint

Disorders of Musculoskeletal Function: Trauma, Infection, and Neoplasms

SECTION I: LEARNING OBJECTIVES

1. Describe the physical agents responsible for soft tissue trauma

2. Differentiate among the three types of soft tissue injuries

3. Compare muscle strains and ligamentous sprains

4. Describe the healing process of soft tissue injuries

5. Differentiate open from closed fractures

6. List the signs and symptoms of a fracture

7. Explain the measures used in treatment of fractures

8. Describe the fracture healing process

9. Differentiate the early complications of fractures from later complications of fracture healing

10. Explain the implications of bone infection

11. Differentiate among osteomyelitis due to spread from a contaminated wound, hematogenous osteomyelitis, and osteomyelitis due to vascular insufficiency in terms of etiologies, manifestations, and treatment

12. Cite the characteristics of chronic osteomyelitis

13. Describe the most common sites of tuberculosis of the bone

14. Define *osteonecrosis*

15. Cite four major causes of osteonecrosis

16. Characterize the blood supply of bone and relate it to the pathologic features of the condition

17. Describe the methods used in diagnosis and treatment of the condition

18. Differentiate between the properties of benign and malignant bone tumors

19. Contrast osteogenic sarcoma, Ewing sarcoma, and chondrosarcoma in terms of the most common age groups and anatomic sites that are affected

20. List the primary sites of tumors that frequently metastasize to the bone

21. State the three primary goals for treatment of metastatic bone disease

SECTION II: ASSESSING YOUR UNDERSTANDING

Activity A *Fill in the blanks.*

1. A broad spectrum of _____ injuries result from numerous physical forces, including blunt tissue trauma, disruption of tendons and ligaments, and fractures of bony structures.

2. Unintentional _____ are the number one cause of nonfatal injuries in all age groups.

3. _____ injuries include contusions, hematomas, and lacerations.

4. A _____ is a stretching injury to a muscle or a musculotendinous unit caused by mechanical overloading.

5. A _____ usually is caused by abnormal or excessive movement of the joint.

6. A _____ involves the displacement or separation of the bone ends of a joint with loss of articulation.

7. _____ bodies are small pieces of bone or cartilage within a joint space.

8. _____ injuries and impingement disorders can result from a number of causes, including excessive use, a direct blow, or stretch injury, usually involving throwing or swinging, as with baseball pitchers or tennis players.

9. Meniscus injury commonly occurs as the result of a _____ injury from a sudden or sharp pivot or a direct blow to the knee, as in hockey, basketball, or football.

10. _____ of the hip commonly result from the knee being struck while the hip and knee are in a flexed position.

11. Grouped according to cause, fractures can be divided into three major categories: fractures caused by _____, fatigue or stress fractures, and _____ fractures.

12. A _____ fracture occurs in bones that already are weakened by disease or tumors.

13. The signs and symptoms of a _____ include pain, tenderness at the site of bone disruption, swelling, loss of function, deformity of the affected part, and abnormal mobility.

14. _____ is another method for achieving immobility and maintaining alignment of the bone ends and maintaining the reduction, particularly if the fracture is unstable or comminuted.

15. _____ are skin bullae and blisters representing areas of epidermal necrosis with separation of epidermis from the underlying dermis by edema fluid.

16. Because of inactivity and restrictions in weight-bearing, the individual with a lower extremity fracture is at risk for the development of venous _____, which includes pulmonary embolism and deep venous thrombosis.

17. The _____ syndrome refers to a constellation of clinical manifestations resulting from the presence of fat droplets in the small blood vessels of the lung or other organs after a long bone fracture or other major trauma.

18. _____ osteomyelitis symptoms include pain, immobility, and muscle atrophy; joint swelling, mild fever, and leukocytosis also may occur.

19. _____, or death of a segment of bone, is a condition caused by the interruption of blood supply to the marrow, medullary bone, or cortex.

20. Malignant bone tumors, such as _____, grow rapidly and can spread to other parts of the body through the bloodstream or lymphatics.

21. _____ bone tumors usually are limited to the confines of the bone, have well-demarcated edges, and are surrounded by a thin rim of sclerotic bone.

22. A _____ is a tumor composed of hyaline cartilage.

23. _____, a malignant tumor of cartilage that can develop in the medullary cavity or peripherally, is the second most common form of malignant bone tumor.

Activity B *Consider the following figure.*

In the figure above, label the type of fracture:

- impacted
- butterfly
- comminuted
- transverse
- oblique
- segmental
- spiral

Activity C *Match the key terms in Column A with their definitions in Column B.*

Column A

_____ **1.** Subluxation

_____ **2.** Malunion

_____ **3.** Contusion

_____ **4.** Compound fracture

_____ **5.** Menisci

_____ **6.** Hematoma

_____ **7.** Chondro-malacia

_____ **8.** Laceration

_____ **9.** Greenstick fracture

_____ **10.** Osteomyelitis

Column B

a. A partial dislocation

b. Acute or chronic infection of the bone

c. Bone fragments have broken through the skin

d. Injury in which the skin is torn or its continuity is disrupted

e. Healing of bone with deformity, angulation, or rotation

f. Large area of local hemorrhage

g. Softening of the articular cartilage

h. A partial break in bone continuity that resembles that seen when a young sapling is broken

i. Area becomes ecchymotic (i.e., black and blue) because of local hemorrhage

j. C-shaped plates of fibrocartilage that are superimposed between the condyles of the femur and tibia

Activity D

1. Put the following events of healing a bone fracture into the proper order in the boxes below.

a. Development of fibrin meshwork within the hematoma

b. Replacement of callus with mature bone

c. Formation of fibro cartilaginous callus

d. Remodeling of bone

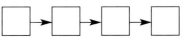

Activity E *Briefly answer the following.*

1. What joints are most commonly involved in sprain type injuries?

_____

_____

_____

2. What is the normal healing process of a sprain? What are some of the greatest concerns?

_____

_____

_____

3. What is the structure of the rotator cuff and how is it usually injured?

_____

_____

_____

4. When someone "breaks a hip" what is usually occurring?

_____

_____

_____

5. What is compartment syndrome and how does it relate to bone tissue?

_____

_____

_____

6. What are the manifestations of osteomyelitis?

_____

_____

_____

7. What is the pathogenesis of osteonecrosis?

_____

_____

_____

8. What are the general characteristics of bone tumors?

_____

_____

_____

9. What is metastatic bone disease?

_____

_____

_____

SECTION III: APPLYING YOUR KNOWLEDGE

Activity F *Consider the following scenario and answer the questions.*

A 15-year-old boy is brought to the emergency department after an injury playing football. The doctor suspects an injury to the meniscus of the knee.

1. As his nurse, what orders would you expect to receive to confirm the suspected diagnosis?

_____

_____

2. The diagnosis of torn meniscus is confirmed. What would the first-line treatment be for this type of injury?

_____

_____

_____

3. The client asks what will happen if his knee does not heal right. The correct answer would include what?

_____

_____

_____

SECTION IV: PRACTICING FOR NCLEX

Activity G *Answer the following questions.*

1. Where do overuse injuries commonly occur?
   a. Knee
   b. Wrist
   c. Neck
   d. Fingers

2. Match the injury to its definition.

Injury	Definition
____ 1. Contusion	a. The ligaments may be incompletely torn or, as in a severe sprain, completely torn or ruptured
____ 2. Hematoma	
____ 3. Laceration	b. An injury in which the skin is torn or its continuity is disrupted
____ 4. Puncture wounds	c. A stretching injury caused by mechanical overloading
____ 5. Strain	d. Blood accumulates and exerts pressure on nerve endings
____ 6. Sprain	e. Displacement or separation of the bone ends of a joint with loss of articulation
____ 7. Dislocation	f. Provide the setting for growth of anaerobic bacteria
	g. The skin overlying the injury remains intact

3. Shoulder and rotator cuff injuries usually occur from trauma or overuse. What orders would be given for conservative treatment of an injured shoulder? Mark all that apply.

   a. Anesthetic injections

   b. Physical therapy

   c. Corticosteroid injections

   d. Anti-inflammatory agents

   e. Pain medicine

4. Hip injuries include dislocations and fractures of the hip. Why is hip dislocation considered a medical emergency?

   a. The dislocation causes great pain

   b. Avascular necrosis can result from the dislocation

   c. The longer the hip is dislocated, the less chance of putting it back in place

   d. Dislocation interrupts the blood supply to the femoral head

5. At times, fractures of long bones need enhancement to promote healing. What can be done to induce bone formation and repair bone defects?

   a. The use of steroids to induce bone growth

   b. The use of growth factors to induce bone growth

   c. The use of vibration therapy to induce bone growth

   d. The use of physical therapy to induce bone growth

6. Determining the extent of the injury when a fracture occurs is important. It is also important to obtain a thorough history. What is important to determine during the history taking? Mark all that apply.

   a. Anyone else in family susceptible to fractures

   b. Recognition of symptoms

   c. Any treatment initiated

   d. Mechanism of injury

   e. What patient has eaten

7. Match the complication with the definition.

Complication of Fracture	Definition
____ 1. Fracture blisters	a. Areas of epidermal necrosis with separation of epidermis from the underlying dermis by edema fluid
____ 2. Compartment syndrome	b. Reflex sympathetic dystrophy
____ 3. Complex regional pain syndrome	c. A condition of increased pressure within a limited space (e.g., abdominal and limb compartments) that compromises the circulation and function of the tissues within the space

8. Fat emboli syndrome (FES) can occur after a fracture of a long bone. What are the clinical features of FES?

   a. Petechiae on soles of feet and palms of hands

   b. Respiratory insufficiency

   c. Encephalopathy

   d. Global neurologic deficits

9. Osteomyelitis is an infection of the bone. Chronic osteomyelitis is complicated by a piece of infected dead bone that has separated from the living bone. How long does the initial intravenous (IV) antibiotic therapy last for chronic osteomyelitis?

   a. 4 weeks

   b. 8 weeks

   c. 12 weeks

   d. 6 weeks

10. Tuberculosis can spread from the lungs into the musculoskeletal system. What is the most common site in the skeletal system for tuberculosis to be found?

   a. Spine

   b. Ankles

   c. Shoulders

   d. Hips

11. Osteonecrosis is a condition where part of a bone dies because of the interruption of its blood supply. What is the most common cause of osteonecrosis other than fracture?

   a. Vessel injury

   b. Prior steroid therapy

   c. Radiation therapy

   d. Embolism

12. Osteosarcoma is an aggressive malignancy of the bone. What is the primary clinical feature of osteosarcoma?

   a. Pain, worse during the day

   b. Erythema in the overlaying skin

   c. Nighttime awakening

   d. Soreness in nearest joint

13. Metastatic bone disease is a frequent disorder. It occurs at a time when primary tumors in the lungs, breasts, and prostate seed themselves (metastasize) to the musculoskeletal system. What are the primary goals of treatment for metastatic bone disease? Mark all that apply.

   a. Prevent pathologic fractures

   b. Cure the disease

   c. Promote survival with maximum functioning

   d. Prevent ischemia to the bone segment

   e. Maintain mobility and pain control

Disorders of Musculoskeletal Function: Developmental and Metabolic Disorders

SECTION I: LEARNING OBJECTIVES

1. Describe the function of the epiphyseal growth plate in skeletal growth

2. Describe common torsional deformities that occur in infants and small children, proposed mechanisms of development, diagnostic methods, and treatment

3. Define genu varum and genu valgum

4. List the problems that occur because of defective tissue synthesis in osteogenesis imperfecta

5. Characterize the abnormalities associated with developmental dysplasia of the hip and methods of diagnosis and treatment

6. Describe the treatment for a newborn with clubfoot

7. Define the term *osteochondroses* and describe the pathology and symptomatology of Legg-Calvé-Perthes disease and Osgood-Schlatter disease

8. Describe the pathology associated with a slipped capital femoral epiphysis and explain why early treatment is important

9. Differentiate between congenital, idiopathic, and neuromuscular scoliosis

10. Cite the origin of osteoclasts and osteoblasts and describe their functions in bone remodeling

11. Describe the function of the RANK ligand/RANK receptor, and the osteoprotegerin-blocking molecule in the regulation of bone remodeling

12. Describe risk factors that contribute to the development of osteoporosis and relate them to the prevention of the disorder

13. Describe the primary features of osteoporotic bone

14. Explain the methods used in the diagnosis of osteoporosis

15. Describe the actions of medications used in the treatment of osteoporosis

16. Compare the pathogenesis and manifestations of osteomalacia and rickets

17. Characterize the cause and manifestations of Paget disease

SECTION II: ASSESSING YOUR UNDERSTANDING

Activity A *Fill in the blanks.*

1. _____ disorders may develop because of normal growth and developmental processes due to hereditary or congenital influences.

2. The long bones of the skeleton, which grow at a relatively rapid rate, are provided with a specialized structure called the _____.

3. The _____ that accompanies joint laxity, coupled with the _____ forces exerted on the limbs during growth, is responsible for a number of variants seen in young children.

4. _____ disease is a developmental deformity of the medial half of proximal tibial epiphysis that results in a progressive varus angulation below the knee.

5. The most common anomaly of the toes or fingers is _____ or the presence of an extra digit on the hand or foot.

6. Osteogenesis imperfecta is a hereditary disease characterized by defective synthesis of _____.

7. Developmental _____ of the hip is an abnormality in hip development that leads to a wide spectrum of hip problems in infants and children, including hips that are unstable, malformed, subluxated, or dislocated.

8. Maternal smoking is associated with the occurrence of _____, and the risk increases enormously when combined with a family history.

9. The primary pathologic feature of Legg-Calvé-Perthes disease is an _____ of the bone and marrow involving the epiphyseal growth center in the femoral head.

10. _____ disease involves microfractures in the area where the patellar tendon inserts into the tibial tubercle, which is an extension of the proximal tibial epiphysis.

11. When appropriately stimulated by growth factors, such as bone morphogenic proteins (BMPs), fibroblast growth factor (FGF), platelet–derived growth factor (PDGF), insulin-like growth factor, and transforming growth factor-β(TGF-β), _____

undergo cell division and differentiate into osteoblasts.

12. _____ is characterized by a reduction in bone mass greater than expected for age, race, or sex that occurs because of a decrease in bone formation, inadequate bone mineralization, or excessive bone deossification.

13. _____ is a metabolic bone disease characterized by a loss of mineralized bone mass causing increased porosity of the skeleton and susceptibility to fractures.

14. _____ osteoporosis, which is caused by an estrogen deficiency, is manifested by a loss of cancellous bone and a predisposition to fractures of the vertebrae and distal radius.

15. _____ osteoporosis is associated with many conditions, including endocrine disorders, malabsorption disorders, malignancies, alcoholism, and certain medications.

16. _____ is a generalized bone condition in which there is inadequate mineralization of bone.

17. A form of osteomalacia called _____ occurs in persons with chronic renal failure.

18. Rickets is a metabolic bone disorder, characterized by a failure or delay in _____ of the cartilaginous growth plate in children whose epiphyses have not yet fused.

19. Paget disease is characterized by focal areas of excessive bone _____ and disorganized osteoid formation.

20. The bones most often affected in _____ disease are the femur, pelvis, humerus, and tibia.

Activity B *Match the key terms in Column A with their definitions in Column B.*

Column A

_____ 1. Pes planus

_____ 2. Genu varum

_____ 3. Osteomalacia

_____ 4. Femoral torsion

_____ 5. Scoliosis

_____ 6. Femoral anteversion

Column B

a. Lateral deviation of the spinal column

b. Outward bowing of the knees >1 inch when the medial malleoli of the ankles are touching

c. Softening of the bones without loss of bone tissue

_____ **7.** Syndactyly

_____ **8.** Internal tibial torsion

_____ **9.** RANKL

_____ **10.** Genu valgum

d. Expressed by osteoblasts and their immature precursors and is necessary for osteoclast differentiation and function

e. Abnormal variations in hip rotation

f. Deformity in which there is decreased space between the knees

g. Rotation of the tibia that makes the feet appear to turn inward

h. Flat footedness

i. Simple webbing of the fingers or toes

j. 80 to 90 degrees of internal rotation of the hip in the prone position

Activity C *Briefly answer the following.*

1. What factors have a negative impact on epiphyseal growth?

_____

_____

_____

2. What is toeing-in and toeing-out?

_____

_____

_____

3. What are the clinical manifestations of osteogenesis imperfecta?

_____

_____

_____

4. What are the different types of scoliosis? Explain what is known about each type.

_____

_____

_____

5. How do osteoclasts and osteoblasts achieve bone metabolism?

_____

_____

_____

6. What is the pathogenesis of osteoporosis?

_____

_____

_____

7. What are the clinical manifestations of osteoporosis?

_____

_____

_____

SECTION III: APPLYING YOUR KNOWLEDGE

Activity D *Consider the following scenario and answer the questions.*

You admit to your floor a 60-year-old man with Paget disease. His symptoms include vertigo, nerve palsies in the upper extremities, and mental deterioration. He asks what drugs he will be given while he is hospitalized.

1. What drugs would the nurse include in her explanation?

_____

_____

_____

SECTION IV: PRACTICING FOR NCLEX

Activity E *Answer the following questions.*

1. Torsional deformities can be natural in infants. When a malalignment does not correct itself, or is not corrected by the time the child reaches the age of 10 to 12, a torsional deformity or malalignment becomes problematic. What is a problem that can occur with femoral anteversion?

a. Patellar subluxation

b. Toeing-in

c. Toeing-out

d. Metatarsus adductus

2. Genu varum and genu valgum, bowlegs and knock-knees, during infancy and toddler-hood, are common findings. They usually correct themselves once the child becomes weight-bearing on the lower extremities. When it does not self-correct, what can genu valgum cause?

a. Gait awkwardness

b. Subluxation

c. Metatarsus adductus

d. Radial torsion

3. Osteogenesis imperfecta is the most common hereditary bone disease. What are the manifestations of osteogenesis imperfecta? Mark all that apply.

a. Triangular appearance to face

b. Thick bones in lower extremities

c. Blue or gray sclera

d. Thick skin

e. Scoliosis

4. Congenital clubfoot is usually corrected non-surgically during the first few weeks of life. Once the correction is made, how is it maintained?

a. The Ponseti method of periodic stretching

b. Galeazzi splints worn for 6 months

c. Denis Browne splint worn for 3 months

d. Ortolani method of periodic stretching

5. Legg-Calvé-Perthes disease is an osteonecrotic disease of the proximal (capital) femoral epiphysis. What does treatment involve? Mark all that apply.

a. Assistive devices

b. Periods of rest

c. Abduction braces

d. Weight-bearing braces

e. Adduction braces

6. Osgood-Schlatter disease is a disease that strikes children between the ages of 11 and 15. This disease involves microfractures, where the patellar tendon inserts into the tibial tubercle. What is Osgood-Schlatter disease characterized by?

a. Pain in the hip

b. Thinning of the patellar tendon

c. Pain in knee at rest

d. Thickening of patellar tendon

7. Scoliosis is an abnormal curvature of the spine. Why is it first noticed?

a. Because of the deformity it causes

b. Because the child cannot stand straight

c. Because of the pain it causes

d. Because the child cannot walk straight

8. Osteoporosis is a disease caused by demineralization of bone. What is the clinical method of choice for diagnosing osteoporosis?

a. Serum calcium levels

b. Dual-energy x-ray absorptiometry (DXA) of the spine and hip

c. Magnetic resonance imaging (MRI) of the chest cavity and femur

d. Body mass index (BMI)

9. Osteomalacia is a bone disease caused by one of two reasons: inadequate calcium absorption or phosphate deficiency. In the elderly, what is the least expensive and most effective long-term treatment for osteomalacia?

a. Pharmacologic replacement of calcium and vitamin D

b. Intravenous (IV) phosphorus

c. Vitamin D rich diet and exposure to mid-day sun

d. Increased calcium and phosphorus in diet

10. Adult rickets can result from several disorders. It can also have a pharmacologic basis for its onset. Which medication can cause rickets in an adult?

a. Cephalosporins

b. Sulfur-based antibiotics

c. Sodium-sparing diuretics

d. Aluminum-sparing antacids

59

Disorders of the Musculoskeletal Function: Rheumatic Disorders

SECTION I: LEARNING OBJECTIVES

1. Characterize the common characteristics of the different systemic autoimmune rheumatic disorders

2. Describe the pathologic changes that may be found in the joint of a person with rheumatoid arthritis

3. List the extra-articular manifestations of rheumatoid arthritis

4. Describe the immunologic process that occurs in systemic lupus erythematosus

5. List four major organ systems that may be involved in systemic lupus erythematosus

6. Describe the manifestations of systemic sclerosis

7. Cite a definition of the seronegative spondyloarthropathies

8. Cite the primary features of ankylosing spondylitis

9. Describe how the site of inflammation differs in spondyloarthropathies from that in rheumatoid arthritis

10. Contrast and compare ankylosing spondylitis, reactive arthritis, and psoriatic arthritis in terms of cause, pathogenesis, and clinical manifestations

11. Compare rheumatoid arthritis and osteoarthritis in terms of joint involvement, level of inflammation, and local and systemic manifestations

12. Describe the pathologic joint changes associated with osteoarthritis

13. Characterize the treatment of osteoarthritis

14. Relate the metabolism and elimination of uric acid to the pathogenesis of crystal-induced arthropathy

15. State why asymptomatic hyperuricemia is a laboratory finding and not a disease

16. Describe the clinical manifestations, diagnostic measures, and methods used in the treatment of gouty arthritis

17. List three types of juvenile arthritis and differentiate among their major characteristics

18. Name one rheumatic disease that affects only the elderly population

SECTION II: ASSESSING YOUR UNDERSTANDING

Activity A *Fill in the blanks.*

1. The cause of _____ remains uncertain, but evidence points to a genetic predisposi-

tion and the development of joint inflammation that is immunologically mediated.

2. It has been suggested that rheumatoid arthritis is initiated in a genetically predisposed individual by the activation of a _____ response to an immunologic trigger, such as a microbial agent.

3. Systemic lupus erythematosus (SLE) is a _____ disease that can affect virtually any organ system, including the musculoskeletal system.

4. Almost all persons with _____ develop polyarthritis and Raynaud phenomenon, a vascular disorder characterized by reversible vasospasm of the arteries supplying the fingers.

5. _____ is a chronic, systemic inflammatory disease of the joints of the axial skeleton manifested by pain and progressive stiffening of the spine.

6. The reactive _____ can be defined as sterile inflammatory joint disorders that are distant in time and place from the initial inciting infective process.

7. _____ is considered a clinical manifestation of reactive arthritis that may be accompanied by extra-articular symptoms such as uveitis, bowel inflammation, and carditis.

8. Arthritis that is associated with an inflammatory bowel disease usually is considered an _____ arthritis because the intestinal disease is directly involved in the pathogenesis.

9. _____, the most prevalent form of arthritis, is a leading cause of disability and pain in the elderly.

10. Popularly known as _____ arthritis, osteoarthritis (OA) is characterized by significant changes in both the composition and mechanical properties of cartilage.

11. _____ syndrome includes acute arthritis with recurrent attacks of severe articular and periarticular inflammation; tophi or the accumulation of crystalline deposits in articular surfaces, bones, soft tissue, and cartilage; gouty nephropathy or renal impairment; and uric acid kidney stones.

12. _____, which is characterized by synovitis, can influence epiphyseal growth by stimulating growth of the affected side.

13. Children with _____ may present with constitutional symptoms, including fever, malaise, anorexia, and weight loss, just as do adults.

14. Juvenile _____ is an inflammatory myopathy primarily involving skin and muscle and it is associated with a characteristic rash.

15. _____ is the most common complaint of elderly persons.

16. _____ is by far the most common form of arthritis among the elderly.

17. _____ is an inflammatory condition of unknown origin characterized by aching and morning stiffness in the cervical regions and shoulder and pelvic girdle areas.

Activity B *Consider the following figure.*

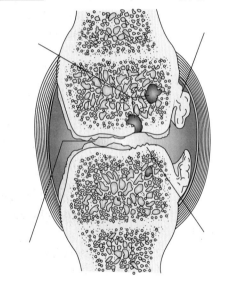

In the figure above, locate the following joint changes seen in osteoarthritis.

- joint space narrows
- erosion of cartilage and bone
- osteophyte development
- bone cysts

Activity C *Match the key terms in Column A with their definitions in Column B.*

Column A	Column B
____ **1.** Spondyloarthropathies	**a.** Autoimmune disease of connective tissue characterized by excessive collagen deposition
____ **2.** Reactive arthritis	
____ **3.** Systemic lapis erythematosus	**b.** Bone spurs

____ **4.** Joint mice

____ **5.** Scleroderma

____ **6.** Osteophytes

____ **7.** Ankylosing spondylitis

____ **8.** Baker cyst

____ **9.** Polymyalgia rheumatica

____ **10.** Gout

c. Multisystem inflammatory disorders that primarily affect the axial skeleton

d. An inflammatory erosion of the sites where tendons and ligaments attach to bone

e. Result from the presence of a foreign substance in the joint tissue

f. Inflammatory condition marked by antinuclear antibodies

g. Enlargement of the bursa in the popliteal area behind the knee

h. Disorder of the muscles and joints, typically of older persons, characterized by pain and stiffness, affecting both sides of the body, and involving the shoulders, arms, neck, and buttock areas

i. Uric acid crystals are found in the joint cavity

j. Fragments of cartilage and bone often become dislodged, creating free-floating osteocartilaginous bodies

Activity D

1. Put the following processes involved in rheumatoid arthritis in proper sequence.

a. Inflammatory response

b. Recruitment of inflammatory cells

c. Destruction of articular cartilage

d. Complement fixation

e. T cell-mediated response

f. Release of enzymes and prostaglandins

g. RF antigen/IgG interaction

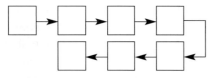

Activity E *Briefly answer the following.*

1. What is the pathogenesis of rheumatoid arthritis?

_____

_____

_____

2. What causes the degradation of a joint in rheumatoid arthritis?

_____

_____

_____

3. What are the musculoskeletal manifestations of systemic lupus erythematosus (SLE)?

_____

_____

_____

4. What are the typical joint changes seen in osteoarthritis?

_____

_____

_____

5. What is the pathogenesis of primary and secondary gout?

_____

_____

_____

SECTION III: APPLYING YOUR KNOWLEDGE

Activity F *Consider the following scenario and answer the questions.*

A 5-year-old girl is brought to the clinic by her mother because she "just isn't feeling well." While taking the history, you note a weight loss of 5 pounds during the past year and complaints of malaise. The child's growth chart shows she is in the 20th percentile for height. During the physical examination, the physician notes pain in three joints, hepatosplenomegaly and lymph adenopathy. The suspected diagnosis is juvenile idiopathic arthritis (JIA). The mother asks you what JIA is.

1. What information would you include in your response?

_____

_____

_____

2. What confirmative test would you expect to see ordered?

_____

_____

_____

SECTION IV: PRACTICING FOR NCLEX

Activity G *Answer the following questions.*

1. Joint destruction in rheumatoid arthritis (RA) occurs by an obscure process. The cellular changes, however, have been documented. Place the process in the correct order.
   a. Vasodilation
   b. Joint swelling
   c. Neutrophils, macrophages and lymphocytes arrive
   d. Lysosomal enzymes released
   e. Immune complexes phagocytized
   f. Inflammatory response
   g. Reactive hyperplasia of synovial cells and subsynovial tissues
   h. Increased blood flow to joint
   i. Destructive changes in joint cartilage

2. Systemic lupus erythematosus (SLE) has been called the great imitator because it can affect many different body systems. What is one of the most commonly occurring symptoms in the early stages of SLE?
   a. Arthritis
   b. Avascular necrosis
   c. Rupture of the Achilles tendon
   d. Classic malar rash

3. Scleroderma is an autoimmune disease of connective tissue that is characterized by hardening of the skin. What diseases do most people with scleroderma develop? Mark all that apply.
   a. Dumping syndrome
   b. Chronic diarrhea
   c. Polyarthritis
   d. Raynaud phenomenon
   e. Chronic vasoconstriction

4. Polymyositis and dermatomyositis are chronic inflammatory myopathies that commonly manifest systemically. What is the treatment of choice for these myopathies?
   a. Muscle relaxants
   b. Corticosteroids
   c. IgG
   d. Nonsteroidal anti-inflammatory drugs (NSAIDs)

5. Ankylosing spondylitis is a disease that typically manifests in late adolescence and early adulthood. What is characteristic of the pain in ankylosing spondylitis?
   a. Worse when active
   b. Worse when sitting
   c. Worse when resting or lying in bed
   d. Worse when standing

6. Reiter syndrome is a reactive arthropathy. What disease is Reiter syndrome associated with?
   a. Pelvic inflammatory disease
   b. Gonorrhea
   c. Syphilis
   d. Human immunodeficiency virus (HIV)

7. A seronegative inflammatory arthropathy is psoriatic arthritis. What drug has been found to be beneficial in controlling both the psoriasis and the arthritis in these patients?
   a. Etanercept
   b. Acetaminophen
   c. Interferon B
   d. Econazole

8. Osteoarthritis (OA) is the most common cause of arthritis and a significant cause of disability in the elderly. What joint changes occur in OA? Mark all that apply.

a. Creation of spurs

b. Loss of synovial fluid

c. Loss of articular cartilage

d. Inflammation of cartilage

e. Synovitis

9. Gout, or gouty arthritis, cannot be diagnosed on the basis of hyperuricemia. What is the diagnostic criterion for gout?

a. Finding of tophaceous deposits

b. Finding of monosodium urate crystals in the synovial fluid

c. Finding of sodium urate crystals in the tissues

d. Finding of urate crystal deposits in the synovial fluid

10. Elderly patients need special consideration in the treatment of the arthritic diseases. Non-steroidal anti-inflammatory drugs (NSAIDs), a first-line group of drugs used in the general population for arthritic diseases, may not be well tolerated by the elderly. What side effects of NSAIDs might be seen in the elderly?

a. Malaise

b. Lethargy

c. Sleeplessness

d. Mania

Structure and Function of the Skin

SECTION I: LEARNING OBJECTIVES

1. Describe the protective functions of skin

2. Characterize the changes in a keratinocyte from its inception in the basal lamina to its arrival on the outer surface of the skin

3. List the four specialized cells of the epidermis and describe their functions

4. Describe the structure and function of the dermis and subcutaneous layers of skin

5. Describe the following skin appendages and their functions: sebaceous gland, eccrine gland, apocrine gland, nails, and hair

6. Characterize the skin in terms of sensory and immune functions

7. Describe the following skin rashes and lesions: macule, patch, papule, plaque, nodule, tumor, wheal, vesicle, bulla, and pustule

8. Describe the characteristics and causes of blisters, calluses, and corns

9. Cite two physiologic explanations for pruritus

10. Describe the causes and treatment of dry skin

11. State common variations found in dark skin

SECTION II: ASSESSING YOUR UNDERSTANDING

Activity A *Fill in the blanks.*

1. The skin, also called the _____, is one of the largest and most versatile organs of the body, accounting for approximately 16% of the body's weight.

2. Variations are found in the properties of the skin, such as the _____ of skin layers, the distribution of sweat glands, and the number and size of hair follicles.

3. The _____ covers the body, and it is specialized in areas to form the various skin appendages: hair, nails, and glandular structures.

4. The top or surface layer of the skin, the _____, consists of dead, keratinized cells.

5. _____ produce keratin, a complex protein that that forms the surface of the skin, is also the structural protein of the hair, and nails.

6. _____ are pigment-synthesizing cells that are located at or in the basal layer.

7. Exposure to the sun's ultraviolet rays increases the production of _____, causing tanning to occur.

8. _____ cells are potent antigen-presenting cells.

9. The _____ is involved in skin disorders that cause bullae or blister formation.

10. The dermis supports the _____ and serves as its primary source of nutrition.

11. The receptors for touch, pressure, heat, cold, and pain are widely distributed in the _____.

12. The _____ layer of the dermis is supplied with free nerve endings that serve as nociceptors and thermoreceptors.

13. _____ sweat glands are simple tubular structures that originate in the dermis and open directly to the skin surface.

14. _____ sweat glands open through a hair follicle and are found primarily in the axillae and groin.

15. Hair is a _____ structure that is pushed upward from the hair follicle.

16. The nails are hardened _____ plates, called fingernails and toenails, which protect the fingers and toes and enhance dexterity.

17. A _____ is a vesicle or fluid-filled papule.

18. A _____ is a hyperkeratotic plaque of skin caused by chronic pressure or friction.

19. _____ are small, well-circumscribed, conical, keratinous thickenings of the skin.

20. Dry skin, also called _____, may be a natural occurrence, as in the drying of skin associated with aging, or it may be symptomatic of underlying systemic disease or skin disorder such as contract dermatitis.

Activity B   *Consider the following figures.*

1. In the figure above, locate and label the following structures:

- nerve ending
- sebaceous gland
- blood vessel
- arrector pili muscle
- dermis
- sweat gland
- papillae
- epidermis

f. Inner layer of skin

g. Mechanoreceptors

h. Immune cells

i. Transformation from viable cells to the dead cells of the stratum corneum

j. Provide sensory information

Activity D *Briefly answer the following.*

1. What are the vital functions of the skin?

_____

_____

_____

2. What are the layers of the epidermis?

_____

_____

_____

3. How is it that a person with albinism cannot synthesize melanin?

_____

_____

_____

4. What is the relationship between melanin and different colors of skin?

_____

_____

_____

5. Describe the structure and function of sebaceous glands.

_____

_____

_____

6. How does an itch differ from pain?

_____

_____

_____

2. In the figure above, locate and label the following structures:

- epidermis
- hair papilla
- dermis
- hair shaft
- arrector pili
- sebaceous gland
- keratinized cells
- hair follicle
- dermal blood vessels

Activity C *Match the key terms in Column A with their definitions in Column B.*

Column A

_____ **1.** Keratinocytes

_____ **2.** Merkel cells

_____ **3.** Keratinization

_____ **4.** Epidermis

_____ **5.** Papillary dermis

_____ **6.** Langerhans' cells

_____ **7.** Dermis

_____ **8.** Ruffini corpuscles

_____ **9.** Melanin

_____ **10.** Reticular dermis

Column B

a. Consists of collagen fibers and ground substance

b. Responsible for skin color, tanning, and protecting against ultraviolet radiation

c. Outer layer of skin

d. Produce a fibrous protein called keratin, which is essential to the protective function

e. Complex meshwork of three-dimensional collagen bundles interconnected with large elastic fibers and ground substance

SECTION III: APPLYING YOUR KNOWLEDGE

Activity E *Consider the following scenario and answer the questions.*

You are the nurse preparing an educational event for the local chapter of the Parent-Teacher Association (PTA). You have been asked to speak on skin disorders.

1. What information would you include about dark-skinned people?

_____

_____

_____

SECTION IV: PRACTICING FOR NCLEX

Activity F *Answer the following questions.*

1. Among the skin's known protective functions is that it serves as an immunologic barrier. What cells detect foreign antigens?

   a. Langerhans' cells
   b. Merkel cells
   c. Keratinocytes
   d. Melanocytes

2. Match the cells of the epidermis with their description or function.

Cell	Description or Function
____ 1. Keratino-cytes	a. Thought to be neuroendocrine cells
____ 2. Melanocytes	b. Pigment-synthesizing cells
____ 3. Merkel cells	c. Replaces lost skin cells
____ 4. Langerhans cells	d. Immunologic cells

3. The basement membrane separates the epithelium from the underlying connective tissue. It is a major site of what is found in skin disease?

   a. Melanocytes
   b. Complement deposition
   c. Lamina lucida
   d. Type IV collagen

4. The pars reticularis is characterized by what?

   a. Dendritic cells
   b. Its color
   c. Three-dimensional collagen bundles
   d. Its immunologic function

5. Why is the subcutaneous tissue considered part of the skin? Mark all that apply.

   a. Eccrine glands extend to this layer
   b. The keratinocytes are formed in the subcutaneous tissue
   c. Skin diseases can involve the subcutaneous tissue
   d. The Merkel cells are formed in the subcutaneous tissue
   e. Deep hair follicles can be found in the subcutaneous tissue

6. Sebaceous glands excrete a mixture that lubricates the hair and skin. What is this mixture called?

   a. Sweat
   b. Chalasia
   c. Cerumen
   d. Sebum

7. Fingernails and toenails, unlike hair, grow continuously. The nail plate itself is nearly transparent and acts as a window for viewing what?

   a. The amount of oxygen in the blood
   b. The color of the blood in the subcutaneous tissue
   c. The health of the nail plate
   d. The color of the stratum corneum

8. When a degeneration of the epidermal cells occurs, layers of the skin separate because of a disruption of the intercellular junctions. When this occurs what is formed?

   a. Lichenifications
   b. Vesicles
   c. Petechiae
   d. Pressure ulcer

9. Pruritus, or the itch sensation, is a byproduct of almost all skin disorders. However, we can itch without having a skin disorder. Itch then can be local or central in our bodies. Where is it postulated that a central "itch center" exists?

   a. Pons

   b. Medulla oblongata

   c. Somatosensory cortex

   d. Sensory area of the cerebrum

10. The first-line treatment for dry skin is a moisturizing agent. How do these agents work?

    a. Decreasing pruritus

    b. Penetrating the lipid barrier of the skin

    c. Increasing transepidermal water loss

    d. Repairing the skin barrier

Disorders of Skin Integrity and Function

SECTION I: LEARNING OBJECTIVES

1. Describe common pigmentary disorders of the skin

2. Relate the behavior of fungi to the production of superficial skin lesions associated with tinea or ringworm

3. State the cause and describe the appearance of impetigo and ecthyma

4. Compare the viral causes, manifestations, and treatments of verrucae, herpes simplex, and herpes zoster lesions

5. Compare acne vulgaris, acne conglobata, and rosacea in terms of appearance and location of lesions

6. Describe the pathogenesis of acne vulgaris and relate it to measures used in treating the disorder

7. Differentiate allergic and contact dermatitis and atopic and nummular eczema

8. Describe the differences and similarities between erythema multiforme minor, Stevens-Johnson syndrome, and toxic epidermal necrolysis

9. Define the term *papulosquamous* and use the term to describe the lesions associated with psoriasis, pityriasis rosea, and lichen planus

10. Relate the life cycle of *Sarcoptes scabiei* to the skin lesions seen in scabies

11. Use knowledge of the life cycles of *Pediculus humanus corporis* and *Pediculus humanus capitis* to explain the lesions associated with body, head, and pubic lice

12. Describe the three types of ultraviolet radiation and relate them to sunburn, aging skin changes, and the development of skin cancer

13. Describe the manifestations and treatment of sunburn

14. State the properties of an effective sunscreen

15. Compare the tissue involvement in first, second-degree full-thickness, and third-degree burns

16. State how the rule of nine is used in determining the body surface area involved in a burn

17. Cite the determinants for grading burn severity using the American Burn Association classification of burns

18. Describe the systemic complications of burns

19. Describe the major considerations in treatment of burn injury

20. Cite two causes of pressure ulcers

21. Explain how shearing forces contribute to ischemic skin damage

22. List four measures that contribute to the prevention of pressure ulcers

23. Describe the origin of nevi and state their relationship to skin cancers

24. Compare the appearance and outcome of basal cell carcinoma, squamous cell carcinoma, and malignant melanoma

25. Differentiate a hemangioma of infancy from a port-wine stain in terms of appearance and outcome

26. Describe the manifestations and probable causes of diaper dermatitis, prickly heat, and cradle cap

27. Describe the distinguishing features of rashes associated with the following infectious childhood diseases: roseola infantum, rubeola, rubella, and varicella

28. Characterize the physiologic changes of aging skin

29. Describe the appearance of skin tags, keratoses, lentigines, and vascular lesions that are commonly seen in the elderly

SECTION II: ASSESSING YOUR UNDERSTANDING

Activity A *Fill in the blanks.*

1. _____ skin disorders include pigmentary skin disorders, infectious processes, acne, rosacea, papulosquamous dermatoses, allergic disorders and drug reactions, and arthropod infestations.

2. An absence of _____ production results in vitiligo or albinism.

3. _____ is a genetic disorder in which there is complete or partial congenital absence of pigment in the skin, hair, and eyes, which is found in all races.

4. _____ are free-living, saprophytic plantlike organisms; certain strains of which are considered part of the normal skin flora.

5. _____ is a yeastlike fungus that is a normal inhabitant of the gastrointestinal tract, mouth, and vagina.

6. Primary _____ infections are superficial skin infections, such as impetigo or ecthyma.

7. _____ is common, superficial bacterial infections caused by staphylococci or group A β-hemolytic *streptococci* that appears as a

small vesicle or pustule or as a large bulla on the face or elsewhere on the body.

8. _____ is a deeper infection affecting the dermis and subcutaneous tissues.

9. _____ and _____ occur on the soles of the feet and palms of the hands, respectively.

10. Herpes _____ is an acute, localized vesicular eruption distributed over a dermatomal segment of the skin.

11. _____ is a disorder of the pilosebaceous unit.

12. _____ consists of a mixture of free fatty acids, triglycerides, diglycerides, monoglycerides, sterol esters, wax esters, and squalene.

13. Noninflammatory acne lesions consist of _____; _____ are plugs of material that accumulate in sebaceous glands that open to the skin surface and _____ are pale, slightly elevated papules with no visible orifice.

14. _____ acne lesions consist of papules, pustules, nodules, and, in severe cases, cysts.

15. Hypersensitivity _____ are usually characterized by epidermal edema with separation of epidermal cells; they include irritant contact dermatitis, allergy contact dermatitis, atopic and nummular eczema, urticaria, and drug-induced skin eruptions.

16. _____ dermatitis results from a cell-mediated, type IV hypersensitivity response brought about by sensitization to an allergen.

17. The lesions of _____ eczema are coin-shaped papulovesicular patches mainly involving the arms and legs.

18. Acute immunologic _____ is commonly the result of an IgE-mediated immune reaction that usually occurs within 1 hour of exposure to an antigen.

19. _____ drugs are usually responsible for localized contact dermatitis types of rashes, whereas _____ drugs cause generalized skin lesions.

20. _____ dermatoses are a group of skin disorders characterized by scaling papules and plaques.

21. _____ is a relatively common chronic, pruritic disease that involves inflammation and papular eruption of the skin and mucous membranes.

22. Lichen simplex chronicus is a localized lichenoid, pruritic dermatitis resulting from _____ rubbing and scratching.

23. A mite, *Sarcoptes scabiei*, which burrows into the epidermis, causes _____.

24. _____ commonly referred to as *sunburn rays* are responsible for nearly all the skin effects of sunlight, including *photoaging*—the wrinkles, pigmentary changes, dryness, and loss of skin tone that occurs with, and is enhanced by, exposure to sunlight.

25. Some drugs are classified as _____ drugs because they produce an exaggerated response to ultraviolet light when the drug is taken in combination with sun exposure.

26. _____ is caused by excessive exposure of the epidermal and dermal layers of the skin to ultraviolet radiation, resulting in an erythematous inflammatory reaction.

27. _____ are typically classified according to the depth of involvement as first-degree, second-degree, and third-degree

28. _____ victims often are confronted with hemodynamic instability, impaired respiratory function, hypermetabolic response, major organ dysfunction, and sepsis.

29. Pressure ulcers are _____ lesions of the skin and underlying structures caused by unrelieved pressure that impairs the flow of blood and lymph.

30. Another form of nevi, the _____, is important because of its capacity to transform to malignant melanoma.

31. Malignant melanoma is a malignant tumor of the _____.

32. Severe, blistering sunburns in early childhood and intermittent intense sun exposures contribute to increased susceptibility to _____ in young and middle-aged adults.

33. _____, which is a neoplasm of the nonkeratinizing cells of the basal layer of the epidermis, is the most common skin cancer in white-skinned people.

34. _____ are the second most frequently occurring malignant tumors of the outer epidermis.

35. Pigmented _____ represent abnormal migration or proliferation of melanocytes seen in infants.

36. _____ of infancy are generally benign vascular tumors produced by proliferation of the endothelial cells.

37. _____ represent slow-growing capillary malformations that grow proportionately with the child and persist throughout life.

38. _____ is a form of contact dermatitis that is caused by an interaction with several factors, including prolonged contact of the skin with a mixture of urine and feces.

39. _____ results from constant maceration of the skin because of prolonged exposure to a warm, humid environment.

40. _____ is a greasy crust or scale formation on the scalp that is usually attributed to infrequent and inadequate washing of the scalp.

Activity B   *Match the key terms in Column A with their definitions in Column B.*

1.

Column A	Column B
____ 1. Herpes simplex virus	a. Pain that persists longer than 1 to 3 months after the resolution of herpes zoster rash
____ 2. Vitiligo	
____ 3. Postherpetic neuralgia	b. Responsible for cold sore
____ 4. Sermatophytid	c. Superficial mycoses
____ 5. Melasma	d. Warts that are common benign papillomas caused by DNA-containing human papillomaviruses
____ 6. *Ecthyma*	
____ 7. Verrucae	
____ 8. *Dermatophytoses*	
____ 9. *Tinea capitis*	e. Sudden appearance of white patches on the skin
____ 10. Shingles	f. Darkened macules on the face

g. Allergic reaction during an acute episode of a fungal infection

h. Ulcerative form of impetigo

i. Caused by infection of herpes zoster

j. Ringworm of the scalp

2.

Column A	Column B
____ **1.** Pediculosis	**a.** Comedones form primarily on the face and neck and, to a lesser extent, on the back, chest, and shoulders.
____ **2.** Acne vulgaris	
____ **3.** Psoriasis	
____ **4.** Acne conglobata	**b.** Disorder characterized the development of edematous wheals accompanied by intense itching
____ **5.** Decubitus ulcers	
____ **6.** Rosacea	**c.** Thickening of the skin associated with rosacea
____ **7.** Urticaria	**d.** Bed sore
____ **8.** Nevi	**e.** Comedones, papules, pustules, nodules, abscesses, cysts, and scars occur on the back, buttocks, and chest.
____ **9.** Rhinophyma	
____ **10.** Hyperkeratosis	
	f. Mole
	g. Erythema (flushing and redness) on the central face and across the cheeks, nose, or forehead
	h. Infestation with lice
	i. Increased epidermal cell turnover with marked epidermal thickening
	j. Chronic inflammatory skin disease characterized by circumscribed red, thickened plaques with an overlying silvery-white scale

Activity C *Briefly answer the following.*

1. What is the cause and symptomology of albinism?

_____

_____

_____

2. What is the mechanism of skin irritation with a fungal infection?

_____

_____

_____

3. What are the types of tinea capitis and what are the mechanisms of irritation?

_____

_____

_____

4. What is the port of entry for cellulitis infections? What are the most common symptoms?

_____

_____

_____

5. Herpes simplex virus (HSV)-1 virus will have episodic recurrences. What is the mechanism of recurrence? What are the signs and symptoms of recurrence?

_____

_____

_____

6. What are the factors believed to contribute to the development of acne?

_____

_____

_____

7. What is atopic dermatitis and how does it affect adults differently than infants?

_____

_____

_____

8. What is thought to be the cause of psoriasis?

_____

_____

_____

9. What is scabies and why does it itch?

_____

_____

_____

10. What is the hypothesized mechanism of skin damage brought about by UVB rays?

_____

_____

_____

11. What are the steps recommended to protect a patient from UV exposure?

_____

_____

_____

12. Why are severe burns an immediate medical emergency?

_____

_____

_____

13. Describe the two main types of basal cell carcinoma

_____

_____

_____

SECTION III: APPLYING YOUR KNOWLEDGE

Activity D *Consider the following scenario and answer the questions.*

A 17-year-old with second- and third-degree burns on his trunk, arms, and neck is brought to the emergency department (ED). In the ED, he is being stabilized for shipment to the nearest burn unit.

1. The mother asks why her son must be sent to another hospital. You explain that the patient is at high risk for complications from his burns. To what does the massive loss of skin tissue predispose him?

_____

_____

_____

2. The parents ask what specific complication can occur because of the burns their son has. Your correct response would include what?

_____

_____

_____

SECTION IV: PRACTICING FOR NCLEX

Activity E *Answer the following questions.*

1. Match the skin disorder with its description.

Skin Disorder	Description
____ **1.** Vitiligo	**a.** Darkened macules on the face
____ **2.** Albinism	**b.** Sudden appearance of white patches on the skin
____ **3.** Melasma	**c.** A genetic disorder in which complete or partial congenital absence of pigment in the skin, hair, and eyes is found, which occurs in all races.

2. Human bodies have, as endemic organisms, both yeast (*Candida albicans*) and molds. What is used as a confirmatory diagnostic test is used when a fungus invades the skin?

a. Potassium hydroxide (KOH) preparations

b. The Forest light

c. Tinea preparations

d. Sodium chloride (Na^+Cl^-) preparations

3. Match the bacterial or viral skin infection with its preferred treatment.

Skin Infection

___ 1. Impetigo

___ 2. Ecthyma

___ 3. Cellulitis

___ 4. Verrucae

___ 5. Herpes simplex virus (HSV-1)

___ 6. Herpes simplex virus (HSV-2)

___ 7. Herpes zoster

Preferred Treatment

a. Systemic antibiotics

b. Bactroban or systemic antibiotics

c. Acyclovir

d. Oral acyclovir

e. Penciclovir cream

f. Oral and intravenous (IV) antibiotics

g. A keratolytic agent

4. Acne vulgaris is typically an infection in the adolescent population. What topical agent used in the treatment of acne is both an antibacterial and a comedolytic?

a. Alcohol
b. Benzoyl peroxide
c. Bactroban
d. Resorcinol

5. Rosacea is a chronic inflammatory process that occurs in middle-aged and older adults. What are common manifestations of rosacea? Mark all that apply.

a. Swelling of the eyelid
b. Heat sensitivity
c. Burning eyes
d. Telangiectasia
e. Erythema

6. Allergic contact dermatitis is a common inflammation of the skin. It produces lesions in the affected areas. What do these lesions look like?

a. Papules
b. Papulosquamous pustules
c. Vesicles
d. Ulcers

7. Atopic dermatitis, or eczema, occurs at all ages and in all races. What happens in black-skinned people who have eczema?

a. Hyperpigmentation of skin
b. Papules cover the area affected
c. Erythema is a prominent symptom
d. Loss of pigmentation from lichenified skin

8. In severe Stevens-Johnson syndrome and toxic epidermal necrolysis, hospitalization is requiree. When large areas of the skin are lost what IV medication may speed-up the healing process?

a. Immunoglobulin
b. Broad-spectrum antibiotics
c. Diflucan
d. Corticosteroids

9. What disease has primary lesions that have a silvery scale over thick red plaques?

a. Pityriasis rosea
b. Psoriasis vulgaris
c. Lichen planus
d. Lichen simplex chronicus

10. What skin disease manifests with lesions on the skin and oral lesions that look like milky white lacework?

a. Eczema
b. Psoriasis
c. Lichen planus
d. Pityriasis rosea

11. Scabies infections are caused by mites that burrow under the skin. They are usually easily treated by bathing with a mite-killing agent and leaving it on for 12 hours. When scabies are resistant to the mite-killing agent what oral drug is prescribed?

a. Clindomycin
b. Interferon B
c. Potassium hydroxide
d. Ivermectin

12. Pressure ulcers can occur quickly in the elderly and in those who are immobile. What is a method for preventing pressure ulcers?

a. Preventing dehydration
b. Frequent position changes
c. Use of water-based skin moisturizers
d. Infrequent changing of incontinent patients

13. Nevi are benign tumors of the skin. One type of nevi is important because of its capacity to transform to malignant melanoma. What type of nevus is this?

a. Nevocellular
b. Compound nevi
c. Dysplastic
d. Dermal

14. Malignant melanomas are metastatic tumors of the skin. In the past decades, the incidence of malignant melanoma has grown. This is related to more exposure to UV light, such as tanning salons. What are risk factors for developing malignant melanoma?

    a. Freckles across the bridge of the nose

    b. Blistering sunburns after age 20

    c. Palmar nevi

    d. Presence of actinic keratoses

15. Basal cell carcinoma is the most common skin cancer in white-skinned people. Although the treatment goal that is most important is elimination of the lesion, it is also important to maintain the function and cosmetic effect. What treatment is used for basal cell carcinoma?

    a. Curettage with electrodesiccation

    b. Systemic chemotherapy

    c. Topical chemotherapy

    d. Simple radiographic radiation

16. Squamous cell carcinoma in light-skinned people is a red scaling, keratotic, slightly elevated lesion with an irregular border, usually with a shallow chronic ulcer. How do the lesions appear in black-skinned people?

    a. Keratotic lesions with rolling, irregular borders

    b. Hyperpigmented nodules

    c. Hypopigmented nodules

    d. Lichenous plaques with silvery scales

17. Hemangiomas of infancy are small, red lesions that are noticed shortly after birth and grow rapidly. What is the treatment of choice for hemangiomas of infancy?

    a. Surgical excision

    b. Laser surgery

    c. No treatment

    d. Chemotherapy

18. Rubella, or 3-day measles, is a childhood disease caused by a togavirus. Because rubella can be easily transmitted and, because it is dangerous to the fetus if contracted by pregnant women early in their gestational period, immunization is required. What type of vaccine is the rubella vaccine?

    a. Attenuated virus vaccine

    b. Antibody/antigen vaccine

    c. Dead virus vaccine

    d. Live virus vaccine

19. Lentigines are skin lesions common in the elderly. A type of lentigine is tan to brown in color with benign spots. Lentigines are removed because they are considered precursors to skin cancer. How are lentigines removed?

    a. Cryotherapy

    b. Chemotherapy

    c. Bleaching agents

    d. Curettage

Answers

CHAPTER 1 CONCEPTS OF HEALTH AND DISEASE

SECTION II: ASSESSING YOUR UNDERSTANDING

Activity A

1. altered health
2. health
3. disease
4. risk factors
5. Congenital defects
6. acquired
7. diagnosis
8. Subclinical disease, Clinical disease
9. Epidemiology
10. Prevalence, incidence

Activity B

1. b	**2.** g	**3.** f	**4.** c	**5.** e
6. h	**7.** d	**8.** a	**9.** i	**10.** j

Activity C

1.

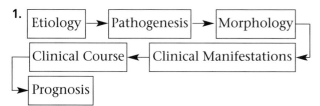

Activity D

1. Pathophysiology is the study of the disease process and the body's response to disease. Physiology is the study of normal bodily process, and pathology is the study of the disease manifestations. Pathophysiology can be viewed as a combination of physiology and pathology.
2. The clinical course of a disease describes the evolution of the disease process. In acute conditions, the disease is usually rapid in onset and quite severe. Consequently, though, acute conditions are often self-limiting. Chronic disease states, however, run a continuous course and present with aggravations and remissions.
3. Congenital conditions are present at birth and result from genetic disturbances, environmental effects, or a combination of genetic and environmental causes. Acquired defects, conversely, are brought about by conditions following birth.
4. Syndromes are the collection of signs, symptoms, and manifestations of the disease. Sequelae are injuries that come as a secondary result of the disease.
5. The importance of risk factors lies in their providing a window into developing disease. It is possible to avoid risky behavior and therefore lower the chances of developing the disease. Risk factors are determined from studying a controlled population where most of the habits and practices are similar. Some of the most prominent studies are the Framingham Study (coronary heart disease), the Nurses' Health Study (breast cancer), and the Nun's Study (Alzheimer disease).

SECTION III: APPLYING YOUR KNOWLEDGE

Activity E

1. Epidemiology
   Incidence and prevalence of diseases
   Morbidity and mortality statistics
   Natural history of a disease and its risk factors
   Prognosis
   Prevention
2. The nurse should explain that evidence-based practice and evidence-based practice guidelines are mechanisms that use the current best scientific findings (evidence) to make decisions about the health care of individuals. They are based on the expertise of the individual practitioner integrated with the evidence

gathered from a systematic review of credible research studies. Practice guidelines may take the form of algorithms, which are step-by-step methods for solving a problem, written directives, or a combination thereof.

SECTION IV: PRACTICING FOR NCLEX
Activity F

1. a. *Rationale:* Most disease states do not have a single cause but instead stem from a number of factors. Some disease states are complicated and hard to diagnose, such as multiple sclerosis, whereas some are simple, straightforward, and easy to diagnose, such as a broken leg.

2. d. *Rationale:* Epidemiology is the study of patterns of disease, such as the spread of a disease in an epidemic. It has also emerged as a science to study the risk factors in multifactorial diseases, such as heart disease and cancer. Scientology is a religion. Morphology refers to the fundamental structure or form of cells or tissues. Histology deals with the study of the cells and extracellular matrix of body tissues.

3. c. *Rationale:* Morbidity and mortality statistics provide information about the functional effects (morbidity) and death-producing (mortality) characteristics of a disease. Morbidity statistics do address the effects a disease has on a person's life and the long-term consequences of the disease state, but morbidity and mortality statistics taken together have a broader scope. Neither morbidity nor mortality statistics address recovery rates from a disease or treatment modalities for a disease. Although mortality does address the causes of death in a given population, morbidity does not address the impact the disease state has on the family.

4. a, b, c. *Rationale:* Clinical practice guidelines are systematically developed statements intended to inform practitioners and clients in making decisions about health care for specific clinical circumstances. They should review and weigh various outcomes, both positive and negative, and make recommendations. Guidelines are different from systematic reviews. They can take the form of algorithms, which are step-by-step methods for solving a problem, written directives for care, or a combination thereof. Nothing takes the place of either written orders by the doctor or the nursing care plan. These are man-

dated by The Joint Commission (as well as the laws of most states in the case of written orders by the doctor) and used in every health care institution in the United States.

5. a. *Rationale:* Secondary prevention detects disease early in its course when it is still asymptomatic and treatment measures can effect a cure or stop the disease from progressing. Most secondary prevention is undertaken in clinical settings. Tertiary prevention goes beyond treating the presenting problem. Tertiary prevention programs are located within health care systems and involve the services of a number of different types of health care professionals. Primary prevention is often accomplished outside the health care system at the community level.

6. c. *Rationale:* A syndrome is a compilation of signs and symptoms (e.g., chronic fatigue syndrome) that are characteristic of a specific disease state. Complications are possible adverse extensions of a disease or outcomes from treatment. Sequelae are lesions or impairments that follow or are caused by a disease. There is no name for a group of disease states that all have the same cause.

7. c. *Rationale:* The natural history of a disease refers to the way the disease will run its course and the expected outcome of the disease process if medical intervention is not undertaken. Prognosis is the term used to designate the probable outcome and prospect of recovery from a disease. Morbidity describes the effects an illness has on a person's life. It is concerned with the incidence of disease as well as its persistence and long-term consequences. Conditions suspected of contributing to the development of a disease are called risk factors.

8. d. *Rationale:* The pathogenesis of a disease is the mechanism by which an etiologic factor causes the disease. Etiology is what sets the disease process in motion, or what causes the disease. Risk factors are multiple factors that predispose to a particular disease.

9. d. *Rationale:* A black eye is usually indicative of an unfortunate accident and could be a sign that a caregiver would see. However, a green thumb is a mythical ability usually assigned to a good gardener. The other choices are either subjective symptoms (reported by the patient) or objective signs (observed by the caregiver) of disease states.

10. b, c. *Rationale:* Standardization relies on the use of written standards, reference measurement

procedures, and reference materials. In vitro diagnostic devices and laboratory equipment are regulated by the U.S. Food and Drug Administration (FDA) and are, of themselves, standardized. Standardization does not need FDA approval. However, new reagents, test kits, and clinical laboratory instruments must meet standardization guidelines mandated by law and obtain FDA approval before they can be marketed in the United States.

CHAPTER 2 CONCEPTS OF ALTERED HEALTH IN CHILDREN

SECTION II: ASSESSING YOUR UNDERSTANDING

Activity A

1. growth and development
2. growth, morphogenesis, differentiate
3. Apgar score
4. injuries during birth
5. respiratory distress syndrome
6. Colic
7. 3–3.5 kg, 6 cm
8. decreases
9. lesions
10. obesity

Activity B

1. Small for gestational age
2. Appropriate for gestational age

Activity C

| 1. h | 2. i | 3. c | 4. j | 5. f |
| 6. a | 7. b | 8. e | 9. g | 10. d |

Activity D

1. Gestational age is divided into prenatal and postnatal assessment. Prenatal assessment of gestational age mostly includes careful menstrual history, physical milestones during pregnancy such as uterine size, detection of fetal heart rate, and fetal movements. Advanced prenatal tests for maturity include ultrasound and amniotic fluid studies. Postnatal assessment of gestational age is done by examination of external physical and neuromuscular characteristics alone or in combination using the Dubowitz or Ballard methods.
2. Due to the force put on the infant during the birth process and the movement of the fetus through the pelvic outlet, the clavicle will often fracture. This is more common in large for gestational age infants.

3. Surfactant reduces surface tension by interrupting hydrogen bonds in the fluid that coats the interior surface of the alveoli. This prevents the alveoli from collapsing and allows them to inflate.
4. The most common risk factors include sleeping in the prone position, prematurity and low birth weight, African American or Native American race, and exposure to environmental cigarette smoke, as well as young age of the mother, lack of or inadequate prenatal care, and smoking or substance use during pregnancy.
5. Organic failure to thrive is the result of a physiologic cause that prevents the infant from obtaining or using nutrients. An example of organic failure to thrive is inadequate growth of an infant with deficient energy reserve because of a congenital defect that makes feeding difficult. Failure of any organ system can cause an organic failure to thrive.
6. Jaundice and hyperbilirubinemia are considered pathologic if their time and pattern of appearance and duration vary significantly from that of physiologic jaundice. The greatest risk associated with hyperbilirubinemia is the development of bilirubin encephalopathy, a neurologic syndrome resulting from deposition of unconjugated bilirubin in the basal ganglia.

SECTION III: APPLYING YOUR KNOWLEDGE

Activity E

1. Primary teeth are lost and replaced by permanent teeth at this stage. There is a high incidence of dental caries during late childhood that is related to inadequate dental care and a high amount of dietary sugar. Children in the early part of this stage may not be as effective at brushing their teeth and may require adult assistance, but may be reluctant to accept parental help.
2. Many chronic health problems are first diagnosed during middle to late childhood. Specific learning disabilities can also be identified at this time. Infections with bacterial and fungal agents are a common problem in childhood.
3. The major task is the development of industry or accomplishment. Failure to meet this task results in a sense of inferiority or incompetence, which can impede further progress.

SECTION IV: PRACTICING FOR NCLEX

Activity F

1. b. *Rationale:* A standard is established for the height, weight, and age of children by sampling a specific population. Statistics from that sample are used to account for variations (called standard deviations) from the "norm" or "average" of the population sampled. Statistically, a child who falls within 1 standard deviation of the norm (or mean for that population) is the same in height and weight as 68% of other 2-year-old children. A child who is the same height and weight as 75% of other 2-year-old children would fall within 2 standard deviations of the norm. A child who is considered small and underweight would fall 3 standard deviations below the mean, and a toddler who is tall and overweight would fall 3 standard deviations above the norm, or mean.

2. d. *Rationale:* There are two main periods of fetal development. The first is the embryonic period, which begins during the second week after fertilization and ends during the eighth week after fertilization. The other answers describe blocks of time in the early stage of pregnancy.

3. a. *Rationale:* An infant is considered term when born between the beginning of the 38th week and completion of the 41st week. A child born at 36 or 37 weeks would be considered preterm. Weight is not a measurement used to decide whether an infant is term.

4. a. *Rationale:* Psychosomatic disorders may manifest during adolescence. Common health problems experienced by adolescents that may be psychosomatic in origin include headache, stomachache, and insomnia. Dental caries occur frequently in middle to late childhood, and leg and skeletal pain are not common complaints of adolescence.

5. c. *Rationale:* It is believed that infants who are considered small for gestational age have depleted hepatic glycogen stores. Brown fat is found near the heart and blood vessels that supply the kidneys and brain and is believed to play a role in maintaining the temperature of these organs during the environmental change that occurs at birth. If the pancreas produces too much insulin for the infant's body requirement, then the infant is usually large for gestational age. When an infant's pancreas does not produce enough insulin for the body's requirements, the infant is diagnosed as insulin-dependent diabetic and would be hyperglycemic.

6. d. *Rationale:* Allergic reactions cause asthma, which frequently manifests for the first time during middle childhood. Cerebral palsy is a disease process with which the child is usually born. Nephrotic syndrome occurs most commonly in children younger than 3 years, whereas pneumonia can occur anytime across the life span.

7. a. *Rationale:* The anterior fontanel is open and palpable until about 18 months to 2 years of age; the smaller fontanels are replaced by bone by the end of the first year. The bones of the child's skull are solidified by 2 years of age, not 3 years of age.

8. b. *Rationale:* Because of the immaturity of the immune system in children of this age, they are at risk for communicable diseases such as chickenpox, the common cold, influenza, and intestinal tract infections. Diaper rash and croup are not communicable diseases, and a urinary tract infection is not transmitted from one child to another.

9. c. *Rationale:* Women are routinely tested for GBS prior to delivery. If they test positive for GBS infection, they are treated with antibiotics during the intrapartal period to help prevent transmission of the bacteria to the newborn. After delivery, infants are treated prophylactically with antibiotics, unless they test positive for GBS themselves. Then they are given a full course of IV antibiotics to prevent sepsis.

10. c. *Rationale:* An increased risk of SIDS is associated with sleeping in the prone position and smoking or substance use during pregnancy. Other risk factors include being Native American or African American; the Asian race is not associated with an increased risk of SIDS. Exposure to environmental cigarette smoke is also a risk factor; however, placing the infant on its back to sleep is recommended to decrease the incidence of SIDS, and breast-feeding has not been identified as a risk for SIDS.

11. a, b, c, d. *Rationale:* Complications that may occur when an infant is large for gestational age include asphyxia during birth and mechanical difficulties that cause trauma during the birth process. They are also at risk for hypoglycemia and polycythemia due to their increased size.

12. a, b, c. *Rationale:* The information to include in an educational event for women having their first babies is information about gestational age and what it means. It should also include information about intrauterine growth retardation, which can occur at any time during the pregnancy. An infant who is small for gestational age weighs less than 90% of all other infants.

13. height. *Rationale:* Sex hormones not only initiate the growth spurt, but also stop it by causing bone maturity, which means that the skeleton ceases to grow.

CHAPTER 3 CONCEPTS OF ALTERED HEALTH IN OLDER ADULTS

SECTION II: ASSESSING YOUR UNDERSTANDING

Activity A

1. 65 to 74, 75 to 84, 85+
2. intrinsic
3. Stochastic
4. telomerase
5. oxidative free radical
6. Collagen
7. vertebral column
8. systolic
9. elastic recoil
10. Presbycusis
11. Xerostomia
12. achlorhydria
13. glomerular filtration
14. Katz
15. inhibit
16. depressed
17. stroke
18. Dementia
19. Delirium
20. total body water

Activity B

1. b	**2.** e	**3.** d	**4.** c	**5.** g
6. h	**7.** i	**8.** a	**9.** f	**10.** j

Activity C

1. The slow steady oxidation of the structures of the epithelial lining of the arterioles results in cellular injury. The constant assault results in adaptation, scarring, and overall thickening of the blood vessel. This reduces the compliance and results in increased systolic pressure.
2. The changes seen in aging are the result of a slow steady decrease in physiological activity, whereas disease is the loss of function due to a pathological process.
3. The somatic mutation theory of aging states that the longevity and function of cells in various tissues of the body are determined by a double-stranded DNA molecule and its specific repair enzymes. DNA undergoes continuous change in response to both exogenous agents and intrinsic processes. Aging may result from conditions that produce mutations in DNA or deficits in DNA repair mechanisms.
4. There is a reduction in muscle size and strength that is related to a loss of muscle fibers and a reduction in the size of the existing fibers. There is a decline in high-speed performance and reaction time because of a decrease in type II muscle fibers. Impairments in the nervous system can also cause movements to slow. However, type I muscle fibers, which offer endurance, are believed to remain consistent with age.
5. Alterations in vision and hearing impairment impair sensory input, increasing the risk for falls. Input from the skeletal muscles is also integrated to help control balance. As the neuronal signaling degrades the ability to send and interpret, sensory data input decreases, which increases the likelihood of falling.
6. Dementia is a general decrease in cognitive abilities without a known pathology. Alzheimer disease is associated with discrete changes in the cellular structure and enzyme activity of neurons.

SECTION III: APPLYING YOUR KNOWLEDGE

Activity D

1. The nurse should respond that an unstable gait is only one of the reasons a person falls. The daughter should see that her father gets his vision and hearing checked. Age- and disease-related alterations in vision and hearing can contribute to an elderly person falling. Medications can also cause elderly people to fall, so the daughter should know what medications her father is taking and their side effects. She should check the environment her father lives in and remove any objects he could trip on, such as scatter rugs or electrical cords that cross an area used as a walkway. She should also make sure his shoes fit properly.
2. The nurse should assess for depression because these are common signs of depression in elderly patients. Depression is often seen in

older people, especially if they have suffered many losses related to aging, such as the death of friends, diminished hearing or vision, decreased mobility, or illness or injury.

SECTION IV: PRACTICING FOR NCLEX
Activity E

1. a. *Rationale:* Skin disorders are common among the older adult population and can include skin cancers, keratoses (i.e., warty lesions), xerosis (i.e., excessive dryness), dermatitis, and pruritus (i.e., generalized itching). The term xenobiotic refers to a chemical compound foreign to a given biological system, and xenomas are tumors that develop on skin infested with certain parasites.

2. d. *Rationale:* As a person ages, there are changes in cardiac function in the body. There is an increase, not a decrease, in systemic vascular resistance and left ventricular afterload, as well as a decrease in the maximal heart rate and maximal cardiac output. The heart becomes less responsive to β-adrenergic stimulation and circulating catecholamines.

3. a. *Rationale:* Speech discrimination, or the ability to distinguish among words that are near-homonyms or to distinguish words spoken by several different speakers, is often impaired. Elderly people who are hearing impaired do not repeat themselves because of a hearing loss nor do they speak slower or softer then their peers who are not hearing impaired. They also do not shout unnecessarily due to a hearing impairment.

4. b. *Rationale:* Smell is a protective mechanism, and persons who cannot smell may be at risk for exposure to environmental hazards. For example, people who cannot smell smoke would be at particular risk if a fire broke out. Taking the wrong medication would be more apt to occur due to visual problems. Living in unhealthy and unclean conditions is not caused by a decline in the ability to either taste or smell. An elderly person who has lost some of their ability to taste or smell may be at risk for eating raw food that has spoiled but not at risk for eating food that is not cooked properly.

5. d. *Rationale:* Dementia affects memory, language, visuospatial ability, and cognition (i.e., abstraction, calculation, judgment, problem solving). It does not affect the physi-

cal changes in the body that occur with aging.

6. d. *Rationale:* Serum creatinine, a byproduct of muscle metabolism, is often used as a measure of GFR. The decline in GFR that occurs with aging is not accompanied by an equivalent increase in serum creatinine levels because the production of creatinine is reduced as muscle mass declines with age. Serum creatinine levels do not increase with age and neither does the GFR. Although GFR decreases with age, serum creatinine levels do not.

7. a. *Rationale:* Urge incontinence is an irritative, not an obstructive symptom of BPH. The other irritative symptoms include urinary frequency, nocturia, and urinary urgency. The obstructive symptoms of BPH include hesitancy in initiation of stream, a diminished force of urine stream, urinary retention, and postvoid dribbling.

8. d. *Rationale:* According to the American Psychiatric Association's *Diagnostic and Statistical Manual of Mental Disorders* (DSM-IV-TR), the criteria for the diagnosis and treatment of a major depression include at least five of the following symptoms during the same 2-week period, with at least one of the symptoms being depressed mood or anhedonia (i.e., loss of interest or pleasure): depressed or irritable mood; loss of interest or pleasure in usual activities; appetite and weight changes; sleep disturbance; psychomotor agitation or retardation; fatigue and loss of energy; feelings of worthlessness, self-reproach, or excessive guilt; diminished ability to think or concentrate; and suicidal ideation, plan, or attempt.

9. b. *Rationale:* Currently, the diagnosis of Alzheimer disease is one of exclusion. That is, no specific diagnostic tests can confirm or rule out the diagnosis. The Mini-Mental State Examination, developed in 1975, is a screening tool that gives a brief, quick picture of a person's cognitive ability. It is not meant to be used as the sole diagnostic tool to confirm or rule out dementia in any patient. A complete metabolic panel run on a patient's blood can confirm the presence of hyperlipidemia, which is believed to be a possible indication of vascular dementia. Although auscultation of bruits in the carotid arteries indicates a decrease in blood flow to the brain because of a narrowing of the carotids, it is not diagnostic of dementia in any form.

10. b. *Rationale:* One of the many concerns surrounding the medication of the elderly

population is polypharmacy because it increases the risk of drug interactions and adverse drug reactions. Being prescribed multiple drugs has also been found to decrease the patient's compliance with drug regimens. Psychotropic drugs administered to older adults with dementia may cause an increase in any confusion they are experiencing. Nonsteroidal anti-inflammatory medications given to an older adult with hypertension can cause an increase in blood pressure. Beta-blocking agents administered to an individual with chronic obstructive pulmonary disease may induce bronchoconstriction.

11. 1-d, 2-b, 3-a, 4-c. *Rationale:* Medications are an important and potentially correctable cause of instability and falls. Centrally acting medications, such as sedatives and hypnotics, have been associated with an increase in the risk of falling and injury. Diuretics can cause volume depletion, electrolyte disturbances, and fatigue, predisposing a person to falls. Antihypertensive drugs can cause fatigue, orthostatic hypotension, and impaired alertness, contributing to the risk of falls.

12. c. *Rationale:* Because of the serious implications of medication use in the elderly, strategies to enhance therapeutic effects and prevent harm need to be used. Careful evaluation of the need for the medication by the health care provider is the first step. Once decided, analysis of the individual's current medication regimen and disease states is necessary to prevent drug–drug interactions, drug–disease interactions, and adverse responses. Dosing should be at the low end, and frequency of drug administration should be kept to a minimum to simplify the routine and enhance compliance. Timing the dose to a specific activity of daily living (e.g., "take with breakfast") can also improve compliance, as can special packaging devices such as pill boxes and blister packs. The cost of medications is another important factor for older adults living on reduced, fixed incomes. Choosing less expensive products of equal efficacy can increase compliance. The importance of educating the individual about the medication cannot be overemphasized. Health care professionals need to provide verbal and written information on the principles of medication use and on the specific medications being used.

13. a, c. *Rationale:* Atrophy of the gastric mucosa and a decrease in the ability to secrete intrin-

sic factor can cause malabsorption of vitamin B_{12}. Vitamin B_{12} is essential in the maturation of red blood cells and, without it, pernicious anemia, a macrocytic anemia, can occur. A lack of vitamin B_{12} can also affect the central nervous system, causing peripheral neuropathies. It is a lack of intrinsic factor that causes the lack of vitamin B_{12} in the body, not the other way around, and a lack of vitamin B_{12} can cause ataxia, which is an impaired ability to coordinate movement, not an improvement in coordination.

14. a, b, d. *Rationale:* Depression can be a symptom of a medical condition, such as pancreatic cancer, hypothyroidism or hyperthyroidism, pneumonia and other infections, congestive heart failure, dementia, and stroke. Hypocholesteremia does not have depression as a symptom.

15. b, c, d. *Rationale:* A decrease in bladder capacity, in bladder and sphincter tone, and in the ability to inhibit detrusor (i.e., bladder muscle) contractions, combined with the nervous system's increased variability to interpret bladder signals, can cause incontinence. Impaired mobility and a slower reaction time can also aggravate incontinence. Of particular importance is the role of pharmaceuticals, such as long-acting sedatives and hypnotics, psychotropics, and diuretics, as a cause of transient urinary incontinence. Aging causes a decrease in the ability to inhibit the detrusor contractions rather than increasing the patient's ability to inhibit the contractions.

CHAPTER 4 CELL AND TISSUE CHARACTERISTICS

SECTION II: ASSESSING YOUR UNDERSTANDING

Activity A

1. Protoplasm
2. eukaryotic, prokaryotic
3. DNA, RNA, proteins
4. protein
5. Rough
6. Golgi
7. Lysosomes
8. peroxides
9. respiration, ATP
10. microtubules
11. microfilaments
12. peripheral

13. epithelial, connective, muscle, neuronal
14. ion
15. muscle, neural

Activity B

1.

1. b	**2.** h	**3.** f	**4.** j	**5.** d
6. a	**7.** e	**8.** g	**9.** i	**10.** c

2.

1. j	**2.** f	**3.** b	**4.** g	**5.** d
6. e	**7.** h	**8.** i	**9.** c	**10.** a

Activity C

$$7 \rightarrow 4 \rightarrow 1 \rightarrow 5 \rightarrow 6 \rightarrow 2 \rightarrow 3$$

Activity D

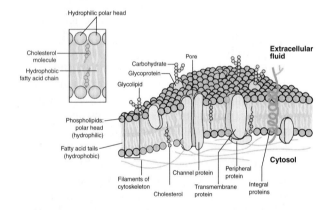

Activity E

1. The three protein complexes are (a) cyclins, (b) cyclin-dependent kinases, and (c) anaphase-promoting complex. The central components of the cell cycle control system are the cyclin-dependent kinases (CDKs), whose activity depends on their association with the regulatory units called cyclins. The anaphase-promoting complex allows for progression through the cell cycle via destruction of previous CDK complexes. Each molecule functions under variable concentrations.

2. In ischemia and hypoxia (an anoxia), the cells do not receive enough oxygen. As a result, the electron transport chain cannot pass electrons from complex to complex. Proton pumping slows or is halted, and the proton gradient decreases, resulting in a decreased production, or a complete lack, of ATP. With no ATP, the cell cannot maintain normal functioning (e.g., membrane potential, transport) and begins to malfunction.

3. Individual cells produce extracellular matrix proteins that form a basement membrane where cells can form anchors. Cells will then form connections between each other via cell junctions (tight, gap, desmosome, hemidesmosome). This interaction between cytoskeletal elements, the basement membrane, and cellular adhesion is the basis for tissue formation.

4. First messengers can be neurotransmitters, protein hormones and growth factors, steroids, and/or other chemical messengers. They will bind to receptors either on the cell membrane (hydrophilic first messengers) or in the cytoplasm (hydrophobic first messengers). The activation of a receptor via first messenger results in the activation of a second messenger. Cell surface receptors are transmembrane proteins that will activate an array of second messengers (cAMP, G proteins, and tyrosine kinases) that will have direct effects on membrane potential or a host of other cellular functions. Activation of an intracellular receptor involves the activation of a transcription factor that will directly influence the expression of a gene product. The gene product will then have an effect on cellular function.

5. Endocytosis is the process of bringing in large molecules or substances to a cell. Receptor-mediated endocytosis is triggered by a specific ligand. The inflammatory system contains cells (macrophages, neutrophils) that will endocytose dead cell material, bacteria, or foreign material. This process is known as phagocytosis. Exocytosis is the release of large quantities of material, such as the exocytosis of a neurotransmitter.

SECTION III: APPLYING YOUR KNOWLEDGE

Activity F

1. In our bodies, fat is stored in tissue called adipose tissue. Adipose tissue is a special form of connective tissue that helps connect different types of tissue in our body to each other. Adipose cells have big empty spaces in them so they can store large quantities of triglycerides and are the largest storage spaces of energy in the body. The subcutaneous fat we store helps shape our body. It also helps insulate our body because fat is a poor conductor of heat.

   Adipose tissue exists in two forms: unilocular and multilocular. Unilocular (white) adipose tissue is composed of cells in which the fat is contained in a single, large droplet in the cytoplasm. Multilocular (brown) adipose tissue is composed of cells that contain multiple droplets of fat and numerous mitochondria.

We have deposits of brown fat when we are born, but they decrease over time. White fat is the kind we have most of, and it is what we add to our body when we gain weight.

SECTION IV: PRACTICING FOR NCLEX
Activity G

1. a. *Rationale:* Rough ER is studded with ribosomes attached to specific binding sites on the membrane. Proteins produced by the rough ER are usually destined for incorporation into cell membranes and lysosomal enzymes or for exportation from the cell. The rough ER segregates (rather than combines) these proteins from other components of the cytoplasm and modifies their structure for a specific function. Rough ER does not transport anything through the cell membrane. Rough ER is studded with ribosomes; it does not destroy them.

2. b. *Rationale:* Recently, data suggest that the Golgi apparatus has yet another function: It can receive proteins and other substances from the cell surface by a retrograde transport mechanism. Golgi bodies do not produce bile. They produce secretory, not excretory, granules, and they produce large carbohydrate molecules rather than small ones.

3. c. *Rationale:* Although GM$_2$ ganglioside accumulates in many tissues, such as the heart, liver, and spleen, its accumulation in the nervous system and retina of the eye causes the most damage.

4. d. *Rationale:* They do not make energy, but they extract it from organic compounds. Proteasomes are small organelles composed of protein complexes that are believed to be present in both the cytoplasm and the nucleus. They are not formed by mitochondria. Mitochondria contain their own DNA and ribosomes and are self-replicating.

5. a. *Rationale:* The cell membrane is often called the plasma membrane. The nuclear membrane is another type of membrane within the cell. The cell membrane provides receptors for hormones and other biologically active substances; it is not a receptor membrane. A main structural component of the membrane is its lipid bilayer. It is not a bilayer membrane.

6. b. *Rationale:* At the membrane of the cell nucleus, both thyroid and steroid hormones cross into the cell nucleus itself, where they influence DNA activity. Ion-channel–linked receptors transiently open or close ion channels. Thyroid and steroid hormones act within the cell nucleus to increase transcription of mRNA to alter cell function.

7. c. *Rationale:* Each of the two pyruvate molecules formed in the cytoplasm from one molecule of glucose yields another molecule of ATP, which is a special carrier for cellular energy. FAD (flavin adenine dinucleotide) is a coenzyme of protein metabolism that accepts electrons and is reduced. NADH $^+$ H$^+$ is an end product of glycolysis. The electron transport chain oxidizes NADH + H$^+$ and FADH$_2$ and donates the electrons to oxygen, which is reduced to water.

8. d. *Rationale:* Active transport is what occurs when cells use energy to move ions against an electrical or chemical gradient. Passive transport is another term for diffusion. There is no such thing as neutral transport. Cotransport is when the sodium ion and the solute are transported in the same direction

9. a. *Rationale:* Four categories of tissue exist: (a) epithelium, (b) connective (supportive), (c) muscle, and (d) nerve. Binding, connecting, and exothelial tissue are not categories of tissue.

10. b. *Rationale:* These glands are ductless and produce secretions (i.e., hormones) that move directly into the bloodstream. Exocrine glands retain their connection with the surface epithelium from which they originated. This connection takes the form of epithelium-lined tubular ducts through which the secretions pass to reach the surface. Exocytosis occurs when part of the cell membrane ruptures to release particles that are too large to pass through the cell membrane. These cells are ductless, but do not necessarily secrete their contents into the bloodstream.

11. c. *Rationale:* Thin and thick filaments are the two types of muscle fibers that are responsible for muscle contraction. The thin filaments are composed primarily of actin, whereas the thick filaments are composed of myosin. During muscle contraction, the thick myosin and thin actin filaments slide over each other, causing shortening of the muscle fiber, although the length of the individual thick and thin filaments remains unchanged. When activated by ATP, the cross-bridges swivel in a fixed arc, much like the oars of a boat, as they become attached to the actin filament.

During contraction, each cross-bridge undergoes its own cycle of movement, forming a bridge attachment and releasing it, and moving to another site where the same sequence of movement occurs. This pulls the thin and thick filaments past each other. The calcium-calmodulin complex is in smooth muscle. It binds to and activates the myosin-containing thick filaments, which interact with actin.

12. cytoplasm. *Rationale:* When seen under a light microscope, three major components of the cell become evident: the nucleus, the cytoplasm, and the cell membrane.

13. jaundice. *Rationale:* When bilirubin collects within the cells, they take on a yellowish color, which is called jaundice.

14. a, c, d. *Rationale:* The human body has several means of transmitting information between cells. These mechanisms include direct communication between adjacent cells through gap junctions, autocrine and paracrine signaling, and endocrine or synaptic signaling. There is no such thing as express communication between cells.

15. b, c, d. *Rationale:* Nondividing cells, such as neurons and skeletal and cardiac muscle cells, have left the cell cycle and are not capable of mitotic division in postnatal life. The cells that produce mucous are capable of mitotic division. Smooth muscle is often called involuntary muscle because it contracts spontaneously or through activity of the autonomic nervous system.

16. involuntary. *Rationale:* Three types of muscle tissue exist: skeletal, cardiac, and smooth. Smooth muscle is often called involuntary muscle because it contracts without the person willing it to contract.

CHAPTER 5 CELLULAR ADAPTATION, INJURY, AND DEATH

SECTION II: ASSESSING YOUR UNDERSTANDING

Activity A

1. size, number, type
2. housekeeping, differentiation
3. size
4. atrophy
5. increase
6. physiologic
7. hyperplasia
8. compensatory

9. Pathological, nonphysiologic
10. Metaplasia
11. irritation, inflammation
12. dysplasia
13. cancer
14. accumulations
15. Free
16. Hypoxia
17. swelling, fatty
18. Necrosis
19. calcium
20. coagulation

Activity B

Normal cells—Physiologic

Nucleus

Basement membrane

Atrophy—Pathologic

Hypertrophy—Both

Hyperplasia—Both

Metaplasia—Both

Dysplasia—Pathologic

Activity C

1. e **2.** b **3.** d **4.** g **5.** a
6. c **7.** f **8.** i **9.** h **10.** j

Activity D

1. The pathogenesis of dystrophic calcification involves the intracellular and/or extracellular formation of crystalline calcium phosphate. The components of the calcium deposits are derived from the bodies of dead or dying cells as well as from the circulation and interstitial fluid. As tissues die, the calcium crystallizes and deposits form.

2. The five categories of cellular injury are (a) injury from physical agents, (b) radiation injury, (c) chemical injury, (d) injury from biologic agents, and (e) injury from nutritional imbalances.

3. The toxicity of lead is related to its multiple biochemical effects. It has the ability to inactivate enzymes, compete with calcium for incorporation into bone, and interfere with nerve transmission and brain development. Lead exposure in children has been demonstrated to result in neurobehavioral and cognitive deficits.

4. The three major mechanisms of cellular damage are free radical formation, hypoxia and ATP depletion, and disruption of intracellular calcium homeostasis. Multiple pathologies, whether mechanical, chemical, biological, or blunt force, will result in a combination of these mechanisms being activated.

5. Oxidative stress leads to the oxidation of cell components, activation of signal transduction pathways, and changes in gene and protein expression. DNA modification and damage can occur because of oxidative stress. In addition, mitochondrial DNA as a target of oxidation and subsequent cause of mitochondrial dysfunction may be the cause of diseases.

6. As oxygen concentrations fall, oxidative metabolism slows down. To make ATP, the cell reverts to anaerobic metabolism. With a decrease in ATP, the ion distribution is altered and cells will swell. The product of anaerobic metabolism is lactic acid, and as lactic acid accumulates, the pH falls. Low pH will change protein conformation, resulting in total loss of enzyme function.

7. Two basic pathways for apoptosis are the extrinsic pathway, which is death receptor dependent and is under cellular control, and the intrinsic pathway, which is death receptor in-

dependent and results from injury. The execution phase of both pathways is initiated by proteolytic enzymes called caspases.

SECTION III: APPLYING YOUR KNOWLEDGE

Activity E

1. Chemotherapy is a general term that can technically refer to chemical (drug) therapy for any kind of illness. However, in practice, this term usually refers to the pharmacologic treatment of cancer. It is important to remember that all rapidly dividing cells (both normal and cancer cells) are affected by chemotherapy drugs, such as the rapidly dividing normal cells found in mucous membranes, hair follicles, and the components of bone marrow. Antineoplastic drugs, or chemotherapy drugs, are very toxic drugs. They act on the tumor cells because tumor cells divide and produce more tumor cells so rapidly, and while tumor cells are dividing, they are very vulnerable to the destructive actions of the chemotherapy drugs. Some of the normal cells surrounding the tumor are also damaged or destroyed because they are vulnerable while they are dividing to produce new, healthy cells.

SECTION IV: PRACTICING FOR NCLEX

Activity F

1. a. *Rationale:* There are numerous molecular mechanisms mediating cellular adaptation, including factors produced by other cells or by the cells themselves. These mechanisms depend largely on signals transmitted by chemical messengers that exert their effects by altering gene function. In general, the genes expressed in all cells fall into two categories: "housekeeping" genes that are necessary for normal function of a cell, and genes that determine the differentiating characteristics of a particular cell type. In many adaptive cellular responses, the expression of the differentiation genes is altered, whereas that of the housekeeping genes remains unaffected. Thus, a cell is able to change size or form without compromising its normal function. Once the stimulus for adaptation is removed, the effect on expression of the differentiating genes is removed and the cell resumes its previous state of specialized function.

2. b. *Rationale:* Compensatory hypertrophy is the enlargement of a remaining organ or

tissue after a portion has been surgically re-moved or rendered inactive. The body does not enlarge its major organs during times of malnutrition. Gene expression, not actin expression, stimulates the body to increase the muscle mass of the heart. Hypertrophy is not a progressive decrease in the size of anything.

3. c. *Rationale:* Metastatic calcification occurs in normal tissues as the result of increased serum calcium levels (hypercalcemia). Almost any condition that increases the serum cal-cium level can lead to calcification in inap-propriate sites such as the lung, renal tubules, and blood vessels. The major causes of hyper-calcemia are hyperparathyroidism, either pri-mary or secondary to phosphate retention in renal failure; increased mobilization of cal-cium from bone as in Paget disease, cancer with metastatic bone lesions, or immobiliza-tion; and vitamin D intoxication. Diabetes mellitus and hypoparathyroidism do not cause hypercalcemia; therefore, they cannot be a cause of metastatic calcification.

4. d. *Rationale:* The main source of methyl mer-cury exposure is from consumption of long-lived fish, such as tuna and swordfish. Although there is mercury in amalgam fill-ings, the amount of mercury vapor given off by the fillings is very small. Most thermome-ters today are made without mercury. The same holds true for most blood pressure ma-chines.
   Lead in paint is a concern, not mercury.

5. a. *Rationale:* Children are exposed to lead through ingestion of peeling lead paint, by breathing dust from lead paint (e.g., during remodeling), or from playing in contami-nated soil. The lead danger to potters is from the ceramic glaze before it is fired. You do not have to keep children away from everything ceramic. Newsprint contains lead, but you are not exposed to a significant amount of lead when you read the newspaper. You have to work directly with ore to be exposed to toxic levels of lead. Walking through part of a mine on a field trip is not a contributing fac-tor to lead poisoning.

6. b. *Rationale:* In a genetic disorder called xero-derma pigmentosum, an enzyme needed to repair sunlight-induced DNA damage is lack-ing. This autosomal recessive disorder is char-acterized by extreme photosensitivity and a 2,000-fold increased risk of skin cancer in sun-exposed skin. Exposure to sun causes the skin to toughen and become leathery feeling, but not in patches of pink-pigmented skin. Vitiligo is a benign acquired skin disease of unknown cause, consisting of irregular patches of various sizes totally lacking in pig-ment and often having hyperpigmented bor-ders. It can appear in the skin of any race and is not scaly. Photosensitivity is a sign of xero-derma pigmentosum, but this disease in-creases, not decreases, the person's risk of skin cancer.

7. b, c. *Rationale:* Lightning and high-voltage wires that carry several thousand volts pro-duce the most severe damage. In electrical in-juries, the body acts as a conductor of the electrical current.

8. d. *Rationale:* Injury from freezing probably results from a combination of ice crystal for-mation and vasoconstriction. The decreased blood flow leads to capillary stasis and arte-riolar and capillary thrombosis. Edema re-sults from increased capillary permeability. Exposure to low-intensity heat (43°C–46°C), such as occurs with partial-thickness burns and severe heat stroke, causes cell injury by inducing vascular injury. The process of warming tissue that has been frozen or par-tially frozen causes pain. If the pain is bad enough, then medication is given to control the pain. Health team members are always concerned about giving pain medication to someone who might be an addict. Asking whether this is the first time this person has had an injury induced by the cold is appro-priate when taking a health history. How-ever, pointing out that "it is obvious you are a homeless person" is not an appropriate re-mark for the nurse to make. Also not appro-priate is wondering when it will happen again.

9. a. *Rationale:* Destructive changes occur in small blood vessels such as the capillaries and venules. Acute reversible necrosis is repre-sented by such disorders as radiation cystitis, dermatitis, and diarrhea from enteritis. More persistent damage can be attributed to acute necrosis of tissue cells that are not capable of regeneration and chronic ischemia. Neither hunger nor muscle spasms are signs of radia-tion injury.

10. b. *Rationale:* Gram-negative bacilli release en-dotoxins that cause cell injury and increased capillary permeability. Certain bacteria excrete elaborate exotoxins that interfere with cellular production of ATP. Gram-negative bacilli do

not disrupt a cell's ability to replicate. Many gram-negative bacilli cause harm to cells.

11. atrophy. *Rationale:* When confronted with a decrease in work demands or adverse environmental conditions, most cells are able to revert to a smaller size and a lower and more efficient level of functioning that is compatible with survival. This decrease in cell size is called atrophy.

12. 1-a, 2-d, 3-b, 4-c. *Rationale:* Pigments are colored substances that may accumulate in cells. They can be endogenous (i.e., arising from within the body) or exogenous (i.e., arising from outside the body). Icterus, also called *jaundice*, is characterized by a yellow discoloration of tissue due to the retention of bilirubin, an endogenous bile pigment. This condition may result from increased bilirubin production from red blood cell destruction, obstruction of bile passage into the intestine, or toxic diseases that affect the liver's ability to remove bilirubin from the blood. Lipofuscin is a yellow-brown pigment that results from the accumulation of the indigestible residues produced during normal turnover of cell structures. The accumulation of lipofuscin increases with age and is sometimes referred to as the *wear-and-tear pigment*. It is more common in heart, nerve, and liver cells than other tissues and is seen more often in conditions associated with atrophy of an organ. One of the most common exogenous pigments is carbon in the form of coal dust. In coal miners or persons exposed to heavily polluted environments, the accumulation of carbon dust blackens the lung tissue and may cause serious lung disease. The formation of a blue lead line along the margins of the gum is one of the diagnostic features of lead poisoning. Melanin a black or dark brown pigment that occurs naturally in the hair, skin, and iris and choroid of the eye.

13. 1-b, 2-c, 3-a, 4-d. *Rationale:* Cell injury can be caused by a number of agents, including physical agents, chemical agents, biologic agents, and nutritional factors. Among the physical agents that generate cell injury are mechanical forces that produce tissue trauma, extremes of temperature, electricity, radiation, and nutritional disorders. Chemical agents can cause cell injury through several mechanisms: They can block enzymatic pathways, cause coagulation of tissues, or disrupt the osmotic or ionic balance of the cell. Biologic agents differ from other injurious

agents in that they are able to replicate and continue to produce injury. Among the nutritional factors that contribute to cell injury are excesses and deficiencies of nutrients, vitamins, and minerals.

14. a, b, c, d. *Rationale:* Many drugs—alcohol, prescription drugs, over-the-counter drugs, and street drugs—are capable of directly or indirectly damaging tissues. Ethyl alcohol can harm the gastric mucosa, liver, developing fetus, and other organs. Antineoplastic (anticancer) and immunosuppressant drugs can directly injure cells. Other drugs produce metabolic end products that are toxic to cells. Acetaminophen, a commonly used over-the-counter analgesic drug, is detoxified in the liver, where small amounts of the drug are converted to a highly toxic metabolite.

CHAPTER 6 GENETIC CONTROL OF CELL FUNCTION AND INHERITANCE

SECTION II: ASSESSING YOUR UNDERSTANDING

Activity A

1. deoxyribonucleic
2. Ribonucleic
3. proteome
4. purine, pyrimidine
5. complementary
6. 23
7. chromatin, chromosomes
8. triplet
9. mutations
10. haplotype
11. transcription
12. exons
13. translation
14. chaperones
15. expression
16. hedgehog
17. fibroblast
18. phenotype
19. locus, alleles
20. pedigree

Activity B

1.

1. a	2. c	3. b	4. e	5. j
6. f	7. d	8. h	9. g	10. i

2.

1. d	2. a	3. c	4. b	5. e

Activity C

1.

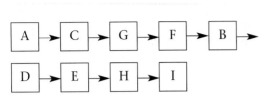

Activity D

1. Mendel discovered the basic pattern of inheritance by conducting carefully planned experiments with garden peas. Experimenting with phenotypic traits in peas, Mendel proposed that inherited traits are transmitted from parents to offspring by means of independently inherited factors, now known as genes, and that these factors are transmitted as recessive and dominant traits from parents to their offspring.

2. Genetic maps use linkage studies to estimate the distances between chromosomal landmarks. They are similar to a road map. Physical maps are similar to a surveyor's map. They make use of cytogenetic and molecular techniques to determine the physical locations of genes on chromosomes.

3. While in metaphase I, chromosomes are paired and condensed. Over time, an interchange of chromatid segments can occur. This process is called crossing over. Crossing over allows for new combinations of genes resulting in an increase in genetic variability. This is a very beneficial process.

4. There are 22 pairs of somatic chromosomes. Half of each pair is received from the female, and the other half is from the male. We then have two sex chromosomes, an X from our mother and, in the case of females, an X from the father for a total of two Xs. Males only have one X chromosome from their mother and one Y chromosome from their father.

5. Gene activator and repressor sites within DNA commonly monitor levels of the synthesized product and regulate gene transcription through a negative feedback mechanism. Expression is also regulated at the transcription level by transcription factors that directly affect protein structure and function

SECTION III: APPLYING YOUR KNOWLEDGE

Activity E

DNA fingerprinting is a technique for comparing the nucleotide sequences of fragments of DNA from different sources. The fragments are obtained by treating the DNA with various enzymes that break DNA strands at specific sites. There is a chance of 1 in 30 billion that two persons who are not monozygotic twins would have identical DNA fingerprints. Because genetic variations are so distinctive, DNA fingerprinting (analysis of DNA sequence differences) can be used to determine family relationships or help identify persons involved in criminal acts.

SECTION IV: PRACTICING FOR NCLEX

Activity F

1. a. *Rationale:* The term proteome is a relatively new term, created to define the complete set of proteins encoded by a genome. A chromosome is any of the threadlike structures in the nucleus of a cell that function in the transmission of genetic information. The terms protogene and nucleotomics are not real words.

2. b. *Rationale:* The two strands of the helix separate, and a complementary molecule is duplicated next to each original strand. Two strands become four strands. During cell division, the newly duplicated double-stranded molecules are separated and placed in each daughter cell by the mechanics of mitosis. As a result, each daughter cell again contains the meaningful strand and the complementary strand joined together as a double helix.

3. c. *Rationale:* Of the 23 pairs of human chromosomes, 22 are called autosomes and are alike in both males and females. The double helix is the shape of the DNA molecule. Ribosomes are areas in a cell that synthesize proteins. Haploid have only one complete set of nonhomologous chromosomes.

4. d. *Rationale:* Rarely, accidental errors in duplication of DNA occur. These errors are called mutations. Ribosomes are areas in a cell that synthesize proteins. Several repair mechanisms exist, and each depends on specific enzymes called endonucleases that

recognize local distortions of the DNA helix, cleave the abnormal chain, and remove the distorted region. Four bases—guanine, adenine, cytosine, and thymine (uracil is substituted for thymine in RNA)—make up the alphabet of the genetic code. A sequence of three of these bases forms the fundamental triplet code used in transmitting the genetic information needed for protein synthesis. This triplet code is called a codon.

5. a. *Rationale:* Polygenic inheritance involves multiple genes at different loci, with each gene exerting a small additive effect in determining a trait. Multifactorial inheritance is similar to polygenic inheritance in that multiple alleles at different loci affect the outcome; the difference is that multifactorial inheritance includes environmental effects on the genes. Monofactorial inheritance is nonexistent, as is collaborative inheritance.

6. b. *Rationale:* When the deletion is inherited from the mother, the infant presents with Angelman ("happy puppet") syndrome. Turner syndrome is a chromosomal anomaly seen in about 1 in 3000 live female births, characterized by the absence of one X chromosome. Down syndrome is a congenital condition characterized by varying degrees of mental retardation and multiple defects. It is the most common chromosomal abnormality of a generalized syndrome and is caused by the presence of an extra chromosome 21 in the G group. Fragile X syndrome is a reproductive disorder characterized by a nearly broken X chromosome, which has a tip hanging by a flimsy thread. It is the most common inherited cause of mental retardation.

7. c. *Rationale:* A recessive trait is one that is expressed only when two homozygous people have a child. A dominant trait is one expressed in either a homozygous or a heterozygous pairing. A single-gene trait and a penetrant trait do not exist. However, single-gene inheritance does exist.

8. d. *Rationale:* The establishment of the International HapMap Project was to map the haplotypes of the many closely related single nucleotide polymorphisms in the human genome and to develop methods for applying the technology of these projects to the diagnosis and treatment of disease. Four bases—

guanine, adenine, cytosine, and thymine (uracil is substituted for thymine in RNA)—make up the alphabet of the genetic code. A sequence of three of these bases forms the fundamental triplet code used in transmitting the genetic information needed for protein synthesis. This triplet code is called a codon. Alternate forms of a gene at the same locus are called alleles.

9. a. *Rationale:* Banding patterns are analyzed to determine whether they match. Four bases—guanine, adenine, cytosine, and thymine (uracil is substituted for thymine in RNA)—make up the alphabet of the genetic code. A sequence of three of these bases forms the fundamental triplet code used in transmitting the genetic information needed for protein synthesis. The small variation in gene sequence (termed a haplotype) is believed to account for the individual differences in physical traits, behaviors, and disease susceptibility. Chromosomes contain all genetic content of the genome.

10. b. *Rationale:* Cloned DNA sequences are usually the compounds used in gene therapy. Messenger RNA carries the instructions for protein synthesis. Sterically stable liposomes are stable liposomes with long circulation times. Sites in the DNA sequence where individuals differ at a single DNA base are called single nucleotide polymorphisms (SNPs, pronounced "snips").

11. haplotype. *Rationale:* As the Human Genome Project progressed, it became evident that the human genome sequence is almost exactly (99.9%) the same in all people. It is the small variation (0.01%) in gene sequence (termed a haplotype) that is believed to account for the individual differences in physical traits, behaviors, and disease susceptibility.

12. b, c, d. *Rationale:* RNA is a single-stranded rather than a double-stranded molecule. Second, the sugar in each nucleotide of RNA is ribose, not deoxyribose. Third, the pyrimidine base thymine in DNA is replaced by uracil in RNA. All cells are supposed to have 23 pairs of chromosomes.

13. insulin. *Rationale:* Recombinant DNA technology has also made it possible to produce proteins that have therapeutic properties.

One of the first products to be produced was human insulin.

14. a, b, c. *Rationale:* A karyotype is a photograph of a person's chromosomes. It is prepared by special laboratory techniques in which body cells are cultured, fixed, and then stained to display identifiable banding patterns. A centromere is the constricted region of a chromosome that joins the two chromatids to each other and attaches to spindle fibers in mitosis and meiosis. Human chromosomes are classified as one of three types, depending on the position of their centromere. Two types of genes, complementary genes, in which each gene is mutually dependent on the other; and collaborative genes, in which two different genes influencing the same trait interact, play a part in multifactorial inheritance.

15. 1-c, 2-a, 3-b, 4-e, 5-d. *Rationale:* The genotype of a person is the genetic information stored in the base sequence triplet code. The phenotype refers to the recognizable traits, physical or biochemical, associated with a specific genotype. Pharmacogenetics is the variability of drug response due to inherited characteristics in individuals. Somatic cell hybridization involves the fusion of human somatic cells with those of a different species (typically, the mouse) to yield a cell containing the chromosomes of both species. Penetrance represents the ability of a gene to express its function. Seventy-five percent penetrance means 75% of persons of a particular genotype present with a recognizable phenotype.

CHAPTER 7 GENETIC AND CONGENITAL DISORDERS

SECTION II: ASSESSING YOUR UNDERSTANDING

Activity A

1. Congenital
2. DNA, chromosomal
3. codominant
4. mutation
5. inherited, spontaneous
6. carrier
7. Marfan
8. recessive
9. 60
10. structure, abnormal
11. Translocation

Activity B *Labeling*

1.

2. The figure represents a simple pedigree for inheritance of an autosomal dominant trait. The colored circle or square represents an affected parent with a mutant gene. An affected parent with an autosomal dominant trait has a 50% chance of passing the mutant gene on to each child regardless of sex.

Activity C

1. h   **2.** c   **3.** e   **4.** a   **5.** g
6. b   **7.** j   **8.** d   **9.** i   **10.** f

Activity D

1. Conditions are inherited as dominant or recessive on one of the autosomal chromosomes or one of the sex chromosomes. If the trait is dominant, the patient will inherit the condition. For a recessive trait to be expressed, both parents must carry the mutation. If the mutation is on the Y chromosome, all male children will be affected; if it is on the X chromosome, about half the offspring may potentially be affected.
2. Multifactorial congenital malformations involve a single organ or tissue derived from the same embryonic developmental field. Second, the risk of recurrence in future pregnancies is increased for the same or a similar defect. Third, the risk increases with increasing incidence of the defect among relatives.
3. Structural changes in chromosomes usually result from breakage in one or more of the chromosomes, followed by rearrangement or deletion of the chromosome parts. Among the factors believed to cause chromosome breakage are exposure to radiation sources, such as x-rays; influence of certain chemicals; extreme changes in the cellular environment; and viral infections.
4. Alterations in sex chromosomes are better tolerated than alterations of autosomal chromosomes because of (a) the inactivation of all but one X chromosome and (b) the modest amount of genetic material that is carried on the Y chromosome.
5. Ova contain the majority of the mitochondria, whereas spermatozoa have very few, if any, so the embryo will inherit most, if not all, of the mitochondria from the mother. The neural and muscular tissues are most affected by mtDNA mutations due to their great dependence on oxidative phosphorylation. These tissues will have numerous mitochondria and suffer from their malfunction.

SECTION III: APPLYING YOUR KNOWLEDGE

Activity E

1. Alcohol passes freely across the placental barrier so concentrations of alcohol in the fetus are at least as high as in the mother. Unlike other agents harmful to the fetus, the harmful effects of alcohol are not restricted to the sensitive period of early gestation but extend throughout pregnancy. Alcohol consumption during pregnancy can cause fetal alcohol syndrome in the baby.
2. Alcohol has widely variable effects on fetal development, ranging from minor abnormalities to fetal alcohol syndrome. There may be prenatal or postnatal growth retardation; central nervous system involvement, including neurologic abnormalities, developmental delays, behavioral dysfunction, intellectual impairment, and skull and brain malformation; and a characteristic set of facial features that include small eye openings, a thin upper lip, and an elongated, flattened midface and philtrum (i.e., the groove in the middle of the upper lip). Each defect can vary in severity, probably reflecting the timing of alcohol consumption in terms of the period of fetal development, amount of alcohol consumed, and hereditary and environmental influences.

SECTION IV: PRACTICING FOR NCLEX

Activity F

1. a. *Rationale:* If the members of a gene pair are identical (i.e., code the exact same gene product), then the person is homozygous, and if the two members are different, then the person is heterozygous. The phenotype is the observable expression of a genotype in terms of morphologic, biochemical, or molecular traits. Although gene expression usually follows a dominant or recessive pattern, it is possible for both alleles (members) of a gene pair to be fully expressed in the heterozygote, a condition called codominance. A gene mutation is a biochemical event such as nucleotide change, deletion, or insertion that produces a new allele. The terms *phenotypic*, *codominant*, and *mutant* are not used to describe a person when referring to the expression of a gene pair.
2. b. *Rationale:* In more than 90% of persons with neurofibromatosis type 1, cutaneous and subcutaneous neurofibromas develop in late childhood or adolescence. The cutaneous neurofibromas, which vary in number from a few to many hundred, manifest as soft, pedunculated lesions that project from the skin. Marfan syndrome affects several organ systems, including the ocular system (eyes), the cardiovascular system (heart and blood

vessels), and the skeletal system (bones and joints). Down syndrome is a congenital condition characterized by varying degrees of mental retardation and multiple defects. Klinefelter syndrome is a condition that occurs in men who have an extra X chromosome in most of their cells. The syndrome can affect different stages of physical, language, and social development. The most common symptom is infertility.

3. c. *Rationale:* Cleft lip with or without cleft palate is one of the most common birth defects. This process is under the control of many genes, and the disturbances in gene expression (hereditary or environmental) at this time may result in cleft lip with or without cleft palate. The defect may also be caused by teratogens (e.g., rubella, anticonvulsant drugs) and is often encountered in children with chromosomal abnormalities.

4. d. *Rationale:* Occasionally, mitotic errors in early development give rise to two or more cell lines characterized by distinctive karyotypes, a condition referred to as mosaicism. A gene mutation is a biochemical event, such as nucleotide change, deletion, or insertion, that produces a new allele. Referring to someone as a "mutant" is a derogatory expression. Monosomy refers to the presence of only one member of a chromosome pair; it is not a term used to denote a person. Having an abnormal number of chromosomes is referred to as aneuploidy; it is not a term used to denote a person.

5. a. *Rationale:* The risk of having a child with Down syndrome increases with maternal age; it is 1 in 1250 at 25 years of age, 1 in 400 at 35 years, and 1 in 100 at 45 years of age. The reason for the correlation between maternal age and nondisjunction is unknown, but is believed to reflect some aspect of aging of the oocyte. Although males continue to produce sperm throughout their reproductive life, females are born with all the oocytes they ever will have. These oocytes may change as a result of the aging process. With increasing age, there is a greater chance of a woman having been exposed to damaging environmental agents such as drugs, chemicals, and radiation. There is no correlation with maternal age and the other syndromes.

6. b. *Rationale:* The embryo's development is most easily disturbed during the period when differentiation and development of the organs are taking place. This time interval, which is often referred to as the period of *organogenesis*, extends from day 15 to day 60 after conception. There are no periods of susceptibility, fetal anomalies, or hormonal imbalance.

7. c. *Rationale:* Teratogenic agents have been divided into three groups: radiation, drugs and chemical substances, and infectious agents. The period of organogenesis, the third trimester, and the second trimester are not teratogenic substances. They are time periods during the pregnancy. Teratogenic substances are not classified as outside, inside, or internal. Although drugs and chemical substances are a class of teratogenic agents, smoking is included in that class as a teratogenic agent. It is not a class unto itself. Bacteria and viruses are considered infectious agents and are therefore teratogenic agents.

8. d. *Rationale:* The acronym TORCH stands for *T*oxoplasmosis, *O*ther, *R*ubella (i.e., German measles), *C*ytomegalovirus, and *H*erpes, which are the agents most frequently implicated in fetal anomalies. Common clinical and pathological manifestations include growth retardation and abnormalities of the brain (microcephaly, hydrocephalus), eye, ear, liver, hematopoietic system (anemia, thrombocytopenia), lungs (pneumonitis), and heart (myocarditis, congenital heart disorders).

9. a. *Rationale:* The birth of a defective child is a traumatic event in any parent's life. Usually, two issues must be resolved. The first deals with the immediate and future care of the affected child, and the second with the possibility of future children in the family having a similar defect.

10. b. *Rationale:* The purpose of prenatal screening and diagnosis is not just to detect fetal abnormalities. Rather, it is meant to provide parents with information needed to make an informed choice about having a child with an abnormality; to provide reassurance and reduce anxiety among high-risk groups; and to allow parents at risk for having a child with a specific defect, who might otherwise forgo having a child, to begin a pregnancy with the assurance that knowledge about the presence or absence of the disorder in the fetus can be confirmed by testing. It is not the object of genetic counseling and prenatal screening to provide information on where to terminate a pregnancy if that is

what the parents choose to do. Prenatal screening cannot be used to rule out all possible fetal abnormalities. It is limited to determining whether the fetus has (or probably has) designated conditions indicated by late maternal age, family history, or well-defined risk factors.

11. 1-a, 2-b, 3-c, 4-d, 5-e. *Rationale:* A single mutant gene may be expressed in many different parts of the body. Marfan syndrome, for example, is a defect in connective tissue that has widespread effects involving skeletal, eye, and cardiovascular structures. In autosomal dominant disorders, a single mutant allele from an affected parent is transmitted to an offspring regardless of sex. In many conditions, the age of onset is delayed, and the signs and symptoms of the disorder do not appear until later in life, as in Huntington's chorea.

    Tay-Sachs is inherited as an autosomal recessive trait. Fragile X syndrome is a single-gene disorder in which the mutation is characterized by a long repeating sequence of three nucleotides within the fragile X gene.

12. a, b, c. *Rationale:* First, multifactorial congenital malformations tend to involve a single organ or tissue derived from the same embryonic developmental field. Second, the risk of recurrence in future pregnancies is for the same or a similar defect. This means that parents of a child with a cleft palate defect have an increased risk of having another child with a cleft palate, but not with spina bifida. Third, the increased risk (compared with the general population) among first-degree relatives of the affected person is 2% to 7%, and among second-degree relatives, it is approximately one-half that amount. The risk increases with increasing incidence of the defect among relatives. Disorders of multifactorial inheritance can be expressed during fetal life and be present at birth, or they may be expressed later in life.

13. Phenylketonuria. *Rationale:* Phenylketonuria is a rare metabolic disorder that affects approximately 1 in every 15,000 infants in the United States. The disorder, which is inherited as a recessive trait, is caused by a deficiency of the liver enzyme phenylalanine hydroxylase. As a result of this deficiency, toxic levels of the amino acid phenylalanine accumulate in the blood and other tissues.

14. a, d. *Rationale:* The physiologic status of the mother—her hormone balance, her general state of health, her nutritional status, and the drugs she takes—undoubtedly influences the development of the unborn child. Other agents, such as radiation, can cause chromosomal and genetic defects and produce developmental disorders. Neither weather nor air pollution has been linked with fetal abnormalities or developmental disorders.

15. a. *Rationale:* In 1983, the U.S. Food and Drug Administration established a system for classifying drugs according to probable risks to the fetus. According to this system, drugs are put into five categories: A, B, C, D, and X. Drugs in category A are the least dangerous, and categories B, C, and D are increasingly more dangerous. Those in category X are contraindicated during pregnancy because of proven teratogenicity.

CHAPTER 8 NEOPLASIA

SECTION II: ASSESSING YOUR UNDERSTANDING

Activity A

1. differentiation, growth
2. proliferation
3. Differentiation
4. cyclins
5. phosphorylate
6. progenitor
7. Stem
8. Embryonic
9. neoplasm
10. Benign
11. differentiated
12. -oma
13. polyp
14. carcinoma
15. solid tumors, hematologic
16. anaplasia
17. growth factors
18. cadherin-catenin-actin
19. protooncogenes, suppressor
20. Human T-cell leukemia virus type 1
21. 30
22. anorexia-cachexia
23. ulceration, necrosis
24. Anemia
25. biopsy
26. Radiation
27. Chemotherapy

Activity B

Activity C

1.

1. b	**2.** a	**3.** e	**4.** j	**5.** f
6. c	**7.** d	**8.** h	**9.** g	**10.** i

2.

1. d	**2.** f	**3.** e	**4.** h	**5.** b
6. a	**7.** i	**8.** j	**9.** c	**10.** g

Activity D

1.

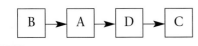

Activity E

1. In terms of cell proliferation, the cells may be divided into three groups: (a) the well-differentiated neurons and cells of skeletal and cardiac muscle that rarely divide and reproduce; (b) the progenitor or parent cell that continues to divide and reproduce, such as blood cells, skin cells, and liver cells; and (c) the undifferentiated stem cells that can be triggered to enter the cell cycle and produce large numbers of progenitor cells when the need arises.

2. Both benign and malignant tumors have lost the ability to suppress growth. As a result, the tumor cells continue to proliferate. Benign tumors are composed of well-differentiated cells and are confined to the area of tissue origin. In contrast, malignant tumors are composed of less differentiated cells that will reenter circulation and establish secondary tumors in another region of the body.

3. The five factors used to describe benign and malignant neoplasm are (a) cell characteristics, (b) rate of growth, (c) manner of growth, (d) capacity to invade and metastasize to other parts of the body, and (e) potential for causing death.

4. Metastasis occurs via lymph channels and blood vessels. When metastasis occurs by way of the lymphatic channels, the tumor cells lodge first in the initial lymph node that receives drainage from the tumor site. If they survive, cancer cells may spread from more distant lymph nodes to the thoracic duct, and then gain access to the blood vasculature. With hematologic spread, the blood-borne cancer cells may enter the venous flow that drains the site of the primary neoplasm. Cancer cells may also enter tumor-associated blood vessels that either infiltrate the tumor or are found at the periphery of the tumor.

5. Cancer cells express abnormal cell surface proteins. Normally, the immune system recognizes these abnormal proteins and destroys the cancerous cell. With a compromised immune system, these abnormalities are missed and allowed to persist in the body.

6. Chemicals will cause cellular transformation either directly (direct reacting agents) or indirectly, only becoming activated via a metabolic process (initiators).

7. Hypermetabolism is the result of the rapidly growing tumor and the increased expression of uncoupling proteins. The first reason is that the tumor uses large quantities of glucose via glycolysis, therefore producing high levels of lactic acid. The lactic acid undergoes the energy-requiring process of gluconeogenesis in order to convert it back to glucose. This process uses large amounts of glucose and wastes large amounts of adenosine triphosphate (ATP). The second reason is the presence of uncoupling proteins. The uncoupling proteins uncouple oxidative phosphorylation, thereby reducing the amount of ATP produced.

8. Paraneoplastic syndromes are characterized by manifestations in sites that are not directly

affected by the disease. Most commonly, manifestations are caused by the elaboration of hormones by cancer cells and others from the production of circulating factors that produce hematopoietic, neurologic, and dermatologic syndromes.

9. Blood tests for tumor markers, cytologic studies and tissue biopsy, endoscopic examinations, ultrasound, x-ray studies, magnetic resonance imaging, computed tomography, and positron emission tomography.

10. The clinical staging of cancer is intended to group patients according to the extent of their disease. Grading of tumors involves the microscopic examination of cancer cells to determine their level of differentiation and the number of mitoses. Cancers are classified as grades I, II, III, and IV, with increasing anaplasia or lack of differentiation. The two basic methods for classifying cancers are *grading* according to the histologic or cellular characteristics of the tumor and *staging* according to the clinical spread of the disease.

SECTION III: APPLYING YOUR KNOWLEDGE

Activity F

1. "To make it better for you, the doctor is going to put a tube just under your skin that the nurses can put your medication in so they won't have to stick you in the hands and arms so many times. You will still get stuck by a needle but it will not be as painful as trying to start IVs in your arms."

2. Because Joe's cancer is found in his blood and bone marrow, surgery cannot be used to cure it. Chemotherapy is the primary treatment for most hematologic and some solid tumors. Chemotherapy is a systemic treatment that enables drugs to reach the site of the tumor as well as other distant sites. Cancer chemotherapeutic drugs exert their effects through several mechanisms. At the cellular level, they exert their lethal action by targeting processes that prevent cell growth and replication. These mechanisms include disrupting the production of essential enzymes; inhibiting DNA, RNA, and protein synthesis; and preventing cell reproduction.

SECTION IV: PRACTICING FOR NCLEX

Activity G

1. a. *Rationale:* Asking whether his tumor will make him die shows that the patient does not understand the educational material he has been given. For unknown reasons, benign tumors have lost the ability to suppress the genetic program for cell proliferation but have retained the program for normal cell differentiation. They do not have the capacity to infiltrate, invade, or metastasize to distant sites.

2. b. *Rationale:* Metastasis occurs by way of the lymph channels (i.e., lymphatic spread) and the blood vessels (i.e., hematogenic spread). In many types of cancer, the first evidence of disseminated disease is the presence of tumor cells in the lymph nodes that drain the tumor area. When metastasis occurs by way of the lymphatic channels, the tumor cells lodge first in the initial lymph node that receives drainage from the tumor site. Once in this lymph node, the cells may die because of the lack of a proper environment, grow into a discernible mass, or remain dormant for unknown reasons. If they survive and grow, the cancer cells may spread from more distant lymph nodes to the thoracic duct, and then gain access to the blood vasculature. Because cancer cells have the ability to shed themselves from the original tumor, they are often found floating in the body fluids around the tumor. Cancer cells neither are moved from one place to another by transporter cells, nor do they form a chain to grow to a new place in the body to form a new tumor.

3. c. *Rationale:* Cancer occurs because of interactions among multiple risk factors or repeated exposure to a single carcinogenic (cancer-producing) agent. Among the traditional risk factors that have been linked to cancer are heredity, hormonal factors, immunologic mechanisms, and environmental agents, such as chemicals, radiation, and cancer-causing viruses. More recently, there has been interest in obesity and type 2 diabetes mellitus as risk factors for a number of cancers. Body type, age, and color of skin have not been identified as risk factors for cancer.

4. d. *Rationale:* Familial adenomatous polyposis of the colon also follows an autosomal dominant inheritance pattern. It is caused by mutation of another tumor suppressor gene, the APC gene. In people who inherit this gene, hundreds of adenomatous polyps may develop, some of which inevitably become malignant. Retinoblastoma is inheritable through an autosomal dominant gene, but only about 40% of retinoblastomas are

inherited. Osteosarcoma and acute lympho-cytic leukemia are not inheritable through an autosomal dominant process.

5. a. *Rationale:* Most known dietary carcinogens occur either naturally in plants (e.g., aflatox-ins) or are produced during food preparation. Among the most potent of the procarcino-gens are the polycyclic aromatic hydrocar-bons. These are of particular interest because they are produced from animal fat in the process of charcoal-broiling meats and are present in smoked meats and fish. Polycyclic aromatic hydrocarbons are also produced in the combustion of tobacco and are present in cigarette smoke. Initiators is another term for procarcinogens. Diethylstilbestrol was a drug that was widely used in the United States from the mid-1940s to 1970 to prevent mis-carriages.

6. b. *Rationale:* Lung cancers, breast cancers, and lymphomas account for about 75% of malig-nant pleural effusions. Complaints of abdom-inal discomfort, swelling and a feeling of heaviness, and an increase in abdominal girth, which reflect the presence of peritoneal effusions or ascites, are the most common presenting symptoms in ovarian cancer, oc-curring in up to 65% of women with the dis-ease.

7. c. *Rationale:* Tumor markers are antigens ex-pressed on the surface of tumor cells or sub-stances released from normal cells in response to the presence of tumor. The serum markers that have proven most useful in clin-ical practice are the human chorionic go-nadotropin, CA 125, prostate-specific antigen, alpha-fetoprotein, carcinoembryonic antigen, and CD blood cell antigens. Deoxyri-bonucleic acid is DNA, which is not a serum tumor marker. Cyclin-dependent kinases (CDKs) come from a family of proteins called cyclins, which control entry and progression of cells through the cell cycle. Cyclins act by complexing with (and thereby activating) proteins called CDKs. They are not serum tumor markers.

8. d. *Rationale:* Growth hormone deficiency in adults is associated with increased prevalence of dyslipidemia, insulin resistance, and car-diovascular mortality. Hypocalcemia is a defi-ciency of calcium in the serum that may be caused by hypoparathyroidism, vitamin D deficiency, kidney failure, acute pancreatitis, or inadequate amounts of plasma magnesium

and protein. It does not result from cancer therapy during childhood.
Hyperinsulinemia is associated with syn-drome X, which is a condition characterized by hypertension with obesity, type 2 diabetes mellitus, hypertriglyceridemia, increased pe-ripheral insulin resistance, hyperinsulinemia, and elevated catecholamine levels.

9. a. *Rationale:* Chemotherapy is more widely used in the treatment of children with cancer than in adults because children tend to better tolerate the acute adverse effects, and in gen-eral, pediatric tumors are more responsive to chemotherapy than adult cancers. Children are very adaptable and tolerate more forms of cancer treatment than do adults. Children do complain about the nausea and vomiting chemotherapy can cause, just like adults. And they do not like losing their hair, just like adults.

10. b. *Rationale:* The combination of select cyto-toxic drugs with radiation has demonstrated a radiosensitizing effect on tumor cells by al-tering the cell cycle distribution, increasing DNA damage, and decreasing DNA repair. Some radiosensitizers are 5-fluorouracil, capecitabine, paclitaxel, gemcitabine, and cis-platin. Doxorubicin is an antitumor antibi-otic, vincristine is a vinca alkaloid, and docetaxel is a taxane.

11. neoplasm. *Rationale:* An abnormal mass of tissue in which the growth exceeds and is un-coordinated with that of the normal tissues is called a neoplasm. Unlike normal cellular adaptive processes such as hypertrophy and hyperplasia, neoplasms do not obey the laws of normal cell growth. They serve no useful purpose, do not occur in response to an ap-propriate stimulus, and continue to grow at the expense of the host.

12. a, c, e. *Rationale:* Malignant neoplasms are less well differentiated and have the ability to break loose, enter the circulatory or lym-phatic systems, and form secondary malig-nant tumors at other sites. They frequently cause suffering and death if untreated or un-controlled. Malignant neoplasms form sec-ondary tumors at sites other than the original tumor site. They are not passed out of the body as waste through the alimentary canal.

13. b, c, e. *Rationale:* Cancer cells differ from nor-mal cells by being immortal with an unlim-ited life span. Cancer cells often lose cell density–dependent inhibition, which is the

cessation of growth after cells reach a particular density. This is sometimes referred to as contact inhibition because cells often stop growing when they come into contact with each other. Another characteristic of cancer cells is the ability to proliferate even in the absence of growth factors. Most cancer cells exhibit a characteristic called genetic instability, which is often considered to be a hallmark of cancer.

14. 1-b, 2-d, 3-c, 4-a. *Rationale:* Cancers for which current screening or early detection has led to improvement in outcomes include those of the breast (breast self-examination, mammography), cervix (Pap smear), colon and rectum (rectal exam, fecal occult blood test, flexible sigmoidoscopy, colonoscopy), prostate (prostate-specific antigen testing, transrectal ultrasonography), and malignant melanoma (self-examination).

15. a, b, d. *Rationale:* With improvement in treatment methods, the number of children who survive childhood cancer is continuing to increase. As these children approach adulthood, there is continued concern that the lifesaving therapy they received during childhood may produce late effects, such as impaired growth, cognitive dysfunction, hormonal dysfunction, cardiomyopathy, pulmonary fibrosis, and risk for second malignancies. Liver failure is not viewed as a late effect of childhood cancer therapy.

CHAPTER 9 STRESS AND ADAPTATION

SECTION II: ASSESSING YOUR UNDERSTANDING

Activity A

1. homeostasis, physiologic
2. Homeostasis
3. negative
4. stress
5. disease
6. hypothalamic-pituitary-adrenocortical, adrenomedullary, sympathetic
7. adapting
8. coping strategy
9. Sleep
10. Alcohol

Activity B

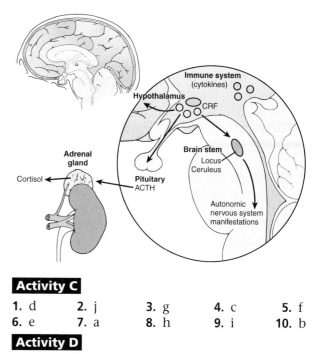

Activity C

1. d	2. j	3. g	4. c	5. f
6. e	7. a	8. h	9. i	10. b

Activity D

1. Negative feedback mechanisms are the primary mechanisms used to maintain homeostasis. The negative feedback mechanism controls blood glucose levels—an increase in blood glucose stimulates an increase in insulin—which enhances the removal of glucose from the blood. When glucose has been taken up by cells and blood glucose levels fall, insulin secretion is inhibited, and glucagon and other counter-regulatory mechanisms stimulate the release of glucose from the liver, which causes the blood glucose to return to normal.

2. The stages of general adaptation syndrome are the alarm stage, the resistance stage, and the exhaustion stage. The *alarm stage* is characterized by a generalized stimulation of the sympathetic nervous system and the hypothalamic-pituitary-adrenocortical axis, resulting in the release of catecholamines and cortisol. During the *resistance* stage, the body selects the most effective and economic channels of defense. During this stage, the increased cortisol levels present during the first stage drop because they are no longer needed. If the stressor is prolonged or overwhelms the ability of the body to defend itself, the exhaustion *stage* ensues, during which resources are depleted and signs of "wear and tear" or systemic damage appear.

3. The results of the coordinated release of these neurohormones include the mobilization of energy, a sharpened focus and awareness, increased cerebral blood flow and glucose utilization, enhanced cardiovascular and respiratory functioning, redistribution of blood flow to the brain and muscles, modulation of the immune response, inhibition of reproductive function, and decrease in appetite.

4. Many organs are functioning at much less than maximum capacity, giving the organ a safety margin. The safety margin for adaptation of most body systems is considerably greater than that needed for normal activities. The red blood cells carry more oxygen than the tissues can use, the liver and fat cells store excess nutrients, and bone tissue stores calcium in excess of that needed for normal neuromuscular function. Many of the body organs, such as the lungs, kidneys, and adrenals, are paired to provide anatomical reserve as well. Both organs are not needed to ensure the continued existence and maintenance of the internal environment. As the body expends greater amounts of energy, athletes are able to tap into these reserves.

5. Physiological symptoms arise from exaggerated sympathetic nervous system activation in response to the traumatic event. Persons with chronic post-traumatic stress disorder (PTSD) have been shown to have increased levels of norepinephrine and increased activity of (α_2-adrenergic receptors. The increases in catecholamines, in tandem with increased thyroid levels in persons with PTSD, are believed to explain some of the intrusive and somatic symptoms of the disorder. In the central nervous system, reactivity of the amygdala and hippocampus and decreased reactivity of the anterior cingulate and orbitofrontal areas are believed to also contribute to PTSD.

SECTION III: APPLYING YOUR KNOWLEDGE
Activity E

1. When eliciting the history of the present illness, the nurse should inquire about the following:
   Primary health problems
   History of substance abuse
   Sleep patterns
   Onset of symptoms

History of life-threatening event
Client's coping strategies

2. Nursing interventions include the following:
   Teaching the family about PTSD
   Using a family-centered approach to care
   Assuring the client of confidentiality
   Validating client's feelings about the trauma
   Allowing the client to tell the story of the trauma
   Assessing the client's ability to meet primary needs
   Identifying other stressors that might affect the client's ability to cope

SECTION IV: PRACTICING FOR NCLEX
Activity F

1. a. *Rationale:* The body's control systems regulate cellular function, control life processes, and integrate functions of the different organ systems. Homeostatic control systems do not feed cells when they are under stress, do not act on invading organisms, and do not shut down the body at death.

2. b. *Rationale:* A homeostatic control system consists of a collection of interconnected components that function to keep a physical or chemical parameter of the body relatively constant. An organ system is a group of organs that function together to accomplish necessary functions in the body; for example, the cardiovascular system provides blood to all the body's components. Biochemical messengers are in the brain; they are not control systems. Neuroendocrine systems are control systems that help regulate the body's response to stress. Neurovascular systems do not aid in the control of homeostasis in the body.

3. c. *Rationale:* Selye contended that many ailments, such as various emotional disturbances, mildly annoying headaches, insomnia, upset stomach, gastric and duodenal ulcers, certain types of rheumatic disorders, and cardiovascular and kidney diseases, appear to be initiated or encouraged by the "body itself because of its faulty adaptive reactions to potentially injurious agents." Psychotic disorders are not caused by stress. Osteogenesis refers to the origin of bone tissue; this is not due to stress. Sarcomas are a type of cancer. There is no such thing as osteogenesis sarcomas. Infections in the head and neck are caused by bacterial or viral invaders of the body; they are not due to stress.

4. d. *Rationale:* The results of the coordinated release of these neurohormones include the mobilization of energy, sharpened focus and awareness, increased cerebral blood flow and glucose utilization, enhanced cardiovascular and respiratory functioning, redistribution of blood flow to the brain and muscles, modulation of the immune response, inhibition of reproductive function, and decrease in appetite.

5. a. *Rationale:* Diseases of the cardiovascular, gastrointestinal, immune, and neurologic systems, as well as depression, chronic alcoholism and drug abuse, eating disorders, accidents, and suicide, have all been linked to the chronic and excessive activation of the stress response.

6. b. *Rationale:* The response to physiologic disturbances that threaten the integrity of the internal environment is specific to the threat; the body usually does not raise the body temperature when an increase in heart rate is needed. In contrast, the response to psychological disturbances is not regulated with the same degree of specificity and feedback control; instead, the effect may be inappropriate and sustained. No systems in the body are regulated by a positive feedback system. In cardiovascular physiology, the baroreflex or baroreceptor reflex is one of the body's homeostatic mechanisms for maintaining blood pressure. It has nothing to do with the body's response to a psychological threat.

7. c. *Rationale:* The ability of body systems to increase their function given the need to adapt is known as the physiologic reserve. Many of the body organs, such as the lungs, kidneys, and adrenals, are paired to provide anatomic reserve as well. Both organs are not needed to ensure the continued existence and maintenance of the internal environment. Genetic endowment, physiologic reserve, and health status are all coping mechanisms, but they do not affect the body's need to survive when one organ out of a pair is missing.

8. c. *Rationale:* The configuration of significant others that constitutes the social network functions to mobilize the resources of the person; these friends, colleagues, and family members share the person's tasks and provide monetary support, materials and tools, and guidance in improving problem-solving capabilities. Social networks cannot protect the person from other internal stressors.

9. d. *Rationale:* In persons with limited coping abilities, either because of physical or mental health, the acute stress response may be detrimental. This is true of persons with preexisting heart disease in whom the overwhelming sympathetic behaviors associated with the stress response can lead to arrhythmias. The acute stress response is not necessarily going to be detrimental to the client who has undergone the resection of a brain tumor, the client who is schizophrenic and off medication, or the client who has a broken femur.

10. a. *Rationale:* PTSD is an example of chronic activation of the stress response as the result of experiencing a severe trauma. In this disorder, memory of the traumatic event seems to be enhanced. Flashbacks of the event are accompanied by intense activation of the neuroendocrine system. Chronic renal insufficiency, schizophrenia, and post delivery depression in a new mother are not the result of chronic activation of the stress response following a severe trauma.

11. multicellular. *Rationale:* A multicellular organism is able to survive only as long as the composition of the internal environment is compatible with the survival needs of the individual cells.

12. eustress. *Rationale:* Selye suggested that mild, brief, and controllable periods of stress could be perceived as positive stimuli to emotional and intellectual growth and development. These periods of stress are called eustress.

13. b, d. *Rationale:* The treatment of stress should be directed toward helping people avoid coping behaviors that impose a risk to their health and providing them with alternative stress-reducing strategies. Nonpharmacologic methods used for stress reduction are relaxation techniques, guided imagery, music therapy, massage, and biofeedback.

14. 1-b. *Rationale:* Corticotropin-releasing factor is a small peptide hormone found in both the hypothalamus and extrahypothalamic structures, such as the limbic system and the brain stem. It is both an important endocrine regulator of pituitary and adrenal activity and a neurotransmitter involved in autonomic nervous system activity, metabolism, and behavior.

   2-d. *Rationale:* The sympathetic nervous system manifestation of the stress reaction has been called the fight-or-flight response. This is the most rapid of the stress responses and represents the basic survival response of our primitive ancestors when confronted with the perils of the wilderness and its inhabitants.

3-c. *Rationale:* The term allostasis has been used by some investigators to describe the physiological changes in the neuroendocrine, autonomic, and immune systems that occur in response to either real or perceived challenges to homeostasis. The persistence and/or accumulation of these allostatic changes (e.g., immunosuppression, activation of the sympathetic nervous and renin-angiotensin-aldosterone systems) has been called an "allostatic load," and this concept has been used to measure the cumulative effects of stress on humans.

4-a. *Rationale:* The hallmark of the stress response, as first described by Selye, is the endocrine–immune interactions (i.e., increased corticosteroid production and atrophy of the thymus) that are known to suppress the immune response. In concert, these two components of the stress system, through endocrine and neurotransmitter pathways, produce the physical and behavioral changes designed to adapt to acute stress.

15. a, b, c. *Rationale:* The most significant arguments for interaction between the neuroendocrine and immune systems derive from evidence that the immune and neuroendocrine systems share common signal pathways (i.e., messenger molecules and receptors), that hormones and neuropeptides can alter the function of immune cells, and that the immune system and its mediators can modulate neuroendocrine function. These systems do not need each other to function.

CHAPTER 10 ALTERATIONS IN TEMPERATURE REGULATION

SECTION II: ASSESSING YOUR UNDERSTANDING

Activity A

1. 36.0–37.5
2. hypothalamus
3. Metabolism
4. pilomotor
5. fever
6. cyclic adenosine monophosphate
7. Kupffer
8. neurogenic fever
9. intermittent fever

10. 15
11. PFAPA
12. Aspirin and NSAIDs, prostaglandin E_2
13. elderly
14. Hyperthermia
15. heat index
16. salt, water
17. hypothermia
18. anesthetic, hypothermia
19. heart rate, cardiac output

Activity B

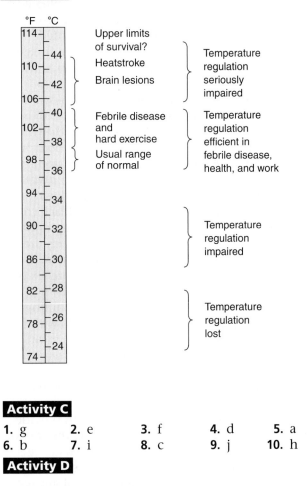

Activity C

1. g	2. e	3. f	4. d	5. a
6. b	7. i	8. c	9. j	10. h

Activity D

B → D → C → A

Activity E

1. Most of the body's heat is produced by the deeper core tissues (i.e., muscles and viscera), which are insulated from the environment and protected against heat loss by an outer shell of subcutaneous tissues and skin

2. During the *first* or *prodromal* period, there are nonspecific complaints such as mild headache and fatigue, general malaise, and

aches and pains. During the *chill*, there is the uncomfortable sensation of being chilled and the onset of generalized shaking. Vasoconstriction and piloerection usually precede the onset of shivering. At this point, the skin is pale and covered with goose flesh. There is a feeling of being cold and an urge to put on more clothing or covering and to curl up in a position that conserves body heat. When the shivering has caused the body temperature to reach the new set-point of the temperature control center, the shivering ceases, and a sensation of warmth develops. At this point, the *third stage* or *flush* begins, during which cutaneous vasodilation occurs and the skin becomes warm and flushed. The *fourth*, or *defervescence*, stage of the febrile response is marked by the initiation of sweating.

3. Infants and young children have decreased immunologic function and are more commonly infected with virulent organisms. In addition, the mechanisms for controlling temperature are not as well developed in infants as they are in older children and adults.

4. Muscle exertion continued for long periods in warm weather can result in excessive heat loads. Elderly persons and those with cardiovascular disease are at increased risk for hyperthermia due to inactive cooling responses. Drugs that increase muscle tone and metabolism or reduce heat loss will impair thermoregulation. Infants and small children who are left in a closed car for even short periods in hot weather are potential victims of hyperthermia.

5. Drugs can interfere with heat dissipation; they can alter temperature regulation by the hypothalamic centers, act as direct pyrogens, injure tissues directly, or induce an immune response.

6. Malnutrition decreases the fuel available for heat generation, and loss of body fat decreases tissue insulation. Alcohol and sedative drugs dull mental awareness to cold and impair judgment to seek shelter or put on additional clothing. Alcohol also inhibits shivering. Persons with cardiovascular disease, cerebrovascular disease, spinal cord injury, and hypothyroidism are also predisposed to hypothermia. Elderly and inactive persons living in inadequately heated quarters are particularly vulnerable to hypothermia.

7. *Passive external rewarming* is done by removing the person from the cold environment, covering with a blanket, supplying warm fluids, and allowing rewarming to occur at the person's own pace. *Active external rewarming* involves immersing the person in warm water, using forced air warming systems, or placing heating pads or hot water bottles on the surface of the body, including the extremities. *Active core rewarming* can be done by instilling warmed fluids into the gastrointestinal tract; peritoneal dialysis; extracorporeal blood warming, in which blood is removed from the body and passed through a heat exchanger and then returned to the body; or inhalation of an oxygen mixture warmed to 42°C to 46°C.

SECTION III: APPLYING YOUR KNOWLEDGE
Activity F

1. *Rationale:* When obtaining the history of the present illness, the nurse should inquire about the following:
   - Onset of illness
   - Any known exposure to infectious or communicable disease
   - Immunization history for pneumonia and flu
   - History of having pneumonia or flu
   - Fever
   - Sore throat
   - Lethargy
   - Malaise
   - Poor appetite
   - Vomiting
   - Diarrhea
   - Cough
   - Shortness of breath
   - Chest pain or joint pain
   - Smoking

2. *Rationale:* The nurse should perform the following physical examinations:
   - Measure temperature, respiratory rate, pulse, and blood pressure
   - Assess the mouth and throat for erythema or lesions
   - Auscultate the lungs and heart for any adventitious sounds
   - Percuss the lung fields to assess for tenderness
   - Observe the patient's affect and energy level
   - Observe whether there is any discharge from the nose, or a cough or respiratory difficulty
   - Assess O_2 saturation and capillary refill
   - Assess hydration status by inspecting oral mucosa and eyes
   - Palpate the skin to assess temperature, moisture, texture, and turgor

- Palpate the lymph nodes and note any that are swollen and tender
- Observe the teeth

SECTION IV: PRACTICING FOR NCLEX

Activity G

1. a. *Rationale:* Temperature-sensitive ion channels, identified as a subset of the transient receptor potential family (thermoTRPs) present in peripheral and central sensory neurons, are activated by innocuous (warm and cool) and noxious (hot and cold) stimuli. Strong and weak and unpleasant and pleasant are not types of stimuli that influence the regulation of body temperature. Hot and cold are considered noxious stimuli.

2. b. *Rationale:* Hyperthermia occurs when the set-point of the body is unchanged, but the mechanisms that control body temperature are ineffective in maintaining body temperature within a normal range during situations when heat production outpaces the ability of the body to dissipate that heat. A body temperature of either 37.6°C or 39.5°C is considered a fever, the same as when the set-point of the body is raised.

3. c. *Rationale:* Exogenous pyrogens, such as bacterial products, bacterial toxins, or whole microorganisms, induce host cells to produce fever-producing mediators called endogenous pyrogens. "Outer" and "set-point" pyrogens do not exist.

4. d. *Rationale:* A fever that has its origin in the central nervous system is sometimes referred to as a neurogenic fever. Neurogenic fevers are characterized by a high temperature that is resistant to antipyretic therapy and is not associated with sweating.
Temperatures that go up and down for no apparent reason and variable temperatures are not neurogenic fevers.

5. a. *Rationale:* The diving reflex triggers apnea and circulatory shunting to establish a heart-brain circulation. In children, the diving reflex along with the rapid cooling process may account for the surprisingly high survival rate after submersion. The diving reflex is greatly diminished in adults. The Moro reflex is a normal mass reflex in a young infant (up to 3 to 4 months of age) elicited by a sudden loud noise, consisting of flexion of the legs, an embracing posture of the arms, and usually a brief cry. The Bainbridge reflex is a cardiac reflex in which stimulation of stretch receptors in the wall of the left atrium causes an increased pulse rate. The oculocephalic reflex is a test of the integrity of brain stem function that involves moving the patient's head quickly and noting whether the eyes lag behind the head movement and then slowly assume the midline position.

6. b. *Rationale:* FUO is defined as a temperature elevation of 38.3°C (101°F) or higher that is present for 3 weeks or longer. Among the causes of FUO are malignancies (i.e., lymphomas, metastases to the liver and central nervous system); infections such as HIV or tuberculosis, or abscessed infections; and drug fever. Disseminated intravascular coagulation and pulmonary and femoral artery emboli do not cause FUO.

7. c. *Rationale:* Familial Mediterranean fever, an autosomal recessive disease, is characterized by an early age of onset (<20 years) of acute episodic bouts of peritonitis and high fever with an average duration of less than 2 days. In some cases, pleuritis, pericarditis, and arthritis are present.

8. d. *Rationale:* Aspirin can cause Reye syndrome in children; therefore, the Centers for Disease Control and Prevention, U.S. Food and Drug Administration, and American Academy of Pediatrics Committee on Infectious Diseases advise against the use of aspirin and other salicylates in children with influenza or chickenpox. Münchhausen syndrome is an unusual psychiatric condition characterized by habitual pleas for treatment and hospitalization for a symptomatic but imaginary acute illness. Guillain-Barré syndrome is an idiopathic, peripheral polyneuritis that occurs 1 to 3 weeks after a mild episode of fever associated with a viral infection or with immunization. Angelman syndrome is an autosomal recessive syndrome characterized by jerky puppetlike movements, frequent laughter, mental and motor retardation, a peculiar open-mouthed facial expression, and seizures.

9. a. *Rationale:* Infants with fever may not necessarily appear ill. In infants younger than 3 months, a mild elevation in temperature (i.e., rectal temperature of 38°C [100.4°F]) can

indicate serious infection that requires immediate medical attention. Signs of toxicity include lethargy, poor feeding, hypoventilation, poor tissue oxygenation, and cyanosis.

10. b. *Rationale:* Heat stroke is a severe, life-threatening failure of thermoregulatory mechanisms resulting in an excessive rise in body temperature—a core temperature greater than 40°C (104°F). The resulting local and systemic inflammatory responses may result in acute respiratory distress syndrome, acute renal failure, disseminated intravascular clotting, multiorgan dysfunction, and rhabdomyolysis. Hyperthermia is also known to cause edema and microhemorrhages in the brain. Rhabdomyoma is a tumor of striated muscle.

11. b, c, d. *Rationale:* Drugs can interfere with (not cause) heat dissipation; they can alter temperature regulation by the hypothalamic centers, act as direct pyrogens, injure tissues directly, or induce an immune response.

12. pilomotor. *Rationale:* Contraction of the pilomotor muscles of the skin aids in heat conservation by reducing the surface area available for heat loss.

13. d. *Rationale:* The physiologic behaviors that occur during the development of fever can be divided into four successive stages: a prodrome; a chill, during which the temperature rises; a flush; and defervescence.

14. a, b, c. *Rationale:* The methods of fever treatment focus on modifications of the external environment intended to increase heat transfer from the internal to the external environment, support of the hypermetabolic state that accompanies fever, protection of vulnerable body organs and systems, and treatment of the infection or condition causing the fever.

15. a, b, c, d. *Rationale:* Malignant hyperthermia is an autosomal dominant metabolic disorder in which heat generated by uncontrolled skeletal muscle contraction can produce severe and potentially fatal hyperthermia. The syndrome is most frequently associated with the halogenated anesthetic agents and the depolarizing muscle relaxant succinylcholine. There are also various nonoperative precipitating factors, including trauma, exercise, environmental heat stress, and infection. The condition is particularly dangerous in a young person who has a large muscle mass to generate heat.

CHAPTER 11 ACTIVITY TOLERANCE AND FATIGUE

SECTION II: ASSESSING YOUR UNDERSTANDING

Activity A

1. Physical activity
2. Aerobic
3. resistance
4. $\dot{V}O_2$max
5. cardiac output
6. Frank-Starling
7. Muscle strength
8. Fast-twitch
9. atrophy
10. creatine kinase
11. gastrointestinal tract
12. glutamine
13. stress-related
14. decline
15. intolerance
16. fatigue
17. Acute
18. bed rest
19. deep vein thrombosis
20. cardiac output, pneumonia, kidney stones

Activity B

1. j	2. g	3. e	4. b	5. c
6. a	7. f	8. d	9. i	10. h

Activity C

1. The physiologic and psychological benefits of exercise are cardiopulmonary fitness; increased muscle strength, flexibility, and endurance; availability of energy substrates to meet the increased energy demands imposed by increased physical activity; and motivation and mental endurance.

2. Increases in blood flow increase shear stress and result in several beneficial functions, such as the production of vasodilators, antioxidants, and anticoagulants. This contributes to improved endothelial cell function, which results in vasodilation, inhibition of platelet activation, and increased fibrinolysis, thus leading to improved patency of the vasculature and maintenance of blood flow and vessel patency. Adaptation to exercise also induces angiogenesis, with an increased growth of vessels to support blood flow to the exercising muscle.

3. In terms of skeletal muscle function, there is a decrease in muscle mass and strength, flexibility and range of joint movement, and

muscle endurance. There is a decrease in size of the individual muscles that occurs with aging, particularly beyond 60 years of age. Muscle strength and mass reportedly decline 30% to 50% between ages 30 and 80 years, with loss of muscle mass accounting for most of the decrease observed in muscle strength. Muscle mass loss is subordinate to an age-related denervation of type II fibers, which removes the trophic effect on the fibers, leading to atrophy. Type I fiber collaterals expand to some of the denervated type II fiber areas in an attempt to lessen muscle fiber loss. This leads to an increase in type I motor neuron units at the expense of type II fibers, resulting in a reduction in muscle mass and muscle strength.

4. Acute fatigue and chronic fatigue are the result of a decrease in the ability to generate muscle contractions. Acute fatigue is rapid in onset and resolves with rest. In contrast to acute fatigue, chronic fatigue has an insidious onset, is typically perceived as being unusually intense relative to the amount of activity performed, lasts longer than 1 month, has a cumulative effect, and is not relieved by cessation of activity.

5. The pathogenesis of CFS include infections, psychological disorders, a dysfunction in the hypothalamic-pituitary-adrenal axis, or an alteration in the autonomic nervous system. Despite much research and the development of several theories, the underlying pathophysiology of CFS remains elusive. Many people with CFS attribute the onset of their disease to an influenzalike infection. Symptoms are changing and variable among patients. As a result, there are no biologic markers for CFS.

6. The mechanism of orthostatic intolerance following bed rest involves multiple factors, including a decrease in vascular volume, a decline in skeletal muscle pump function, reduced sympathetic innervation of the resistance vessels, and resetting of the baroreceptors that control blood pressure.

SECTION III: APPLYING YOUR KNOWLEDGE
Activity D

1. A holistic approach should be taken when caring for persons who are immobile or require prolonged periods of bed rest. Interventions and treatment should include actions that

address the person's physical and psychosocial needs. The goals of care for the immobilized person include structuring a safe environment in which the person is not at risk for complications; providing diversional activities to offset problems with sensory deprivation; and preventing complications of bed rest by implementing an interdisciplinary plan of care that includes repositioning schedules, prophylactic interventions to prevent deep vein thrombosis, and consultation with various disciplines to provide a comprehensive approach to care and treatment.

2. The concerns of his caregiver are as follows:
   - Cardiovascular changes, including venous stasis, a redistribution of blood volume, and deep vein thrombosis
   - Water and sodium diuresis; the loss of water and sodium results in an increase in hematocrit, hemoglobin, and red cell mass owing to the loss of plasma volume
   - Postural intolerance
   - Changes in lung volumes and the mechanics of breathing that can contribute to respiratory complications, such as atelectasis, accumulation of secretions, hypoxemia, and pneumonia
   - Prolonged bed rest affects the renal system by altering the composition of body fluids and predisposing to the development of kidney stones; bed rest may also predispose to urinary tract infections and urinary incontinence because of positional changes and difficulty in emptying the bladder
   - Loss of strength; muscles atrophy, change shape and appearance, and shorten when immobilized
   - Metabolic and endocrine changes
   - Gastrointestinal responses, including loss of appetite, slowed rate of absorption, and distaste for food combine to contribute to nutritional hypoproteinemia
   - Pressure sores
   - Psychosocial changes, including depression and social isolation

SECTION IV: PRACTICING FOR NCLEX
Activity E

1. d. *Rationale:* Skeletal muscle consists of two distinct types of muscle fibers based on differences in their size, speed, contractile properties, endurance, and metabolic

characteristics: red (dark) slow-twitch (type I) and white (light) fast-twitch (type II) muscle fibers. Periods of sustained inactivity, such as prolonged immobility or bed rest, primarily affect slow-twitch fibers, which quickly decondition.

2. c. *Rationale:* Persons with congestive heart failure (CHF) typically experience symptoms of breathlessness, exertional fatigue, and exercise intolerance, resulting in atrophy of skeletal muscles. When these individuals engage in exercise, there is a shift toward using fast-twitch muscle fibers. This causes an early dependence on anaerobic metabolism and excessive intramuscular acidification that leads to increased fatigability. The increased reliance on anaerobic metabolism and subsequent vasoconstrictor response can also lead to an increase in afterload work for an already compromised left ventricle.

3. d. *Rationale:* Because of the effects of exercise training on vascular function and angiogenesis, it has been proposed as a mechanism for improving blood flow and decreasing exercise-related leg pain (claudication) in persons with peripheral vascular disease(PVD). The vastus lateralis is the large muscle on the lateral thigh. Weight training will strengthen this muscle, but is not recommended for people with PVD. Isometric exercise does not increase the endurance of the heart. Aerobic exercise does not decrease respiratory stress.

4. a. *Rationale:* With sufficient training, the body adapts by increasing the rate of sweat production. As temperature regulation improves with training, the trained person begins to sweat sooner, often within 1 to 2 minutes of the start of exercise. Sweat production begins even before the core temperature rises, and a cooling effect is initiated soon after the start of exercise; the sweat produced is more dilute than that produced by a nontrained person. Sweat normally contains large amounts of sodium chloride; production of a dilute sweat allows evaporative cooling to take place while sodium chloride is conserved.

5. b. *Rationale:* Maximal heart rate decreases 6 to 10 beats/minute/decade, and it is this decrease in heart rate that is believed to contribute to a decreased cardiac output. Although there is a natural decrease in lung capacity as a person ages, it does not contribute to decreased cardiac output. The resistance of major blood vessels does not

decrease cardiac output. There is a natural decrease in muscle strength in the elderly, not a decrease in the peripheral blood vessels. Even with a decrease in peripheral blood vessels, it would not cause a decreased cardiac output.

6. c. *Rationale:* This type of fatigue is common among persons with forced immobility, musculoskeletal disorders such as arthritis, neuromuscular disorders such as multiple sclerosis, and wasting syndromes such as HIV/AIDS.

7. d. *Rationale:* The deconditioning responses to the inactivity of immobility and bed rest affect all body systems. One of the important factors to keep in mind is the rapidity with which the changes occur and the length of time required to overcome these effects.

8. a. *Rationale:* Muscle atrophy and disuse not only contribute to wasting and weakening of muscle tissue, but also play a role in the development of joint contractures. A contracture is the abnormal shortening of muscle tissue and connective tissue, rendering the muscle highly resistant to stretch.

9. b. *Rationale:* To be classified as CFS, the fatigue must be clinically evaluated, cause severe mental and physical exhaustion, and result in a significant reduction in the individual's premorbid activity level. In addition, there must be evidence of the concurrent occurrence of four of the following symptoms: sore throat, tender cervical or axillary lymph nodes, muscle pain, multijoint pain without swelling or redness, headaches, unrefreshing sleep, and postexertional malaise lasting more than 24 hours. The fatigue and concurrent symptoms must be of 6 months' duration or longer.

10. c. *Rationale:* The immune system is also subject to physiologic changes associated with bed rest or immobility. Research demonstrates that there is an increase in interleukin (IL)-1, IL-6, and tumor necrosis factor-alpha production. An increase in these mediators has been associated with hyperinflammatory reactions and tissue injury or wasting.

11. resistance. *Rationale:* In isometric, or resistance, exercise, sustained muscle contraction is generated against an immovable load with no change in length of the involved muscle group or joint movement.

12. c. *Rationale:* The role of the respiratory system during exercise is to increase the rate of oxygen and carbon dioxide exchange. This takes place through a series of physiologic

responses. With exercise, the respiratory rate increases four- to fivefold, tidal volume increases five- to sevenfold, and minute ventilation (respiratory rate × tidal volume) increases up to 20 to 30 times its resting value. With the increase in cardiac output, a greater volume of blood under slightly increased pressure is delivered to the pulmonary vessels in the lungs. This results in the opening of more pulmonary capillary beds, producing better alveolar perfusion and more efficient exchange of oxygen and carbon dioxide.

13. ergometry. *Rationale:* Ergometry is a procedure for determining physical performance capacity.

14. a, b, c, e. *Rationale:* After a period of bed rest and assumption of the supine position, the cardiovascular system exhibits changes that reflect the loss of gravitational and exercise stimuli. These changes include (a) a redistribution and change in blood volume, (b) increased cardiac workload, (c) orthostatic hypotension, and (d) venous stasis with the potential for development of deep venous thrombosis.

15. Wolff's. *Rationale:* According to Wolff's law, the density of bone is directly proportional to the stress placed on it.

CHAPTER 12 BLOOD CELLS AND THE HEMATOPOIETIC SYSTEM

SECTION II: ASSESSING YOUR UNDERSTANDING

Activity A

1. hematocrit
2. 90%, 6.5%, 2%
3. liver
4. Albumin
5. cells
6. hemoglobin
7. Carbonic anhydrase
8. granulocytes
9. Neutrophils
10. eosinophils
11. immune
12. thymus
13. monocytes, macrophages
14. megakaryocytes
15. constant

Activity B

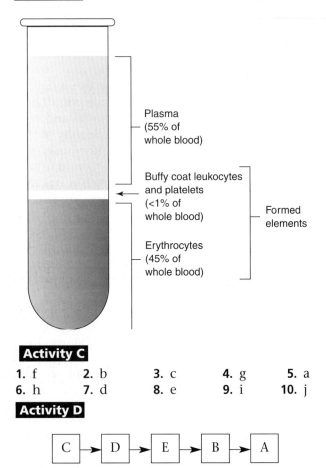

Plasma (55% of whole blood)

Buffy coat leukocytes and platelets (<1% of whole blood)

Formed elements

Erythrocytes (45% of whole blood)

Activity C

| 1. f | 2. b | 3. c | 4. g | 5. a |
| 6. h | 7. d | 8. e | 9. i | 10. j |

Activity D

C → D → E → B → A

Activity E

1. The lifelong potential for proliferation and self-renewal of stem cells makes them an indispensable and lifesaving source of reserve cells for the entire hematopoietic system. Several levels of differentiation lead to the development of committed unipotential cells, which are the progenitors for each blood cell type. They serve as an unending reserve of cells.

2. When a person trains at high elevations, the partial pressure of O_2 is low, resulting in systemic hypoxia. The body responds by releasing erythropoietin, which stimulates red blood cell production. After some time, the body will return to normal oxygenation. When the person then returns to lower elevations to race or train, the body has a greater oxygen-carrying capacity and can perform at a higher level.

SECTION III: APPLYING YOUR KNOWLEDGE

Activity F

1. The nurse can tell Sally that growth factors help make her new bone marrow grow faster. The rationale behind this answer is that growth factors are used to increase peripheral stem cells for transplantation and to accelerate cell proliferation after bone marrow engraftment.

SECTION IV: PRACTICING FOR NCLEX

Activity G

1. a. *Rationale:* There are three types of globulins: the alpha globulins that transport bilirubin and steroids, the beta globulins that transport iron and copper, and the gamma globulins that constitute the antibodies of the immune system. Alpha globulins transport bilirubin and steroids. Beta globulins transport iron and copper. Autoantibodies are immunoglobulins that recognize an antigen on that person's own tissue.

2. b. *Rationale:* The erythrocytes, or red blood cells, are the most numerous of the formed elements. They are small, biconcave disks with a large surface area and can easily deform to move through the small capillaries of the circulatory system. They contain the oxygen-carrying protein, hemoglobin, which functions in the transport of oxygen. The neutrophils are primarily responsible for maintaining normal host defenses against invading bacteria and fungi, cell debris, and a variety of foreign substances. Eosinophils constitute 1% to 3% of the total number of white blood cells and increase in number during allergic reactions and parasitic infections. In allergic reactions, it is believed that they release enzymes or chemical mediators that detoxify the agents associated with allergic reactions. In parasitic infections, the eosinophils use surface markers to attach themselves to the parasite and then release hydrolytic enzymes that kill it. The leukocytes, or white blood cells, constitute only 1% of the total blood volume. They originate in the bone marrow and circulate throughout the lymphoid tissues of the body. Leukocytes are crucial to our defense against disease. They are responsible for the immune response that protects against disease-causing microorganisms; they identify and destroy cancer cells, and they participate in the inflammatory response and wound healing.

3. c. *Rationale:* Pluripotent stem cells with their lifelong potential for proliferation and self-renewal are an indispensable and lifesaving source of reserve cells for the entire hematopoietic system. Several levels of differentiation lead to the development of committed unipotential cells, which are the progenitors for each blood cell type. These cells are referred to as colony-forming units.

4. d. *Rationale:* Sources of the stem cells include bone marrow, peripheral blood, and umbilical cord blood. All replenish the recipient with a normal population of pluripotent stem cells. Immature embryonic cells do not necessarily contain stem cells. Immature neural cells are not stem cells. Yellow bone marrow does not make blood cells, so it would not contain stem cells.

5. a. *Rationale:* Cytokines, such as the interleukins, interferons, and tumor necrosis factor, support the proliferation of stem cells and the development of lymphocytes, and act synergistically to aid the multiple functions of the colony-stimulating factors. B-cell growth factor, T-cell growth factor, colony-stimulating factors, and transforming growth factor are all cytokines that stimulate the growth and production of new blood cells.

6. b. *Rationale:* The erythrocyte sedimentation rate is a screening test for monitoring the fluctuations in the clinical course of a disease. In anticoagulated blood, red blood cells aggregate and sediment to the bottom of a tube. The rate of fall of the aggregates is accelerated in the presence of fibrinogen and other plasma proteins that are often increased in inflammatory diseases.

7. c. *Rationale:* Usually, the posterior iliac crest is used in all persons older than 12 to 18 months of age. Other sites include the anterior iliac crest, sternum, and spinous processes T10 through L4. The sternum is not commonly used in children because the cavity is too shallow, and there is danger of mediastinal and cardiac perforation.

8. d. *Rationale:* Under normal conditions, the numbers and total mass for each type of circulating blood cell remain relatively constant. The blood cells are produced in different numbers according to needs and regulatory factors. This regulation of blood cells is believed to be at least partially controlled by hormonelike growth factors called

cytokines. The immune system does not regulate the number of each type of blood cell. The hematopoietic system is the system in which the blood cells are made, but it does not regulate the number of each type of cell. Pluripotent stem cells are the precursors to every type of cell.

9. a. *Rationale:* Peripheral blood stem cells are harvested from the blood after the administration of a cytokine growth factor that increases the quantity and migration of the cells from the bone marrow. HLA is the abbreviation for human leukocyte antigen and is what is matched in umbilical cord blood. It does not increase either the quantity or the migration of peripheral blood stem cells. Platelets are a rich source of growth factors, but they do not, by themselves, increase either the quantity or the migration of peripheral blood stem cells. There is a human growth hormone but not a human growth factor.

10. b. *Rationale:* The genes for most hematopoietic growth factors have been cloned, and their recombinant proteins have been generated for use in a wide range of clinical problems. They are used to treat bone marrow failure caused by chemotherapy or aplastic anemia, the anemia of kidney failure and cancer, hematopoietic neoplasms, infectious diseases such as AIDS, and congenital and myeloproliferative disorders. Autoimmune disorders, Parkinson disease, and Huntington disease are not anemic disorders, so the recombinant proteins have not been used in the treatment of these diseases.

11. heat. *Rationale:* Because water has a high capacity to hold heat, plasma can absorb and distribute much of the heat that is generated in the body.

12.

Protein	Percent	Purpose
Albumin	54	Contributes to the plasma osmotic pressure and maintenance of blood volume; buffer
Globulins	38	Transporters and antibodies
Fibrinogen	7	Key factor in blood clotting

Rationale: Albumin is the most abundant and comprises approximately 54% of the plasma proteins. It does not pass through the pores in the capillary wall to enter the interstitial fluid, and, therefore, contributes to the plasma osmotic pressure and maintenance of blood volume. Albumin also serves as a carrier for certain substances and acts as a blood buffer. The globulins comprise approximately 38% of plasma proteins. There are three types of globulins: the *alpha globulins* that transport bilirubin and steroids, the *beta globulins* that transport iron and copper, and the *gamma globulins* that constitute the antibodies of the immune system. Fibrinogen comprises approximately 7% of the plasma proteins and is a key factor in blood clotting. The remaining 1% of the circulating proteins is comprised of hormones, enzymes, complement, and carriers for lipids.

13.

Abbreviation	Definition
Hgb	Measurement of hemoglobin
Hct	Measurement of hematocrit
MCV	Mean corpuscular volume
MCHC	Mean corpuscular hemoglobin concentration
MCH	Mean cell hemoglobin

Rationale: Measurement of hemoglobin, hematocrit, mean corpuscular volume (MCV), mean corpuscular hemoglobin concentration (MCHC), and mean cell hemoglobin (MCH) is usually included in the CBC.

14. a, b. *Rationale:* Blood is made up of plasma, plasma proteins, fixed elements or blood cells, and substances such as hormones, enzymes, electrolytes, and byproducts of cellular waste. Ascites is an accumulation of intraperitoneal fluid containing large amounts of protein and electrolytes. Bile is a secretion of the liver that is stored in the gallbladder.

15. a, c, d. *Rationale:* Bone marrow and peripheral blood transplants may be derived from the patient (autologous) or from a histocompatible donor (allogeneic). A heterologous donor has incompatible tissue types.

CHAPTER 13 DISORDERS OF HEMOSTASIS

SECTION II: ASSESSING YOUR UNDERSTANDING

Activity A

1. hemostasis
2. nucleus
3. actin, myosin
4. growth factors
5. ADP, TXA$_2$
6. coagulation cascade
7. liver
8. disseminated intravascular coagulation
9. Hypercoagulability
10. Smoking
11. thrombocytosis
12. protein C
13. coagulation
14. Bleeding
15. thrombocytopenia
16. Platelet
17. Immune
18. Thrombocytopathia
19. X-linked
20. clotting factors
21. scurvy
22. disseminated intravascular coagulation

Activity B

1.

2.

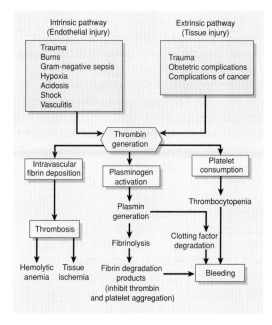

Activity C

1. c	2. g	3. i	4. e	5. a
6. f	7. j	8. h	9. d	10. b

Activity D

Activity E

1. The five stages of hemostasis are (a) vessel spasm, which constricts the vessel and reduces blood flow; (b) formation of the platelet plug, which initiates platelet contact with subendothelial tissue; c) blood coagulation via fibrin polymerization; (d) clot retraction in order to squeeze out serum; and (e) clot dissolution by fibrinolysis by plasminogen.
2. Platelets are attracted to a damaged vessel wall, become activated, and change from smooth disks to spiny spheres, exposing glycoprotein receptors on their surfaces. Platelet adhesion requires a protein molecule called von Willebrand factor, which is produced by the endothelial cells of blood vessels and circulates in the blood as a carrier protein for coagulation factor VIII. Adhesion to the vessel subendothelial layer occurs when the platelet

receptor binds to von Willebrand factor at the injury site, linking the platelet to exposed collagen fibers.

3. The intrinsic pathway, which is a relatively slow process, begins in the circulation with the activation of factor XII, which is activated as blood comes in contact with collagen in the injured vessel wall. The extrinsic pathway, which is a much faster process, begins with trauma to the blood vessel or surrounding tissues and the release of tissue factor, an adhesive lipoprotein released from the subendothelial cells. The terminal steps in both pathways are the same: the activation of factor X and the conversion of prothrombin to thrombin.

4. These drugs act as haptens and induce antigen-antibody response and formation of immune complexes that cause platelet destruction by complement-mediated lysis. In persons with drug-associated thrombocytopenia, there is a rapid fall in the platelet count within 2 to 3 days of resuming a drug or 7 or more days (i.e., the time needed to mount an immune response) after starting a drug for the first time.

5. Activation through the extrinsic pathway occurs with liberation of tissue factors, associated with obstetric complications, trauma, bacterial sepsis, and cancers. The intrinsic pathway may be activated through extensive endothelial damage with activation of factor XII. Disseminated intravascular coagulation begins with massive activation of the coagulation sequence as a result of unregulated generation of thrombin, resulting in systemic formation of fibrin. In addition, levels of all major anticoagulants are reduced. The microthrombi that result cause vessel occlusion and tissue ischemia. Multiple organ failure may ensue. Clot formation consumes all available coagulation proteins and platelets, and severe hemorrhage results.

SECTION III: APPLYING YOUR KNOWLEDGE
Activity F

1. Prevent bleeding and make the environment as safe as possible.
2. When teaching families and clients about hemophilia, the nurse would include information on
   - Measures for controlling bleeding.
   - Limiting local joint damage.

- Ways to be active without injuring themselves.
- How to cope with the disorder.
- Referrals to a genetic counselor.
- Local support groups.

The nurse also provides home care.

SECTION IV: PRACTICING FOR NCLEX
Activity G

1. a. *Rationale:* Platelet adhesion requires a protein molecule called von Willebrand factor. This factor is produced by the endothelial cells of blood vessels and circulates in the blood as a carrier protein for coagulation factor VIII. The release of growth factors results in the proliferation and growth of vascular endothelial cells, smooth muscle cells, and fibroblasts, and is important in vessel repair. Ionized calcium contributes to vasoconstriction. Platelet factor 4 is a heparin-binding chemokine.

2. b. *Rationale:* The coagulation process results from the activation of what has traditionally been designated the intrinsic or the extrinsic pathways. The intrinsic pathway, which is a relatively slow process, begins in the circulation with the activation of factor XII. The extrinsic pathway, which is a much faster process, begins with trauma to the blood vessel or surrounding tissues and the release of tissue factor, an adhesive lipoprotein released from the subendothelial cells. The terminal steps in both pathways are the same: the activation of factor X and the conversion of prothrombin to thrombin. All other answers do not exist in the formation of clots.

3. a. *Rationale:* The anticoagulant drugs warfarin and heparin are used to prevent thromboembolic disorders, such as deep vein thrombosis and pulmonary embolism. Warfarin acts by decreasing prothrombin and other procoagulation factors. It alters vitamin K in a manner that reduces its ability to participate in synthesis of the vitamin K–dependent coagulation factors in the liver.

4. b. *Rationale:* Heparin binds to antithrombin III, causing a conformational change that increases the ability of antithrombin III to inactivate thrombin, factor Xa, and other clotting factors. By promoting the inactivation of clotting factors, heparin ultimately suppresses the formation of fibrin. Heparin does not bind to factors X and Xa. Heparin does not inactivate factor VIII.

5. b. *Rationale:* Platelets, through the action of their actin and myosin filaments, also contribute to clot retraction. Clot retraction therefore requires large numbers of platelets, and failure of clot retraction is indicative of a low platelet count. Factor Xa is necessary factor in blood coagulation. It does not cause failure of clot retraction.

6. c. *Rationale:* The common underlying causes of secondary thrombocytosis include tissue damage due to surgery, infection, cancer, and chronic inflammatory conditions such as rheumatoid arthritis and Crohn disease. Lyme disease, caused by a tick bite, does not cause thrombocytosis. Hirschsprung disease and megacolon are the same thing, and they are not inflammatory conditions.

7. a. *Rationale:* A reduction in platelet number, also referred to as *thrombocytopenia*, is an important cause of generalized bleeding. Thrombocytopenia usually refers to a decrease in the number of circulating platelets to a level less than 100,000/μL. The greater the decrease in the platelet count, the greater the risk of bleeding. Thrombocytopenia can result from a decrease in platelet production, increased sequestration of platelets in the spleen, or decreased platelet survival.

8. b. *Rationale:* Hemophilia A is an X-linked recessive disorder that primarily affects males. Approximately 90% of persons with hemophilia produce insufficient quantities of factor VIII. The prevention of trauma is important in persons with hemophilia.

9. c. *Rationale:* In persons with bleeding disorders caused by vascular defects, the platelet count and results of other tests for coagulation factors are normal. A shift to the left indicates an infectious or inflammatory process, not a clotting disorder. A lack of iron indicates iron-deficiency anemia, not a clotting disorder. A normal hematocrit indicates a normal number of packed red blood cells, not a clotting disorder.

10. a. *Rationale:* Disseminated intravascular coagulation is a paradox in the hemostatic sequence and is characterized by widespread coagulation and bleeding in the vascular compartment. It is not a primary disease but occurs as a complication of a wide variety of conditions, including disease or injury such as septicemia, acute hypotension, poisonous snakebites, neoplasms, obstetric emergencies, severe trauma, extensive surgery, and hemorrhage.

11. c. *Rationale:* Hemostasis is divided into five stages: (a) vessel spasm, (b) formation of the platelet plug, (c) blood coagulation or development of an insoluble fibrin clot, (d) clot retraction, and (e) clot dissolution.

12. intravascular

13. Heparin

14. a, b, c, e. *Rationale:* Platelets that adhere to the vessel wall release growth factors that cause proliferation of smooth muscle and thereby contribute to the development of atherosclerosis. Smoking, elevated levels of blood lipids and cholesterol, hemodynamic stress, diabetes mellitus, and immune mechanisms may cause vessel damage, platelet adherence, and, eventually, thrombosis.

15. a, c, e. *Rationale:* In disseminated intravascular coagulation, microemboli may obstruct blood vessels and cause tissue hypoxia and necrotic damage to organ structures, such as the kidneys, heart, lungs, and brain. As a result, common clinical signs may be due to renal, circulatory, or respiratory failure; acute bleeding ulcers; or convulsions and coma. A form of hemolytic anemia may develop when red blood cells are damaged as they pass through vessels partially blocked by thrombus.

CHAPTER 14 DISORDERS OF RED BLOOD CELLS

SECTION II: ASSESSING YOUR UNDERSTANDING

Activity A

1. biconcave, cell membrane
2. iron
3. nucleus
4. 4
5. glycolytic
6. methemoglobin
7. red blood cell count
8. hematocrit
9. mean corpuscular hemoglobin concentration
10. Anemia
11. hypoxia
12. Hemolytic
13. sickle cell, thalassemias
14. Spherocytosis
15. β-thalassemias, α-thalassemias
16. G6PD
17. Iron-deficiency
18. chronic blood loss
19. Megaloblastic

20. Pernicious
21. Aplastic anemia
22. Polycythemia
23. oxygen
24. conjugate
25. anemia

Activity B

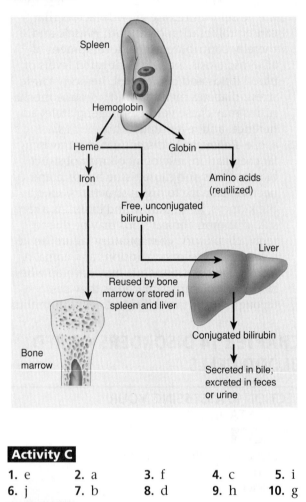

Activity C

| 1. e | 2. a | 3. f | 4. c | 5. i |
| 6. j | 7. b | 8. d | 9. h | 10. g |

Activity D

1. The hemoglobin molecule is composed of two pairs of structurally different α and β polypeptide chains. Each polypeptide chain consists of a globin (protein) portion and heme unit, which surrounds an atom of iron that binds oxygen. Thus, each molecule of hemoglobin can carry four molecules of oxygen. The binding that occurs is cooperative, or allosteric. When one oxygen molecule binds, it makes it easier for the next to bind. The process also works in reverse.

2. A group of large phagocytic cells found in the spleen, liver, bone marrow, and lymph nodes facilitates the destruction of red blood cells (RBCs). These phagocytic cells recognize old and defective RBCs, and then ingest and destroy them in a series of enzymatic reactions. During these reactions, the amino acids from the globulin chains and iron from the heme units are salvaged and reused. The bulk of the heme unit is converted to bilirubin, which is insoluble in plasma and attaches to plasma proteins for transport. Bilirubin is removed from the blood by the liver and conjugated with glucuronide to render it water soluble so that it can be excreted in the bile.

3. The three categories of anemic effects are (a) manifestations of impaired oxygen transport and the resulting compensatory mechanisms, (b) reduction in red blood cell indices and hemoglobin levels, and (c) signs and symptoms associated with the pathologic process that is causing the anemia.

4. Premature destruction of the cells due to the rigid nondeformable membrane occurs in the spleen, causing hemolysis and anemia due to a decrease in red blood cell numbers. Vessel occlusion, a complex process involving an interaction among the sickle cells, endothelial cells, leukocytes, platelets, and other plasma proteins, will interrupt blood flow. The adherence of sickle cells to the vessel endothelium causes endothelial activation with liberation of inflammatory mediators and substances that increase platelet activation and promote blood coagulation.

5. Exposure to high doses of radiation, chemicals, and toxins that suppress cellular activity directly or through immune mechanisms are the standard cancer treatments. Chemotherapy and irradiation commonly result in bone marrow depression, which causes anemia, thrombocytopenia, and neutropenia. Identified toxic agents, including benzene, the antibiotic chloramphenicol, and the alkylating agents and antimetabolites used in the treatment of cancer, will decrease bone marrow of stem cells, thus affecting the production of red blood cells.

6. Viscosity rises exponentially with the hematocrit and interferes with cardiac output and blood flow. Hypertension is common, and there may be complaints of headache, dizziness, inability to concentrate, and some difficulty with hearing and vision because of decreased cerebral blood flow. Venous stasis gives rise to a plethoric appearance or dusky redness, even cyanosis, particularly of the lips, fingernails, and mucous membranes. Because of the increased concentration of blood cells,

the person may experience itching and pain in the fingers or toes, and the hypermetabolism may induce night sweats and weight loss.

7. Hyperbilirubinemia in the neonate is treated with phototherapy or exchange transfusion. Phototherapy is more commonly used to treat jaundiced infants and reduce the risk of kernicterus. Exposure to fluorescent light in the blue range of the visible spectrum (420- to 470-nm wavelength) reduces bilirubin levels. Bilirubin in the skin absorbs the light energy and is converted to a structural isomer that is more water soluble and can be excreted in the stool and urine. Hyperbilirubinemia in the neonate is treated with phototherapy or exchange transfusion. Phototherapy is more commonly used to treat jaundiced infants and reduce the risk of kernicterus. Exposure to fluorescent light in the blue range of the visible spectrum (420- to 470-nm wavelength) reduces bilirubin levels. Bilirubin in the skin absorbs the light energy and is converted to a structural isomer that is more water soluble and can be excreted in the stool and urine.

SECTION III: APPLYING YOUR KNOWLEDGE

Activity E

1. During a blood transfusion, the nurse and Mrs. McFee will watch for the following symptoms:
   - Sensation of heat along the vein while the transfusion is going in
   - Urticaria
   - Headache
   - Pain in the low back
   - Chills
   - Fever
   - Chest pain
   - Abdominal cramps
   - Nausea
   - Vomiting
   - Tachycardia
   - Hypotension
   - Dyspnea

   The most feared and lethal transfusion reaction is the destruction of donor red blood cells by reaction with antibody in the recipient's serum. This immediate hemolytic reaction is usually caused by ABO incompatibility.
2. Most transfusion reactions result from administrative errors or misidentification, and care should be taken to correctly identify the recipient and the transfusion source.

SECTION IV: PRACTICING FOR NCLEX

Activity F

1. a. *Rationale:* When red blood cells (RBCs) age and are destroyed in the spleen, the iron from their hemoglobin is released into the circulation and returned to the bone marrow for incorporation into new RBCs or to the liver and other tissues for storage. Iron is not bound to RBCs in the liver. Iron does not bind with oxygen in the lung without first being incorporated into an RBC. Iron is stored in tissues of the body, but not for strength, only for its oxygen-binding capacity.

2. d. *Rationale:* The plasma-insoluble form of bilirubin is referred to as unconjugated bilirubin, and the water-soluble form as conjugated bilirubin. Serum levels of conjugated and unconjugated bilirubin can be measured in the laboratory and are reported as direct and indirect, respectively.

3. a. *Rationale:* Hyperbilirubinemia, an increased level of serum bilirubin, is a common cause of jaundice in the neonate. A benign, self-limited condition, it is most often related to the developmental state of the neonate. Rarely, cases of hyperbilirubinemia are pathologic and may lead to kernicterus and serious brain damage.

4. b. *Rationale:* It takes about 5 days for the progeny of stem cells to fully differentiate, an event marked by increased reticulocytes in the blood. If the bleeding is controlled and sufficient, iron stores are available. The red blood cell concentration returns to normal within 3 to 4 weeks.

5. c. *Rationale:* Chronic blood loss does not affect blood volume, but instead leads to iron-deficiency anemia when iron stores are depleted. It is commonly caused by gastrointestinal bleeding and menstrual disorders. Because of compensatory mechanisms, patients are commonly asymptomatic until the hemoglobin level is less than 8 g/dL. The red blood cells (RBCs) that are produced have too little hemoglobin, giving rise to microcytic hypochromic anemia. Macrocytic anemia is when the RBCs are larger than normal. Hyperchromic means the cells are a darker color red then they should be.

6. d. *Rationale:* Hemolytic anemia is characterized by the premature destruction of red blood cells (RBCs), the retention in the body of iron and the other products of hemoglobin

destruction, and an increase in erythro-poiesis. Almost all types of hemolytic anemia are distinguished by normocytic and normochromic RBCs.

7. d. *Rationale:* In hemolytic anemia, intravascular hemolysis is less common than extravascular hemolysis and occurs as a result of complement fixation in transfusion reactions, mechanical injury, or toxic factors. It is characterized by hemoglobinemia, hemoglobinuria, jaundice, and hemosiderinuria. Spherocytosis is the most common inherited disorder of the red blood cell membrane and is not associated with hemolytic anemia.

8. b. *Rationale:* Therapy for aplastic anemia in the young and severely affected includes stem cell replacement by bone marrow or peripheral blood transplantation. Histocompatible donors supply the stem cells to replace the patient's destroyed marrow cells. A liver transplant will not produce new blood cells for the body. Spleen transplants are not done and would not produce new blood cells for the body.

9. a. *Rationale:* Chronic renal failure almost always results in anemia, primarily because of a deficiency of erythropoietin. Unidentified uremic toxins and retained nitrogen also interfere with the actions of erythropoietin, and red blood cell production and survival. Hemolysis and blood loss associated with hemodialysis and bleeding tendencies also contribute to the anemia of renal failure. Fibrinogen is essential for blood clotting, not oxygen transportation.

10. c. *Rationale:* Erythroblastosis fetalis, or hemolytic disease of the newborn, occurs in Rh-positive infants of Rh-negative mothers who have been sensitized. The Rh-negative mother usually becomes sensitized during the first few days after delivery, when fetal Rh-positive red blood cells from the placental site are released into the maternal circulation. Because the antibodies take several weeks to develop, the first Rh-positive infant of an Rh-negative mother is usually not affected. There is no such thing as microcytic or macrocytic disease of the newborn, or is there a hemolytic iron-deficiency anemia.

11. vitamin B_{12}. *Rationale:* Pernicious anemia is believed to result from immunologically mediated, possibly autoimmune, destruction of the gastric mucosa. The resultant chronic atrophic gastritis is marked by loss of parietal cells and production of antibodies that interfere with binding of vitamin B_{12} to intrinsic factor.

12. a, b, d. *Rationale:* Factors associated with sickling and vessel occlusion include cold, stress, physical exertion, infection, and illnesses that cause hypoxia, dehydration, or acidosis.

13. 1-c, 2-a, 3-b. *Rationale:* Red blood cell (RBC) indices are used to differentiate types of anemias by size or color of RBCs. The mean corpuscular volume (MCV) reflects the volume or size of the RBCs. The MCV falls in microcytic (small cell) anemia and rises in macrocytic (large cell) anemia. Some anemias are normocytic (i.e., cells are of normal size or MCV). The *mean* corpuscular hemoglobin concentration is the concentration of hemoglobin in each cell.

14. a, b. *Rationale:* In anemia, the oxygen-carrying capacity of hemoglobin is reduced, causing tissue hypoxia. Tissue hypoxia can give rise to fatigue, weakness, dyspnea, and sometimes angina. Hypoxia of brain tissue results in headache, faintness, and dim vision. The redistribution of the blood from cutaneous tissues or a lack of hemoglobin causes pallor of the skin, mucous membranes, conjunctiva, and nail beds. Tachycardia and palpitations may occur as the body tries to compensate with an increase in cardiac output Ruddy skin and bradycardia are not signs or symptoms of anemia.

15. a, b, e. *Rationale:* Primary polycythemia, or polycythemia vera, is a neoplastic disease of the pluripotent cells of the bone marrow characterized by an absolute increase in total red blood cell mass accompanied by elevated white blood cell and platelet counts. It is most commonly seen in men with a median age of 62 years, but may occur at any age. In addition, early findings include splenomegaly and depletion of iron stores. Hypertension is common, and there may be complaints of headache, dizziness, inability to concentrate, and some difficulty with hearing and vision because of decreased cerebral blood flow. Venous stasis gives rise to a plethoric appearance or dusky redness, even cyanosis, particularly of the lips, fingernails, and mucous membranes.

16. transfusion. *Rationale:* Persons who are homozygous for the trait (thalassemia major) have severe, transfusion-dependent anemia that is evident at 6 to 9 months of age when the hemoglobin switches from HbF to HbA. If transfusion therapy is not started early in life, severe growth retardation occurs in children with the disorder.

CHAPTER 15 DISORDERS OF WHITE BLOOD CELLS AND LYMPHOID TISSUES

SECTION II: ASSESSING YOUR UNDERSTANDING

Activity A

1. granulocytes
2. thymus
3. plasma
4. natural killer
5. myeloid, lymphoid
6. thymus, spleen
7. CD4$^+$, CD8$^+$
8. aplastic
9. alloantibodies
10. neutropenia
11. Infectious mononucleosis
12. Leukemias
13. Lymphomas
14. B-
15. nodular, lymphocyte
16. Hodgkin lymphoma
17. leukemias
18. lymphocytic
19. leukemia
20. Acute leukemias
21. lymphocytic, monocytic
22. Chronic leukemias
23. B lymphocytes
24. lymphocytosis
25. Philadelphia
26. Plasma cell dyscrasias
27. bone
28. M protein

Activity B

1. e	2. d	3. b	4. a	5. f
6. h	7. i	8. c	9. g	10. j

Activity C

1. Neutrophils migrate to sites of infection, where they engulf, digest, and destroy microorganisms. Thus, a decrease in the number of neutrophils places a person at risk for infection. The risk for and severity of neutropenia-associated infection are directly proportional to the absolute neutrophil count and duration of the neutropenia (defined as a circulating neutrophil count of less than 1500 /mL)
2. The Epstein-Barr virus (EBV) initially penetrates the nasopharyngeal, oropharyngeal, and salivary epithelial cells. It then spreads to the underlying oropharyngeal lymphoid tissue, and, more specifically, to B lymphocytes, all of which have receptors for EBV. Infection of the B cells may take one of two forms—it may kill the infected B cell, or it may become incorporated into its genome. The B cells that harbor the EBV genome proliferate in the circulation and produce the well-known heterophil antibodies that are used for the diagnosis of infectious mononucleosis. The resultant destruction of B cells and production of large T cells result in enlarged lymph nodes, particularly in the cervical, axillary, and groin areas. Hepatitis and splenomegaly are common manifestations of the disease and are believed to be immune mediated.
3. The manifestations of non-Hodgkin lymphoma depend on lymphoma type and the stage of the disease. Persons with indolent or slow-growing lymphomas usually present with painless lymphadenopathy due to increased cell filtering, which may be isolated or widespread. The indolent lymphomas are usually disseminated at the time of diagnosis, and bone marrow involvement is frequent. Many low-grade lymphomas eventually transform into more aggressive forms of lymphoma/leukemia. Persons with intermediate or more aggressive forms of lymphoma usually present with symptoms such as fever, drenching night sweats, or weight loss. Frequently, there is increased susceptibility to bacterial, viral, and fungal infections, as well as a poor humoral antibody response.
4. First, it usually arises in a single node or chain of nodes, whereas non-Hodgkin lymphoma frequently originates at extranodal sites and spreads to anatomically contiguous nodes. Second, Hodgkin lymphoma is characterized by the presence of large, atypical, mononuclear tumor cells called Reed-Sternberg cells. The cells, which frequently constitute less than 1% of the total cell population, are a diagnostic hallmark of the disease.
5. The incidence of leukemia among persons who have been exposed to high levels of radiation is unusually high. An increased incidence of leukemia is also associated with exposure to benzene and the use of antitumor drugs. Leukemia may occur as a second cancer after aggressive chemotherapy for other cancers. The existence of a genetic predisposition to develop acute leukemia is suggested by the increased leukemia incidence among a number of congenital disorders. In individuals with

Down syndrome, the incidence of acute leukemia is ten times that of the general population. Also, there are numerous reports of multiple cases of acute leukemia occurring within the same family.

6. Both are characterized by an abrupt onset of symptoms, including fatigue resulting from anemia; low-grade fever, night sweats, and weight loss due to the rapid proliferation and hypermetabolism of the leukemic cells; bleeding because of a decreased platelet count; and bone pain and tenderness due to bone marrow expansion. Infection results from neutropenia. Generalized lymphadenopathy, splenomegaly, and hepatomegaly caused by infiltration of leukemic cells occur in all acute leukemias but are more common in acute lymphocytic leukemia (ALL). In addition to the common manifestations of acute leukemia, infiltration of malignant cells in the skin, gums, and other soft tissue is particularly common in the monocytic form of acute myelogenous leukemia (AML). The leukemic cells may also cross the blood-brain barrier and establish sanctuary in the central nervous system (CNS). CNS involvement is more common in ALL than AML and is more common in children than adults. Signs and symptoms of CNS involvement include cranial nerve palsies, headache, nausea, vomiting, papilledema, and, occasionally, seizures and coma. Leukostasis and blood clotting are seen in severe cases.

7. The early chronic stage is marked by leukocytosis, anemia, and thrombocytopenia. Splenomegaly and hepatomegaly are often present. The accelerated phase of chronic myelogenous leukemia (CML) is characterized by enlargement of the spleen, resulting in a feeling of abdominal fullness and discomfort. An increase in basophil count and more immature cells in the blood or bone marrow confirm transformation to the accelerated phase. Symptoms such as low-grade fever, night sweats, bone pain, and weight loss develop because of rapid proliferation and hypermetabolism of the leukemic cells. Bleeding and easy bruising may arise from dysfunctional platelets. The terminal blast crisis phase of CML represents evolution to acute leukemia and is characterized by an increasing number of myeloid precursors, especially blast cells, in the blood. Constitutional symptoms become more pro-

nounced during this period, and splenomegaly may increase significantly. Isolated infiltrates of leukemic cells can involve the skin, lymph nodes, bones, and central nervous system.

8. The cause of multiple myeloma is unknown. Risk factors are believed to include chronic immune stimulation, autoimmune disorders, exposure to ionizing radiation, and occupational exposure to pesticides or herbicides. Myeloma has been associated with exposure to Agent Orange during the Vietnam War. A number of viruses have been associated with the pathogenesis of myeloma. There is a 4.5-fold increase in the likelihood of developing myeloma for persons with HIV.

SECTION III: APPLYING YOUR KNOWLEDGE
Activity D

1. The causes of leukemia are really unknown. We do know that the event or events causing the leukemias exert their effects through disruption or dysregulation of genes that normally regulate blood cell development, blood cell stability, or both.

2. Treatment of acute lymphocytic leukemia consists of a number of chemotherapeutic agents designed to achieve remission followed by high doses of chemotherapy given to patients who have achieved remission with their induction therapy. This part of Lucy's treatment is designed to reduce the number of cancer cells in her body even more once remission has been achieved. Then, in an attempt to cure her, she will receive lower doses of chemotherapy over a long period of time.

SECTION IV: PRACTICING FOR NCLEX
Activity E

1. a. *Rationale:* A small population of cells called pluripotent stem cells are capable of providing progenitor cells, or parent cells, for myelopoiesis and lymphopoiesis, processes by which myeloid and lymphoid blood cells are made. Unipotent cells are the progenitors for each of the blood cell types and come from pluripotent stem cells. Multipotential progenitor cells act as parent cells for multiple types of blood cells. Myeloproliferative cells do not exist.

2. b. *Rationale:* The portion of the cortex between the medullary and superficial cortex is called the paracortex. The region contains most of the T cells in the lymph-nodes. The B-cell–dependent cortex consists of two types of follicles: immunologically inactive follicles, called primary follicles, and active follicles that contain germinal centers called secondary follicles. There is no primary cortex in the lymph nodes.

3. d. *Rationale:* Severe congenital neutropenia, or Kostmann syndrome, is characterized by an arrest in myeloid maturation at the promyelocyte stage of development, resulting in an absolute neutrophil count of less than 200 cells/μL. The disorder is characterized by severe bacterial infections. Kostmann syndrome is not characterized by bone marrow disorders, viral infections, or autoimmune disorders.

4. a. *Rationale:* The incidence of drug-induced neutropenia has increased significantly over the past few decades and is attributed primarily to a wider use of drugs in general and, more specifically, to the use of chemotherapeutic drugs in the treatment of cancer.

5. b. *Rationale:* Hepatitis and splenomegaly are common manifestations of infectious mononucleosis and are believed to be immune mediated. Hepatitis is characterized by hepatomegaly, nausea, anorexia, and jaundice. Although discomforting, it is usually a benign condition that resolves without causing permanent liver damage. The spleen may be enlarged two to three times its normal size, and rupture of the spleen is an infrequent complication. Cranial nerve palsies, not peripheral nerve palsies, can occur. Lymph nodes do not rupture. Severe bacterial infections are complications of Kostmann syndrome.

6. c. *Rationale:* Non-Hodgkin lymphomas (NHLs) represent the cancer with the second fastest rate of increase in the United States and the most commonly occurring hematologic cancer. Neoplasms of immature B cells include lymphoblastic leukemia/lymphoma (i.e., acute lymphocytic leukemia). They are not classed as NHLs. Mantle cell lymphoma is one of the mature B-cell lymphomas.

7. d. *Rationale:* Endemic Burkitt lymphoma is the most common childhood cancer (peak ages 3–7 years) in Central Africa, often beginning in the jaw. It occurs in regions of Africa where both Epstein-Barr virus and malaria infection are common. Neither herpes zoster nor streptococcal infections are associated with endemic Burkitt lymphoma.

8. a. *Rationale:* Although acute lymphoblastic leukemia and acute myelogenous leukemia are distinct disorders, they typically present with similar clinical features. Both are characterized by an abrupt onset of symptoms, including fatigue resulting from anemia; low-grade fever, night sweats, and weight loss due to the rapid proliferation and hypermetabolism of the leukemic cells; bleeding because of a decreased platelet count; and bone pain and tenderness due to bone marrow expansion. Polycythemia is an increase in the erythrocytes in the blood. It is not an indication of leukemia.

9. b. *Rationale:* Diagnosis of multiple myeloma is based on clinical manifestations, blood tests, and bone marrow examination. The classic triad of bone marrow plasmacytosis (more than 10% plasma cells), lytic bone lesions, and either the serum M-protein spike or the presence of Bence-Jones proteins in the urine is definitive for a diagnosis of multiple myeloma. Oligoclonal bands are indicative of multiple sclerosis, and BCR-ABL fusion protein is found in chronic myelogenous leukemia.

10. c. *Rationale:* Hypogammaglobulinemia is common in chronic lymphocytic leukemia, especially in persons with advanced disease. An increased susceptibility to infection reflects an inability to produce specific antibodies and abnormal activation of complement. The most common infectious organisms are those that require opsonization for bacterial killing, such as *Streptococcus pneumoniae, Staphylococcus aureus,* and *Haemophilus influenzae.* Acne rosacea, *Pseudomonas aeruginosa,* and *Escherichia coli* are not infectious agents common in clients with chronic lymphocytic leukemia.

11. lyse

12. c. *Rationale:* The alimentary canal, respiratory passages, and genitourinary systems are guarded by accumulations of lymphatic tissue that are not enclosed in a capsule. This form of lymphatic tissue is called diffuse lymphatic tissue or MALT because of its association with mucous membranes. Lymphocytes are found in the subepithelial of these tissues. Lymphomas can arise from MALT as well as lymph node tissue. The cardiovascular system and the central nervous system do not have MALT.

13. b, c, d. *Rationale:* The existence of a genetic predisposition to develop acute leukemia is suggested by the increased leukemia incidence among a number of congenital disorders, including Down syndrome, neurofibromatosis, and Fanconi anemia. Neither Cushing syndrome nor Prader-Willi syndrome are genetic disorders.

14. a, c, e. *Rationale:* Massive necrosis of malignant cells can occur during the initial phase of treatment. This phenomenon, known as tumor lysis syndrome, can lead to life-threatening metabolic disorders, including hyperkalemia, hyperphosphatemia, hyperuricemia, hypomagnesemia, hypocalcemia, and acidosis, with the potential for causing acute renal failure.

15. radiation. *Rationale:* As the cure rate for Hodgkin lymphoma has risen and longer-term follow-up data became available, the importance of the late effects of treatment, including secondary malignancies, has become more apparent. Because these malignancies have mainly been attributed to radiation therapy, studies are being conducted to determine the lowest effective radiation dose.

CHAPTER 16 MECHANISMS OF INFECTIOUS DISEASE

SECTION II: ASSESSING YOUR UNDERSTANDING

Activity A

1. commensalism
2. infection
3. parasitic
4. opportunistic
5. transmissible neurodegenerative
6. Viruses
7. prokaryotes
8. Staining
9. spirochetes
10. mycoplasmas
11. fungal
12. yeasts, molds
13. feces
14. prodromal stage
15. acute stage
16. convalescent period
17. -*itis*
18. -*emia*
19. Virulence
20. exotoxins

Activity B

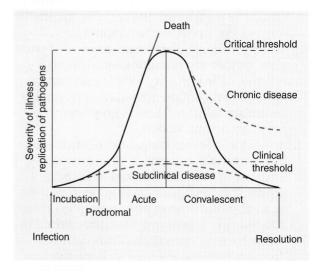

Activity C

1.

1. b	**2.** f	**3.** d	**4.** g	**5.** a
6. e	**7.** c	**8.** h	**9.** i	**10.** j

2.

1. f	**2.** a	**3.** j	**4.** e	**5.** c
6. d	**7.** b	**8.** h	**9.** g	**10.** i

Activity D

1.

Activity E

1. Viruses are incapable of replication outside a living cell. They must penetrate a susceptible living cell and use the biosynthetic machinery of the cell to produce viral progeny. Not every viral agent causes lysis and death of the host cell during the course of replication. Some viruses enter the host cell and insert their genome into the host cell chromosome, where it remains in a latent, nonreplicating state for long periods without causing disease. Under the appropriate stimulation, the virus undergoes active replication and produces symptoms of disease months to years later.

2. The portal of entry refers to the process by which a pathogen enters the body, gains access to susceptible tissues, and causes disease. Among the potential modes of transmission are penetration, direct contact, ingestion, and inhalation. In terms of pathophysiology, symptoms are the outward expression of the

struggle between invading organisms and the retaliatory inflammation and immune responses of the host.

3. The course of any infectious disease can be divided into several distinguishable stages after the point of time in which the potential pathogen enters the host. These stages are the incubation period, the prodromal stage, the acute stage, the convalescent stage, and the resolution stage. The stages are based on the progression and intensity of the host's symptoms over time. The duration of each phase and the pattern of the overall illness can be specific for different pathogens, thereby aiding in the diagnosis of an infectious disease.

4. The goal of treatment for an infectious disease is complete removal of the pathogen from the host and the restoration of normal physiologic function to damaged tissues. When an infectious process gains the upper hand and therapeutic intervention is essential, the choice of treatment may be medicinal using antimicrobial agents; immunologic with antibody preparations, vaccines, or substances that stimulate and improve the host's immune function; or surgical by removing infected tissues.

5. Potential agents of bioterrorism have been categorized into three levels (A, B, C) based on risk of use, transmissibility, invasiveness, and mortality rate. The agents considered to be in the highest biothreat level—plague, tularemia, smallpox, and hemorrhagic fever—are category A. The category B agents include agents of food- and waterborne disease, agents of zoonotic infections, and viral encephalitides. Category C agents are defined as emerging pathogens and potential risks for the future, even though many of these organisms are causes of ancient diseases such as tuberculosis and tickborne fever viruses.

SECTION III: APPLYING YOUR KNOWLEDGE
Activity F

1. An antibiotic is considered bactericidal if it causes irreversible and lethal damage to the bacterial pathogen and bacteriostatic if its inhibitory effects on bacterial growth are reversed when the agent is eliminated.

2. The drugs used to treat HIV infections are not antibiotics or antiviral agents. They are classified as antiretroviral agents. These drugs are acyclovir, ganciclovir, vidarabine, ribavirin, zidovudine, lamivudine, didanosine, stavudine, zalcitabine, nevirapine, efavirenz, and delavirdine.

SECTION IV: PRACTICING FOR NCLEX
Activity G

1. a. *Rationale:* A parasitic relationship is one in which only the infecting organism benefits from the relationship and the host either gains nothing from the relationship or sustains injury from the interaction. If the host sustains injury or pathologic damage in response to a parasitic infection, the process is called an infectious disease. Mutual and commensal relationships do not harm the human body. Communicable diseases can be passed from one human to another; they are not parasitic.

2. b. *Rationale:* The *Rickettsiaceae* are accidentally transmitted to humans through the bite of the arthropod (i.e., vector) and produce a number of potentially lethal diseases, including Rocky Mountain spotted fever and epidemic typhus. Viruses, *Chlamydiaceae*, and *Anaplasmataceae* do not cause either epidemic typhus or Rocky Mountain spotted fever.

3. c. *Rationale:* SARS was recognized in the Guangdong province in southern China beginning in November 2002. The illness was highly transmissible, as evidenced by the first recognized occurrence in Taiwan. Four days after returning to Taiwan from work in the Guangdong province, a businessman developed a febrile illness and was admitted to a local hospital. Within 1 month, a large nosocomial outbreak of SARS was documented to have affected ~3000 people in Taipei City, Taiwan. Since the SARS outbreak began in China and crossed continental borders for the first time, it was classified as not only an epidemic but also a pandemic. Regional and endemic mean the same thing, a specific area where the disease occurs. Nosocomial is an infection acquired in a health care facility.

4. d. *Rationale:* Symptomatology refers to the collection of signs and symptoms expressed by the host during the disease course. This is also known as the clinical picture or disease presentation. The virulence of the disease is its power to produce the disease. The source of the disease is the place where it came from. The diagnosis of the disease is the naming of the disease process in the body.

5. a. *Rationale:* The diagnosis of an infectious disease requires two criteria: the recovery of a

probable pathogen or evidence of its presence from the infected sites of a diseased host, and accurate documentation of clinical signs and symptoms compatible with an infectious process. Culture and sensitivity are the growing of microorganisms outside the body and the testing to see what kills it. Identifying a microorganism by microscopic appearance and Gram stain reaction are not the criteria for diagnosis. Serology, an indirect means of identifying infectious agents by measuring serum antibodies in the diseased host, and the quantification of those antibodies, an antibody titer, are not criteria for diagnosis.

6. b. *Rationale:* Potential agents of bioterrorism have been categorized into three levels (A, B, C) based on risk of use, transmissibility, invasiveness, and mortality rate.

7. c. *Rationale:* Aided by a global market and the ease of international travel, the past 5 years have witnessed the importation or emergence of a host of novel infectious diseases. During the late summer and early fall of 1999, West Nile virus (WNV) was identified as the cause of an epidemic involving 56 patients in the New York City area. This outbreak, which led to seven deaths (primarily in the elderly), marked the first time that WNV had been recognized in the Western hemisphere since its discovery in Uganda nearly 60 years earlier. Coxsackie diseases, caused by the Coxsackie virus; respiratory syncytial disease, better known as RSV; and hand, foot, and mouth disease are not considered global diseases.

8. d. *Rationale:* The course of any infectious disease can be divided into several distinguishable stages after the point of time in which the potential pathogen enters the host. These stages are the incubation period, the prodromal stage, the acute stage, the convalescent stage, and the resolution stage. There are no postacute, subacute, or postdromal stages to a disease.

9. a. *Rationale:* An abscess is a localized pocket of infection composed of devitalized tissue, microorganisms, and the host's phagocytic white blood cells: in essence, a stalemate in the infectious process. A pimple is a small papule or pustule. A lesion is a pathologic change in body tissue. Acne is a disease of the skin.

10. c. *Rationale:* Other exotoxins that have gained notoriety include the Shiga toxins produced by *E. coli* O157:H7 and other select strains. The ingestion of undercooked ham-

burger meat or unpasteurized fruit juices contaminated with this organism produces hemorrhagic colitis and a sometimes fatal illness called hemolytic uremic syndrome, characterized by vascular endothelial damage, acute renal failure, and thrombocytopenia. *E. coli* does not cause nephritic syndrome, hemolytic thrombocytopenia, or neuroleptic malignant syndrome.

11. prions. *Rationale:* Prions, protein particles that lack any kind of a demonstrable genome, have been found to cause pathologic processes in humans. The various prion-associated diseases produce very similar symptomatology and pathology in the host and are collectively called transmissible neurodegenerative diseases.

12. Congenital. *Rationale:* When an infectious disease is transmitted from mother to child during gestation or birth, it is classified as a congenital infection.

13. 1-c, 2-a, 3-d, 4-b

14. a, c, d, e. *Rationale:* Virulence factors are substances or products generated by infectious agents that enhance their ability to cause disease. Although the number and type of microbial products that fit this description are numerous, they can generally be grouped into four categories: toxins, adhesion factors, evasive factors, and invasive factors. Prodromal means occurring first or prior to a specific event. It is not a virulence factor.

15. a, d, e. *Rationale:* A number of factors produced by microorganisms enhance virulence by evading various components of the host's immune system. Extracellular polysaccharides, including capsules, slime, and mucous layers, discourage engulfment and killing of pathogens by the host's phagocytic white blood cells. Phospholipases and collagenases are enzymes that are invasive virulence factors.

CHAPTER 17 INNATE AND ADAPTIVE IMMUNITY

SECTION II: ASSESSING YOUR UNDERSTANDING

Activity A

1. immune system
2. allergies, autoimmune
3. innate
4. Adaptive
5. antigens

6. Humoral
7. Cell-mediated
8. macrophages
9. neutrophils, macrophages
10. Neutrophils
11. macrophage
12. B, T
13. Natural killer cells
14. Dendritic
15. Chemokines
16. colony-stimulating factors
17. epithelial
18. pathogens
19. Opsonization
20. Antigens
21. immunoglobulins
22. Humoral
23. CD4$^+$ helper T cell (T_H)
24. Regulatory
25. bone marrow, thymus
26. spleen

Activity B

The figure is a schematic model of an immunoglobulin G molecule showing the constant and variable regions of the light and dark chains. Each immunoglobulin is composed of two identical light (L) chains and two identical heavy (H) chains to form a Y-shaped molecule. The two forked ends of the immunoglobulin molecule bind antigen and are called *Fab* (i.e., antigen-binding) fragments, and the tail of the molecule, which is called the *Fc* fragment, determines the biologic properties that are characteristic of a particular class of immunoglobulins. The amino acid sequence of the heavy and light chains shows constant (C) regions and variable (V) regions. The *constant regions* have sequences of amino acids that vary little among the antibodies of a particular class of immunoglobulin. The constant regions allow separation of immunoglobulins into classes (e.g., IgM, IgG) and allow each class of antibody to interact with certain effectors cells and molecules. The *variable regions* contain the antigen-binding sites of the molecule. The wide variation in the amino acid sequence of the variable regions seen from antibody to antibody allows this region to recognize its complementary epitope. A unique amino acid sequence in this region determines a distinctive three-dimensional pocket that is complementary to the antigen, allowing recognition and binding.

Activity C

1.

1. c	2. j	3. f	4. h	5. e
6. d	7. a	8. b	9. i	10. g

2.

1. g	2. d	3. f	4. e	5. a
6. b	7. c	8. h	9. j	10. i

Activity D

1. Although cells of both innate and adaptive immune systems communicate critical information by cell-to-cell contact, many interactions and effector responses depend on the secretion of short-acting soluble molecules called cytokines. One type of cytokine, chemokines, direct leukocyte movement and migration, and another group of cytokines, the colony-stimulating factors, promote the proliferation and differentiation of bone marrow progenitor cells. Chemokines give the cells of the immune system the ability to act systemically as one.

2. The innate immune system consists of the epithelial barriers, phagocytic cells (mainly neutrophils and macrophages), natural killer cells, and several plasma proteins, including those of the complement system. These mechanisms are present in the body before an encounter with an infectious agent and are rapidly activated by microbes before the development of adaptive immunity. The activation and regulation of inflammation is also a major job of innate immunity.

3. These phagocytic cells were recruited during an inflammatory response to recognize and kill infectious invaders. The early responding innate immune cell is the neutrophil, followed shortly by the more efficient, multifunctional macrophage. They are activated to engulf and digest microbes that attach to their cell membrane. Once the cell is activated and the microbe is ingested, the cell generates digestive enzymes, toxic oxygen, and nitrogen intermediates (i.e., hydrogen peroxide or nitric oxide) through metabolic pathways. The phagocytic killing of microorganisms helps contain infectious agents.

4. There are three pathways for recognizing microorganisms that result in activation of the complement system: the classical, the lectin, and the alternative pathway. The reactions of the complement systems are divided into three phases: (a) initiation or activation, (b) amplification of inflammation, and (c) membrane attack response.

5. The MHC molecules involved in self-recognition and cell-to-cell communication fall into two classes: class I and class II. Class I MHC molecules are cell surface glycoproteins that interact with the antigen receptor-foreign peptide complex and the CD8 molecule on T cytotoxic lymphocytes. MHC-I molecules are found on nearly all nucleated cells in the body and thereby are capable of alerting the immune system of any cell changes due to viruses, intracellular bacteria, or cancer.

6. Macrophages are key members of the mononuclear phagocytic system that engulf and digest microbes and other foreign substances. The monocytes migrate from the blood to various tissues, where they mature into the major tissue phagocyte, the macrophages. As the general scavenger cells of the body, the macrophage can be fixed in a tissue or can be free to migrate from an organ to lymphoid tissues. The tissue macrophages are scattered in connective tissue or clustered in organs such as the lung (i.e., alveolar macrophages), liver (i.e., Kupffer cells), spleen, lymph nodes, peritoneum, central nervous system (i.e., microglial cells), and other areas. Macrophages are activated to engulf and break down complex antigens into peptide fragments for association with class II MHC molecules. Macrophages can then present these complexes to the helper T cell so that self–nonself recognition and activation of the immune response can occur.

7. The immunoglobulins have been divided into five classes: IgG, IgA, IgM, IgD, and IgE.

   I. IgG—protects against bacteria, toxins, and viruses in body fluids and activates the complement system
   II. IgA—serves as a primary defense against local infections in mucosal tissues
   III. IgM—is first circulating immunoglobulin to appear in response to an antigen
   IV. IgD—serves as an antigen receptor for initiating the differentiation of B cells
   V. IgE—is involved in inflammation, allergic responses, and combating parasitic infections

8. Active immunity is acquired through immunization or actually having a disease. It is active because it depends on a response to the antigen by the person's immune system. Due to memory, the immune system is usually able to react within hours to subsequent exposure to the same agent because of the presence of memory B and T lymphocytes and circulating antibodies. Passive immunity is immunity transferred from another source. An infant receives passive immunity naturally from the transfer of antibodies from its mother in utero and through a mother's breast milk.

SECTION III: APPLYING YOUR KNOWLEDGE

Activity E

1. The nurse will be sure to mention the following key points:

   • Every baby is born with passive immunity.
   • The baby receives antibodies from the mother through placenta and colostrum.
   • Passive immunity lasts up to 6 months.
   • Passive immunity is replaced by immunity received from immunizations.

SECTION IV: PRACTICING FOR NCLEX

Activity F

1. a. *Rationale:* The major components of innate immunity are the skin and mucous membranes; phagocytic cells (mainly neutrophils and macrophages); specialized lymphocytes called natural killer (NK) cells; and several plasma proteins, including the proteins of the complement system. Adaptive, humoral, and cell-mediated immunity do not use NK cells.

2. b. *Rationale:* The actions of cytokines are often pleiotropic and redundant. Cytokines are not described as rapid and self-limiting, cell specific and targeted, or dendritic and morphologic.

3. c. *Rationale:* The T lymphocytes (T cells) are generated from stem cells in the bone marrow. They complete their maturation in the thymus and function in the peripheral tissues to produce cell-mediated immunity and aid in antibody production.

4. d. *Rationale:* Activation of macrophages ensures enhanced phagocytic, metabolic, and enzymatic potential, resulting in more efficient destruction of infected cells. This type of defense is important against intracellular pathogens such as *Mycobacterium* species and *Listeria monocytogenes*. Contact dermatitis due to a poison ivy reaction or sensitivity to dyes is an example of delayed or cell-mediated hypersensitivity caused by hapten-carrier complexes. Blood transfusions do not cause hypersensitivity reactions by hapten-carrier complexes.

5. a. *Rationale:* Passive immunity can also be artificially provided by the transfer of antibodies produced by other people or animals. Some protection against infectious disease can be provided by the injection of hyperimmune serum, which contains high concentrations of antibodies for a specific disease, or immune serum or gamma-globulin, which contains a pool of antibodies from many individuals providing protection against numerous infectious agents. Immunizations and allergy shots are examples of active immunity. Exposure to poison ivy can be the cause of a hypersensitivity reaction; it is not immunity.

6. b. *Rationale:* Self-regulation is an essential property of the immune system. An inadequate immune response may lead to immunodeficiency, but an inappropriate or excessive response may lead to conditions varying from allergic reactions to autoimmune diseases. All answers are autoimmune diseases except for Huntington disease.

7. c. *Rationale:* The term tolerance is used to define the ability of the immune system to be nonreactive to self-antigens while producing immunity to foreign agents. All other responses have nothing to do with the recognition of and tolerance to self-antigens.

8. d. *Rationale:* Cord blood does not normally contain IgM or IgA. If present, these antibodies are of fetal origin and represent exposure to intrauterine infection.

9. a. *Rationale:* Aging is characterized by a declining ability to adapt to environmental stresses. One of the factors believed to contribute to this problem is a decline in immune responsiveness. This includes changes in cell-mediated and humoral immune responses. Elderly persons tend to be more susceptible to infections, have more evidence of autoimmune and immune complex disorders than younger persons, and have a higher incidence of cancer. None of the other answers are true or acceptable.

10. b. *Rationale:* Among the functions of the innate immune system is the induction of a complex cascade of events known as the inflammatory response. Recent evidence suggests that inflammation plays a key role in the pathogenesis of a number of disorders, such as atherosclerosis and coronary artery disease, bronchial asthma, type 2 diabetes mellitus, rheumatoid arthritis, multiple sclerosis, and systemic lupus erythematosus.

Osteoporosis is the abnormal loss of bone tissue and density. Osteogenesis imperfecta is a genetic disease causing multiple bone fractures in a newborn. Hydronephrosis is a condition of the kidney causing distension of the pelvis and calyces due to an obstruction in the ureter that does not enable urine to pass.

11. Antigens
12. 1-d, 2-e, 3-a, 4-c, 5-b
13. epithelial
14. b, c. *Rationale:* Although cells of both innate and adaptive immune systems communicate critical information about the invading microbe or pathogen by cell-to-cell contact, many interactions and effector responses depend on the secretion of chemical mediators (cytokines, chemokines, and colony-stimulating factors). Virulence factors define how much power an organism has to produce disease. Coxiella are organisms that cause Q fever.

15. b, e. *Rationale:* The T and B lymphocytes are the only cells in the body capable of specifically recognizing different antigenic determinants of microbial agents and other pathogens and therefore responsible for two defining characteristics of adaptive immunity, specificity and memory. Phagocytes, dendritic cells, and natural killer cells all participate in innate immunity.

CHAPTER 18 INFLAMMATION, TISSUE REPAIR, AND WOUND HEALING

SECTION II: ASSESSING YOUR UNDERSTANDING

Activity A
1. Inflammation
2. rubor, tumor, calor, dolor
3. systemic
4. Acute, chronic
5. vascular, cellular
6. leukocytosis
7. Monocyte/macrophages
8. Vascular
9. leukocytes
10. cell-to-cell
11. cell migration
12. chemokines
13. metabolic burst
14. coagulation, complement
15. dilation, permeability

16. eicosanoid
17. prostaglandins
18. cyclooxygenase
19. omega-3 fatty acids
20. Complement
21. kinin, smooth muscle, pain
22. tumor necrosis factor-α
23. superoxide, hydrogen peroxide, hydroxyl
24. endothelial cell damage
25. exudates
26. penetrate deeply, spread rapidly
27. CRP (C-reactive protein)
28. parenchymal, stromal
29. Labile cells
30. stabile
31. Granulation
32. collagen, fibroblast
33. premature infant

Activity B

1. The figure depicts the cyclooxygenase and lipoxygenase pathways and sites where the corticosteroids and nonsteroidal anti-inflammatory drugs (NSAIDs) exert their action.

    Inflammation is essential to the first phase of wound healing, and immune mechanisms prevent infections that impair wound healing. Among the conditions that impair inflammation and immune function is administration of corticosteroid drugs. Release of arachidonic acid by phospholipases initiates a series of complex reactions that lead to the production of inflammatory mediators. The cyclooxygenase pathway culminates in the synthesis of prostaglandins, and the lipoxygenase pathway culminates in the synthesis of the leukotrienes. Aspirin and the NSAIDs reduce inflammation by inactivating the first enzyme in the cyclooxygenase pathway for prostaglandin synthesis.

Activity C

1. c	2. a	3. i	4. f	5. j
6. g	7. b	8. h	9. d	10. e

Activity D

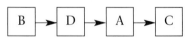

Activity E

1. These signs are rubor (redness), tumor (swelling), calor (heat), and dolor (pain). The rubor is the result of increased blood flow due to histamine release. The tumor, or swelling, is due to an increased permeability of blood vessels due to histamine and other long-term vasoactive mediators. The calor, or heat, is the result of increased perfusion of the tissues at the wound site. Dolor, or pain, is due to bradykinin, prostaglandins, and histamine effects on sensory nerve endings.

2. Acute inflammation is the early (almost immediate) reaction of local tissues and their blood vessels to injury. It typically occurs before adaptive immunity becomes established and is aimed primarily at removing the injurious agent and limiting the extent of tissue damage. Acute inflammation can be triggered by a variety of stimuli, including infections, immune reactions, blunt and penetrating trauma, physical or chemical agents, and tissue necrosis from any cause. In contrast to acute inflammation, chronic inflammation is self-perpetuating and may last for weeks, months, or even years. It may develop as the result of a recurrent or progressive acute inflammatory process or from low-grade, smoldering responses that fail to evoke an acute response.

3. The first pattern is an immediate transient response, which occurs with minor injury. It develops rapidly after injury and is usually reversible and of short duration. Typically, this type of leakage affects venules 20 to 60 mm in diameter, leaving capillaries and arterioles unaffected. The second pattern is an immediate sustained response, which occurs with more serious types of injury and continues for several days. It affects all levels of the microcirculation and is usually due to direct damage of the endothelium by injurious stimuli. The third pattern is a delayed hemodynamic response in which the increased permeability begins after a delay of 2 to 12 hours, lasts for several hours or even days, and involves venules as well as capillaries. A delayed response often accompanies radiation types of injuries.

4. Phagocytosis involves three distinct steps: (a) recognition and adherence, (b) engulfment, and (c) intracellular killing. Phagocytosis is initiated by recognition and binding of particles by specific receptors on the surface of phagocytic cells. Microbes can be bound directly to the membrane of the phagocytic cells by several types of pattern recognition receptors or indirectly by receptors that recognize microbes coated with carbohydrate-binding lectins, antibody, and/or complement.

Endocytosis is accomplished through cytoplasmic extensions that surround and enclose the particle in a membrane-bound phagocytic vesicle. Intracellular killing of pathogens is accomplished through several mechanisms, including toxic oxygen and nitrogen products, lysozymes, proteases, and defensins.

5. Mediators can be classified by function: (a) those with vasoactive and smooth muscle–constricting properties such as histamine, arachidonic acid metabolites, and platelet-activating factor; (b) plasma proteases that activate members of the complement system, coagulation factors of the clotting cascade, and vasoactive peptides of the kinin system; (c) chemotactic factors such as complement fragments and chemokines; and (4) reactive molecules and cytokines liberated from leukocytes, which when released into the extracellular environment can affect the surrounding tissue and cells.

6. The types of chronic inflammation are nonspecific and granulomatous. Nonspecific chronic inflammation involves a diffuse accumulation of macrophages and lymphocytes at the site of injury. Ongoing chemotaxis causes macrophages to infiltrate the inflamed site, where they accumulate owing to prolonged survival and immobilization. These mechanisms lead to fibroblast proliferation, with subsequent scar formation that in many cases replaces the normal connective tissue or the functional parenchymal tissues of the involved structures. A granulomatous lesion is a small, 1- to 2-mm lesion in which there is a mass of epithelioid cells surrounded by lymphocytes. Granulomatous inflammation is associated with foreign bodies and with microorganisms that are poorly digested and usually not easily controlled by other inflammatory mechanisms.

7. The acute phase response includes changes in the concentrations of plasma proteins, skeletal muscle catabolism, negative nitrogen balance, elevated erythrocyte sedimentation rate, and increased numbers of leukocytes. These responses are generated by the release of cytokines that affect the thermoregulatory center in the hypothalamus to produce fever. The metabolic changes provide amino acids that can be used in the immune response and for tissue repair. In general, the acute phase response serves to coordinate the various changes in body activity to enable an optimal host response.

8. Depending on the extent of tissue loss, wound closure and healing occur by primary or secondary intention. Small or "clean" wounds (e.g., a surgical incision) are an example of healing by primary intention. Larger wounds that have a greater loss of tissue and contamination heal by secondary intention. Healing by secondary intention is slower than healing by primary intention and results in the formation of larger amounts of scar tissue.

SECTION III: APPLYING YOUR KNOWLEDGE
Activity F

1. After an injury, the body initiates what is called the inflammatory response. This means that the body sends cells and fluids that are specific to destroying infectious organisms and healing the injury to the site of the wound. What you are seeing on the bandages is a serous exudate from the plasma in the circulatory system that has responded to the burn injury.

2. The body's response to an injury activates many different types and kinds of cells. This response is called the acute phase response, and some of the cells that are released during this response act on the central nervous system. Their actions can cause outward manifestations of their work, such as anorexia, somnolence, and malaise.

SECTION IV: PRACTICING FOR NCLEX
Activity G

1. a. *Rationale:* The classic description of inflammation has been handed down through the ages. In the first century AD, the Roman physician Celsus described the local reaction of injury in terms now known as the cardinal signs of inflammation. These signs are rubor (redness), tumor (swelling), calor (heat), and dolor (pain). In the second century AD, the Greek physician Galen added a fifth cardinal sign, functio laesa (loss of function).

   Altered level of consciousness is not a cardinal sign of inflammation. Sepsis and fever are systemic signs of infection.

2. b, c, e. *Rationale:* Eosinophils, basophils, and mast cells produce lipid mediators and cytokines that induce inflammation. They are particularly important in inflammation associated with immediate hypersensitivity reactions and allergic disorders. Neutrophils and macrophages are white blood cells that

respond to inflammation and destroy invading bacteria. They do not induce inflammation.

3. b. *Rationale:* Chronic inflammation involves the proliferation of fibroblasts instead of exudates. As a result, the risk of scarring and deformity is usually greater than in acute inflammation. Chronic inflammation is not the persistent destruction of healthy tissue. Typically, agents that cause chronic inflammation do not penetrate deeply or spread rapidly. Acute inflammation, not chronic, is the result of allergic reactions.

4. b, d, e. *Rationale:* Wound healing is commonly divided into three phases: (a) the inflammatory phase, (b) the proliferative phase, and (c) the maturational or remodeling phase. There is no activation or nutritional phase in wound healing.

5. c. *Rationale:* An increase in tissue oxygen tension by hyperbaric oxygen enhances wound healing by a number of mechanisms, including the increased killing of bacteria by neutrophils, impaired growth of anaerobic bacteria, and promotion of angiogenesis and fibroblast activity. Eosinophil activity is not affected by hyperbaric treatment of wounds.

6. b. *Rationale:* Animal and human bites are particularly troublesome in terms of infection. The animal inflicting the bite, the location of the bite, and the type of injury are all important determinants of whether the wound becomes infected. Approximately 28% to 80% of all cat bites become infected. Dog bites, for unclear reasons, become infected only approximately 3% to 18% of the time. Bites inflicted by children are usually superficial and seldom become infected, whereas bites inflicted by adults have a much higher rate of infection.

7. c. *Rationale:* The child has a greater capacity for repair than the adult but may lack the reserves needed to ensure proper healing. This lack of reserves is evidenced by an easily upset electrolyte balance, sudden elevation or lowering of temperature, and rapid spread of infection. The neonate and small child may have an immature immune system with no antigenic experience with organisms that contaminate wounds. The younger the child, the more likely that the immune system is not fully developed. The skin of a neonate or a small child is not as fragile as the skin of an elderly person.

8. c. *Rationale:* Infection impairs all dimensions of wound healing. It prolongs the inflammatory phase, impairs the formation of granulation tissue, and inhibits proliferation of fibroblasts and deposition of collagen fibers. All wounds are contaminated at the time of injury. Although body defenses can handle the invasion of microorganisms at the time of wounding, badly contaminated wounds can overwhelm host defenses. Trauma and existing impairment of host defenses can also contribute to the development of wound infections.

9. c. *Rationale:* Histamine causes dilation of arterioles and increases the permeability of venules. It acts at the level of the microcirculation by binding to histamine 1 receptors on endothelial cells and is considered the principal mediator of the immediate transient phase of increased vascular permeability in the acute inflammatory response. Arachidonic acid is a 20-carbon unsaturated fatty acid found in phospholipids of cell membranes. Release of arachidonic acid by phospholipases initiates a series of complex reactions that lead to the production of the eicosanoid family of inflammatory mediators (prostaglandins, leukotrienes, and related metabolites). Fibroblasts and cytokines are not the principal mediator of the transient phase of an acute inflammatory response.

10. a. *Rationale:* The most prominent systemic manifestations of inflammation include the acute phase response, alterations in white blood cell count (leukocytosis or leukopenia), and fever. A widening pulse pressure is not indicative of systemic inflammation, and thrombocytopenia is a hematologic disorder, not an indication of systemic inflammation.

CHAPTER 19 DISORDERS OF THE IMMUNE RESPONSE

SECTION II: ASSESSING YOUR UNDERSTANDING

Activity A

1. immune
2. Immunodeficiency
3. innate
4. adaptive
5. humoral, cellular
6. X
7. pyogenic
8. maternal
9. antibody
10. kidney
11. malignancies

12. CD4$^+$ helper, CD8$^+$ cytotoxic
13. T lymphocytes
14. combined immunodeficiency
15. severe combined immunodeficiency
16. boys
17. complement
18. secondary
19. degranulation
20. respiratory burst
21. Hypersensitivity
22. allergic reactions
23. Anaphylaxis
24. atopic
25. rhinitis
26. type II
27. ADCC
28. Type III
29. Serum
30. Arthus reaction
31. type IV reactions
32. contact dermatitis
33. transplantation
34. autologous, syngeneic, allogeneic
35. Graft-versus-host-disease
36. Autoimmune
37. self-tolerance
38. autoantibodies

Activity B

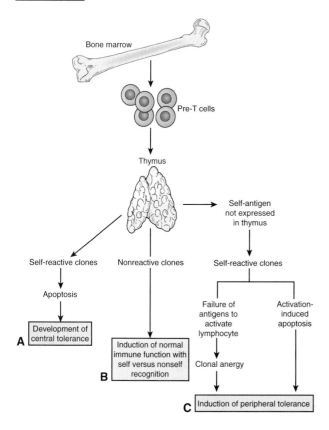

Activity C

1. e	**2.** h	**3.** l	**4.** a	**5.** f
6. m	**7.** d	**8.** k	**9.** i	**10.** c
11. n	**12.** j	**13.** g	**14.** B	**15.** o

Activity D

Activity E

1. A primary deficiency or immunodeficiency is congenital or inherited. Secondary immunodeficiency is acquired.

2. During the first few months of life, infants are protected from infection by IgG antibodies that have been transferred from the maternal circulation during fetal life. An infant's level of maternal IgG gradually declines over a period of approximately 6 months. Concomitant with the loss of maternal antibody, the infant's immature humoral immune system begins to function, and between the ages of 1 and 2 years, the child's antibody production reaches adult levels. Once the level of maternal antibodies drops, the infant is susceptible to infection.

3. Type I hypersensitivity reactions begin with mast cell or basophil sensitization. During the sensitization or priming stage, allergen-specific IgE antibodies attach to receptors on the surface of mast cells and basophils. With subsequent exposure, the sensitizing allergen binds to the cell-associated IgE and triggers a series of events that ultimately lead to degranulation of the sensitized mast cells or basophils, causing release of their preformed mediators. Mast cells are also the source of lipid-derived membrane products (e.g., prostaglandins, leukotrienes) and cytokines that participate in the continued response to the allergen.

4. In direct cell-mediated cytotoxicity, CD8$^+$ cytolytic T lymphocytes (CTLs) directly kill the antigen-presenting target cells. In viral infections, CTL responses can lead to tissue injury by killing infected target cells even if the virus itself has no cytotoxic effects. Because CTLs cannot distinguish between cytopathic and noncytopathic viruses, they kill virtually all infected cells regardless of whether the infection is harmful. Delayed-type hypersensitivity reactions occur in response to soluble protein antigens and primarily involve antigen-presenting cells such as macrophages and CD4$^+$ helper T cells of the T$_H$1 type. During

the reaction, T_H1 cells are activated and secrete an array of cytokines that recruit and activate monocytes, lymphocytes, fibroblasts, and other inflammatory cells. These T-cell–mediated responses require the synthesis of effector molecules and take 24 to 72 hours to develop, which is why they are called delayed-type hypersensitivity disorders.

5. Severe combined immunodeficiency (SCID) is the result of genetic mutations that lead to absence of all T- and B-cell function and, in some cases, a lack of natural killer cells. Affected infants have a disease course that resembles AIDS, with failure to thrive, chronic diarrhea, and opportunistic infections. Survival beyond the first year of life is rare without prompt immune reconstitution through bone marrow or hematopoietic stem cell transplantation. Early diagnosis is critical because the chances of successful treatment are highest in infants who have not experienced severe opportunistic infections. There is also hope that gene therapy will someday be available, for some, if not all, forms of SCID.

SECTION III: APPLYING YOUR KNOWLEDGE

Activity F

1. The correct response would include information about the antinuclear antibodies test. The basis for most serologic assays is the demonstration of antibodies directed against tissue antigens or cellular components. For example, a child with chronic or acute history of fever, arthritis, and a macular rash along with high levels of antinuclear antibody has a probable diagnosis of systemic lupus erythematous. The detection of autoantibodies in the laboratory is usually accomplished by one of three methods: indirect fluorescent antibody assays, enzyme-linked immunosorbent assay, or particle agglutination of some kind.
2. Medications used in the treatment of systemic lupus erythematous include corticosteroids (prednisone) and immunosuppressive (cytotoxic) agents (azathioprine, cyclophosphamide, methotrexate).

SECTION IV: PRACTICING FOR NCLEX

Activity G

1. c. *Rationale:* During the first few months of life, infants are protected from infection by IgG antibodies that have been transferred from the maternal circulation during fetal life. IgA, IgM, IgD, and IgE do not normally cross the placenta.
2. a, b, c, d. *Rationale:* Medications that cause reversible secondary hypogammaglobulinemia include the disease-modifying antirheumatic drugs; corticosteroid agents; and the antiepileptic drugs, phenytoin and carbamazepine. Interferon-beta 1a drugs are used in the treatment of autoimmune disorders.
3. a. *Rationale:* In general, persons with cell-mediated immunodeficiency disorders have infections or other clinical problems that are more severe than antibody disorders. Children with defects in this branch of the immune response rarely survive beyond infancy or childhood, unless immunologic reconstitution is achieved through bone marrow transplantation. In DiGeorge syndrome, children who survive the immediate neonatal period may have recurrent or chronic infections because of impaired T-cell immunity. Children may also have an absence of immunoglobulin production, caused by a lack of helper T-cell function. X-linked immunodeficiency with hyper-IgM, the X-linked immunodeficiency of hyper-IgM, also known as the hyper-IgM syndrome, is characterized by low IgG and IgA levels with normal or, more frequently, high IgM concentrations. X-linked agammaglobulinemia is a primary humeral immunodeficiency disorder. Y-linked agammaglobulinemia does not exist.
4. b. *Rationale*: Disorders that affect both B and T lymphocytes, with resultant defects in both humoral and cell-mediated immunity, fall under the broad classification of combined immunodeficiency syndrome. A single mutation in any one of the many genes that influence lymphocyte development or response, including lymphocyte receptors, cytokines, or major histocompatibility antigens, could lead to combined immunodeficiency.
5. c. *Rationale:* Ataxia-telangiectasia is a complex syndrome of neurologic, immunologic, endocrinologic, hepatic, and cutaneous abnormalities. Pierre-Robin syndrome, Angelman syndrome, and Adair-Dighton syndrome are not immunologic deficiencies.
6. a. *Rationale:* Disorders caused by immune responses are collectively referred to as hypersensitivity reactions. Antigens cause allergic reactions. Mediator response action and allergen stimulating reaction have nothing to do with hypersensitivity reactions.

Copyright © 2009, Wolters Kluwer Health l Lippincott Williams & Wilkins. *Study Guide for Pathophysiology: Concepts of Altered Health States, 8e.*

7. b. *Rationale:* Anaphylaxis is a systemic life-threatening hypersensitivity reaction characterized by widespread edema, vascular shock secondary to vasodilation, and difficulty breathing. It is not called an antigen reaction or an Arthus reaction.

8. c. *Rationale:* Serum sickness is a systemic immune complex disorder that is triggered by the deposition of insoluble antigen-antibody (IgM, IgG, and, occasionally, IgA) complexes in blood vessels, joints, heart, and kidney tissue. This is not anti-immune disease, systemic lupus erythematosus, or antigen-antibody sickness.

9. d. *Rationale:* Cornstarch powder is applied to the gloves during the manufacturing process to prevent stickiness and give the gloves a smooth feel. The cornstarch glove powder has an important role in the allergic response. Latex proteins are readily absorbed by glove powder and become airborne during removal of the gloves. Baking powder is not used inside gloves. Pieces of latex that become airborne and latex proteins that attach to clothing are not significant contributors to the incidence of latex allergy.

10. antidonor. *Rationale:* When preformed antidonor antibodies are present, rejection occurs immediately after transplantation.

11. a, b, d. *Rationale:* Because autoimmunity does not develop in all persons with genetic predisposition, it appears that other factors such as a "trigger event" interact to precipitate the altered immune state. The event or events that trigger the development of an autoimmune response are unknown. It has been suggested that the "trigger" may be a virus or other microorganism, a chemical substance, or a self-antigen from a body tissue that has been hidden from the immune system during development.

CHAPTER 20 ACQUIRED IMMUNODEFICIENCY SYNDROME

SECTION II: ASSESSING YOUR UNDERSTANDING

Activity A
1. HIV, immunosuppression, opportunistic
2. retrovirus
3. sexual, blood-to-blood, perinatally
4. Sexual
5. blood

6. percutaneous inoculation; needle stick
7. CD4+ T lymphocytes, macrophages, dendritic
8. antibody-producing B lymphocytes, cell-mediated
9. interrupt
10. CD4+ T
11. Opportunistic
12. bacterial pneumonia, tuberculosis
13. Wasting
14. lipodystrophy
15. low-risk; risk-free
16. antibody
17. western blot
18. DNA
19. decrease, eradicate
20. depression, anxiety
21. Polymerase chain reaction testing

Activity B
1. h 2. e 3. i 4. c 5. a
6. f 7. b 8. d 9. g

Activity C
The steps of viral replication are as follows:
1. Binding of the virus to the CD4+ T cell
2. Attachment and uncoating of the virus, allowing the genetic material to enter the host cell
3. DNA synthesis via reverse transcriptase
4. Integration into the host DNA
5. Transcription of viral DNA into mRNA
6. Translation of mRNA into a protein
7. Cleavage of protein product into separate proteins for new viruses
8. Assemblage of new HIV

Activity D
1. HIV replication involves the killing of the CD4+ T cell and the release of copies of HIV into the bloodstream. These virions invade other CD4+ T cells, allowing the infection to progress. Every day, millions of infected CD4+ T cells are destroyed, releasing billions of viral particles into the bloodstream; nearly all CD4+ T cells are replaced; and nearly all viral particles are destroyed. As the years progress, the CD4+ cell count gradually decreases through this process, and the number of viruses detected in the blood of persons infected with HIV increases, resulting in decreased activation of B and T cells.
2. The three phases are the primary infection phase, chronic asymptomatic or latency phase, and overt AIDS phase. In the primary

infection phase, the signs and symptoms (e.g., fever, malaise, fatigue) usually appear 1 to 4 weeks after exposure to HIV and last 7 to 10 days. After several weeks, the immune system acts to control viral replication and reduces the viral load to a stable level. In the chronic asymptomatic phase, which lasts about 10 years, the patient is symptom free. Slowly, the $CD4^+$ cell count drops from 1000 cells/_L to 200 cells/μL. In the overt AIDS phase, $CD4^+$ counts are below 200 cells/μL. The risk of opportunistic infections and death increases significantly.

3. The goal of HAART is sustained suppression of HIV replication, resulting in an undetectable viral load and an increasing $CD4^+$ cell count. In general, antiviral therapies are prescribed to slow the progression to AIDS and improve the overall survival time of persons with HIV infection.

4. Reverse transcriptase inhibitors inhibit HIV replication by acting on the enzyme reverse transcriptase by either blocking elongation or copying. Protease inhibitors bind to the protease enzyme and inhibit its action, preventing the cleavage of the polyprotein chain into individual proteins, which would be used to construct the new virus. Entry inhibitors prevent HIV from entering or fusing with the $CD4^+$ cell, thus blocking HIV from inserting its genetic information into the $CD4^+$ T cell. Integrase inhibitors block the integration step of the viral cycle, thus preventing the ability of HIV's genome to integrate into the host's genome.

5. Infected women may transmit the virus to their offspring in utero, during labor and delivery, or through breast milk. The risk of transmission is increased if the mother has advanced HIV disease, prolonged time from rupture of membranes to delivery, if the mother breast-feeds the child, or if there is increased exposure of the fetus to maternal blood.

SECTION III: APPLYING YOUR KNOWLEDGE

Activity E

1. The nurse should include the following:
   - Information on lab tests that will need to be done:
     - Viral load testing every 3–4 months
     - $CD4^+$ cell count every 3–4 months

   - Tests for opportunistic infections
     - Complete blood count
     - Sedimentation rate
     - Culture and sensitivity tests
   - U.S. Department of Health and Human Services Guidelines for the treatment of HIV/AIDS
   - HAART
   - Antiviral drugs and what they are used for
   - Treatment of opportunistic infections as/when they occur
   - Support for psychosocial issues

2. The evaluation will include a complete history, physical evaluation, and baseline laboratory tests, and a plan of care will be developed based on symptoms, viral load, and cell count. Routine follow-up care of a stable, asymptomatic HIV-infected patient should include a history and physical examination along with $CD4^+$ cell count and viral load testing every 3 to 4 months. Persons who are symptomatic may need to be seen more frequently.

SECTION IV: PRACTICING FOR NCLEX

Activity F

1. b, c, d. *Rationale:* HIV is transmitted from one person to another through sexual contact, blood-to-blood contact, or perinatally. It is not transmitted through casual contact. Several studies involving more than 1,000 uninfected, nonsexual household contacts with persons with HIV infection (including siblings, parents, and children) have shown no evidence of casual transmission. HIV is not spread by mosquitoes or other insect vectors.

2. b, h, a, e, f, g, c, d. *Rationale:* Replication of HIV occurs in eight steps. The first step involves the binding of the virus to the $CD4^+$ T cell. The second step allows for the internalization of the virus. The third step consists of DNA synthesis. The fourth step is called integration. The fifth step involves transcription of the double-stranded viral DNA to form a single-stranded messenger RNA (mRNA) with the instructions for building new viruses. The sixth step includes translation of mRNA. The seventh step is called cleavage. Finally, during the eighth step, the proteins and viral RNA are assembled into new HIV viruses and released from the $CD4^+$ T cell.

3. a. *Rationale:* The typical course of HIV is defined by three phases, which usually occur over a period of 8 to 12 years. The three phases are the primary infection phase, chronic asymptomatic or latency phase, and overt AIDS phase. There is no identified conversion phase.

4. b. *Rationale:* Opportunistic infections involve common organisms that normally do not produce infection unless there is impaired immune function. Although a person with AIDS may live for many years after the first serious illness, as the immune system fails, these opportunistic illnesses become progressively more severe and difficult to treat.

5. c. *Rationale:* The most common causes of respiratory disease in persons with HIV infection are bacterial pneumonia, *Pneumocystis carinii* pneumonia (PCP), and pulmonary tuberculosis. The best predictor of PCP is a CD4$^+$ cell count below 200 cell/μL, and it is at this point that prophylaxis with trimethoprim-sulfamethoxazole (or an alternative agent in the case of adverse reactions to sulfa compounds) is strongly recommended. Trimethobenzamide, triamterene, and trimipramine are drugs that are not used as prophylactics against opportunistic respiratory infections in people with HIV/AIDS.

6. a, c, e. *Rationale:* More than 50% of people with skin lesions also have gastrointestinal lesions. Gastrointestinal tract Kaposi sarcoma is often asymptomatic, but can cause pain, bleeding, or obstruction. Rectal burning and diarrhea are not symptoms of Kaposi sarcoma of the gastrointestinal tract.

7. c. *Rationale:* Because there is no cure for HIV or AIDS, adopting riskfree or low-risk behavior is the best protection against the disease. Abstinence or a long-term, mutually monogamous sexual relationship between two uninfected partners is the best way to avoid HIV infection and other sexually transmitted diseases. Correct and consistent use of latex condoms can provide protection from HIV by not allowing contact with semen or vaginal secretions during intercourse. Natural or lambskin condoms do not provide the same protection from HIV as latex because of the larger pores in the material. Only water-based lubricants should be used with condoms because petroleum (oil-based) products weaken the structure of the latex.

8. b. *Rationale:* The HIV antibody test procedure consists of screening with an enzyme immunoassay (EIA), also known as enzyme-linked immunoabsorbent assay (ELISA), followed by a confirmatory test, the western blot assay, which is performed if the EIA is positive. The complete metabolic panel cannot diagnose HIV/AIDS. The diagnostic test for HIV/AIDS is the ELISA, not the ALEA. The confirmatory test for HIV/AIDS is not the eastern blot test.

9. c. *Rationale:* Because different drugs act on different stages of the replication cycle, optimal treatment includes a combination of at least two to three drugs, often referred to as HAART. The goal of HAART is sustained suppression of HIV replication, resulting in an undetectable viral load and an increasing CD4$^+$ cell count. The other treatments are not used in the treatment of HIV/AIDS.

10. a. *Rationale:* In 1997, wasting became an AIDS-defining illness. The syndrome is common in persons with HIV infection or AIDS. Wasting is characterized by involuntary weight loss of at least 10% of baseline body weight in the presence of diarrhea, more than two stools per day, or chronic weakness and fever. This diagnosis is made when no other opportunistic infections or neoplasms can be identified as causing these symptoms. Beal syndrome and WAGAR syndrome are not identified with HIV/AIDS. AIDS is not a recognized syndrome.

11. a, b, c. *Rationale:* These reactions may be influenced by inadequate information, fear of contagion, shame, prejudices, and condemnation of risk behaviors. Acknowledging a diagnosis of HIV or AIDS may be the first indication to family and colleagues of an otherwise hidden lifestyle (i.e., homosexuality, drug use). This increases the strain on relationships with important support persons. Shock is a common reaction people have when they are diagnosed with HIV, often followed by anger at themselves or others and denial or guilt. In addition to the fear and grief associated with death, the person with HIV or AIDS may also experience uncertainty and may feel helpless, hopeless, stigmatized, and out of control. Acceptance of the lifestyle may also have occurred prior to the diagnosis of HIV/AIDS.

12. b. *Rationale:* The risk of transmission is increased if the mother has advanced HIV

disease, as evidenced by low CD4+ cell counts, high levels of HIV in the blood (high viral load), prolonged time from rupture of membranes to delivery, or breast-feeds the child, or if there is increased exposure of the fetus to maternal blood.

CHAPTER 21 STRUCTURE AND FUNCTION OF THE CARDIOVASCULAR SYSTEM

SECTION II: ASSESSING YOUR UNDERSTANDING

Activity A

1. oxygen, waste, hormones
2. pulmonary, systemic
3. pulmonary
4. systemic
5. low
6. atria, ventricles
7. same
8. volume, pressure
9. hemodynamics
10. large
11. Viscosity
12. Turbulent
13. thicker
14. distensibility
15. aortic, pulmonic
16. precedes
17. elastic
18. Diastole
19. stroke volume
20. ejection
21. cardiac output
22. cardiac reserve
23. Frank-Starling
24. heart rate
25. tunica adventitia, tunica media, tunica intima
26. arterial pressure pulse
27. decreases
28. central venous pressure
29. Valves
30. Autoregulation
31. hyperemia
32. anastomotic
33. microcirculation
34. capillary pores
35. colloidal osmotic
36. medulla oblongata
37. sympathetic, parasympathetic
38. Cushing reflex

Activity B

1.

2.

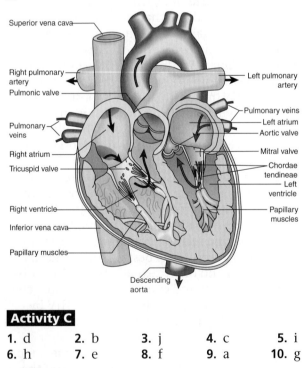

Activity C

1. d	2. b	3. j	4. c	5. i
6. h	7. e	8. f	9. a	10. g

Activity D

1. The most important factors governing the flow of blood in the cardiovascular system are pressure, resistance, and flow. Blood flow (F) through a vessel or series of blood vessels is determined

by the pressure difference (ΔP) between the two ends of a vessel (the inlet and the outlet) and the resistance (R) that blood must overcome as it moves through the vessel (F = ΔP/R).

2. This is because, even though each individual capillary is very small, the total cross-sectional area of the systemic capillaries greatly exceeds the cross-sectional area of other parts of the circulation. Because of this large surface area, the slower movement of blood allows ample time for exchange of nutrients, gases, and metabolites between the tissues and the blood.

3. The anatomic arrangement of the actin and myosin filaments in the myocardial muscle fibers is such that the tension or force of contraction is dependent on the degree to which the muscle fibers are stretched just before the ventricles begin to contract. The maximum force of contraction and cardiac output is achieved when venous return produces an increase in left ventricular end diastolic filling (i.e., preload) such that the muscle fibers are stretched about two and one-half times their normal resting length. When the muscle fibers are stretched to this degree, there is optimal overlap of the actin and myosin filaments needed for maximal contraction.

4. Sympathetic innervation via α-adrenergic receptors is excitatory in that they produce vasoconstriction; β-adrenergic receptors are inhibitory in that they produce vasodilation. Smooth muscle contraction and relaxation also occur in response to local tissue factors, such as lack of oxygen, increased hydrogen ion concentrations, and excess carbon dioxide. Nitric oxide acts locally to produce smooth muscle relaxation and regulate blood flow.

5. The factors that travel in the bloodstream that will regulate blood flow are as follows:

- Norepinephrine—potent vasoconstrictor
- Epinephrine—mild vasoconstriction or dilation, depending on the receptor type found in target tissue
- Angiotensin II—powerful vasoconstrictor
- Histamine—powerful vasodilator and can increase permeability
- Serotonin—vasoconstrictor
- Bradykinin—vasodilator
- Prostaglandins—vasodilator or vasoconstrictor, depending on type of prostaglandin

SECTION III: APPLYING YOUR KNOWLEDGE
Activity E

1. You would give this client nitroglycerin and calcium channel blocking drugs to reverse the spasm of the artery.

SECTION IV: PRACTICING FOR NCLEX
Activity F

1. a. *Rationale:* The total blood volume is a function of age and body weight, ranging from 85 to 90 mL/kg in the neonate and from 70 to 75 mL/kg in the adult.

2. b. *Rationale:* The blood vessels and the blood vessel itself constitute resistance to flow. A helpful equation for understanding the relationship between resistance, blood vessel diameter (radius), and blood viscosity factors that affect blood flow was derived by the French physician Poiseuille more than a century ago. The other laws do not address resistance to flow.

3. b. *Rationale:* Compliance refers to the total quantity of blood that can be stored in a given portion of the circulation for each millimeter rise in pressure. Compliance reflects the distensibility of the blood vessel. Wall tension, laminar blood flow, and resistance are not major factors in the distensibility of the blood vessel.

4. c. *Rationale:* The Cushing reflex is a special type of central nervous system (CNS) reflex resulting from an increase in intracranial pressure (ICP). When the ICP rises to levels that equal intraarterial pressure, blood vessels to the vasomotor center become compressed, initiating the CNS ischemic response. The purpose of this reflex is to produce a rise in arterial pressure to levels above ICP so that the blood flow to the vasomotor center can be reestablished. If the ICP rises to the point that the blood supply to the vasomotor center becomes inadequate, vasoconstrictor tone is lost, and the blood pressure begins to fall. The elevation in blood pressure associated with the Cushing reflex is usually of short duration and should be considered a protective homeostatic mechanism. The brain and other cerebral structures are located within the rigid confines of the skull, with no room for expansion, and any increase in ICP tends to compress the blood vessels that supply the brain.

5. c. *Rationale:* In clinical practice, the measurement of the cardiac forms of troponin T and troponin I are used in the diagnosis of myocardial infarction. Troponin C is not diagnostic of a myocardial infarction. Troponin A is not one of the troponin complexes.

6. d. *Rationale:* Approximately 60% of the stroke volume is ejected during the first quarter of systole, and the remaining 40% is ejected during the next two quarters of systole. Little blood is ejected from the heart during the last quarter of systole, although the ventricle remains contracted.

7. a. *Rationale:* With peripheral arterial disease, there is a delay in the transmission of the reflected wave so that the pulse decreases rather than increases in amplitude.

8. b. *Rationale:* The efficiency of the heart as a pump is often measured in terms of cardiac output (CO), or the amount of blood the heart pumps each minute. The CO is the product of the stroke volume (SV) and the heart rate (HR), and can be expressed by the equation: $CO = SV \times HR$. AV stands for atrioventricular, and EF stands for ejection fraction. Neither is part of the equation for CO.

9. b, c, d, e. *Rationale:* The heart's ability to increase its output according to body needs mainly depends on four factors: the preload, or ventricular filling; the afterload, or resistance to ejection of blood from the heart; cardiac contractility; and the heart rate. Cardiac reserve does not add to the heart's ability to increase its output.

10. d. *Rationale:* The fact that nitric oxide is released into the vessel lumen (to inactivate platelets) and away from the lumen (to relax smooth muscle) suggests that it protects against both thrombosis and vasoconstriction. Nitroglycerin, which is used in treatment of angina, produces its effects by releasing nitric oxide in vascular smooth muscle of the target tissues. None of the other answers are released by nitroglycerin.

11. a. *Rationale:* The osmotic pressure caused by the plasma proteins in the blood tends to pull fluid from the interstitial spaces back into the capillary. This pressure is termed colloidal osmotic pressure to differentiate the osmotic effects of the plasma proteins, which are suspended colloids, from the osmotic effects of substances such as sodium and glucose, which are dissolved crystalloids.

12. c. *Rationale:* The lymph capillaries drain into larger lymph vessels that ultimately empty into the right and left thoracic ducts. The thoracic ducts empty into the circulation at the junctions of the subclavian and internal jugular veins. The lymphatic system only joins the vascular system in one place, so no other answer is accurate.

13. b. *Rationale:* The medullary cardiovascular neurons are grouped into three distinct pools that lead to sympathetic innervation of the heart and blood vessels and parasympathetic innervation of the heart. The first two, which control sympathetic-mediated acceleration of heart rate and blood vessel tone, are called the vasomotor center. The third, which controls parasympathetic-mediated slowing of heart rate, is called the cardioinhibitory center.

CHAPTER 22 DISORDERS OF BLOOD FLOW IN THE SYSTEMIC CIRCULATION

SECTION II: ASSESSING YOUR UNDERSTANDING

Activity A

1. blood vessels
2. endothelium
3. vasoconstriction, dilation
4. ischemia
5. Infarction
6. cholesterol
7. cholesterol, triglyceride
8. lipoproteins
9. lipolytic
10. small intestine, liver
11. Chylomicrons
12. bad cholesterol
13. low-density lipoprotein receptors, scavenger
14. atherosclerosis
15. good cholesterol
16. coronary heart disease
17. genetic
18. secondary
19. lower, elevate
20. Atherosclerosis
21. hypercholesterolemia
22. Cigarette smoking
23. inflammation
24. C-reactive protein
25. Homocysteine
26. free radicals
27. vasculitides
28. embolus
29. Thromboangiitis obliterans

30. Raynaud phenomenon
31. aneurysm
32. asymptomatic, rupture
33. hemorrhage
34. valves
35. deep vein thrombosis
36. Venous insufficiency
37. stasis of blood, increased blood coagulability, vessel wall injury

Activity B

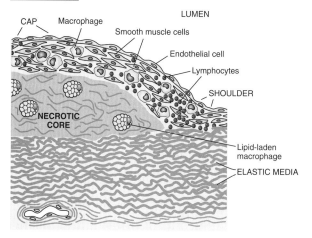

Activity C

1. h	**2.** i	**3.** g	**4.** j	**5.** d
6. a	**7.** f	**8.** c	**9.** e	**10.** b

Activity D

Following is the sequence of events of atherosclerotic pathogenesis:

1. Endothelial injury
2. Foam cell formation
3. Development of fatty streak
4. Formation of fibrofatty plaque
5. Complicated lesion

Activity E

1. Once believed to be nothing more than a lining for blood vessels, it is now known that the endothelium is a versatile, multifunctional tissue that plays an active role in controlling vascular function. As a semipermeable membrane, the endothelium controls the transfer of molecules across the vascular wall. The endothelium also plays a role in the control of platelet adhesion and blood clotting, modulation of blood flow and vascular resistance, metabolism of hormones, regulation of immune and inflammatory reactions, and elaboration of factors that influence the growth of other cell types, particularly vascular smooth muscle cells.

2. High-calorie diets increase the production of very low-density lipoprotein (VLDL) with triglyceride elevation and high conversion of VLDL to low-density lipoprotein (LDL). Excess ingestion of cholesterol may reduce the formation of LDL receptors and thereby decrease LDL removal. Diets that are high in triglycerides and saturated fats increase cholesterol synthesis and suppress LDL receptor activity. In diabetes mellitus and the metabolic syndrome, typical dyslipidemia is seen with elevation of triglycerides, low high-density lipoprotein, and minimal or modest elevation of LDL.

3. Lipid-lowering drugs work in several ways, including decreasing cholesterol production, decreasing cholesterol absorption from the intestine, or removing cholesterol from the bloodstream. Drugs that act directly to decrease cholesterol levels also have the beneficial effect of further lowering cholesterol levels by stimulating the production of additional low-density lipoprotein receptors.

4. The seven signs and symptoms of acute arterial occlusion are (a) pistol shot (acute onset), (b) pallor, (c) polar (cold), (d) pulselessness, (e) pain, (f) paresthesia, and (g) paralysis.

5. Ischemia due to vasospasm causes changes in skin color that progress from pallor to cyanosis, a sensation of cold, and changes in sensory perception, such as numbness and tingling. After the ischemic episode, there is a period of hyperemia with intense redness, throbbing, and paresthesias. In severe, progressive cases usually associated with Raynaud phenomenon, trophic changes may develop. The nails may become brittle, and the skin over the tips of the affected fingers may thicken. Ulceration and superficial gangrene of the fingers, although infrequent, may occur.

6. During muscle contraction, which is similar to systole, valves in the communicating channels close to prevent backward flow of blood into the superficial system, as blood in the deep veins is moved forward by the action of the contracting muscles. During muscle relaxation, which is similar to diastole, the communicating valves open, allowing blood from the superficial veins to move into the deep veins.

SECTION III: APPLYING YOUR KNOWLEDGE

Activity F

1. The nurse would expect to receive the following orders from the physician: CT and MRI

scans, aortic angiography, and trans-esophageal echocardiography

2. The priority nursing action is to give medication to lower the blood pressure. A large-bore IV would be started, and IV sodium nitroprusside would be given along with a β-adrenergic blocking drug.

SECTION IV: PRACTICING FOR NCLEX

Activity G

1. 1-f, 2-e, 3-b, 4-a, 5-d, 6-c. *Rationale:* Disturbances in blood flow can result from pathologic changes in the vessel wall (i.e., atherosclerosis, vasculitis), acute vessel obstruction due to thrombus or embolus, vasospasm (i.e., Raynaud phenomenon), or abnormal vessel dilation (i.e., arterial aneurysms or varicose veins).

2. a, d. *Rationale:* There are two sites of lipoprotein synthesis: the small intestine and the liver. The chylomicrons, which are the largest of the lipoprotein molecules, are synthesized in the wall of the small intestine. The liver synthesizes and releases very low-density lipoprotein and high-density lipoprotein. The large intestine and the pancreas play no part in synthesizing lipoprotein.

3. a. *Rationale:* Many types of primary hypercholesterolemia have a genetic basis. There may be a defective synthesis of the apoproteins, a lack of receptors, defective receptors, or defects in the handling of cholesterol in the cell that are genetically determined. For example, the low-density lipoprotein (LDL) receptor is deficient or defective in the genetic disorder known as familial hypercholesterolemia (type 2A). This autosomal dominant type of hyperlipoproteinemia results from a mutation in the gene specifying the receptor for LDL. Although heterozygotes commonly have an elevated cholesterol level from birth, they do not develop symptoms until adult life, when they often develop xanthomas (i.e., cholesterol deposits) along the tendons and atherosclerosis appears. Myocardial infarction (MI) before 40 years of age is common. Homozygotes are much more severely affected; they have cutaneous xanthomas in childhood and may experience MI by as early as 1 to 2 years of age. Homozygotic cutaneous xanthoma and adult onset hypercholesterolemia (type 1A) are not known diseases. Causes of secondary hyperlipoproteinemia include obesity with high-calorie intake and diabetes mellitus. It does not have a genetic basis.

4. b. *Rationale:* The cause or causes of atherosclerosis have not been determined with certainty. Epidemiologic studies have, however, identified predisposing risk factors, which include a major risk factor of hypercholesterolemia. Other risk factors include increasing age, family history of premature coronary heart disease, and male gender.

5. c. *Rationale:* Temporal arteritis (i.e., giant cell arteritis), the most common of the vasculitides, is a focal inflammatory condition of medium-size and large arteries. It predominantly affects branches of arteries originating from the aortic arch, including the superficial temporal, vertebral, ophthalmic, and posterior ciliary arteries. Neither polyarteritis nodosa nor Raynaud disease are the most common of the vasculitides. Varicose veins are not vasculitides.

6. c. *Rationale:* Acute arterial occlusion is a sudden event that interrupts arterial flow to the affected tissues or organ. Most acute arterial occlusions are the result of an embolus or a thrombus. Other answers are not appropriate for the nurse to give the client.

7. a, d. *Rationale:* Raynaud disease or phenomenon is a functional disorder caused by intense vasospasm of the arteries and arterioles in the fingers and, less often, the toes. There are two types of Raynaud disease: primary and secondary. The secondary type, called Raynaud phenomenon, is associated with other disease states or known causes of vasospasm. Raynaud phenomenon is associated with previous vessel injury, such as frostbite, occupational trauma associated with the use of heavy vibrating tools, collagen diseases, neurologic disorders, and chronic arterial occlusive disorders. The initial diagnosis is based on history of vasospastic attacks supported by other evidence of the disorder. Treatment measures are directed toward eliminating factors that cause vasospasm and protecting the digits from trauma during an ischemic episode. Abstinence from smoking and protection from cold are priorities. The presenting symptoms of this patient do not support a diagnosis of, or treatment for, arterial thrombosis or peripheral artery disease.

8. c, d. *Rationale:* Abdominal aortic aneurysms can involve any part of the vessel circumference (saccular) or extend to involve the entire circumference (fusiform). Berry aneurysms

typically occur in the circle of Willis. Dissecting aneurysms are false aneurysms and typically occur in the thoracic aorta. Aneurysms can occur at the bifurcation of a blood vessel but are not termed "bifurcating aneurysms."

9. b. *Rationale:* Sclerotherapy, which is often used in the treatment of small residual varicosities, involves the injection of a sclerosing agent into the collapsed superficial veins to produce fibrosis of the vessel lumen. Surgical treatment consists of removing the varicosities and the incompetent perforating veins, but it is limited to persons with patent deep venous channels. Sclerotherapy produces fibrosis of the vessel lumen. There is no fibrotherapy for varicose veins. There is no Trendelenburg therapy for varicose veins. There is a Trendelenburg test that is diagnostic for primary or secondary varicose veins.

10. d. *Rationale:* In 1846, Virchow described the triad that has come to be associated with venous thrombosis: stasis of blood, increased blood coagulability, and vessel wall injury. Inflammation is a symptom of venous thrombosis, not a risk factor. Decreased venous blood flow can occur because of venous thrombosis; if the thrombus does not completely obstruct the vein, it is not a risk factor. Hypocoagulability would not cause a thrombus to form.

CHAPTER 23 DISORDERS OF BLOOD PRESSURE REGULATION

SECTION II: ASSESSING YOUR UNDERSTANDING

Activity A

1. Arterial
2. systolic, diastolic
3. pulse pressure
4. mean arterial pressure
5. cardiac output, peripheral vascular resistance
6. vessel constriction, fluid retention
7. equilibrium
8. kidneys, sodium, water
9. Primary, secondary
10. 140 mm Hg, 90 mm Hg
11. constitutional
12. left ventricle
13. nephrosclerosis
14. ischemic, hemorrhage
15. 140/90 mm Hg
16. Diuretics
17. β_1-adrenergic
18. calcium channel receptor-blocking
19. systole
20. secondary
21. oral contraceptive
22. Malignant
23. Preeclampsia-eclampsia
24. orthostatic hypotension.
25. Antihypertensive, psychotropic

Activity B

1. Mechanisms of blood pressure regulation. The solid lines represent the mechanisms for renal and baroreceptor control of blood pressure through changes in cardiac output and peripheral vascular resistance. The dashed lines represent the stimulus for regulation of blood pressure by the baroreceptors and the kidneys.

2.

Assumption of the upright position

Activity C

1. i.	**2.** h	**3.** d	**4.** j	**5.** a
6. b	**7.** e	**8.** g	**9.** f	**10.** c

Activity D

1. Decrease in blood pressure
2. Stimulation of juxtaglomerular apparatus
3. Release of renin
4. Conversion of angiotensinogen to angiotensin I
5. Conversion of angiotensin I to angiotensin II by angiotensin-converting enzyme
6. Increased vascular resistance, release of aldosterone
7. Na$^+$ retention, stimulation of ADH release
8. Water retention

Activity E

1. Short-term regulation is accomplished through the cardiovascular center of the autonomic nervous system, baroreceptors, and chemoreceptors. The cardiovascular center transmits parasympathetic impulses to the heart through the vagus nerve and sympathetic impulses to the heart and blood vessels through the spinal cord and peripheral sympathetic nerves. The baroreceptors are pressure-sensitive receptors located in the walls of blood vessels and the heart. They respond to changes in the stretch of the vessel wall by sending impulses to cardiovascular centers in the brain stem to effect appropriate changes in heart rate and vascular smooth muscle tone. The arterial chemoreceptors are chemosensitive cells that monitor the oxygen, carbon dioxide, and hydrogen ion content of the blood.

2. Most acute kidney disorders result in decreased urine formation, retention of salt and water, and hypertension. Renovascular hypertension refers to hypertension caused by reduced renal blood flow and activation of the renin-angiotensin-aldosterone mechanism. The reduced renal blood flow that occurs with renovascular disease causes the affected kidney to release excessive amounts of renin, increasing circulating levels of angiotensin II. Angiotensin II, in turn, acts as a vasoconstrictor to increase peripheral vascular resistance and as a stimulus for increased aldosterone levels and sodium retention by the kidney.

3. Decreases in blood pressure are sensed by the juxtaglomerular apparatus, which releases renin. Renin, an enzyme, will react with its substrate angiotensinogen in circulation to form angiotensin I. Angiotensin I is converted to angiotensin II by angiotensin-converting enzyme, which is found on epithelial cells. Angiotensin II is a potent vasoconstrictor; it stimulates the release of ADH and aldosterone. ADH will increase water retention in the kidney, and aldosterone will increase Na$^+$ retention, which will facilitate water resorption. This effectively increases peripheral resistance and increases vascular volume.

4. Among the aging processes that contribute to an increase in blood pressure is stiffening of the large arteries, particularly the aorta. With aging, the elastin fibers in the walls of the arteries are gradually replaced by collagen fibers that render the vessels stiffer and less compliant. Decreased baroreceptor sensitivity, increased peripheral vascular resistance, and decreased renal blood flow also contribute.

SECTION III: APPLYING YOUR KNOWLEDGE

Activity F

1. The following assessments need to be made in further evaluating this patient: (a) history to elicit symptoms, especially dizziness and history of syncope and falls; medical conditions such as diabetes mellitus; use of prescription and over-the-counter drugs; and symptoms of autonomic nervous system dysfunction (i.e., erectile or bladder dysfunction); (b) physical examination to document blood pressure in both arms and the heart rate while in supine, sitting, and standing positions, noting especially the occurrence of symptoms; and (c) noninvasive, 24-hour ambulatory blood pressure monitoring

2. Treatment of orthostatic hypotension is usually directed toward alleviating the cause or, if this is not possible, toward helping people learn ways to cope with the disorder and prevent falls and injuries. Medications that predispose to postural hypotension should be avoided. Correcting the fluid deficit and trying a different antihypertensive medication are examples of measures designed to correct the cause.

3. We would teach your father to do things such as sitting on the edge of the bed for a few minutes and moving his legs before getting up; avoiding alcohol and vigorous exercise in a warm environment; using diuretics in moderation; and exerting himself only to the point where he is ready to sweat or lose body fluids. It might also be necessary for him to learn to wear tight-fitting elastic support hose or an

abdominal support garment to help prevent pooling of blood in the lower extremities and abdomen.

SECTION IV: PRACTICING FOR NCLEX
Activity G

1. c. *Rationale:* At normal heart rates, mean arterial pressure can be estimated by adding one-third of the pulse pressure to the diastolic pressure (i.e., diastolic blood pressure pulse pressure/3).

2. a, b, e. *Rationale:* The constitutional risk factors include a family history of hypertension, race, and age-related increases in blood pressure. Another factor that is believed to contribute to hypertension is insulin resistance and the resultant hyperinsulinemia that occurs in metabolic abnormalities such as type 2 diabetes. Lifestyle factors can contribute to the development of hypertension by interacting with other risk factors. These lifestyle factors include high salt intake, excessive calorie intake and obesity, excessive alcohol consumption, and low intake of potassium. Although stress can raise blood pressure acutely, there is less evidence linking it to chronic elevations in blood pressure. Smoking and a diet high in saturated fats and cholesterol, although not identified as primary risk factors for hypertension, are independent risk factors for coronary heart disease and should be avoided.

3. d. *Rationale:* Like adrenal medullary cells, the tumor cells of a pheochromocytoma produce and secrete the catecholamines, epinephrine and norepinephrine. The hypertension that develops is a result of the massive release of these catecholamines. Their release may be paroxysmal rather than continuous, causing periodic episodes of headache, excessive sweating, and palpitations. Headache is the most common symptom and can be quite severe. Nervousness, tremor, facial pallor, weakness, fatigue, and weight loss occur less frequently. Marked variability in blood pressure between episodes is typical.

4. a. *Rationale:* Because chronic hypertension is associated with autoregulatory changes in coronary artery, cerebral artery, and kidney blood flow, care should be taken to avoid excessively rapid decreases in blood pressure, which can lead to hypoperfusion and ischemic injury. Therefore, the goal of initial treatment measures should be to obtain a partial reduction in blood pressure to a safer, less critical level, rather than to normotensive levels.

5. b. *Rationale:* Cerebral vasoconstriction is probably an exaggerated homeostatic response designed to protect the brain from excesses of blood pressure and flow. The regulatory mechanisms are often insufficient to protect the capillaries, and cerebral edema frequently develops. As it advances, papilledema (i.e., swelling of the optic nerve at its point of entrance into the eye) ensues, giving evidence of the effects of pressure on the optic nerve and retinal vessels. The patient may have headache, restlessness, confusion, stupor, motor and sensory deficits, and visual disturbances. In severe cases, convulsions and coma follow. Lethargy, nervousness, and hyperreflexia are not signs or symptoms of cerebral edema in malignant hypertension.

6. c. *Rationale:* Liver damage, when it occurs, may range from mild hepatocellular necrosis with elevation of liver enzymes to the more ominous Hemolysis, Elevated Liver function tests, and Low Platelet count (HELLP) syndrome that is associated with significant maternal mortality.

7. d. *Rationale:* Hypertension in infants is associated most commonly with high umbilical catheterization and renal artery obstruction caused by thrombosis. Cerebral vascular bleeds, coarctation of the aorta, and pheochromocytoma can raise blood pressure; however, they are not the most common cause of hypertension in an infant.

8. a. *Rationale:* Among the aging processes that contribute to an increase in blood pressure are a stiffening of the large arteries, particularly the aorta; decreased baroreceptor sensitivity; increased peripheral vascular resistance; and decreased renal blood flow.

9. b. *Rationale:* Pseudohypertension should be suspected in older persons with hypertension in whom the radial or brachial artery remains palpable but pulseless at higher cuff pressures. The presenting parameters of the patient are not compatible with essential, orthostatic, or secondary hypertension.

10. c. *Rationale:* The renin-angiotensin-aldosterone system plays a central role in blood pressure regulation. Angiotensin II has two major functions in the rennin-angiotensin-aldosterone system and acts as both a short- and a long-term regulation of blood pressure. It is a strong vasoconstrictor, especially of the

arterioles regulating blood pressure in the short term. However, its second major action, the stimulation of aldosterone secretion from the adrenal gland, is the end of the renin-angiotensin-aldosterone loop. The aldosterone that is secreted notifies the kidneys to stop production or rennin (the negative feedback in the loop) and contributes to the long-term regulation of blood pressure by increasing salt and water retention by the kidney.

CHAPTER 24 DISORDERS OF CARDIAC FUNCTION

SECTION II: ASSESSING YOUR UNDERSTANDING

Activity A

1. pericardium
2. frictional
3. pericarditis
4. effusion
5. tamponade
6. constrictive
7. atherosclerosis
8. metabolic activity, autoregulatory
9. increased activity
10. 12-lead ECG
11. Echocardiography
12. Atherosclerosis
13. stable, unstable
14. chronic ischemic heart disease, acute coronary syndrome
15. T-wave inversion, ST-segment elevation, development of an abnormal Q wave
16. resting membrane potential
17. troponin assays
18. Acute ST-segment
19. 20 to 40
20. ventricular remodeling
21. vagal
22. nitroglycerin
23. Atherectomy
24. papillary muscle
25. Stable angina
26. exertion, emotional
27. genetic
28. mixed
29. hypertrophic cardiomyopathy
30. Dilated
31. Polyarthritis
32. neurologic
33. valves
34. stenosis

35. regurgitation
36. prolapse
37. stenosis
38. regurgitation
39. fetal heart
40. blood, cyanosis, pulmonary
41. acyanotic
42. ventricular septal
43. Kawasaki

Activity B

Activity C

1.

1. i	**2.** h	**3.** c	**4.** d	**5.** a
6. f	**7.** g	**8.** b	**9.** e	**10.** j

2.

1. g	**2.** e	**3.** b	**4.** h	**5.** a
6. f	**7.** c	**8.** j	**9.** i	**10.** d

Activity D

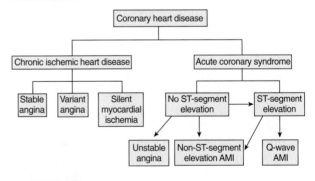

Activity E

1. The pericardial cavity has little reserve volume, so small additions of fluid increase the pericardial pressure. Right heart filling pressures are lower than the left, and increases in pericardial fluid pressure will result in decreased right-side filling.
2. Myocardial oxygen supply is determined by the coronary arteries, capillary inflow, and ability of hemoglobin to transport and

deliver oxygen to the heart muscle. Important factors in the transport and delivery of oxygen include the fraction of inspired oxygen in the blood and the number of red blood cells with normal functioning hemoglobin. There are three major determinants of myocardial oxygen demand (MVO_2): the heart rate, myocardial contractility, and myocardial wall stress or tension. The heart rate is the most important factor in myocardial oxygen demand for two reasons: (a) as the heart rate increases, myocardial oxygen consumption or demand also increases; and (b) subendocardial coronary blood flow is reduced because of the decreased diastolic filling time with increased heart rates.

3. On rupture, lipid core provides a stimulus for platelet aggregation and thrombus formation. Both smooth muscle and foam cells in the lipid core contribute to the expression of tissue factor in unstable plaques. Once exposed to blood, tissue factor initiates the extrinsic coagulation pathway, resulting in the local generation of thrombin and deposition of fibrin.

4. Biomarkers for acute coronary syndrome include cardiac-specific troponin I and troponin T, myoglobin, and creatine kinase MB. As the myocardial cells become necrotic, their intracellular enzymes begin to diffuse into the surrounding interstitium and then into the blood.

5. The pathophysiology is divided into three phases: development of the unstable plaque that ruptures, the acute ischemic event, and the long-term risk of recurrent events that remain after the acute event. Inflammation plays a prominent role in plaque instability, with inflammatory cells releasing cytokines that cause the fibrous cap to become thinner and more vulnerable to rupture. The acute ischemic event can be caused by an increase in myocardial oxygen demand precipitated by tachycardia or hypertension, or, more commonly, by a decrease in oxygen supply related to a reduction in coronary lumen diameter due to platelet-rich thrombi or vessel spasm.

6. The extent of the infarct depends on the location and extent of occlusion, amount of heart tissue supplied by the vessel, duration of the occlusion, metabolic needs of the affected tissue, extent of collateral circulation, and other factors such as heart rate, blood pressure, and cardiac rhythm. An infarct may involve the endocardium, myocardium, epicardium, or a combination of these.

7. The term reperfusion refers to reestablishment of blood flow through use of fibrinolytic therapy, percutaneous coronary intervention, or coronary artery bypass grafting. Early reperfusion (within 15–20 minutes) after onset of ischemia can prevent necrosis and improve myocardial perfusion in the infarct zone. Reperfusion after a longer interval can salvage some of the myocardial cells that would have died owing to longer periods of ischemia. It may also prevent microvascular injury that occurs over a longer period.

8. Cardiomyopathy is a heterogeneous group of diseases of the myocardium associated with mechanical and/or electrical dysfunction that usually exhibit inappropriate ventricular hypertrophy or dilatation and are due to a variety of causes that frequently are genetic. Cardiomyopathies are either confined to the heart or part of generalized systemic disorders, often leading to cardiovascular death or progressive heart failure–related disability.

9. Rheumatic heart disease is a complication of immune-mediated response to group A streptococcal throat infection. The acute stage of rheumatic fever includes history of an initiating streptococcal infection and subsequent involvement of the connective tissue elements of the heart, blood vessels, joints, and subcutaneous tissues. The recurrent phase usually involves extension of the cardiac effects of the disease. The chronic phase of rheumatic fever is characterized by permanent deformity of the heart valves.

10. Blood typically shunts across the ductus from the higher pressure left side to the lower pressure right side. A murmur is typically detected within days or weeks of birth. The murmur is loudest at the second left intercostal space, continuous through systole and diastole, and has a characteristic machinery sound. A widened pulse pressure is common due to the continuous runoff of aortic blood into the pulmonary artery.

11. Tetralogy of Fallot consists of four associated defects: (a) a ventricular septal defect involving the membranous septum and the anterior portion of the muscular septum; (b) dextroposition or shifting to the right of the aorta; (c) obstruction or narrowing of the pulmonary outflow channel, including pulmonic valve stenosis, a decrease in the size of the pulmonary trunk, or both; and (d) hypertrophy of the right ventricle because of the

increased work required to pump blood through the obstructed pulmonary channels.

SECTION III: APPLYING YOUR KNOWLEDGE

Activity F

1. Classic symptoms of a STEMI include:
   - Abrupt onset and pain as the significant symptom.
   - Pain that is typically severe, crushing, and usually substernal.
   - Pain that radiates to the left arm, neck, or jaw.
   - Pain that is not relieved by rest or nitroglycerin.
   - Gastrointestinal distress, including nausea and vomiting.
   - Fatigue and weakness, especially of the arms and legs.
   - Tachycardia, anxiety, restlessness, and feelings of impending doom.
   - Pale, cool, moist skin.
2. The emergency department goals of management for a patient with a STEMI are:
   - Identification of persons who are candidates for reperfusion therapy.
   - Evaluation of the person's chief complaint, typically chest pain, along with other associated symptoms to differentiate acute coronary syndrome from other diagnoses.
   - Institution of a monitor: a 12-lead ECG should be obtained and read by a physician within 10 minutes of arrival to the emergency department.
   - Administration of oxygen, aspirin, nitrates, pain medications, antiplatelet and anticoagulant therapy, β-adrenergic blocking agents, and an angiotensin-converting enzyme inhibitor.
   - Administration of immediate reperfusion therapy with a thrombolytic agent or percutaneous coronary intervention for persons with ECG evidence of infarction.

SECTION IV: PRACTICING FOR NCLEX

Activity G

1. a. *Rationale:* The pain is typically worse with deep breathing, coughing, swallowing, and positional changes because of changes in venous return and cardiac filling. All other answers make the pain worse.
2. b. *Rationale:* A key diagnostic finding is pulsus paradoxus, or an exaggeration of the normal variation in the systemic arterial pulse volume with respiration. None of the other answers occur in cardiac tamponade.
3. c. *Rationale:* Kussmaul's sign is an inspiratory distention of the jugular veins caused by the inability of the right atrium, encased in its rigid pericardium, to accommodate the increase in venous return that occurs with inspiration. None of the other physiologic signs occur in constrictive pericarditis.
4. a, c, e. *Rationale:* The major determinants of plaque vulnerability to disruption include the size of the lipid-rich core, the stability and thickness of its fibrous cap, the presence of inflammation, and lack of smooth muscle cells. A decrease in blood pressure and coronary blood flow are not determinants of plaque vulnerability to rupture.
5. d. *Rationale:* The troponin assays have high specificity for myocardial tissue and have become the primary biomarker for the diagnosis of myocardial infarction (MI). The troponin complex, which is part of the actin filament, consists of three subunits (i.e., TnC, TnT, TnI) that regulate calcium-mediated actin-myosin contractile process in striated muscle. TnI and TnT, which are present in cardiac muscle, begin to rise within 3 hours after the onset of MI and may remain elevated for 7 to 10 days after the event. This is especially adventitious in the late diagnosis of MI. The other blood work may be ordered, but not to confirm the diagnosis of MI.
6. b, d. *Rationale:* Unstable angina (UA)/non–ST-segment elevation myocardial infarction (NSTEMI) is classified as either low or intermediate risk of acute MI, the diagnosis of which is based on the clinical history, ECG pattern, and serum biomarkers. The other answers are not diagnostic of UA/NSTEMI.
7. a. *Rationale:* The principal biochemical consequence of MI is the conversion from aerobic to anaerobic metabolism with inadequate production of energy to sustain normal myocardial function. As a result, a striking loss of contractile function occurs within 60 seconds of onset. None of the other answers occur.
8. b. *Rationale:* Although a number of analgesic agents have been used to treat the pain of STEMI, morphine is usually the drug of choice. It is indicated if chest pain is unrelieved with oxygen and nitrates. The reduction in anxiety that accompanies the administration of morphine contributes to

a decrease in restlessness and autonomic nervous system activity, with a subsequent decrease in the metabolic demands of the heart. Morphine does not cause a feeling of depression to the patient.

9. c. *Rationale:* If blood flow can be restored within the 20- to 40-minute time frame, loss of cell viability does not occur or is minimal.

10. d. *Rationale:* Angina pectoris is usually precipitated by situations that increase the work demands of the heart, such as physical exertion, exposure to cold, and emotional stress. The pain is typically described as a constricting, squeezing, or suffocating sensation. It is usually steady, increasing in intensity only at the onset and end of the attack. Changing positions abruptly does not cause an attack of angina pectoris.

11. a. *Rationale:* Serum biochemical markers for myocardial infarction are normal in patients with chronic stable angina. All other answers are tests used in the diagnosis of angina.

12. Hypertrophic cardiomyopathy—genetic
Left ventricular noncompaction—genetic
Myocarditis—acquired
Dilated cardiomyopathy—mixed
Peripartum cardiomyopathy—acquired

13. b. *Rationale:* Alcoholic cardiomyopathy is the single most common identifiable cause of DCM in the United States and Europe. The other answers are incorrect.

14. c. *Rationale:* The intracardiac vegetative lesions also have local and distant systemic effects. The loose organization of these lesions permits the organisms and fragments of the lesions to form emboli and travel in the bloodstream, causing cerebral, systemic, or pulmonary emboli. Prevention of the valves of the heart from either opening or closing completely is not a systemic effect of the lesions. Fragmentation of the lesions does not make them larger.

15. d. *Rationale:* It is believed that antibodies directed against the M protein of certain strains of streptococci cross-react with glycoprotein antigens in the heart, joint, and other tissues to produce an autoimmune response through a phenomenon called molecular mimicry. None of the other answers are correct.

16. a. *Rationale:* Persons with palpitations and mild tachyarrhythmias or increased adrenergic symptoms, as well as those with chest dis-

comfort, anxiety, and fatigue, often respond to therapy with the β-adrenergic blocking drugs. None of the other types of drugs are used in the treatment of mitral valve prolapse to relieve symptoms or prevent complications.

17. b. *Rationale:* Heart failure manifests itself as tachypnea or dyspnea at rest or on exertion. For the infant, this most commonly occurs during feeding. The other answers are incorrect.

18. c. *Rationale:* The degree of obstruction may be dynamic and can increase during periods of stress, causing hypercyanotic attacks ("tet spells"). None of the other answers occur in association with tetralogy of Fallot or tet spells.

CHAPTER 25 DISORDERS OF CARDIAC CONDUCTION AND RHYTHM

SECTION II: ASSESSING YOUR UNDERSTANDING

Activity A

1. pacemaker
2. interrupts
3. circumflex
4. Purkinje system
5. Depolarization
6. Repolarization
7. absolute refractory period
8. ECG
9. frontal or vertical, horizontal
10. lead specific
11. rhythm, impulse conduction
12. automaticity
13. reentry
14. paroxysmal supraventricular tachycardias
15. sinus rhythm
16. Premature atrial contractions
17. bundle of His
18. sawtooth
19. Atrial fibrillation
20. torsade de pointes
21. premature ventricular contraction
22. Ventral tachycardia
23. quivers
24. Heart block
25. First
26. Ischemic
27. Catecholaminergic polymorphic
28. pacemaker, cardioversion, defibrillation

Activity B

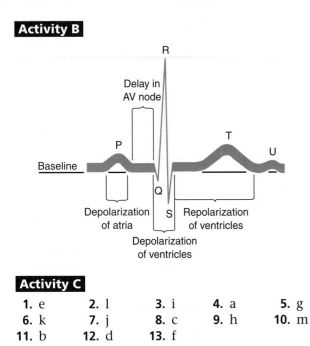

Activity C

1. e	2. l	3. i	4. a	5. g
6. k	7. j	8. c	9. h	10. m
11. b	12. d	13. f		

Activity D

1. Sinoatrial node depolarization
2. Atrioventricular node depolarization
3. Bundle of His
4. Bundle branches
5. Purkinje fibers

Activity E

1. The point at which the Na$^+$ channels open is called the depolarization threshold. When the cell has reached this threshold, a rapid influx of Na$^+$ occurs. This rapid influx of Na$^+$ produces a rapid, positively directed change in the transmembrane potential, resulting in the electrical spike and overshoot during phase 0 of the action potential. The rapid depolarization that comprises phase 0 is responsible for the QRS complex on the ECG. Depolarization of a cardiac cell causes adjacent cells to depolarize, stimulating a wave of depolarization across the heart, cell by cell. Phase 1 occurs at the peak of the action potential and signifies inactivation of the fast Na$^+$ channels with an abrupt decrease in sodium permeability. Phase 2 represents the plateau of the action potential. K$^+$ permeability is low. An influx of Ca^{++} into the cell contributes to the phase 2 plateau. The phase 2 plateau coincides with the ST segment of the ECG. During the phase 3 repolarization period, the slow Ca^{++} channels close, and the influx of Ca^{++} and Na$^+$ ceases. There is a sharp rise in K$^+$ permeabil-

ity, contributing to the rapid outward movement of K$^+$ and reestablishment of the resting membrane potential. Phase 4 represents the resting membrane potential. Phase 4 corresponds to diastole.

2. There are several forms of reentry: anatomic, functional, and reflective. Anatomic reentry consists of an excitation wave that travels in a set pathway. Functional reentry depends on the local differences in conduction velocity. Reflection is another form of reentry that can occur in parallel pathways of myocardial tissue or the Purkinje network.

3. Anticoagulant medications may be used to prevent embolic stroke, and medications may be used to control the ventricular rate in persons with persistent atrial fibrillation. Cardioversion may be considered when pulmonary edema or unstable cardiac status is present.

4. Long QT syndrome can be caused by various agents and conditions that reduce the magnitude of outward repolarizing potassium currents, enhance the magnitude of the inward depolarizing sodium and calcium currents, or both. Thus, there is delayed repolarization of the ventricles with development of early depolarizing afterpotentials that initiate the arrhythmia.

5. The exercise stress test elicits the body's response to measured increases in acute exercise. This technique provides information about changes in heart rate, blood pressure, respiration, and perceived level of exercise. It is useful in determining exercise-induced alterations in hemodynamic response and ECG ischemic-type ST segment changes, and can detect and classify disturbances in cardiac rhythm and conduction associated with exercise. These changes are indicative of a poorer prognosis in persons with known coronary disease and recent myocardial infarction.

6. Antiarrhythmic drugs act by modifying disordered formation and conduction of impulses that induce cardiac muscle contraction. Class I medications block fast sodium channels, thus slowing depolarization. Class II drugs are β-adrenergic blocking drugs that act by blunting the effect of sympathetic nervous system stimulation on the heart, thereby inhibiting calcium channel opening, and thus decreasing rate and contractility. Class III drugs act by inhibiting the potassium current and repolarization, thereby extending the action potential and refractory period. Class IV drugs act by blocking

the slow calcium channels, reducing the force of myocardial contractility, and thereby decreasing myocardial oxygen demand.

SECTION III: APPLYING YOUR KNOWLEDGE

Activity F

1. The drugs of choice for atrial fibrillation are anticoagulant medications and medications such as digitalis and beta blockers used to control the ventricular rate of the heart.

2. The treatment used to convert atrial fibrillation to sinus rhythm is cardioversion. Complications of this treatment include an increased risk of thromboembolism.

SECTION IV: PRACTICING FOR NCLEX

Activity G

1. a. *Rationale:* Persons with acute coronary syndrome are at risk for developing extension of an infarcted area, ongoing myocardial ischemia, and life-threatening arrhythmias. Research has revealed that 80% to 90% of ECG-detected ischemic events are clinically silent. Thus, ECG monitoring is more sensitive than a patient's report of symptoms for identifying transient ongoing myocardial ischemia. Other answers are incorrect.

2. b. *Rationale:* Today, it is accepted that a more optimal rhythm is respiratory sinus arrhythmia. Respiratory sinus arrhythmia is a cardiac rhythm characterized by gradual lengthening and shortening of RR intervals. This variation in cardiac cycles is related to intrathoracic pressure changes that occur with respiration and resultant alterations in autonomic control of the sinoatrial node. The other answers do not cause the variation in cardiac cycles related to respiratory sinus arrhythmia.

3. c. *Rationale:* Sick sinus syndrome is a term that describes a number of forms of cardiac impulse formation and intraatrial and atrioventricular conduction abnormalities. In children, the syndrome is most commonly associated with congenital heart defects, particularly following corrective cardiac surgery.

4. a, b, c. *Rationale:* The treatment of atrial fibrillation depends on its cause, recency of onset, and persistence of the arrhythmia. The size of the pulse deficit and the atrial rate are not variables in treatment of atrial fibrillation.

5. d. *Rationale:* The long QT syndrome (LQTS) is characterized by prolongation of the QT interval that may result in a characteristic type of polymorphic ventricular tachycardia called torsade de pointes and sudden cardiac death. Torsade de pointes (twisting or rotating around a point) is a specific type of ventricular tachycardia. The term refers to the polarity of the QRS complex, which swings from positive to negative and vice versa. The QRS abnormality is characterized by large bizarre polymorphic multiformed QRS complexes that vary, often from beat to beat, in amplitude and direction, as well as in rotation of the complexes around the isoelectric line. Medications linked to LQTS include digitalis, antiarrhythmic agents (e.g., amiodarone, procainamide, quinidine), verapamil (calcium channel blocker), haloperidol (antipsychotic agent), and erythromycin (antibiotic).

6. a. *Rationale:* A distinguishing feature of second-degree atrioventricular block is that conducted P waves relate to QRS complexes with recurring PR intervals; that is, the association of P waves with QRS complexes is not random. The other answers are not correct.

7. d. *Rationale:* The disorder typically manifests in adulthood with very incomplete penetrance, and a high percentage of mutation carriers are asymptomatic. Cardiac events typically occur during sleep or rest. Cardiac events during exercise, on arising in the morning, and just before bedtime at night are not indicative of Brugada syndrome.

8. a, d. *Rationale:* Holter monitoring is useful for documenting arrhythmias, conduction abnormalities, and ST segment changes.

9. a. *Rationale:* This technique provides information about changes in heart rate, blood pressure, respiration, and perceived level of exercise. It is useful in determining exercise-induced alterations in hemodynamic response and ECG ischemic-type ST segment changes, and can detect and classify disturbances in cardiac rhythm and conduction associated with exercise. Exercise stress tests do not determine any of the other answers.

10.

Drug	Use	Class
Procainamide	Supraventricular and ventricular arrhythmias	Class IA
Atenolol	Supraventricular arrhythmias and tachyarrhythmias	Class II
Amiodarone	Treatment of serious ventricular arrhythmias	Class III
Diltiazem	Slowing the sinoatrial node pacemaker and inhibiting conduction in the atrioventricular node	Class IV
Lidocaine	Treating ventricular arrhythmias only	Class IB

11. b. *Rationale:* Ablation therapy is used for treating recurrent, life-threatening supraventricular and ventricular tachyarrhythmias. Ablative therapy may be performed by catheter or surgical techniques. It involves localized destruction, isolation, or excision of cardiac tissue that is considered to be arrhythmogenic. Ablation therapy does not involve open heart surgery. It neither excises ischemic cardiac tissue nor reestablishes conductivity in areas of mild infarct.

CHAPTER 26 HEART FAILURE AND CIRCULATORY SHOCK

SECTION II: ASSESSING YOUR UNDERSTANDING

Activity A

1. Heart failure
2. coronary artery disease, hypertension, valvular
3. large
4. Cardiac output
5. sympathetic, parasympathetic
6. stroke volume
7. Ejection fraction
8. decrease
9. normal
10. compensatory mechanisms
11. Frank-Starling
12. contractile, volume overload, pressure overload
13. diastolic
14. compress, increase, delay
15. tachycardia

16. side
17. peripheral edema
18. hepatic
19. Left ventricular failure
20. left
21. High-output failure
22. Low-output failure
23. C-reactive protein
24. myocardial hypertrophy
25. acute heart failure
26. Paroxysmal nocturnal
27. Acute pulmonary edema
28. brain
29. right
30. oxygenation
31. ventricular
32. brain natriuretic peptide
33. left ventricular
34. Circulatory shock
35. myocardial infarction
36. Hypovolemic
37. Vasodilatory
38. neurogenic shock
39. immune
40. Structural
41. Aging

Activity B

1.

1. j	2. f	3. d	4. i	5. c
6. b	7. e	8. a	9. g	10. h

2.

1. g	2. c	3. a	4. d	5. b
6. f	7. h	8. e		

3.

1. c	2. e	3. b	4. d	5. a

Activity C

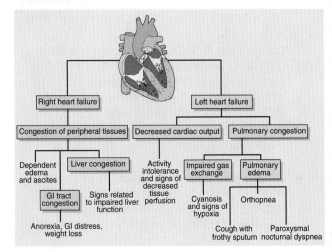

Activity D

1. A number of factors determine cardiac contractility by altering the systolic Ca^{++} levels. Catecholamines increase Ca^{++} entry into the cell by phosphorylation of the Ca^{++} channels via a cAMP-dependent protein kinase. Another mechanism that can modulate inotropy is the Na^+/Ca^+ exchange pump and the ATPase-dependent Ca^{++} pump on the myocardial cell membrane. These pumps transport Ca^{++} out of the cell, thereby preventing the cell from becoming overloaded with Ca^{++}. If Ca^{++} extrusion is inhibited, the rise in intracellular Ca^{++} can increase inotropy.

2. With both systolic and diastolic ventricular dysfunction, compensatory mechanisms are usually able to maintain adequate resting cardiac function until the later stages of heart failure. Therefore, cardiac function measured at rest is a poor clinical indicator of the extent of cardiac impairment because cardiac output may be relatively normal at rest.

3. With diastolic dysfunction, blood is unable to move freely into the left ventricle, causing an increase in intraventricular pressure at any given volume. The elevated pressures are transferred backward from the left ventricle into the atria and pulmonary venous system, causing a decrease in lung compliance that increases the work of breathing and evokes symptoms of dyspnea. Cardiac output is decreased because of a decrease in the volume (preload) available for adequate cardiac output. Inadequate cardiac output during exercise may lead to fatigue of the legs and the accessory muscles of respiration.

4. The many compensatory mechanisms of the cardiovascular system work in the following ways; however, they only serve to make heart failure worse:
   - Frank-Starling mechanism: increases inotropy, but eventually increases metabolic demand of cardiac tissue
   - Activation of the sympathetic nervous system: increases inotropy, but increases wall tension and metabolic demand
   - Renin-angiotensin-aldosterone mechanism: increases blood volume and maintains cardiac output, but eventually increases wall tension
   - Natriuretic peptides: inhibits sympathetic and renal compensation and decreases work of heart, but inactivation results in decreased cardiac output

   - Myocardial hypertrophy and remodeling: cardiomyocyte hypertrophy and increased inotropy, but demands more oxygen and increases metabolic needs

5. The signs and symptoms include shortness of breath and other respiratory manifestations, fatigue and limited exercise tolerance, fluid retention and edema, cachexia and malnutrition, and cyanosis. Persons with severe heart failure may exhibit diaphoresis and tachycardia. These signs are the result of decreased tissue perfusion and resultant hypoxia.

6. Diuretics promote the excretion of fluid and help sustain cardiac output and tissue perfusion by reducing preload and allowing the heart to operate at a more optimal part of the Frank-Starling curve.

7. In severe shock, cellular metabolic processes are essentially anaerobic due to the decreased availability of oxygen. Excess amounts of lactic acid accumulate in the cellular and extracellular compartments, limited amounts of ATP are produced, and normal cell function cannot be maintained. The sodium-potassium membrane pump is impaired, resulting in cellular edema and an increase in the permeability of cell membranes. Mitochondrial activity becomes severely depressed, and lysosomal membranes may rupture, resulting in the release of enzymes that cause further intracellular destruction. This is followed by cell death and the release of intracellular contents into the extracellular spaces. The destruction of the cell membrane activates the arachidonic acid cascade, release of inflammatory mediators, and production of oxygen free radicals that extend cellular damage.

8. The five major complications of severe shock are (a) pulmonary injury, (b) acute renal failure, (c) gastrointestinal ulceration, (d) disseminated intravascular coagulation, and (e) multiple organ dysfunction syndrome.

SECTION III: APPLYING YOUR KNOWLEDGE

Activity E

1. The diagnostic tests the nurse would expect to be ordered for this child would be echocardiograph, chest x-rays, and laboratory studies for anemia and electrolyte imbalances.

2. Drugs used in the treatment of heart failure in infants and children include inotropic agents such as digitalis, diuretics, and vasodilating agents. Medication dosages are based on the child's weight and renal function.

SECTION IV: PRACTICING FOR NCLEX
Activity F

1. 1-f, 2-a, 3-c, 4-b, 5-e, 6-d
2. a, c. *Rationale:* The signs and symptoms of heart failure include shortness of breath and other respiratory manifestations, fatigue and limited exercise tolerance, fluid retention and edema, cachexia and malnutrition, and cyanosis. Persons with severe heart failure may exhibit diaphoresis and tachycardia. A ruddy complexion, bradycardia, and a chronic productive cough are not signs or symptoms of heart failure.
3. a, b, d, e. *Rationale:* Shock is not a specific disease but a syndrome that can occur in the course of many life-threatening traumatic conditions or disease states. It can be caused by an alteration in cardiac function (cardiogenic shock), a decrease in blood volume (hypovolemic shock), excessive vasodilation with maldistribution of blood flow (distributive shock), or obstruction of blood flow through the circulatory system (obstructive shock). Excessive vasoconstriction and hypervolemia are not causes of shock.
4. a, c, e. *Rationale:* Signs and symptoms of cardiogenic shock include indications of hypoperfusion with hypotension, although a preshock state of hypoperfusion may occur with a normal blood pressure. The lips, nail beds, and skin may become cyanotic because of stagnation of blood flow and increased extraction of oxygen from the hemoglobin as it passes through the capillary bed. Mean arterial and systolic blood pressures decrease due to poor stroke volume, and there is a narrow pulse pressure and near-normal diastolic blood pressure due to arterial vasoconstriction. Urine output decreases due to lower renal perfusion pressures and the increased release of aldosterone. Elevation of preload is reflected in a rise in central venous pressure and pulmonary capillary wedge pressure. Neurologic changes, such as alterations in cognition or consciousness, may occur due to low cardiac output and poor cerebral perfusion. The other physiologic occurrences are not signs or symptoms of shock.
5. c. *Rationale:* The treatment of hypovolemic shock is directed toward correcting or controlling the underlying cause and improving tissue perfusion. Ongoing loss of blood must be corrected, such as in surgery. Oxygen is administered to increase oxygen delivery to the tissues. Medications are usually administered intravenously. In hypovolemic shock, the goal of treatment is to restore vascular volume. This can be accomplished through intravenous administration of fluids and blood. The crystalloids (e.g., isotonic saline, Ringer's lactate) are readily available and effective, at least temporarily. Plasma volume expanders (e.g., pentastarch, colloidal albumin) have a high molecular weight, do not necessitate blood typing, and remain in the vascular space for longer periods than the crystalloids, such as dextrose and saline. Blood or blood products (packed or frozen red cells) are administered based on hematocrit and hemodynamic findings. Fluids and blood are best administered based on volume indicators such as central venous pressure and urine output. Vasoactive medications are agents capable of constricting or dilating blood vessels. Considerable controversy exists about the advantages or disadvantages related to the use of these drugs. Generally, vasoconstrictor agents are not used as a primary form of therapy in hypovolemic shock and may be detrimental. These agents are given only when volume deficits have been corrected, yet hypotension persists.
6. a. *Rationale:* In contrast to other shock states due to the loss of blood volume or impaired cardiac function, the heart rate in neurogenic shock is often slower than normal, and the skin is dry and warm. This type of distributive shock is rare and usually transitory. The other answers are not correct.
7. b. *Rationale:* Anaphylaxis is a clinical syndrome that represents the most severe form of systemic allergic reaction. Anaphylactic shock results from an immune-mediated reaction in which vasodilator substances such as histamine are released into the blood. The vascular response in anaphylaxis is often accompanied by life-threatening laryngeal edema and bronchospasm, circulatory collapse, contraction of gastrointestinal and uterine smooth muscle, and urticaria (hives) or angioedema.
8. a. *Rationale:* Although activated neutrophils kill microorganisms, they also injure the endothelium by releasing mediators that increase vascular permeability. In addition, activated endothelial cells release nitric oxide, a potent vasodilator that acts as a key mediator of septic shock.
9. b. *Rationale:* The primary physiologic result of obstructive shock is elevated right heart

pressure due to impaired right ventricular function. The other answers are not correct.

10. c. *Rationale:* The degree of renal damage in shock is related to the severity and duration of shock. None of the other answers relate to the damage to the renal system in shock.

11. c. *Rationale:* Major risk factors for the development of MODS are severe trauma, sepsis, prolonged periods of hypotension, hepatic dysfunction, infarcted bowel, advanced age, and alcohol abuse. Respiratory dysfunction is not a major risk factor in MODS.

12. b. *Rationale:* Structural (congenital) heart defects are the most common cause of heart failure in children. The other answers are not correct.

CHAPTER 27 STRUCTURE AND FUNCTION OF THE RESPIRATORY SYSTEM

SECTION II: ASSESSING YOUR UNDERSTANDING

Activity A

1. gas exchange
2. conducting, respiratory
3. conducting
4. warmed, filtered, moistened
5. mucus
6. glottis
7. hyaline
8. hilum
9. pulmonary lobule
10. alveoli
11. pulmonary
12. lymphatic
13. parasympathetic
14. sympathetic
15. partial pressure
16. pressure difference
17. intrapleural
18. Valsalva
19. compliance
20. tidal volume
21. inspiratory reserve volume (IRV), expiratory reserve volume (ERV)
22. inspiratory capacity
23. vital capacity
24. minute volume
25. Pulmonary, alveolar
26. collapse
27. Dead space
28. mismatching
29. blood
30. Hemoglobin
31. cooperatively
32. pH, carbon dioxide, temperature
33. dissolved carbon dioxide, hemoglobin, bicarbonate
34. pneumotaxic, apneustic
35. chemoreceptors, lung
36. carbon dioxide
37. Dyspnea

Activity B

Trachea

Left primary bronchus

Secondary bronchi

Segmental bronchi

Terminal bronchioles

Activity C

1. f	2. g	3. h	4. b	5. i
6. a	7. c	8. j	9. d	10. e

Activity D

a→c→b→g→f→e→d

Activity E

1. The pleural membrane lines the thoracic cavity and encases the lungs. The outer parietal layer lines the pulmonary cavities and adheres to the thoracic wall, the mediastinum, and the diaphragm. The inner visceral pleura closely covers the lung and is adherent to its surfaces. It is continuous with the parietal pleura at the hilum of the lung, where the major bronchus and pulmonary vessels enter and leave the lung. A thin film of serous fluid separates the two pleural layers, allowing the two layers to glide over each other and yet hold together, so there is no separation between the lungs and the chest wall.

2. During inspiration, the size of the chest cavity increases, the intrathoracic pressure becomes more negative, and air is drawn into the lungs. The diaphragm is the principal muscle of inspiration. When the diaphragm contracts, the abdominal contents are forced downward, and

the chest expands from top to bottom. The external intercostal muscles, which also aid in inspiration, connect to the adjacent ribs and slope downward and forward. When they contract, they raise the ribs and rotate them slightly so that the sternum is pushed forward; this enlarges the chest from side to side and from front to back. The scalene muscles elevate the first two ribs, and the sternocleidomastoid muscles raise the sternum to increase the size of the chest cavity. Expiration is largely passive. It occurs as the elastic components of the chest wall and lung structures that were stretched during inspiration recoil, causing air to leave the lungs as the intrathoracic pressure increases. When needed, the abdominal and the internal intercostal muscles can be used to increase expiratory effort.

3. Pulmonary surfactant forms a monolayer with its hydrophilic surface binding to liquid film on the surface of the alveoli and its hydrophobic surface facing outward toward the gases in the alveolar air. This monolayer interrupts the surface tension that develops at the air–liquid interface in the alveoli, keeping them from collapsing and allowing equal inflation.

4. Gas diffusion in the lung is described by the Fick's law of diffusion. The Fick's law states that the volume of a gas diffusing across the membrane per unit time is directly proportional to the partial pressure difference of the gas (P1 – P2), the surface area (SA) of the membrane, and the diffusion coefficient (D), and is inversely proportional to the thickness (T) of the membrane.

5. Arterial blood is commonly used for measuring blood gases. Venous blood is not used because venous levels of oxygen and carbon dioxide reflect the metabolic demands of the tissues rather than the gas exchange function of the lungs.

6. Coughing is a neurally mediated reflex that protects the lungs from accumulation of secretions and from entry of irritating and destructive substances. It is one of the primary defense mechanisms of the respiratory tract. The cough reflex is initiated by receptors located in the tracheobronchial wall; these receptors are extremely sensitive to irritating substances and to the presence of excess secretions. Afferent impulses from these receptors are transmitted through the vagus to the medullary center, which integrates the cough response.

SECTION III: APPLYING YOUR KNOWLEDGE

Activity F

1. When the oxygen levels in the body drop below a specific set-point, the small blood vessels in the lungs go into a vasoconstrictive state; they squeeze down so very little blood can go through them. This means that no oxygen is exchanged at this point either. This vasoconstriction can occur in a limited part of the lung, or it can occur throughout the lung. This is called generalized hypoxia.

2. Arterial blood gas and pulmonary function tests would be ordered.

SECTION IV: PRACTICING FOR NCLEX

Activity G

1. a, c. *Rationale:* The lungs are the functional structures of the respiratory system. In addition to their gas exchange function, they inactivate vasoactive substances such as bradykinin and convert angiotensin I to angiotensin II. They also serve as a reservoir for blood storage. Heparin-producing cells are particularly abundant in the capillaries of the lung, where small clots may be trapped. The other functions do not occur in the lungs.

2. a. *Rationale:* The bronchial blood vessels are the only ones that can undergo angiogenesis (formation of new vessels) and develop collateral circulation when vessels in the pulmonary circulation are obstructed, as in pulmonary embolism. The development of new blood vessels helps keep lung tissue alive until the pulmonary circulation can be restored. The blood in the bronchiole blood vessels is unoxygenated, so they neither carry oxygen-rich blood to the lung tissues nor participate in gas exchange. Bronchiole blood vessels drain blood into the bronchial veins.

3. 1-b, 2-d, 3-c, 4-a

4. b. *Rationale:* Specifically, lung compliance (C) describes the change in lung volume (ΔV) that can be accomplished with a given change in respiratory pressure (ΔP); thus, $C = \Delta V/\Delta P$. This equation has nothing to do with surface tension, airway resistance, or change in peak expiratory flow.

5. c. *Rationale:* The work of breathing is determined by the amount of effort required to move air through the conducting airways and

by the ease of lung expansion, or compliance. Expansion of the lungs is difficult for persons with stiff and noncompliant lungs; they usually find it easier to breathe if they keep their tidal volume low and breathe at a more rapid rate (e.g., $300 \times 20 = 6,000$ mL) to achieve their minute volume and meet their oxygen needs. In contrast, persons with obstructive airway disease usually find it less difficult to inflate their lungs but expend more energy in moving air through the airways. As a result, these persons take deeper breaths and breathe at a slower rate (e.g., $600 \times 10 = 6,000$ mL) to achieve their oxygen needs. People with chronic obstructive pulmonary disease do not have hyperpneic breathing under normal conditions.

6. c. *Rationale:* The distribution of ventilation between the apex and base of the lung varies with body position and the effects of gravity on intrapleural pressure. Intrapleural pressure impacts the distribution of ventilation, not intrathoracic or alveolar pressures.

7. d. *Rationale:* Generalized hypoxia occurs at high altitudes and in persons with chronic hypoxia due to lung disease and causes vasoconstriction throughout the lung. Prolonged hypoxia can lead to pulmonary hypertension and increased workload on the right heart.

8. a. *Rationale:* Physiologic shunting of blood usually results from destructive lung disease that impairs ventilation or from heart failure that interferes with movement of blood through sections of the lungs. Obstructive lung disease, pulmonary hypertension, and regional hypoxia usually do not cause the physiologic shunting of blood.

9. b. *Rationale:* In the clinical setting, blood gas measurements are used to determine the partial pressure of oxygen and carbon dioxide in the blood. Arterial blood is commonly used for measuring blood gases. Venous blood is not used because venous levels of oxygen and carbon dioxide reflect the metabolic demands of the tissues rather than the gas exchange function of the lungs. The other answers are not correct.

10. a, c, e. *Rationale:* The automatic and voluntary components of respiration are regulated by afferent impulses that are transmitted to the respiratory center from a number of sources. Afferent input from higher brain centers is evidenced by the fact that a person can consciously alter the depth and rate of respiration. Fever, pain, and emotion exert their influence through lower brain centers.

11. d-c-e-a-b. *Rationale:* Coughing itself requires the rapid inspiration of a large volume of air (usually about 2.5 L), followed by rapid closure of the glottis and forceful contraction of the abdominal and expiratory muscles. As these muscles contract, intrathoracic pressures are elevated to levels of 100 mm Hg or more. The rapid opening of the glottis at this point leads to an explosive expulsion of air.

12. d. *Rationale:* Dyspnea is observed in at least three major cardiopulmonary disease states: primary lung diseases, such as pneumonia, asthma, and emphysema; heart disease that is characterized by pulmonary congestion; and neuromuscular disorders, such as myasthenia gravis and muscular dystrophy, that affect the respiratory muscles. Dyspnea is not an identified component of multiple sclerosis.

CHAPTER 28 RESPIRATORY TRACT INFECTIONS, NEOPLASMS, AND CHILDHOOD DISORDERS

SECTION II: ASSESSING YOUR UNDERSTANDING

Activity A

1. Viruses
2. bronchial, obstruct, bacterial
3. upper
4. rhinoviruses
5. Antihistamines
6. Rhinitis, paranasal
7. oxygen
8. hemagglutinin, neuraminidase
9. upper, viral, bacterial
10. vaccination
11. reassortment
12. pneumonia
13. Lobar pneumonia, bronchopneumonia
14. nosocomial
15. immunocompromised
16. Legionnaire
17. mycoplasma
18. Tuberculosis
19. waxy

20. Primary
21. tuberculin skin, x-rays
22. Histoplasmosis
23. Fungal
24. smoking
25. 80%
26. Lung cancers
27. small cell lung cancers (SCLCs)
28. non–small cell lung cancers (NSCLCs)
29. Croup
30. 25th to 28th

Activity B

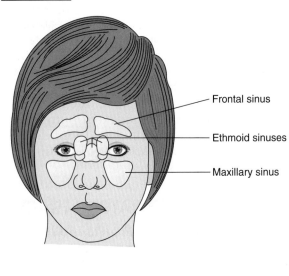

Activity C

1. i	**2.** c	**3.** a	**4.** b	**5.** d
6. j	**7.** e	**8.** f	**9.** g	**10.** h

Activity D

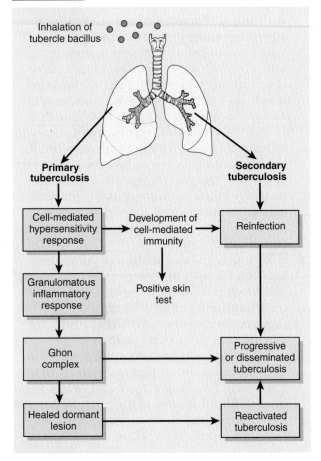

Activity E

1. The fingers are the greatest source of spread, and the nasal mucosa and conjunctival surface of the eyes are the most common portals of entry of the virus. The most highly contagious period is during the first 3 days after the onset of symptoms, and the incubation period is approximately 5 days. Cold viruses have been found to survive for more than 5 hours on the skin and hard surfaces, such as plastic countertops. Aerosol spread of colds, through coughing and sneezing, is much less important than the spread by fingers picking up the virus from contaminated surfaces and carrying it to the nasal membranes and eyes.

2. Contagion results from the ability of the influenza A virus to develop new HA and NA subtypes against which the population is not protected. An antigenic shift, which involves a major genetic rearrangement in either antigen, may lead to epidemic or pandemic infection. Lesser changes, called antigenic drift, find the population partially protected by cross-reacting antibodies.

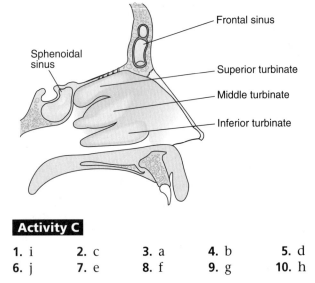

3. Viral pneumonia occurs as a complication of influenza. It typically develops within 1 day after onset of influenza and is characterized by rapid progression of fever, tachypnea, tachycardia, cyanosis, and hypotension. The clinical course of influenza pneumonia progresses rapidly. It can cause hypoxemia and death within a few days of onset. Survivors often develop diffuse pulmonary fibrosis.

4. The lung below the main bronchi is normally sterile, despite frequent entry of microorganisms into the air passages by inhalation during ventilation or aspiration of nasopharyngeal secretions. Bacterial pneumonia results due to loss of the cough reflex, damage to the ciliated endothelium that lines the respiratory tract, or impaired immune defenses. Bacterial adherence also plays a role in colonization of the lower airways. The epithelial cells of critically and chronically ill persons are more receptive to binding microorganisms that cause pneumonia. Other clinical risk factors favoring colonization of the tracheobronchial tree include antibiotic therapy that alters the normal bacterial flora, diabetes, smoking, chronic bronchitis, and viral infection.

5. During the first stage, alveoli become filled with protein-rich edema fluid containing numerous organisms. Marked capillary congestion follows, leading to massive outpouring of polymorphonuclear leukocytes and red blood cells. Because the first consistency of the affected lung resembles that of the liver, this stage is referred to as the "red hepatization" stage. The next stage involves the arrival of macrophages that phagocytose the fragmented polymorphonuclear cells, red blood cells, and other cellular debris. During this stage, which is termed the "gray hepatization" stage, the congestion has diminished, but the lung is still firm. The alveolar exudate is then removed, and the lung returns to normal.

6. *Mycobacterium tuberculosis hominis* is an airborne infection spread by minute, invisible particles called droplet nuclei that are harbored in the respiratory secretions of persons with active tuberculosis. Coughing, sneezing, and talking all create respiratory droplets; these droplets evaporate, leaving the organisms, which remain suspended in the air and are circulated by air currents. Thus, living under crowded and confined conditions increases the risk for spread of the disease.

7. Inhaled droplet nuclei pass down the bronchial tree without settling on the epithelium and are deposited in the alveoli. Soon after entering the lung, the bacilli are phagocytosed by alveolar macrophages, but resist killing, because cell wall lipids of the *Mycobacterium tuberculosis* block fusion of phagosomes and lysosomes. Although the macrophages that first ingest *M. tuberculosis* cannot kill the organisms, they initiate a cell-mediated immune response that eventually contains the infection. As the tubercle bacilli multiply, the infected macrophages degrade the mycobacteria and present their antigens to T lymphocytes. The sensitized T lymphocytes, in turn, stimulate the macrophages to increase their concentration of lytic enzymes and ability to kill the mycobacteria. When released, these lytic enzymes also damage lung tissue. The development of a population of activated T lymphocytes and related development of activated macrophages capable of ingesting and destroying the bacilli constitutes the cell-mediated immune response.

8. Lung cancer is classified as squamous cell lung carcinoma, adenocarcinoma, small cell carcinoma, and large cell carcinoma.

9. The manifestations of lung cancer can be divided into three categories: (a) those due to involvement of the lung and adjacent structures; (b) the effects of local spread and metastasis; and (c) nonmetastatic paraneoplastic manifestations involving endocrine, neurologic, and connective tissue function.

10. Pulmonary immaturity, together with surfactant deficiency, lead to alveolar collapse. The type II alveolar cells that produce surfactant do not begin to mature until approximately the 25th to 28th weeks of gestation, and consequently, many premature infants are born with poorly functioning type II alveolar cells and have difficulty producing sufficient amounts of surfactant. Without surfactant, the large alveoli remain inflated, whereas the small alveoli become difficult to inflate, resulting in respiratory distress syndrome.

SECTION III: APPLYING YOUR KNOWLEDGE

Activity F

1. Diagnostic tests for squamous cell cancer of the lung include chest radiography, bronchoscopy, cytologic studies (Papanicolaou

test) of the sputum or bronchial washings, percutaneous needle biopsy of lung tissue, scalene lymph node biopsy, CT scans, MRI studies, ultrasonography to locate lesions and evaluate the extent of the disease, and positron emission tomography, a noninvasive alternative for identifying metastatic lesions in the mediastinum or distant sites.

2. Treatments used for squamous cell (non–small cell lung cancer [NSCLC]) cancer of the lung include surgery—for the removal of small, localized NSCLC tumors; radiation therapy—a definitive or main treatment modality for palliation of symptoms; and chemotherapy—often using a combination of drugs. A combination of these treatments can also be used.

SECTION IV: PRACTICING FOR NCLEX

Activity G

1. c. *Rationale:* Decongestant drugs (i.e., sympathomimetic agents) are available in over-the-counter nasal sprays, drops, and oral cold medications. These drugs constrict the blood vessels in the swollen nasal mucosa and reduce nasal swelling. Rebound nasal swelling can occur with indiscriminate use of nasal drops and sprays. Oral preparations containing decongestants may cause systemic vasoconstriction and elevation of blood pressure when given in doses large enough to relieve nasal congestion. They should be avoided by persons with hypertension, heart disease, hyperthyroidism, diabetes mellitus, or other health problems.

2. b. *Rationale:* One distinguishing feature of an influenza viral infection is the rapid onset, sometimes in as little as 1 to 2 minutes, of profound malaise. None of the other answers are distinguishing characteristics of an influenza viral infection.

3. c. *Rationale:* Recently, a highly pathogenic influenza A subtype H5N1 was found in poultry in East and Southeast Asian countries. Although the H5N1 strain is highly contagious from one bird to another, the transmission from human to human is relatively inefficient and not sustained. The result is only rare cases of person-to-person transmission. Most cases occur after exposure to infected poultry or surfaces contaminated with poultry droppings. Because infection in humans is associated with high mortality, there exists considerable concern that the H5N1 strain might mutate and initiate a pandemic.

4. a, c, d. *Rationale:* Community-acquired pneumonia may be further categorized according risk of mortality and need for hospitalization based on age, presence of coexisting disease, and severity of illness using physical examination findings and laboratory and radiologic findings. The other answers are not categories used to classify community-acquired pneumonia.

5. d. *Rationale:* Neutropenia and impaired granulocyte function, as occurs in persons with leukemia, chemotherapy, and bone marrow depression, predispose to infections caused by *Staphylococcus aureus, Aspergillus*, gram-negative bacilli, and candida. The other organisms can cause pneumonia, but they are not usually seen in people with neutropenia and impaired granulocyte function.

6. a. *Rationale:* Elderly persons are less likely to experience marked elevations in temperature; in these persons, the only sign of pneumonia may be a loss of appetite and deterioration in mental status. Pleuritic pain, a sharp pain that is more severe with respiratory movements, is common.

7. b. *Rationale:* The pathogenesis of tuberculosis in a previously unexposed immunocompetent person is centered on the development of a cell-mediated immune response that confers resistance to the organism and development of tissue hypersensitivity to the tubercular antigens. The destructive nature of the disease, such as caseating necrosis and cavitation, results from the hypersensitivity immune response rather than the destructive capabilities of the tubercle bacillus. Tuberculosis does not have rapidly progressing pulmonary lesions, nor does it have purulent necrosis or purulent pulmonary lesions.

8. c. *Rationale:* The oral antifungal drugs itraconazole and fluconazole are used for treatment of less severe forms of infection. Intravenous amphotericin B is used in the treatment of persons with progressive disease. Long-term treatment is often required. Bacillus Calmette-Guérin is an attenuated strain of live tubercle vaccine. Rifampin is an oral drug used in the treatment of tuberculosis.

9. d. *Rationale:* The non–small cell lung cancers (NSCLCs) include squamous cell carcinomas, adenocarcinomas, and large cell carcinomas. As with the small cell lung cancers (SCLCs), these cancers have the capacity to synthesize bioactive products and produce paraneoplas-

tic syndromes. NSCLCs do not neutralize bioactive syndromes. In addition, they neither synthesize ACTH nor produce panneoplastic syndromes.

10. a. *Rationale:* The infant with bronchopulmonary dysplasia (BPD) often demonstrates a barrel chest, tachycardia, rapid and shallow breathing, chest retractions, cough, and poor weight gain. Other signs and symptoms listed are not signs and symptoms of BPD.

11. Epiglottitis: Upper airway
Acute bronchiolitis: Lower airway
Asthma: Lower airway
Spasmodic croup: Upper airway
Laryngotracheobronchitis: Upper airway

12. b. *Rationale:* The child with bronchiolitis is at risk for respiratory failure resulting from impaired gas exchange. The other answers are not applicable.

CHAPTER 29 DISORDERS OF VENTILATION AND GAS EXCHANGE

SECTION II: ASSESSING YOUR UNDERSTANDING

Activity A

1. carbon dioxide (CO_2), oxygen (O_2)
2. Ventilation
3. oxygenation, removal of CO_2
4. Hypoxemia
5. hypoxia
6. ventilation, vasoconstriction, red blood
7. Hypercapnia
8. pH, acidosis
9. Pleural effusion
10. Hemothorax
11. inflated
12. expiratory
13. asthma
14. T lymphocyte
15. Chronic obstructive
16. inflammation, fibrosis
17. Emphysema, proteases
18. α_1-antitrypsin
19. hypersecretion of mucus
20. pink puffers
21. blue bloaters
22. Bronchiectasis
23. Cystic fibrosis
24. interstitial
25. collagen, elastic
26. embolism
27. pulmonary embolism
28. Pulmonary hypertension
29. hypoxemia
30. Respiratory failure

Activity B

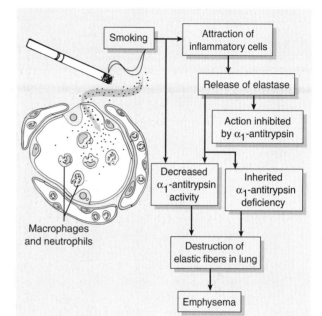

Activity C

1.

1. d	**2.** b	**3.** i	**4.** a	**5.** j
6. e	**7.** f	**8.** g	**9.** h	**10.** c

2.

1. e	**2.** b	**3.** g	**4.** i	**5.** d
6. j	**7.** a	**8.** h	**9.** f	**10.** c

Activity D

1.

Activity E

1. The mechanisms that result in hypoxemia are hypoventilation, impaired diffusion of gases, inadequate circulation of blood through the pulmonary capillaries, and mismatching of ventilation and perfusion.

2. The clinical manifestations of atelectasis include tachypnea, tachycardia, dyspnea, cyanosis, signs of hypoxemia, diminished chest expansion, absence of breath sounds, and intercostal retractions. Both chest expansion and breath sounds are decreased on the affected area. There may be intercostal retraction over the involved area during inspiration.

3. The symptoms of the acute response are caused by the release of chemical mediators from the presensitized mast cells. Mediator release results in the infiltration of inflammatory cells, opening of the mucosal intercellular junctions, and increased access of antigen to submucosal mast cells. There is bronchospasm caused by direct stimulation of parasympathetic receptors, mucosal edema caused by increased vascular permeability, and increased mucus secretions. The late phase response involves inflammation and increased airway responsiveness that prolong the asthma attack. An initial trigger in the late phase response causes the release of inflammatory mediators from mast cells, macrophages, and epithelial cells. These substances induce the migration and activation of other inflammatory cells, which then produce epithelial injury and edema, changes in mucociliary function, and reduced clearance of respiratory tract secretions, and increased airway responsiveness.

4. The two processes that are critical to the pathogenesis of bronchiectasis are airway obstruction and chronic persistent infection, causing damage to the bronchial walls, leading to weakening and dilation.

5. Cystic fibrosis is caused by mutations in a single gene on the long arm of chromosome 7 that encodes for the cystic fibrosis transmembrane regulator (CFTR), which functions as a chloride channel in epithelial cell membranes. Mutations in the CFTR gene render the epithelial membrane relatively impermeable to the chloride ion. The impaired transport of Cl^- ultimately leads to a series of secondary events, including increased absorption of Na^+ and water from the airways into the blood. This lowers the water content of the mucociliary blanket coating the respiratory epithelium, causing it to become more viscid. The resulting dehydration of the mucous layer leads to defective mucociliary function and accumulation of viscid secretions that obstruct the airways and predispose to recurrent pulmonary infections. The obstruction develops from the thick mucus, and recurrent infections damage lung tissue, leading to the development of bronchiectasis.

6. Obstruction of pulmonary blood flow causes reflex bronchoconstriction in the affected area of the lung, wasted ventilation and impaired gas exchange, and loss of alveolar surfactant. Pulmonary hypertension and right heart failure may develop when there is massive vasoconstriction because of a large embolus.

7. Pathologic lung changes include diffuse epithelial cell injury with increased permeability of the alveolar-capillary membrane, which permits fluid, plasma proteins, and blood cells to move out of the vascular compartment into the interstitium and alveoli of the lung. Diffuse alveolar cell damage leads to accumulation of fluid, surfactant inactivation, and formation of a hyaline membrane. The work of breathing becomes greatly increased as the lung stiffens and becomes more difficult to inflate. There is increased intrapulmonary shunting of blood, impaired gas exchange, and hypoxemia despite high supplemental oxygen therapy. Gas exchange is further compromised by alveolar collapse resulting from abnormalities in surfactant production. When injury to the alveolar epithelium is severe, disorganized epithelial repair may lead to fibrosis.

SECTION III: APPLYING YOUR KNOWLEDGE

Activity F

1. Diagnostic tests that the nurse would expect to be ordered to confirm the diagnosis of asthma include spirometry, inhalation challenge tests, and laboratory findings.

2. "A plan of care will be developed with the input of both you and your daughter to encourage independence as it relates to the control of her symptoms, along with measures directed at helping her develop and maintain a positive self-concept."

SECTION IV: PRACTICING FOR NCLEX

Activity G

1.

Mechanism	Outcome
Decreased oxygen in air	Hypoxemia
Inadequate circulation through pulmonary capillaries	Decreased PO_2
Hypoventilation	Decreased PO_2
Disease in respiratory system	Hypoxemia
Mismatched ventilation and perfusion	Decreased PO_2
Dysfunction of neurologic system	Hypoxemia

Rationale: Hypoxemia can result from an inadequate amount of O_2 in the air, disease of the respiratory system, dysfunction of the neurologic system, or alterations in circulatory function. The mechanisms, whereby respiratory disorders lead to a significant reduction in PO_2 are hypoventilation, impaired diffusion of gases, inadequate circulation of blood through the pulmonary capillaries, and mismatching of ventilation and perfusion.

2. a, b, c, e. *Rationale:* Hypercapnia refers to an increase in CO_2 levels. In the clinical setting, four factors contribute to hypercapnia: alterations in CO_2 production, disturbance in the gas exchange function of the lungs, abnormalities in respiratory function of the chest wall and respiratory muscles, and changes in neural control of respiration. A decrease in CO_2 production does not cause hypercapnia.

3. b. *Rationale:* One of the complications of untreated moderate or large hemothorax is fibrothorax—the fusion of the pleural surfaces by fibrin, hyalin, and connective tissue—and, in some cases, calcification of the fibrous tissue, which restricts lung expansion. Calcification of the lung tissue does not occur because of a hemothorax. Neither does pleuritis or an atelectasis.

4. d. *Rationale:* Persons with talc lung are also highly susceptible to the occurrence of pneumothorax. Talc lung may result from inhalation of talc particles, but is more commonly an occurrence of injected or inhaled talc powder that is used as a filler with heroin, methamphetamine, or codeine. Hemothorax, chylothorax, or fibrothorax is not a complication of talc lung.

5. a, b, c. *Rationale:* Treatment of pleuritis consists of treating the underlying disease and inflammation. Analgesics and nonsteroidal anti-inflammatory drugs (e.g., indomethacin) may be used for pleural pain. Although these agents reduce inflammation, they may not entirely relieve the discomfort associated with deep breathing and coughing.

6. c. *Rationale:* If the collapsed area is large, the mediastinum and trachea shift to the affected side. In compression atelectasis, the mediastinum shifts away from the affected lung. None of the other answers are correct.

7. a. *Rationale:* For children younger than 2 years, nebulizer therapy is usually preferred.

Children between 3 and 5 years of age may begin using a metered-dose inhaler with a spacer and holding chamber. The other answers are not correct.

8. b. *Rationale:* The term chronic obstructive pulmonary disease encompasses two types of obstructive airway disease: emphysema, with enlargement of air spaces and destruction of lung tissue; and chronic obstructive bronchitis, with increased mucus production, obstruction of small airways, and a chronic productive cough. Persons with COPD often have overlapping features of both disorders. Asthma and chronic bronchitis have not been identified as components of COPD.

9. c. *Rationale:* In the past, bronchiectasis often followed a necrotizing bacterial pneumonia that frequently complicated measles, pertussis, or influenza. Chickenpox has never been linked to bronchiectasis.

10. d. *Rationale:* In addition to airway obstruction, the basic genetic defect that occurs with CF predisposes to chronic infection with a surprisingly small number of organisms, the most common being *Pseudomonas aeruginosa, Burkholderia cepacia, Staphylococcus aureus,* and *Haemophilus influenzae.* The other disease-causing organisms are not linked to CF.

11. a, b, e. *Rationale:* Important etiologic determinants in the development of the pneumoconioses are the size of the dust particle, its chemical nature and ability to incite lung destruction, and the concentration of dust and the length of exposure to it. The density and biologic nature of the dust particles are not linked to their ability to cause pneumoconioses.

12. a. *Rationale:* Drugs can cause a variety of both acute and chronic alterations in lung function. For example, some of the cytotoxic drugs (e.g., bleomycin, busulfan, methotrexate, cyclophosphamide) used in treatment of cancer cause pulmonary damage as a result of direct toxicity of the drug and by stimulating the influx of inflammatory cells into the alveoli. Amiodarone, a drug used to treat resistant cardiac arrhythmias, is preferentially sequestered in the lung and causes significant pneumonitis in 5% to 15% of persons receiving it. Inderal does not cause a direct toxicity in the lungs.

13. b. *Rationale:* Chest pain, dyspnea, and increased respiratory rate are the most frequent

signs and symptoms of pulmonary embolism. Pulmonary infarction often causes pleuritic pain that changes with respiration; it is more severe on inspiration and less severe on expiration. Neither mediastinal and tracheal shifts nor pericardial pain are signs of a pulmonary infarction.

14. b. *Rationale:* Continued exposure of the pulmonary vessels to hypoxemia is a common cause of pulmonary hypertension. Unlike blood vessels in the systemic circulation, most of which dilate in response to hypoxemia and hypercapnia, the pulmonary vessels constrict. None of the other answers are correct.

15. c. *Rationale:* Management of cor pulmonale focuses on the treatment of the lung disease and heart failure. Low-flow oxygen therapy may be used to reduce the pulmonary hypertension and polycythemia associated with severe hypoxemia caused by chronic lung disease. Low-flow oxygen used in treating cor pulmonale does not stimulate the body to breathe, it does not act in an inhibitory way on the respiratory center in the brain, nor does it reduce the formation of pulmonary emboli.

16. b, d, e. *Rationale:* Clinically, acute lung injury/ARDS is marked by a rapid onset, usually within 12 to 18 hours of the initiating event, of respiratory distress, an increase in respiratory rate, and signs of respiratory failure. Chest radiography shows diffuse bilateral infiltrates of the lung tissue in the absence of cardiac dysfunction. Marked hypoxemia occurs that is refractory to treatment with supplemental oxygen therapy, which results in a decrease in the PF ratio. Many persons with ARDS have a systemic response that results in multiple organ failure, particularly the renal, gastrointestinal, cardiovascular, and central nervous systems. The other answers are not clinical signs of ARDS.

17. d. *Rationale:* Many of the adverse consequences of hypercapnia are the result of respiratory acidosis. Direct effects of acidosis include depression of cardiac contractility, decreased respiratory muscle contractility, and arterial vasodilation. Raised levels of PCO_2 greatly increase cerebral blood flow, which may result in headache, increased cerebral spinal fluid pressure, and sometimes papilledema.

CHAPTER 30 STRUCTURE AND FUNCTION OF THE KIDNEY

SECTION II: ASSESSING YOUR UNDERSTANDING

Activity A

1. kidneys
2. hilus
3. Nephrons
4. cortex
5. renal pyramids
6. aorta
7. glomeruli
8. glomerulus
9. Peritubular capillaries
10. filtrate
11. glomerular filtration rate
12. concentration, basolateral
13. Cotransport
14. proximal
15. renal threshold
16. loop of Henle
17. Na^+-K^+-$2Cl^-$
18. distal convoluted
19. antidiuretic hormone
20. sympathetic
21. clearance
22. Aldosterone
23. sodium
24. bicarbonate, hydrogen
25. Urea
26. erythropoietin
27. Proteinuria
28. specific gravity
29. Creatinine
30. Blood urea nitrogen

Activity B

| 1. e | 2. d | 3. i | 4. a | 5. j |
| 6. g | 7. b | 8. h | 9. f | 10. c |

Activity C

1. Decreased glomerular filtration rate→juxtaglomerular release of renin→ conversion of angiotensinogen to angiotensin I by renin→ conversion of angiotensin I to angiotensin II by angiotensin-converting enzyme→ angiotensin II stimulates release of antidiuretic hormone and aldosterone→ sodium and water retention

Activity D

1. The glomerular capillary membrane is composed of three layers: the capillary endothelial layer, the basement membrane, and the single-celled capsular epithelial layer. The endothelial layer contains many small perforations called fenestrations. The epithelial layer that covers the glomerulus is continuous with the epithelium that lines Bowman's capsule. The cells of the epithelial layer have unusual octopuslike structures that possess a large number of extensions, or foot processes. These foot processes form slit pores through which the glomerular filtrate passes. The basement membrane consists of a homogeneous acellular meshwork of collagen fibers, glycoproteins, and mucopolysaccharides. The spaces between the fibers that make up the basement membrane represent the pores of a filter and determine the size-dependent permeability barrier of the glomerulus.

2. The basic mechanisms of transport across the tubular epithelial cell membrane include active and passive transport mechanisms. Water and urea are passively absorbed along concentration gradients. Sodium, K^+, chloride, calcium, and phosphate ions, as well as urate, glucose, and amino acids, are reabsorbed using primary or secondary active transport mechanisms to move across the tubular membrane. Some substances, such as hydrogen, potassium, and urate ions, are secreted into the tubular fluids.

3. The juxtaglomerular complex is a feedback control system that links changes in the glomerular filtration rate (GFR) with renal blood flow. It is located at the site where the distal tubule extends back to the glomerulus, and then passes between the afferent and efferent arteriole. The distal tubular site that is nearest the glomerulus is characterized by densely nucleated cells called the macula densa. In the adjacent afferent arteriole, the smooth muscle cells of the media are modified as special secretory cells called juxtaglomerular cells. These cells contain granules of inactive renin, an enzyme that functions in the conversion of angiotensinogen to angiotensin. Renin functions by means of angiotensin II to produce vasoconstriction of the efferent arteriole as a means of preventing serious decreases in GFR. Angiotensin II also increases sodium reabsorption indirectly by stimulating aldosterone secretion from the adrenal gland and directly by increasing sodium reabsorption by the proximal tubule cells. The increase in sodium will result in an increase in water retention, which will increase blood volume and, in turn, increase GFR.

4. The actions of atrial natriuretic peptide (ANP) include vasodilation of the afferent and efferent arterioles, which results in an increase in renal blood flow and glomerular filtration rate. ANP inhibits aldosterone secretion by the adrenal gland and sodium reabsorption from the collecting tubules through its action on aldosterone and through direct action on the tubular cells. It also inhibits ADH release from the posterior pituitary gland, thereby increasing excretion of water by the kidneys. ANP also has vasodilator properties.

5. The kidneys function as an endocrine organ in that they produce chemical mediators that travel through the blood to distant sites where they exert their actions. The kidneys participate in control of blood pressure by way of the renin-angiotensin mechanism, in calcium metabolism by activating vitamin D, and in regulating red blood cell production through the synthesis of erythropoietin.

6. By blocking the reabsorption of these solutes, diuretics create an osmotic pressure gradient within the nephron that prevents the passive reabsorption of water. Thus, diuretics cause water and sodium to be retained within the nephron, thereby promoting the excretion of both. The increase in urine flow that a diuretic produces is related to the amount of sodium and chloride reabsorption that it blocks.

SECTION III: APPLYING YOUR KNOWLEDGE

Activity E

1. Tests that the nurse would expect to be ordered to either confirm or deny the diagnosis include urine-specific gravity, urinalysis with culture and sensitivity, urine osmolality, glomerular filtration rate, blood urea nitrogen, and serum electrolytes.

2. A simple flat-plate x-ray will show the kidneys, ureters, and any radiopaque stones that may be in the kidney, ureters, or pelvis.

SECTION IV: PRACTICING FOR NCLEX

Activity F

1. a. *Rationale:* The plasma level at which the substance appears in the urine is called the renal threshold. Renal clearance, renal filtration rate, and renal transport level are not the right answers.

2. b. *Rationale:* With ingestion of a high-protein diet, renal blood flow increases 20% to 30% within 1 to 2 hours. Although the exact mechanism for this increase is uncertain, it is believed to be related to the fact that amino acids and sodium are absorbed together in the proximal tubule (secondary active transport). The same mechanism is believed to explain the large increases in renal blood flow and glomerular filtration rate that occur with high blood glucose levels in persons with uncontrolled diabetes mellitus.

3. Renal clearance is the volume of plasma that is completely cleared each minute of any substance that finds its way into the urine. It is determined by the ability of the substance to be filtered in the glomeruli and the capacity of the renal tubules to reabsorb or secrete the substance. Every substance has its own clearance rate, the units of which are always volume of plasma per unit time. It can be determined by measuring the amount of a substance that is excreted in the urine (i.e., urine concentration × urine flow rate in milliliters per minute) and dividing by its plasma concentration.

4. c. *Rationale:* Small doses of aspirin compete with uric acid for secretion into the tubular fluid and reduce uric acid secretion, and large doses compete with uric acid for reabsorption and increase uric acid excretion in the urine.

5. d. *Rationale:* Alkaline or acid diuresis may be used to increase elimination of drugs in the urine, particularly in situations of drug overdose. The other answers are incorrect

6. a. *Rationale:* Persons with end-stage kidney disease are often anemic because of an inability of the kidneys to produce erythropoietin. This anemia is usually managed by the administration of a recombinant erythropoietin (epoetin alfa) that is produced through DNA technology to stimulate erythropoiesis.

7. b. *Rationale:* The increase in urine flow that a diuretic produces is related to the amount of sodium and chloride reabsorption that it blocks. The other answers are not correct.

8. b. *Rationale:* With diminished renal function, there is a loss of renal concentrating ability, and the urine-specific gravity may fall to levels of 1.006 to 1.010 (usual range is 1.010–1.025 with normal fluid intake). These low levels are particularly significant if they occur during periods that follow a decrease in water intake (e.g., during the first urine specimen on arising in the morning). The other answers are incorrect.

9. d. *Rationale:* Creatinine is freely filtered in the glomeruli, is not reabsorbed from the tubules into the blood, and is only minimally secreted into the tubules from the blood; therefore, its blood values depend closely on the glomerular filtration rate (GFR). A normal serum creatinine level usually indicates normal renal function. In addition to its use in calculating the GFR, the serum creatinine level is used in estimating the functional capacity of the kidneys. If the value doubles, the GFR—and renal function—has probably fallen to one-half its normal state. A rise in the serum creatinine level to three times its normal value suggests that there is a 75% loss of renal function. A blood urea nitrogen level, 24-hour urine test, and urine test of first void in the morning do not tell you about serum creatinine levels.

10. a. *Rationale:* Cystoscopy provides a means for direct visualization of the urethra, bladder, and ureteral orifices. It relies on the use of a cystoscope, an instrument with a lighted lens. None of the other tests provides direct visualization of the bladder, urethra, and ureteral orifices.

CHAPTER 31 DISORDERS OF THE FLUID AND ELECTROLYTE BALANCE

SECTION II: ASSESSING YOUR UNDERSTANDING

Activity A

1. intracellular fluid compartment
2. extracellular fluid compartment
3. Electrolytes
4. nonelectrolytes
5. Diffusion
6. Osmosis
7. Osmolarity, osmolality
8. Na^+
9. osmolar gap

10. Osmotically active
11. Na⁺/K⁺-ATPase
12. Capillary filtration
13. lymphatic system
14. Edema
15. plasma proteins
16. Pitting
17. Third-space fluids
18. insensible water losses
19. kidney
20. effective circulating volume
21. angiotensin II, aldosterone
22. Thirst, antidiuretic hormone
23. Psychogenic polydipsia
24. Diabetes insipidus
25. hyponatremia, hypernatremia
26. hypovolemia
27. Third-space losses
28. isotonic
29. Hyponatremia
30. Normovolemic hypotonic
31. antidiuretic hormone
32. Hypernatremia
33. water
34. Na⁺-K⁺ exchange mechanism
35. resting membrane potential
36. hyperkalemia
37. hypokalemia
38. renal failure
39. excess
40. Vitamin D
41. Magnesium
42. hypocalcemia
43. hypophosphatemia
44. calcium
45. Magnesium

Activity B

Activity C

1.

| **1.** c | **2.** g | **3.** e | **4.** b | **5.** j |
| **6.** f | **7.** a | **8.** h | **9.** d | **10.** i |

2.

| **1.** d | **2.** h | **3.** b | **4.** a | **5.** c |
| **6.** j | **7.** e | **8.** g | **9.** i | **10.** f |

Activity D

Activity E

1. The extracellular fluid (ECF), including blood plasma and interstitial fluids, contains large amounts of sodium and chloride; moderate amounts of bicarbonate; and only small quantities of potassium, magnesium, calcium, and phosphorus. In contrast to the ECF, the intracellular fluid contains almost no calcium; small amounts of sodium, chloride, bicarbonate, and phosphorus; moderate amounts of magnesium; and large amounts of potassium.

2. The forces that control the movement of water between the capillary and interstitial spaces are (a) capillary filtration pressure, which pushes water out of the capillary and into the interstitial spaces; (b) capillary colloidal osmotic pressure, which pulls water back into the capillary; (c) interstitial hydrostatic pressure, which opposes the movement of water out of the capillary; and (d) tissue colloidal osmotic pressure, which pulls water out of the capillary and into the interstitial spaces.

3. Mechanisms that contribute to edema formation include factors that increase the capillary filtration pressure, decrease the capillary colloidal osmotic pressure, increase capillary permeability, or produce obstruction to lymph flow.

4. The major regulator of sodium and water balance is the maintenance of the effective circulating volume, which can be described as that portion of the extracellular fluid that fills the vascular compartment and is "effectively" perfusing the tissues. A low effective circulating volume results in feedback mechanisms that produce an increase in renal and sodium and water retention, as well as a high circulating volume in feedback mechanisms that decreases sodium and water retention.

5. The three types of polydipsia include (a) symptomatic or true thirst, (b) inappropriate or false thirst that occurs despite normal levels of body water and serum osmolality, and (c) compulsive water drinking.

6. There may be a decrease in blood urea nitrogen and hematocrit because of dilution due to expansion of the plasma volume. An increase in vascular volume may be evidenced by distended neck veins, slow-emptying peripheral veins, a full and bounding pulse, and an increase in central venous pressure. When excess fluid accumulates in the lungs (i.e., pulmonary edema), there are complaints of shortness of breath and difficult breathing, respiratory crackles, and a productive cough. Ascites and pleural effusion may occur with severe fluid volume excess.

7. These changes include prolongation of the PR interval, depression of the ST segment, flattening of the T wave, and appearance of a prominent U wave. Normally, potassium leaves the cell during the repolarization phase of the action potential, returning the membrane potential to its normal resting value. Hypokalemia reduces the permeability of the cell membrane to potassium and thus produces a decrease in potassium efflux that prolongs the rate of repolarization and lengthens the relative refractory period. The U wave may normally be present on the ECG but should be of lower amplitude than the T wave. With hypo-kalemia, the amplitude of the T wave decreases as the U-wave amplitude increases.

8. Systemic effects of hypercalcemia are (a) changes in neural excitability, (b) alterations in smooth and cardiac muscle function, and (c) exposure of the kidneys to high concentrations of calcium.

SECTION III: APPLYING YOUR KNOWLEDGE

Activity F

1. "When a patient has burns over a large area of her body, there is a loss of protein in the plasma of the body. There is also injury to the capillaries in the burned area. Large amounts of albumin are moved out of the blood and are lost in the urine. We are working hard to infuse fluid that the body needs with our IV solutions."

2. The nurse knows that the diagnosis of fluid volume deficit is based on these factors:
   - History of conditions that predispose to sodium and water losses
   - Weight loss
   - Intake and output
   - Heart rate
   - Blood pressure
   - Testing for venous refill
   - Capillary refill time

SECTION IV: PRACTICING FOR NCLEX

Activity G

1. a, b, d, e. *Rationale:* The physiologic mechanisms that contribute to edema formation include factors that (a) increase the capillary filtration pressure, (b) decrease the capillary colloidal osmotic pressure, (c) increase capillary permeability, or (d) produce obstruction to lymph flow.

2. 1-d, 2-e, 3-a, 4-c, 5-b

3. a. *Rationale:* The major regulator of sodium and water balance is the maintenance of the effective circulating volume. The other answers are not regulated by the effective circulating volume.

4. b. *Rationale:* Psychogenic polydipsia may be compounded by antipsychotic medications that increase ADH levels and interfere with water excretion by the kidneys. Cigarette smoking, which is common among persons with psychiatric disorders, also stimulates ADH secretion.

5. c. *Rationale:* Other acquired causes of nephrogenic DI are drugs such as lithium and electrolyte disorders such as potassium depletion or chronic hypercalcemia. The other answers are not acquired causes of nephrogenic DI.

6. c. *Rationale:* When this occurs, water moves into the brain cells, causing cerebral edema and potentially severe neurologic impairment. The other cells are not correct.

7. a. *Rationale:* Changes in nerve and muscle excitability are particularly important in the heart, where alterations in plasma potassium can produce serious cardiac arrhythmias and conduction defects. The other answers are not correct.

8. b. *Rationale:* The small, but vital, amount of extracellular fluid, calcium, phosphorus, and magnesium is directly or indirectly regulated by vitamin D and parathyroid hormone. The other answers are not correct.

9. d. *Rationale:* The NPT2 gene is also inhibited by the recently identified hormone phosphatonin. When this hormone is overproduced, as in tumor-induced osteomalacia, marked hypophosphatemia occurs. The other conditions are not caused by hypophosphatemia.

10. a. *Rationale:* Severe hypermagnesemia (>12 mg/dL) is associated with muscle and respiratory paralysis, complete heart block, and cardiac arrest.

CHAPTER 32 DISORDERS OF ACID-BASE BALANCE

SECTION II: ASSESSING YOUR UNDERSTANDING

Activity A

1. 7.35, 7.45
2. pH
3. metabolic
4. volatile, nonvolatile
5. H_2CO_3
6. dietary proteins
7. Henderson-Hasselbalch equation
8. buffer system
9. bone
10. bicarbonate
11. Albumin, plasma globulins
12. H^+, HCO_3^-
13. ammonia
14. Hypokalemia
15. Aldosterone
16. variability
17. anion gap
18. acidosis, alkalosis
19. Compensatory mechanisms
20. Metabolic acidosis
21. lactic
22. ketoacids
23. salicylates

24. alcohol dehydrogenase
25. Chronic kidney
26. HCO_3^-
27. Metabolic alkalosis

28. hypoventilation, hypoxemia
29. acidosis
30. vasodilation
31. alkalosis

Activity B

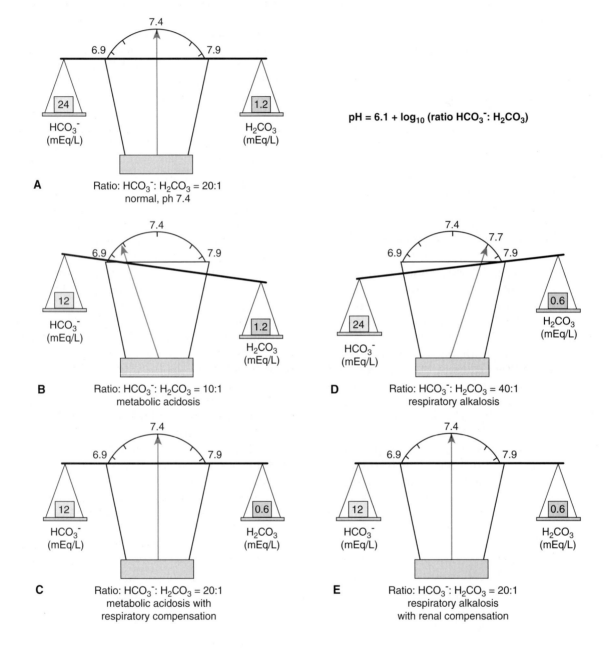

$$pH = 6.1 + \log_{10} (\text{ratio } HCO_3^- : H_2CO_3)$$

A Ratio: HCO_3^- : H_2CO_3 = 20:1
normal, ph 7.4

B Ratio: HCO_3^- : H_2CO_3 = 10:1
metabolic acidosis

D Ratio: HCO_3^- : H_2CO_3 = 40:1
respiratory alkalosis

C Ratio: HCO_3^- : H_2CO_3 = 20:1
metabolic acidosis with
respiratory compensation

E Ratio: HCO_3^- : H_2CO_3 = 20:1
respiratory alkalosis
with renal compensation

Activity C

1. e	**2.** a	**3.** i	**4.** h	**5.** c
6. b	**7.** d	**8.** j	**9.** f	**10.** g

Activity D

1. Carbon dioxide is transported in the body (a) as a dissolved gas; (b) as bicarbonate (HCO_3^-); and (c) as carbaminohemoglobin, bound to amino acids.

2. Excess H^+ ions can be exchanged for Na^+ and K^+ on the bone surface and dissolution of bone minerals with release of compounds, such as sodium bicarbonate ($NaHCO_3$) and calcium carbonate ($CaCO_3$), into the extracellular fluid can be used for buffering excess acids. It has been estimated that as much as 40% of buffering of an acute acid load takes place in bone. The role of bone buffers is even greater in the presence of chronic acidosis. The consequences of bone buffering include demineralization of bone and predisposition to development of kidney stones due to increased urinary excretion of calcium. Persons with chronic kidney disease are at particular risk for reduction in bone calcium due to acid retention.

3. The transcompartmental exchange of H^+ and potassium ions (K^+) provides an important system for regulation of acid-base balance. Both ions are positively charged, and both ions move freely between the intracellular fluid (ICF) and extracellular fluid (ECF) compartments. When excess H^+ is present in the ECF, it moves into the ICF in exchange for K^+ and when excess K^+ is present in the ECF, it moves into the ICF in exchange for H^+. Thus, alterations in potassium levels can affect acid-base balance, and changes in acid-base balance can influence potassium levels.

4. The kidneys play two major roles in regulating acid-base balance. The first is accomplished through the reabsorption of the HCO_3^- that is filtered in the glomerulus so this important buffer is not lost in the urine. The second is through the excretion of H^+ from fixed acids that result from protein and lipid metabolism.

5. There are two types of acid-base disorders: metabolic and respiratory. Metabolic disorders produce an alteration in the plasma HCO_3^- concentration and result from the addition or loss of nonvolatile acid or alkali to or from the extracellular fluids. A reduction in pH due to a decrease in HCO_3^- is called metabolic acidosis, and an elevation in pH due to increased HCO_3^- levels is called metabolic alkalosis. Respiratory disorders involve an alteration in the PCO_2, reflecting an increase or decrease in alveolar ventilation. Respiratory acidosis is characterized by a decrease in pH, reflecting a decrease in ventilation and an increase in PCO_2. Respiratory alkalosis involves an increase in pH, resulting from an increase in alveolar ventilation and a decrease in PCO_2.

6. The manifestations of metabolic acidosis fall into three categories. The first category is signs and symptoms of the disorder causing the acidosis or the primary condition. The second is changes in body function related to recruitment of compensatory mechanisms that contribute to the manifestations. In situations of acute metabolic acidosis, the respiratory system compensates for a decrease in pH by increasing ventilation to reduce PCO_2; this is accomplished through deep and rapid respirations. There may be complaints of difficult breathing or dyspnea with exertion; with severe acidosis, dyspnea may be present even at rest. The third is alterations in cardiovascular, neurologic, and musculoskeletal function resulting from the decreased pH and its effect on protein structure.

7. The signs and symptoms of respiratory alkalosis are associated with hyperexcitability of the nervous system and a decrease in cerebral blood flow. Alkalosis increases protein binding of extracellular calcium. This reduces ionized calcium levels, causing an increase in neuromuscular excitability. A decrease in the CO_2 content of the blood causes constriction of cerebral blood vessels. Because CO_2 crosses the blood-brain barrier rather quickly, the manifestations of acute respiratory alkalosis are usually of sudden onset. The person often experiences lightheadedness, dizziness, tingling, and numbness of the fingers and toes. These manifestations may be accompanied by sweating, palpitations, panic, air hunger, and dyspnea. Because CO_2 provides the stimulus for short-term regulation of respiration, short periods of apnea may occur in persons with acute episodes of hyperventilation.

SECTION III: APPLYING YOUR KNOWLEDGE

Activity E

1. This patient's laboratory values indicate metabolic acidosis.
2. A blood glucose level would be important to rule out diabetes mellitus as a cause of the metabolic acidosis.

SECTION IV: PRACTICING FOR NCLEX

Activity F

1. a. *Rationale:* The H_2CO_3 content of the blood can be calculated by multiplying the partial pressure of CO_2 (PCO_2) by its solubility coefficient, which is 0.03.

2. a, c, e. *Rationale:* The pH of body fluids is regulated by three major mechanisms: (a) chemical buffer systems of the body fluids, which immediately combine with excess acids or bases to prevent large changes in pH; (b) the lungs, which control the elimination of CO_2; and (c) the kidneys, which eliminate H^+ and both reabsorb and generate HCO_3^-. None of the other answers are correct.

3. c. *Rationale:* The renal mechanisms for regulating acid-base balance cannot adjust the pH within minutes as respiratory mechanisms can, but they continue to function for days, until the pH has returned to normal or near-normal range. It is the respiratory system that responds within minutes to return the body's pH near to its normal limits. The rest of the answers are wrong.

4. d. *Rationale:* The total base excess or deficit, also referred to as the whole blood buffer base, measures the level of all buffer systems of the blood—hemoglobin, protein, phosphate, and HCO_3^-. For clinical purposes, base excess or deficit can be viewed as a measurement of bicarbonate excess or deficit.

5. a. *Rationale:* Metabolic disorders produce an alteration in the plasma HCO_3^- concentration and result from the addition or loss of nonvolatile acid or alkali to or from the extracellular fluids. None of the other answers are correct.

6. b. *Rationale:* Often, compensatory mechanisms are interim measures that permit survival while the body attempts to correct the primary disorder. All other answers are wrong.

7. c. *Rationale:* The anion gap is often useful in determining the cause of the metabolic acidosis. None of the other tests are used to determine the cause of metabolic acidosis.

8. d. *Rationale:* A fall in pH to less than 7.0 to 7.10 can reduce cardiac contractility and predispose to potentially fatal cardiac dysrhythmias. No other answer is correct.

9. a, b, c. *Rationale:* Elevated levels of CO_2 produce vasodilation of cerebral blood vessels, causing headache, blurred vision, irritability, muscle twitching, and psychological disturbances. Seizures and psychotic breaks are not signs or symptoms of respiratory acidosis.

10. a. *Rationale:* One of the most common causes of respiratory alkalosis is hyperventilation syndrome, which is characterized by recurring episodes of overbreathing, often associated with anxiety.

CHAPTER 33 DISORDERS OF RENAL FUNCTION

SECTION II: ASSESSING YOUR UNDERSTANDING

Activity A

1. shape, position
2. agenesis
3. Potter syndrome
4. hypoplasia
5. dysplasia
6. multicystic
7. Polycystic
8. autosomal dominant
9. destructive
10. Stagnation
11. Hydronephrosis
12. distention
13. calculi
14. nidus
15. calcium
16. pain
17. second
18. *Escherichia coli*
19. urethra
20. more
21. anatomic, functional
22. Catheter
23. cystitis
24. Glomerulonephritis
25. nephritic, nephrotic
26. Acute nephritic
27. deposition
28. hypercellularity
29. Goodpasture
30. Nephrotic
31. Membranous
32. Buerger
33. basement membrane
34. Renal tubular acidosis
35. HCO_3^-
36. Acute pyelonephritis
37. Wilms tumor
38. hematuria, mass

Activity B

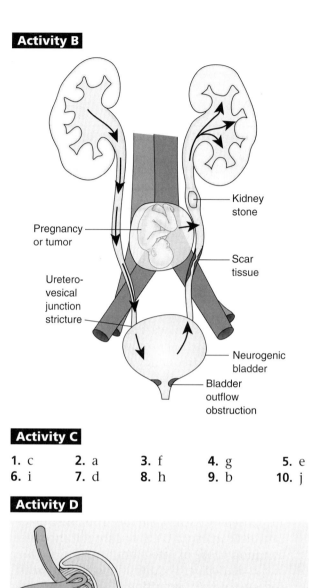

- Kidney stone
- Pregnancy or tumor
- Uretero-vesical junction stricture
- Scar tissue
- Neurogenic bladder
- Bladder outflow obstruction

Activity C

1. c	**2.** a	**3.** f	**4.** g	**5.** e
6. i	**7.** d	**8.** h	**9.** b	**10.** j

Activity D

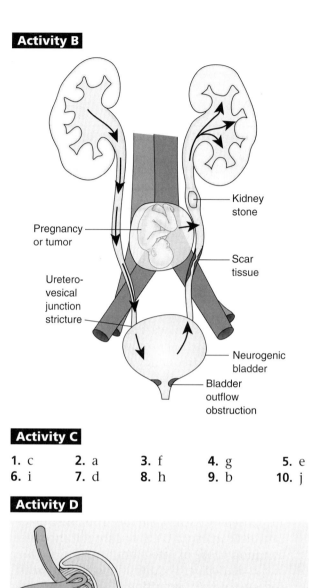

- Glomerular damage
- Increased permeability to proteins Proteinuria ($\geq$ 3.5 g/24 h)
- Hypoproteinemia
- Decreased plasma oncotic pressure
- Compensatory synthesis of proteins by liver
- Edema
- Hyperlipidemia

Activity E

1. The destructive effects of urinary obstruction on kidney structures are determined by the degree (i.e., partial vs. complete, unilateral vs. bilateral) and the duration of the obstruction. The two most damaging effects of urinary obstruction are stasis of urine, which predisposes to infection and stone formation, and progressive dilation of the renal collecting ducts and renal tubular structures, which causes destruction and atrophy of renal tissue.

2. Kidney stone formation requires supersaturated urine and an environment that allows the stone to grow. The risk for stone formation is increased when the urine is supersaturated with stone components (e.g., calcium salts, uric acid, magnesium ammonium phosphate, cystine). Supersaturation depends on urinary pH, solute concentration, ionic strength, and complexation. The greater the concentration of two ions, the more likely they are to precipitate. Complexation influences the availability of specific ions.

3. The risk factors for urinary tract infection are higher:
   - In persons with urinary obstruction and reflux
   - In persons with neurogenic disorders that impair bladder emptying
   - In women who are sexually active
   - In postmenopausal women
   - In men with diseases of the prostate
   - In elderly persons
   - In persons who have undergone catheterization
   - In women with diabetes

4. The host defenses of the bladder include the washout phenomenon, in which bacteria are removed from the bladder and urethra during voiding; the protective mucin layer that lines the bladder and protects against bacterial invasion; and local immune responses. In the ureters, peristaltic movements facilitate the movement of urine from the renal pelvis through the ureters and into the bladder. Immune mechanisms, particularly secretory immunoglobulin A, appear to provide an important antibacterial defense. Phagocytic blood cells further assist in the removal of bacteria from the urinary tract. In women, the normal flora of the periurethral area, which consists of organisms such as lactobacillus, provides defense against the colonization of

uropathic bacteria. In men, the prostatic fluid has antimicrobial properties that protect the urethra from colonization.

5. The cellular changes that occur with glomerular disease include increases in glomerular and/or inflammatory cell number, basement membrane thickening, and changes in noncellular glomerular components.

6. The development of glomerulonephritis follows a streptococcal infection by approximately 7 to 12 days—the time needed for the production of antibodies. The primary infection usually involves the pharynx. Oliguria, which develops as the glomerular filtration rate decreases, is one of the first symptoms. Proteinuria and hematuria follow because of increased glomerular capillary wall permeability. The red blood cells are degraded by materials in the urine, and cola-colored urine may be the first sign of the disorder. Sodium and water retention gives rise to edema (particularly of the face and hands) and hypertension.

7. Widespread thickening of the glomerular capillary basement membrane occurs in almost all persons with diabetes and can occur without evidence of proteinuria. This is followed by a diffuse increase in mesangial matrix, with mild proliferation of mesangial cells. As the disease progresses, the mesangial cells impinge on the capillary lumen, reducing the surface area for glomerular filtration.

8. Drug-related nephropathies involve functional or structural changes in the kidneys that occur after exposure to a drug. Because of their large blood flow and high filtration pressure, the kidneys are exposed to any substance that is in the blood. The kidneys are also active in the metabolic transformation of drugs and therefore are exposed to a number of toxic metabolites. Drugs and toxic substances can damage the kidneys by causing a decrease in renal blood flow, obstructing urine flow, directly damaging tubulointerstitial structures, or producing hypersensitivity reactions.

SECTION III: APPLYING YOUR KNOWLEDGE

Activity F

1. The nurse would expect the following orders: urine analysis, urine culture and sensitivity, and broad-spectrum antibiotic given intravenously.

2. To prevent further contamination by the indwelling catheter, the nurse would maintain a closed drainage system, pay careful attention to perineal hygiene, and practice careful handwashing.

SECTION IV: PRACTICING FOR NCLEX

Activity G

1. a, b, c, e. *Rationale:* Bilateral renal dysplasia causes oligohydramnios and the resultant Potter facies, pulmonary hypoplasia, and renal failure. Multicystic kidneys are a disorder, not the result of a congenital problem.

2. 1-b, 2-a, 3-d, 4-c

3. a. *Rationale:* Urinary tract obstruction encourages the growth of microorganisms and should be suspected in persons with recurrent UTIs. The other answers can cause lower UTIs, but an obstruction would be considered because of the frequency of the infections.

4. b. *Rationale:* Phosphate levels are increased in alkaline urine and magnesium, always present in the urine, and combine to form struvite stones. These stones can increase in size until they fill an entire renal pelvis. Because of their shape, they are often called staghorn stones. The other minerals can form stones, but not staghorn stones.

5. c. *Rationale:* Most uncomplicated lower UTIs are caused by *Escherichia coli*. The other organisms can cause UTIs, but are not the most common cause of infection.

6. b, c, d. *Rationale:* Toddlers often present with abdominal pain, vomiting, diarrhea, abnormal voiding patterns, foul-smelling urine, fever, and poor growth. Toddlers do not typically have frequency in voiding, nor do they complain of burning when they urinate.

7. d. *Rationale:* Group A β-hemolytic streptococci has the ability to seed from one area of the body to another. One area it seeds to is the kidney, where it causes acute postinfectious glomerulonephritis. Other organisms can cause acute postinfectious glomerulonephritis, but they are not the most common cause of the disease.

8. a. *Rationale:* The lesions of diabetic nephropathy most commonly involve the glomeruli and are associated with three glomerular syndromes: nonnephrotic proteinuria, nephrotic syndrome, and chronic renal failure. The other answers are not commonly associated with diabetic nephropathy.

9. b. *Rationale:* The most common causative agents of acute pyelonephritis are gram-negative bacteria, including *Escherichia coli* and *Proteus, Klebsiella, Enterobacter,* and *Pseudomonas*. The other answers are not considered a common causative agent of acute pyelonephritis.

10. c. *Rationale:* The tolerance to drugs varies with age and depends on renal function, state of hydration, blood pressure, and pH of the urine. None of the other answers are correct.

11. d. *Rationale:* The common presenting signs of a Wilms' tumor are a large asymptomatic abdominal mass and hypertension. The tumor is often discovered inadvertently, and it is not uncommon for the mother to discover it while bathing the child. Some children may present with abdominal pain, vomiting, or both. Hypotension, oliguria, and diarrhea are not common presenting signs of a Wilms tumor.

CHAPTER 34 ACUTE RENAL FAILURE AND CHRONIC KIDNEY DISEASE

SECTION II: ASSESSING YOUR UNDERSTANDING

Activity A

1. Acute renal failure
2. prerenal, intrinsic, postrenal
3. Prerenal
4. tubular epithelial
5. blood urea nitrogen
6. Postrenal
7. cause
8. chronic kidney disease
9. 120 to 130
10. creatinine
11. tubulointerstitial, albumin
12. uremic
13. dehydration, overload
14. sodium
15. bone
16. osteodystrophy
17. Hypertension
18. uremia
19. atrophy, demyelination
20. glomerular filtration rate

Activity B

Intrinsic (damage to structures within the kidney)

Prerenal (marked decrease in renal blood flow)

Postrenal (obstruction of urine outflow from the kidney)

Activity C

| 1. b | 2. j | 3. d | 4. g | 5. a |
| 6. e | 7. h | 8. i | 9. f | 10. c |

Activity D

1. Acute tubular necrosis (ATN) is characterized by the destruction of tubular epithelial cells with acute suppression of renal function. ATN can be caused by a variety of conditions, including acute tubular damage due to ischemia, sepsis, nephrotoxic effects of drugs, tubular obstruction, and toxins from a massive infection. Tubular epithelial cells are particularly sensitive to ischemia and are vulnerable to toxins. The tubular injury that occurs in ATN is frequently reversible.

2. The onset or initiating phase, which lasts hours or days, is the time from the onset of the precipitating event until tubular injury occurs. The maintenance phase of acute tubular necrosis is characterized by a marked decrease in the glomerular filtration rate, causing sudden retention of endogenous metabolites, such as urea, potassium, sulfate, and creatinine, that are normally cleared by the kidneys. Fluid retention gives rise to edema, water intoxication, and pulmonary congestion. If the period of oliguria is prolonged, hypertension frequently develops and, with it, signs of uremia. The recovery phase is the period during which repair of renal tissue takes place. Its onset is usually heralded by a gradual increase in urine output and a fall in serum creatinine,

indicating that the nephrons have recovered to the point at which urine excretion is possible.

3. Glomerular filtration rate (GFR) is used to classify chronic kidney disease (CKD) into five stages, beginning with kidney damage with normal or elevated GFR and progressing to CKD and, potentially, kidney failure.

4. As kidney structures are destroyed, the remaining nephrons undergo structural and functional hypertrophy, each increasing its function as a means of compensating for those that have been lost. In the process, each remaining nephron must filter more solute particles from the blood. It is only when the few remaining nephrons are destroyed that the manifestations of kidney failure become evident.

5. The manifestations of chronic kidney disease include an accumulation of nitrogenous wastes; alterations in water, electrolyte, and acid-base balance; mineral and skeletal disorders; anemia and coagulation disorders; hypertension and alterations in cardiovascular function; gastrointestinal disorders; neurologic complications; disorders of skin integrity; and disorders of immunologic function. The point at which these disorders make their appearance and the severity of the manifestations are determined largely by the extent of renal function that is present and the coexisting disease conditions.

6. The anemia of chronic kidney disease is due to several factors, including chronic blood loss, hemolysis, bone marrow suppression due to retained uremic factors, and decreased red blood cell (RBC) production due to impaired production of erythropoietin and iron deficiency. The kidneys are the primary site for the production of the hormone erythropoietin, which controls RBC production. In renal failure, erythropoietin production is usually insufficient to stimulate adequate RBC production by the bone marrow.

7. People with chronic kidney disease tend to have an increased prevalence of left ventricular dysfunction, with both depressed left ventricular ejection fraction, as in systolic dysfunction, and impaired ventricular filling, as in diastolic failure. Multiple factors lead to development of left ventricular dysfunction, including extracellular fluid overload, shunting of blood through an arteriovenous fistula for dialysis, and anemia. Coupled with the hypertension that is often present, they cause increased myocardial work and oxygen demand, with eventual development of heart failure.

Congestive heart failure and pulmonary edema tend to occur in the late stages of kidney failure. Coexisting conditions that have been identified as contributing to the burden of cardiovascular disease include hypertension, anemia, diabetes mellitus, dyslipidemia, and coagulopathies. Anemia, in particular, has been correlated with the presence of left ventricular hypertrophy.

SECTION III: APPLYING YOUR KNOWLEDGE

Activity E

1. The nurse would include the following in discharge teaching to the child and his family: description of the disease process; prognosis; manifestations of the disease, including physical growth and developmental delays; medication regimen, including side effects; and dietary restrictions, including protein, caloric, sodium, and fluid restrictions.

2. Chronic kidney disease is a progressive disorder that can be slowed by adherence to dietary restrictions and medication regimen. The disorder usually progresses to the point where the child needs hemodialysis or peritoneal dialysis, or a kidney transplant. All forms of renal replacement therapy are considered safe in the pediatric population, and renal transplantation is considered the best treatment for a child.

SECTION IV: PRACTICING FOR NCLEX

Activity F

1. a. *Rationale:* The most common indicator of acute renal failure is azotemia, an accumulation of nitrogenous wastes (urea nitrogen, uric acid, and creatinine) in the blood and a decrease in the glomerular filtration rate. The other answers are not common indicators of acute renal failure.

2. a, c, d. *Rationale:* Ischemic ATN occurs most frequently in persons who have major surgery, severe hypovolemia, overwhelming sepsis, trauma, and burns. Hypervolemia and hypertension are not considered contributing factors to ischemic ATN.

3. b. *Rationale:* In clinical practice, GFR is usually estimated using the serum creatinine concentration. The other answers are not used to estimate the GFR.

4. c. *Rationale:* The number one hematologic disorder that accompanies CKD is anemia. The other answers are incorrect.

5. a, b, c. *Rationale:* Uremic pericarditis resembles viral pericarditis in its presentation. This includes all potential complications, up to and including cardiac tamponade. The presenting signs include mild to severe chest pain with respiratory accentuation and a pericardial friction rub. Fever is variable in the absence of infection and is more common in dialysis than uremic pericarditis. Shortness of breath and thromboangiitis are not indicative of uremic pericarditis.

6. d. *Rationale:* Restless leg syndrome is a manifestation of peripheral nerve involvement and can be seen in as many as two-thirds of patients on dialysis. The other answers are not correct.

7. a. *Rationale:* Many persons with chronic kidney disease fail to mount a fever with infection, making the diagnosis more difficult. All of the other answers occur.

8. a, b, c. *Rationale:* The cause of sexual dysfunction in men and women with CKD is unclear. The cause is probably multifactorial and may result from high levels of uremic toxins, neuropathy, altered endocrine function, psychological factors, and medications (e.g., antihypertensive drugs). The other answers do not apply in this situation.

9. b. *Rationale:* Access to the vascular system is accomplished through an external arteriovenous shunt (i.e., tubing implanted into an artery and a vein) or, more commonly, through an internal arteriovenous fistula (i.e., anastomosis of a vein to an artery, usually in the forearm). The other answers are incorrect.

10. c. *Rationale:* At least 50% of the protein intake for clients with CKD should consist of proteins of high biologic value, such as those in eggs, lean meat, and milk, which are rich in essential amino acids. The other sources of protein contribute to high levels of nitrogen.

CHAPTER 35 DISORDERS OF THE BLADDER AND LOWER URINARY TRACT

SECTION II: ASSESSING YOUR UNDERSTANDING

Activity A

1. bladder
2. retroperitoneally, symphysis
3. prostate
4. ureters
5. epithelial lining
6. external sphincter
7. parasympathetic, sympathetic
8. sacral, pelvic nerve
9. pons
10. Cortical
11. β_2-adrenergic
12. α_1 receptors
13. obstruction, incontinence
14. prostate gland
15. store, empty
16. micturition reflex
17. stroke
18. Atony
19. Stress incontinence
20. neurogenic, myogenic
21. transitional
22. hematuria

Activity B

Activity C

1. i	2. f	3. a	4. d	5. j
6. g	7. b	8. e	9. h	10. c

Activity D

1. The bladder is composed of four layers: (a) is an outer serosal layer, which covers the upper surface and is continuous with the peritoneum; (b) a network of smooth muscle fibers called the detrusor muscle; (c) a submucosal layer of loose connective tissue; and (d) an inner mucosal lining of transitional epithelium.

2. The pelvic nerve carries sensory fibers from the stretch receptors in the bladder wall; the pudendal nerve carries sensory fibers from the external sphincter and pelvic muscles; and the hypogastric nerve carries sensory fibers from the trigone area.

3. As bladder filling occurs, ascending spinal afferents relay this information to the micturition center, which also receives important descending information from the forebrain concerning behavioral cues for bladder emptying and urine storage. Descending pathways from the pontine micturition center produce coordinated inhibition or relaxation of the external sphincter. Cortical brain centers enable inhibition of the micturition center in the pons and conscious control of urination. Neural influences from the subcortical centers in the basal ganglia modulate the contractile response. They modify and delay the detrusor contractile response during filling, and then modulate the expulsive activity of the bladder to facilitate complete emptying.

4. The detrusor muscle of the bladder fundus and bladder neck contract down on the urine, the ureteral orifices are forced shut, the bladder neck is widened and shortened as it is pulled up by the globular muscles in the bladder fundus, the resistance of the internal sphincter in the bladder neck is decreased, and the external sphincter relaxes as urine moves out of the bladder.

5. The necessary factors that every child must possess in order to attain conscious control of bladder function are (a) normal bladder growth, (b) myelination of the ascending afferents that signal awareness of bladder filling, (c) development of cortical control and descending communication with the sacral micturition center, (d) ability to consciously tighten the external sphincter to prevent incontinence, (e) and motivation of the child to stay dry.

6. During the early stage of obstruction, the bladder begins to hypertrophy and becomes hypersensitive to afferent stimuli arising from stretch receptors in the bladder wall. The ability to suppress urination is diminished, and bladder contraction can become so strong that it virtually produces bladder spasm. There is further hypertrophy of the bladder muscle, the thickness of the bladder wall may double, and the pressure generated by detrusor contraction will increase to overcome resistance from the obstruction. As the force needed to expel urine from the bladder increases, compensatory mechanisms may become ineffective, causing muscle fatigue before complete emptying can be accomplished.

The inner smooth surface of the bladder is replaced with coarsely woven structures called trabeculae. Small pockets of mucosal tissue commonly develop between the trabecular ridges. These pockets form diverticula, making the patent more susceptible to secondary infections. Along with hypertrophy of the bladder wall, there is hypertrophy of the trigone area and the interureteric ridge, which is located between the two ureters. This causes backpressure on the ureters, the development of hydroureters, and, eventually, kidney damage.

7. The angle between the bladder and the posterior proximal urethra normally is 90 to 100 degrees, with at least one-third of the bladder base contributing to the angle when not voiding. During the first stage of voiding, this angle is lost as the bladder descends. In women, diminution of muscle tone associated with childbirth can cause weakness of the pelvic floor muscles and result in stress incontinence by obliterating the critical posterior urethrovesical angle. In these women, loss of the posterior urethrovesical angle, descent and funneling of the bladder neck, and backward and downward rotation of the bladder occur, so that the bladder and urethra are already in an anatomic position for the first stage of voiding. Any activity that causes downward pressure on the bladder is sufficient to allow the urine to escape involuntarily.

8. The neurogenic theory for overactive bladder postulates that the central nervous system (CNS) functions as an on–off switching circuit for voluntary control of bladder function. Therefore, damage to the CNS inhibitory pathways may trigger bladder overactivity owing to uncontrolled voiding reflexes. Neurogenic causes of overactive bladder include stroke, Parkinson disease, and multiple sclerosis.

9. The overall capacity of the bladder is reduced, as is the urethral closing pressure. Detrusor muscle function also tends to decline with aging; thus, there is a trend toward a reduction in the strength of bladder contraction and impairment in emptying that leads to larger postvoid residual volumes.

SECTION III: APPLYING YOUR KNOWLEDGE

Activity E

1. "In people who have multiple sclerosis, the demyelination of the nerves can cause an interruption in the messages from the brain

and the spinal cord reaching the bladder. This causes a condition known as a neurogenic bladder."

2. The nurse would expect the client to be given an antimuscarinic drug, such as oxybutynin, tolterodine, or propantheline, to decrease detrusor muscle tone and increase bladder capacity.

SECTION IV: PRACTICING FOR NCLEX

Activity F

1. a, c, e. *Rationale:* Disruption of pontine control of micturition, as in spinal cord injury, results in uninhibited spinal reflex–controlled contraction of the bladder without relaxation of the external sphincter, a condition known as detrusor-sphincter dyssynergia. The other answers are not true.
2. a. *Rationale:* As the child grows, the bladder gradually enlarges, with an increase in capacity, in ounces, that approximates the age of the child plus 2. The other answers are not true.
3. b. *Rationale:* Sphincter electromyelogram allows the activity of the striated (voluntary) muscles of the perineal area to be studied. Cystometry measures the ability of the bladder to store urine as well as the pressure of the bladder during filling and emptying. Uroflowmetry measures the flow rate during urination.
4. b. *Rationale:* During the early stage of obstruction, the bladder begins to hypertrophy and becomes hypersensitive to afferent stimuli arising from stretch receptors in the bladder wall. The ability to suppress urination is diminished, and bladder contraction can become so strong that it virtually produces bladder spasm. There is urgency, sometimes to the point of incontinence, and frequency during the day and at night. The other answers are wrong.
5. c. *Rationale:* The most common causes of spastic bladder dysfunction are spinal cord lesions such as spinal cord injury, herniated intervertebral disk, vascular lesions, tumors, and myelitis. The other answers are wrong.
6. d. *Rationale:* With acute overdistention of the bladder, usually no more than 1000 mL of urine is removed from the bladder at one time. The other answers are incorrect.
7. a. *Rationale:* In women, the angle between the bladder and the posterior proximal urethra (i.e., urethrovesical junction) is important to continence. This angle normally is 90 to 100 degrees. The other answers are incorrect.
8. b, c, e. *Rationale:* Among the transient causes of urinary incontinence are recurrent urinary tract infections, medications that alter bladder function or perception of bladder filling and the need to urinate, diuretics and conditions that increase bladder filling, stool impaction, restricted mobility, and confusional states. The other answers are not associated with transient urinary incontinence.
9. b. *Rationale:* Habit training with regularly scheduled toileting—usually every 2 to 4 hours—is often effective. The other answers are incorrect.
10. c. *Rationale:* The intervesicular administration of bacillus Calmette-Guérin vaccine, made from a strain of *Mycobacterium bovis* that was formerly used to protect against tuberculosis, causes a significant reduction in the rate of relapse and prolongs relapsefree interval in persons with cancer in situ. The other drugs are used to treat bladder cancer, but not cancer in situ.

CHAPTER 36 STRUCTURE AND FUNCTION OF THE GASTROINTESTINAL SYSTEM

SECTION II: ASSESSING YOUR UNDERSTANDING

Activity A

1. gastrointestinal system
2. pharyngoesophageal
3. gastroesophageal
4. stomach
5. duodenum, jejunum, ileum
6. jejunum
7. epithelial, mucus
8. Serous
9. mesentery
10. pacemaker
11. enteric
12. Mechanoreceptors, chemoreceptors
13. vagovagal
14. oral, pharyngeal, esophageal
15. small intestine
16. Defecation
17. hormones
18. gastrin
19. Ghrelin
20. Cholecystokinin
21. parietal, vitamin B_{12}
22. pepsinogen
23. gastrin
24. Brunner glands
25. bacteria

26. indigestible dietary residue
27. Digestion
28. Absorption
29. enterocytes
30. brush border enzymes
31. lipase

32. Anorexia
33. Nausea
34. Vomiting

Activity B

1.

Mesentery

Muscularis externa

Longitudinal muscle   Circular muscle

Epithelium
Lamina propria   } Mucosa
Muscularis mucosa

Serosa (mesothelium)

Serosa (connective tissue)

Submucosa

2.

Enterocyte being extruded from a villus

Enterocyte

Vein

Lacteal

Artery

Crypt of Lieberkühn

Activity C

1. c	**2.** e	**3.** b	**4.** f	**5.** g
6. i	**7.** h	**8.** d	**9.** a	**10.** j

Activity D

1. The upper part—the mouth, esophagus, and stomach—acts as an intake source and receptacle through which food passes and in which initial digestive processes take place. The middle portion—the duodenum, jejunum, and ileum—is the place where most digestive and absorptive processes occur. The lower segment—the cecum, colon, and rectum—serves as a storage channel for the efficient elimination of waste.

2. The emptying of the stomach is regulated by hormonal and neural mechanisms. The hormones cholecystokinin and glucose-dependent insulinotropic polypeptide, which are believed in part to control gastric emptying, are released in response to the pH and the osmolar and fatty acid composition of the chyme. Afferent receptor fibers synapse with the neurons in the intramural plexus or trigger intrinsic reflexes by means of vagal or sympathetic pathways that participate in extrinsic reflexes.

3. With segmentation waves, slow contractions of the circular muscle layer occlude the lumen and drive the contents forward and backward. Most of the contractions that produce segmentation waves are local events involving only 1 to 4 cm of intestine at a time. They function mainly to mix the chyme with the digestive enzymes from the pancreas and to ensure adequate exposure of all parts of the chyme to the mucosal surface of the intestine, where absorption takes place. Peristaltic movements are rhythmic propulsive movements designed to propel the chyme along the small intestine toward the large intestine.

4. The incretin effect is the increase in insulin release after an oral glucose load. The two hormones that account for about 90% of the incretin effect are GLP-1, which is released from L cells in the distal small bowel, and GIP, which is released by K cells in the upper gut (mainly, the jejunum). Because increased levels of GLP-1 and GIP can lower blood glucose levels by augmenting insulin release in a glucose-dependent manner (i.e., at low blood glucose levels no further insulin is secreted, minimizing the risk of hypoglycemia), these hormones have been targeted as possible antidiabetic drugs. Moreover, GLP-1 can exert other metabolically beneficial effects, including suppressing glucagon release, slowing gastric emptying, augmenting net glucose clearance, and decreasing appetite and body weight.

5. The first is protection and lubrication. Saliva is rich in mucus, which protects the oral mucosa and coats the food as it passes through the mouth, pharynx, and esophagus. The sublingual and buccal glands produce only mucus-type secretions. The second function of saliva is its protective antimicrobial action. The saliva cleans the mouth and contains the enzyme lysozyme, which has an antibacterial action. Third, saliva contains ptyalin and amylase, which initiate the digestion of dietary starches.

6. The cellular mechanism for hydrochloric acid (HCL) secretion by the parietal cells in the stomach involves the hydrogen (H^+)/potassium (K^+)-adenosine triphosphatase (ATPase) transporter and chloride (Cl^-) channels located on their luminal membrane. During the process of HCL secretion, carbon dioxide (CO_2) produced by aerobic metabolism combines with water (H_2O), catalyzed by carbonic anhydrase, to form carbonic acid (H_2CO_3), which dissociates into H^+ and bicarbonate (HCO_3^-). The H^+ is secreted with Cl^- into the stomach, and the HCO_3^- moves out of the cell and into blood from the basolateral membrane. At the luminal side of the membrane, H^+ is secreted into the stomach via the H^+/K^+-ATPase transporter, and chloride follows H^+ into the stomach by diffusing through Cl^- channels in the luminal membrane.

7. Digestion of starch begins in the mouth with the action of amylase. Pancreatic secretions also contain an amylase. Amylase breaks down starch into several disaccharides, including maltose, isomaltose, and α-dextrins. The brush border enzymes convert the disaccharides into monosaccharides that can be absorbed.

8. Protein digestion begins in the stomach with the action of pepsin. Proteins are broken down further by pancreatic enzymes, such as trypsin, chymotrypsin, carboxypeptidase, and elastase. The pancreatic enzymes are secreted as precursor molecules. Trypsinogen, which lacks enzymatic activity, is activated by an enzyme located on the brush border cells of the duodenal enterocytes. Activated trypsin activates additional trypsinogen molecules and other pancreatic precursor proteolytic enzymes. The amino acids are liberated on the surface of the mucosal surface of the intestine by brush border enzymes that degrade proteins into peptides that are one, two, or three amino acids long. Similar to glucose, many amino acids are transported across the mucosal membrane in a sodium-linked process that uses ATP as an energy source. Some amino acids are absorbed by facilitated diffusion processes that do not require sodium.

SECTION III: APPLYING YOUR KNOWLEDGE
Activity E

1. The gastrointestinal (GI) tract is the largest endocrine gland in the body. Many nerves make the GI tract work. The stomach begins digestion by kneading and churning the food we eat. Food then progresses to the small intestine, where most of the food is digested and absorbed. Our food then goes into the large intestine, where it is compacted into the feces that we expel from our bodies.

SECTION IV: PRACTICING FOR NCLEX
Activity F

1. a. *Rationale:* At the end of the pyloric channel, the circular layer smooth muscle

thickens to form the pyloric sphincter. This muscle serves as a valve that controls the rate of stomach emptying and prevents the regurgitation of intestinal contents back into the stomach. There is no cardiac sphincter in the gastrointestinal tract. The antrum is a portion of the stomach that is the wider, upper portion of the pyloric region. The cardiac orifice is the opening between the esophagus and the stomach.

2. b. *Rationale:* It is in the jejunum and ileum that food is digested and absorbed. The other answers are incorrect.

3. c. *Rationale:* No contraction can occur without an action potential, and an action potential cannot occur unless the slow wave brings the membrane potential to threshold. The other answers are incorrect.

4. d. *Rationale:* The external sphincter is controlled by nerve fibers in the pudendal nerve, which is part of the somatic nervous system and therefore under voluntary control. The other answers are incorrect.

5. a. *Rationale:* Ghrelin is a newly discovered peptide hormone produced by endocrine cells in the mucosal layer of the fundus of the stomach. It displays potent growth hormone–releasing activity and has a stimulatory effect on food intake and digestive function, while reducing energy expenditure. The isolation of this hormone has led to new insights into the gut-brain regulation of growth hormone secretion and energy balance. The other hormones are secreted elsewhere in the gastrointestinal tract.

6. a, b, c, d. *Rationale:* Saliva has three functions. The first is protection and lubrication. Saliva is rich in mucus, which protects the oral mucosa and coats the food as it passes through the mouth, pharynx, and esophagus. The second function of saliva is its protective antimicrobial action. Third, saliva contains ptyalin and amylase, which initiate the digestion of dietary starches. The other answer is incorrect.

7. b. *Rationale:* The major metabolic function of colonic microflora is the fermentation of undigestible dietary residue and endogenous mucus produced by the epithelial cells. The other answers are not their main function.

8. c. *Rationale:* Absorption is accomplished by active transport and diffusion. The other answers are incorrect.

9. d. *Rationale:* A common cause of nausea is distention of the duodenum or upper small intestinal tract. The other answers are not associated with nausea.

10. d. *Rationale:* Serotonin is believed to be involved in the nausea and emesis associated with cancer chemotherapy and radiation therapy. Serotonin antagonists (e.g., granisetron, ondansetron) are effective in treating the nausea and vomiting associated with these stimuli. The other answers are incorrect.

CHAPTER 37 DISORDERS OF GASTROINTESTINAL FUNCTION

SECTION II: ASSESSING YOUR UNDERSTANDING

Activity A

1. esophagus
2. Congenital
3. Dysphagia
4. Hiatal hernia
5. gastroesophageal reflux disease
6. bronchial asthma
7. Reflux esophagitis
8. infant
9. alcohol, tobacco
10. impermeable
11. prostaglandins
12. Gastritis
13. Acute gastritis
14. Chronic gastritis
15. autoantibodies
16. Peptic ulcer
17. hemorrhage, obstruction
18. bleeding ulcers
19. Histamine
20. stress ulcers
21. carcinoma
22. Irritable bowel syndrome
23. Crohn, ulcerative colitis
24. Crohn
25. colon, rectum
26. Nutritional
27. Lieberkühn
28. Cancer
29. bacterial enterocolitis
30. Diverticulosis
31. Diverticulitis
32. appendicitis
33. diarrhea
34. noninflammatory diarrhea
35. Chronic
36. Inflammatory diarrhea

37. Constipation
38. Fecal impaction
39. cephalocaudal
40. Paralytic
41. serous membrane
42. gluten
43. Colonoscopy

Activity B

1.

1. g	**2.** f	**3.** a	**4.** e	**5.** j
6. h	**7.** d	**8.** i	**9.** c	**10.** b

2.

1. c	**2.** g	**3.** a	**4.** b	**5.** e
6. j	**7.** d	**8.** f	**9.** i	**10.** h

Activity C

1. Gastroesophageal reflux disease is believed to be associated with a weak or incompetent lower esophageal sphincter that allows reflux to occur, the irritant effects of the refluxate, and decreased clearance of the refluxed acid from the esophagus after it has occurred. In most cases, reflux occurs during transient relaxation of the esophagus. Gastric distension and meals high in fat increase the frequency of relaxation. Delayed gastric emptying may also contribute to reflux by increasing gastric volume and pressure with greater chance for reflux. Esophageal mucosal injury is related to the destructive nature of the refluxate and the amount of time it is in contact with mucosa. Acidic gastric fluids (pH <4.0) are particularly damaging.

2. Several factors contribute to the protection of the gastric mucosa, including an impermeable epithelial cell surface covering, mechanisms for the selective transport of hydrogen and bicarbonate ions, and the characteristics of gastric mucus. The gastric epithelial cells are connected by tight junctions that prevent acid penetration, and they are covered with an impermeable hydrophobic lipid layer that prevents diffusion of ionized water-soluble molecules. The secretion of hydrochloric acid by the parietal cells of the stomach is accompanied by secretion of bicarbonate ions (HCO_3^-). For every hydrogen ion (H^+) that is secreted, a HCO_3^- is produced, and as long as HCO_3^- production is equal to H^+ secretion, mucosal injury does not occur. Water-insoluble mucus forms a thin, stable gel that adheres to the gastric mucosal surface and provides protection from the proteolytic (protein-digesting) actions of pepsin. It also forms an unstirred layer that traps bicarbonate, forming an alkaline interface between the luminal contents of the stomach and its mucosal surface. The water-soluble mucus is washed from the mucosal surface and mixes with the luminal contents; its viscid nature makes it a lubricant that prevents mechanical damage to the mucosal surface.

3. A peptic ulcer can affect one or all layers of the stomach or duodenum. The ulcer may penetrate only the mucosal surface, or it may extend into the smooth muscle layers. Occasionally, an ulcer penetrates the outer wall of the stomach or duodenum. Spontaneous remissions and exacerbations are common. Healing of the muscularis layer involves replacement with scar tissue. Although the mucosal layers that cover the scarred muscle layer regenerate, the regeneration is often less than perfect, which contributes to repeated episodes of ulceration.

4. Chronic infection with *Helicobacter pylori* appears to serve as a cofactor in some types of gastric carcinomas. The bacterial infection causes gastritis, followed by atrophy, intestinal metaplasia, and carcinoma. This sequence of cellular events depends on both the presence of the bacterial proteins and the host immune response, the latter being influenced by the host genetic background. However, the vast majority of people with *H. pylori* will not develop gastric cancer, and not all *H. pylori* infections increase the risk of gastric cancer, suggesting that other factors must be involved.

5. The condition is believed to result from deregulation of intestinal motor and sensory functions modulated by the central nervous system. Irritable bowel syndrome is characterized by persistent or recurrent symptoms of abdominal pain; altered bowel function; and varying complaints of flatulence, bloatedness, nausea and anorexia, constipation or diarrhea, and anxiety or depression. A hallmark of irritable bowel syndrome is abdominal pain that is relieved by defecation and associated with a change in consistency or frequency of stools. Abdominal pain is usually intermittent, cramping, and in the lower abdomen.

6. According to the currently accepted hypothesis, this normal state of homeostasis is disrupted in

inflammatory bowel disease, leading to unregulated and exaggerated immune responses against bacteria in the normal intestinal flora of genetically susceptible individuals. Thus, as in many other autoimmune disorders, the pathogenesis of Crohn disease and ulcerative colitis involves a failure of immune regulation, genetic predisposition, and an environmental trigger, especially microbial flora.

7. In a manner similar to the small intestine, bands of circular muscle constrict the large intestine. As the circular muscle contracts at each of these points (approximately every 2.5 cm), the lumen of the bowel becomes constricted, so that it is almost occluded. The combined contraction of the circular muscle and the lack of a continuous longitudinal muscle layer cause the intestine to bulge outward into pouches called haustra. Diverticula develop between the longitudinal muscle bands of the haustra, in the area where the blood vessels pierce the circular muscle layer to bring blood to the mucosal layer. An increase in intraluminal pressure in the haustra provides the force for creating these herniations. The increase in pressure is believed to be related to the volume of the colonic contents. The scantier the contents, the more vigorous are the contractions and the greater is the pressure in the haustra.

8. The pathophysiology of constipation can be classified into three broad categories: normal transit constipation, slow transit constipation, and disorders of defecatory or rectal evacuation. Normal transit constipation (or functional constipation) is characterized by perceived difficulty in defecation, and usually responds to increased fluid and fiber intake. Slow transit constipation, which is characterized by infrequent bowel movements, is often caused by alterations in intestinal innervation. Hirschsprung disease is an extreme form of slow transit constipation, in which the ganglion cells in the distal bowel are absent due to a defect that occurred during embryonic development; the bowel narrows at the area that lacks ganglionic cells. Although most persons with this disorder present in infancy or early childhood, some with a relatively short segment of involved colon do not have symptoms until later in life. Defecatory disorders are most commonly due to dysfunction of the pelvic floor or anal sphincter.

9. The cause of colon cancer is unknown, but attention has focused on dietary fat intake, refined sugar intake, fiber intake, and the adequacy of such protective micronutrients as vitamins A, C, and E in the diet. It has been hypothesized that a high level of fat in the diet increases the synthesis of bile acids in the liver, which may be converted to potential carcinogens by the bacterial flora in the colon. Bacterial organisms in particular are suspected of converting bile acids to carcinogens; their proliferation is enhanced by a high dietary level of refined sugars. Dietary fiber is believed to increase stool bulk, and thereby dilute and remove potential carcinogens. Refined diets often contain reduced amounts of vitamins A, C, and E, which may act as oxygen free radical scavengers.

SECTION III: APPLYING YOUR KNOWLEDGE

Activity D

1. "The doctor wants to give you the chemotherapy medicine to try to reduce the size of your tumor so the surgery will not be as extensive as it would be if the surgery were done today."

2. "Even though your cancer has already spread, removing the tumor in your esophagus will make you more comfortable and, hopefully, allow you to live longer than you would without the surgery."

SECTION IV: PRACTICING FOR NCLEX

Activity E

1. a. *Rationale:* The newborn infant with EA/tracheoesophageal fistulae typically has frothing and bubbling at the mouth and nose, episodes of coughing, cyanosis, and respiratory distress. The other answers are not associated with EA as signs and symptoms of the defect.

2. b. *Rationale:* Esophageal acid clearance can be retarded in cases of severe erosive esophagitis where gastroesophageal reflux and a large hiatal hernia coexist. The other answers are incorrect.

3. c. *Rationale:* Tilting of the head to one side and arching of the back may be noted in children with severe reflux. Early satiety is another indication of gastroesophageal reflux, but not coupled with consolable crying. The other answers are not correct.

4. a, c, e. *Rationale:* The stomach lining is usually impermeable to the acid it secretes, a property that allows the stomach to contain acid and pepsin without having its wall digested. Several factors contribute to the protection of the gastric mucosa, including an impermeable epithelial cell surface covering, mechanisms for the selective transport of hydrogen and bicarbonate ions, and the characteristics of gastric mucus. These mechanisms are collectively referred to as the gastric mucosal barrier. The other answers are incorrect.

5. d. *Rationale: Helicobacter pylori* gastritis can be a chronic infection that can lead to gastric atrophy, peptic ulcer, and is associated with increased risk of gastric adenocarcinoma and low-grade B-cell gastric lymphoma mucosa-associated lymphoid tissue (MALToma). The other answers are incorrect.

6. a. *Rationale:* Diagnostic procedures for peptic ulcer include history taking, laboratory tests, radiologic imaging, and endoscopic examination. The other answers are not expected orders for a suspected peptic ulcer.

7. a, c. *Rationale:* Diagnosis of gastric cancer is accomplished by means of a variety of techniques, including barium x-ray studies, endoscopic studies with biopsy, and cytologic studies (e.g., Papanicolaou [Pap] smear) of gastric secretions. Cytologic studies can prove particularly useful as routine screening tests for persons with atrophic gastritis or gastric polyps. CT and endoscopic ultrasonography are often used to delineate the spread of a diagnosed stomach cancer. Pap smears are done on gastric secretions, but not by the nurse. A lower gastrointestinal study would be of no value in diagnosing this client. A tech does not do an endoscopic ultrasound.

8. b. *Rationale:* A hallmark of irritable bowel syndrome is abdominal pain that is relieved by defecation and associated with a change in consistency or frequency of stools. Nausea, altered bowel function, and diarrhea are also symptoms of irritable bowel syndrome, but not combined with abdominal pain that is unrelieved by defecation. A bowel impaction is not a symptom of irritable bowel syndrome.

9. c. *Rationale:* A characteristic feature of Crohn disease is the sharply demarcated, granulomatous lesions that are surrounded by normal-appearing mucosal tissue. When the lesions are multiple, they are often referred to as skip lesions because they are interspersed between what appear to be normal segments of the bowel.

10. d. *Rationale:* Rotavirus infection typically begins after an incubation period of less than 24 hours, with mild to moderate fever and vomiting, followed by onset of frequent watery, stools. The fever and vomiting usually disappear on about the second day, but the diarrhea continues for 5 to 7 days. Dehydration may develop rapidly, particularly in infants. The other answers are incorrect.

11. a. *Rationale:* One of the most common complaints of diverticulitis is pain in the lower left quadrant, accompanied by nausea and vomiting, tenderness in the lower left quadrant, a slight fever, and an elevated white blood cell count. Both B and D describe a suspected appendicitis, and C describes symptoms of a peptic ulcer.

12. b, c, d. *Rationale:* Noninflammatory diarrhea is associated with large-volume watery and nonbloody stools, periumbilical cramps, bloating, nausea, and/or vomiting. The other answers are incorrect.

13. b. *Rationale:* One of the most important manifestations of peritonitis is the translocation of extracellular fluid into the peritoneal cavity (through weeping or serous fluid from the inflamed peritoneum) and into the bowel because of bowel obstruction. The other answers are incorrect.

14. c. *Rationale:* The primary treatment of celiac disease consists of removal of gluten and related proteins from the diet. No other answer is correct.

15. d. *Rationale:* To reduce the likelihood of false-positive tests, persons are instructed to avoid nonsteroidal antiinflammatory drugs such as ibuprofen and aspirin for 7 days prior to testing, to avoid vitamin C in excess of 250 mg from either supplements or citrus fruits for 3 days before testing, and to avoid red meats for 3 days before testing. The other answers are incorrect.

CHAPTER 38 DISORDERS OF HEPATOBILIARY AND EXOCRINE PANCREAS FUNCTION

SECTION II: ASSESSING YOUR UNDERSTANDING

Activity A

1. accessory
2. artery, portal vein
3. hepatic portal vein
4. bile
5. albumin
6. cholesterol, bile
7. fat
8. triglycerides
9. emulsifying, micelles
10. Cholestasis
11. bile
12. Hemolytic
13. Conjugation
14. Phase 1 reactions
15. CYP gene
16. Phase 2 reactions
17. toxic metabolites
18. Cholestatic
19. Hepatitis
20. injection drug, blood transfusions, high-risk sexual behavior
21. Autoimmune
22. Intrahepatic
23. Secondary
24. fatty
25. Cirrhosis
26. Portal hypertension
27. increased, dilatation
28. Ascites
29. Spontaneous bacterial peritonitis
30. hepatorenal
31. encephalopathy
32. liver cancer
33. gallbladder
34. Cholecystokinin
35. cholesterol, bilirubin
36. cholecystitis
37. exocrine
38. pancreatitis
39. Chronic pancreatitis
40. cigarette smoking

Activity B

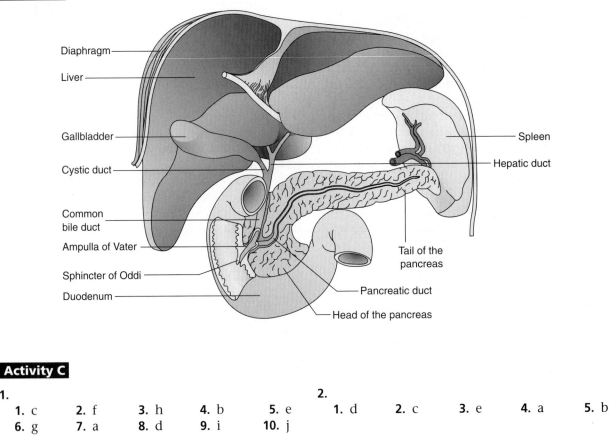

Diaphragm
Liver
Gallbladder
Cystic duct
Common bile duct
Ampulla of Vater
Sphincter of Oddi
Duodenum
Spleen
Hepatic duct
Tail of the pancreas
Pancreatic duct
Head of the pancreas

Activity C

1.

1. c	**2.** f	**3.** h	**4.** b	**5.** e
6. g	**7.** a	**8.** d	**9.** i	**10.** j

2.

1. d	**2.** c	**3.** e	**4.** a	**5.** b

Activity D

1.

Amino acids Glycerol Lactic acid

→ Gluconeogenesis →

Glucose ←→ Glycogen

Triglycerides

Bloodstream

2.

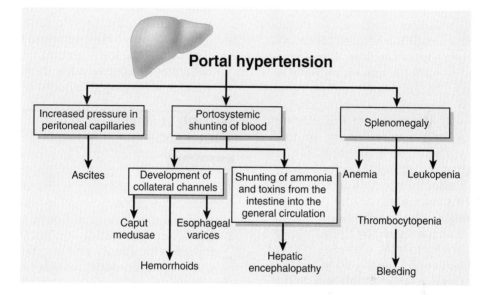

Activity E

1. The liver is one of the most versatile and active organs in the body. It produces bile; metabolizes hormones and drugs; synthesizes proteins, glucose, and clotting factors; stores vitamins and minerals; changes ammonia produced by deamination of amino acids to urea; and converts fatty acids to ketones. The liver degrades excess nutrients and converts them into substances essential to the body. In its capacity for metabolizing drugs and hormones, the liver serves as an excretory organ.

2. A number of mechanisms are implicated in the pathogenesis of cholestasis. Primary biliary cirrhosis and primary sclerosing cholangitis are caused by disorders of the small intrahepatic canaliculi and bile ducts. In the case of extrahepatic obstruction caused by conditions such as cholelithiasis, common duct strictures, or obstructing neoplasms, the effects begin with increased pressure in the large bile ducts. Genetic disorders involving the transport of bile into the canaliculi can also result in cholestasis.

3. The four major causes of jaundice are excessive destruction of red blood cells, impaired uptake of bilirubin by the liver cells, decreased conjugation of bilirubin, and obstruction of bile flow in the canaliculi of the hepatic lobules or in the intrahepatic or extrahepatic bile ducts. From an anatomic standpoint, jaundice can be categorized as prehepatic, intrahepatic, and posthepatic.

4. Elevated serum enzyme tests usually indicate liver injury earlier than other indicators of liver function. The key enzymes are alanine aminotransferase (ALT) and aspartate aminotransferase (AST), which are present in liver cells. ALT is liver specific, whereas AST is derived from organs other than the liver. In most cases of liver damage, there are parallel

rises in ALT and AST. The most dramatic rise is seen in cases of acute hepatocellular injury.

5. The clinical course of viral hepatitis involves a number of syndromes, including asymptomatic infection with only serologic evidence of disease, acute hepatitis, the carrier state without clinically apparent disease or with chronic hepatitis, and chronic hepatitis with or without progression to cirrhosis, with rapid onset of liver failure. Not all hepatotoxic viruses provoke each clinical syndrome.

6. The metabolic end products of alcohol metabolism (e.g., acetaldehyde, free radicals) are responsible for a variety of metabolic alterations that can cause liver injury. Acetaldehyde, for example, has multiple toxic effects on liver cells and liver function. The metabolism of alcohol leads to chemical attack on certain membranes of the liver. Acetaldehyde is known to impede the mitochondrial electron transport system, which is responsible for oxidative metabolism and generation of ATP; as a result, the hydrogen ions that are generated in the mitochondria are shunted into lipid synthesis and ketogenesis. Binding of acetaldehyde to other molecules impairs the detoxification of free radicals and synthesis of proteins. Acetaldehyde also promotes collagen synthesis and fibrogenesis.

7. Fatty liver is characterized by the accumulation of fat in hepatocytes, a condition called steatosis. The liver becomes yellow, enlarges owing to excessive fat accumulation, and is characterized by inflammation and necrosis of liver cells. Alcoholic hepatitis is the intermediate stage between fatty changes and cirrhosis. It is often seen after an abrupt increase in alcohol intake and is common in "spree" drinkers. Alcoholic cirrhosis is the result of repeated bouts of drinking-related liver injury and designates the onset of end-stage alcoholic liver disease. The gross appearance of the early cirrhotic liver is one of fine, uniform nodules on its surface.

8. Cirrhosis is characterized by diffuse fibrosis and conversion of normal liver architecture into nodules containing proliferating hepatocytes encircled by fibrosis. The formation of nodules represents a balance between regenerative activity and constrictive scarring. The fibrous tissue that replaces normally functioning liver tissue forms constrictive bands that disrupt flow in the vascular channels and biliary duct systems of the liver. The disruption of vascular channels predisposes to portal hypertension and its complications, obstruction of biliary channels and exposure to the destructive effects of bile stasis, and loss of liver cells, leading to liver failure.

9. An increase in capillary pressure due to portal hypertension and obstruction of venous flow through the liver, salt and water retention by the kidney, and decreased colloidal osmotic pressure due to impaired synthesis of albumin by the liver. Diminished blood volume (i.e., underfill theory) and excessive blood volume (i.e., overfill theory) have been used to explain the increased salt and water retention by the kidney.

10. With the gradual obstruction of venous blood flow in the liver, the pressure in the portal vein increases, and large collateral channels develop between the portal and systemic veins that supply the lower rectum. The dilation of the collaterals between the inferior and internal iliac veins may give rise to hemorrhoids.

SECTION III: APPLYING YOUR KNOWLEDGE

Activity F

1. The nurse would expect serum aminotransferase, liver biopsy, complete blood count, and complete metabolic panel to be ordered.

2. Interferons, nucleotide and nucleotide analog antiretroviral agents, and pegylated interferon α-2a might be ordered for this patient.

SECTION IV: PRACTICING FOR NCLEX

Activity G

1. a. *Rationale:* Kupffer cells are reticuloendothelial cells that are capable of removing and phagocytizing old and defective blood cells, bacteria, and other foreign material from the portal blood as it flows through the sinusoid. Langerhans cells are stellate dendritic cells found mostly in the stratum spinosum of the epidermis. Epstein's cells do not exist. Davidoff cells are large granular epithelial cells found in intestinal glands.

2. b. *Rationale:* The morphologic features of cholestasis depend on the underlying cause. Common to all types of obstructive and hepatocellular cholestasis is the accumulation of bile pigment in the liver. The other answers are incorrect.

3. c. *Rationale:* Usually, only a small amount of bilirubin is found in the blood; the normal

level of total serum bilirubin is 0.1 to 1.2 mg/dL. The other answers are incorrect.

4. d. *Rationale:* Because of the greater activity of the drug-metabolizing enzymes in the central zones of the liver, these agents typically cause centrilobular necrosis. The other answers are incorrect.

5. a. *Rationale:* The earliest symptoms are unexplained pruritus or itching, weight loss, and fatigue, followed by dark urine and pale stools. The other answers are not indicative of primary biliary cirrhosis.

6. b. *Rationale:* When the capacity of the liver to export triglyceride is saturated, excess fatty acids contribute to the formation of fatty liver.

7. c. *Rationale:* Because of the many limitations in sodium restriction, the use of diuretics has become the mainstay of treatment for ascites. A paracentesis may be done if the diuretics do not correct the problem. A thoracentesis would never be done for ascites. DDAVP is given to decrease urine output, not increase it.

8. d. *Rationale:* Diagnostic methods include ultrasound, CT scans, and MRI. Liver biopsy may be used to confirm the diagnosis. The serum α-fetoprotein can be indicative of liver cancer, but it is not confirmatory. An endoscopy is of no value. An ultrasound of the liver is not confirmatory for liver cancer.

9. a. *Rationale:* Gallbladder sludge (thickened gallbladder mucoprotein with tiny trapped cholesterol crystals) is believed to be a precursor of gallstones. The other answers are incorrect.

10. b. *Rationale:* Serum amylase and lipase are the laboratory markers most commonly used to establish a diagnosis of acute pancreatitis, whereas cholesterol and triglycerides are not used as such.

11. c. *Rationale:* In pancreatic cancer, the most significant and reproducible environmental risk factor is cigarette smoking. The other answers are incorrect.

CHAPTER 39 ALTERATIONS OF NUTRITIONAL STATUS

SECTION II: ASSESSING YOUR UNDERSTANDING

Activity A

1. Nutritional status
2. Metabolism
3. ATP
4. basal metabolic rate

5. voluntary physical activity
6. adipose
7. Leptin
8. recommended dietary allowance
9. Percent daily value
10. Proteins
11. nitrogen
12. elevate, lower
13. increase, decrease
14. carbohydrates
15. Vitamins
16. Minerals
17. Fiber
18. hypothalamus
19. glucose
20. Anthropometric
21. body mass index
22. circumference
23. Obesity
24. fat distribution
25. Weight cycling
26. increased
27. Bariatric surgery
28. pediatric
29. Malnutrition, starvation
30. starvation
31. marasmus
32. recurrent

Activity B

1.
| 1. f | 2. d | 3. b | 4. h | 5. i |
| 6. c | 7. a | 8. g | 9. j | 10. e |

2.
| 1. f | 2. c | 3. b | 4. a | 5. g |
| 6. d | 7. e | | | |

Activity C

1. There are two types of adipose tissue: white fat and brown fat. White fat is the prevalent form. At body temperature, the lipid content of fat cells exists as an oil of triglycerides. Triglycerides have the highest caloric content of all nutrients and are an efficient form of energy storage. Fat cells synthesize triglycerides from dietary fats and carbohydrates. When calorie intake is restricted for any reason, fat cell triglycerides are broken down, and the resultant fatty acids and glycerol are released as energy sources. Brown fat differs from white fat in terms of its thermogenic capacity or ability to produce heat. Brown fat, the site of diet-induced thermogenesis and nonshivering thermogenesis, is found primarily in early

neonatal life in humans and in animals that hibernate. In humans, brown fat decreases with age, but is still detectable in the sixth decade. This small amount of brown fat has a minimal effect on energy expenditure.

2. Bioimpedance is performed by attaching electrodes at the wrist and ankle that send a harmless current through the body. The flow of the current is affected by the amount of water in the body. Because fatfree tissue contains virtually all water and conducting electrolytes, measurements of the resistance (i.e., impedance) to current flow can be used to estimate the percentage of body fat present.

3. Nongenetic causes of obesity are family eating patterns, inactivity because of labor-saving devices and time spent on the computer and watching television, reliance on the automobile for transportation, easy access to food, energy density of food, increased consumption of sugar-sweetened beverages, and increasing portion sizes. The obese may be greatly influenced by the availability of food, the flavor of food, time of day, and other cues. The composition of the diet may also be a causal factor, and the percentage of dietary fat independent of total calorie intake may play a part in the development of obesity. Psychological factors include using food as a reward, comfort, or means of getting attention. Eating may be a way to cope with tension, anxiety, and mental fatigue. Some persons may overeat and use obesity as a means of avoiding emotionally threatening situations.

4. The causes of anorexia appear to be multifactorial, with determinants that include genetic influence; personality traits of perfectionism and compulsiveness; anxiety disorders; family history of depression and obesity; and peer, familial, and cultural pressures with respect to appearance. The *DSM-IV-TR* diagnostic criteria for anorexia nervosa are (a) a refusal to maintain a minimally normal body weight for age and height (e.g., at least 85% of minimal expected weight or BMI ≥ 17.5); (b) an intense fear of gaining weight or becoming fat; (c) a disturbance in the way one's body size, weight, and shape is perceived; and (d) amenorrhea (in girls and women after menarche). Other psychiatric disorders often coexist with anorexia nervosa, including major depression or dysthymia and obsessive-compulsive disorder. Alcohol and substance abuse may also be present, more often among those with binging-purging type of anorexia nervosa.

5. The criteria to diagnose bulimia nervosa are (a) recurrent binge eating (at least two times per week for 3 months); (b) inappropriate compensatory behaviors such as self-induced vomiting, abuse of laxatives or diuretics, fasting, or excessive exercise that follow the binge eating episode; (c) self-evaluation that is unduly influenced by body shape and weight; and (d) a determination that the eating disorder does not occur exclusively during episodes of anorexia nervosa.

6. Binge eating is characterized by recurrent episodes of binge eating at least 2 days per week for 6 months and at least three of the following: (a) eating rapidly; (b) eating until becoming uncomfortably full; (c) eating large amounts when not hungry; (d) eating alone because of embarrassment; and (e) disgust, depression, or guilt because of eating episodes.

SECTION III: APPLYING YOUR KNOWLEDGE

Activity D

1. Questions include the following:
   - Do you consider yourself a perfectionist?
   - Do you do things compulsively?
   - Is there a family history of obesity?
   - Is anyone in your family overweight?
   - Does anyone in your family have an anxiety disorder?
   - Does anyone in your family have a history of depression?
2. Criteria include the following:
   - Refusal to maintain a minimally normal body weight for age and height
   - An intense fear of gaining weight or becoming fat
   - A disturbance in the way one's body size, weight, and shape is perceived
   - Amenorrhea (in girls and women after menarche)

SECTION IV: PRACTICING FOR NCLEX

Activity E

1. 1-e, 2-c, 3-b, 4-d, 5-a
2. a, c, e. *Rationale:* The factors secreted by adipose tissue are termed adipokines and include leptin, certain cytokines (e.g., tumor necrosis factor-α), growth factors, and adiponectin (important in insulin resistance).
3. a. *Rationale:* An estimated average requirement is the intake that meets the estimated nutrient need of half of the persons in a

specific group. The adequate intake (AI) is set when there is not enough scientific evidence to estimate an average requirement. The recommended dietary allowance (RDA) defines the intakes that meet the nutrient needs of almost all healthy persons in a specific age and gender group. The dietary reference intake includes a set of at least four nutrient-based reference values—the estimated average requirement, the AI, the RDA, and the tolerable upper intake level.

4. b. *Rationale:* The Food and Nutrition Board has set an acceptable macronutrient distribution range for fat of no less than 20% to prevent the fall of HDL cholesterol associated with very low-fat diets. The other answers are incorrect.

5. c. *Rationale:* Centers in the hypothalamus also control the secretion of several hormones (e.g., thyroid and adrenocortical hormones) that regulate energy balance and metabolism. Cholecystokinin and glucagon-like peptide-1 are intestinal hormones. Ghrelin is secreted mostly in the stomach.

6. d. *Rationale:* The body mass index (BMI) uses height and weight to determine healthy weight. It is calculated by dividing the weight in kilograms by the height in meters squared (BMI = weight [kg]/height [m^2]). The other answers are incorrect.

7. a. *Rationale:* The obesity type is determined by dividing the waist by the hip circumference. The other answers are incorrect.

8. b. *Rationale:* Compared with women, men tend to experience less pressure to engage in behaviors such as self-induced vomiting or laxative use when overeating, less of a subjective sense of loss of control when binge eating, and a greater tendency to use compulsive exercise rather than purging for weight control.

9. b. *Rationale:* Pediatricians are now beginning to see hypertension, dyslipidemia, type 2 diabetes, and psychosocial stigma in obese children and adolescents. The other answers are not correct.

10. c. *Rationale:* The hospitalized patient often finds eating a healthful diet difficult and commonly has restrictions on food and water intake in preparation for tests and surgery. Pain, medications, special diets, and stress can decrease appetite. Even when the patient is well enough to eat, being alone in a room where unpleasant treatments may be given is not conducive to eating. The other answers are not correct.

CHAPTER 40 MECHANISMS OF ENDOCRINE CONTROLS

SECTION II: ASSESSING YOUR UNDERSTANDING

Activity A

1. hormones
2. nervous, immune
3. paracrine
4. autocrine
5. free, bound
6. high-affinity receptors
7. receptors
8. Lipid-soluble
9. hypothalamus
10. master gland
11. metabolites, hormone levels

Activity B

1. c	**2.** a	**3.** e	**4.** d	**5.** b
6. f	**7.** g			

Activity C

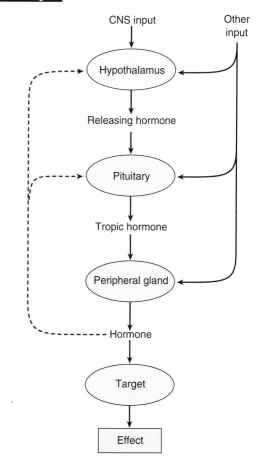

Activity D

1. Hormones are generally thought of as chemical messengers transported in body fluids. They are highly specialized organic molecules produced by endocrine organs that exert their action on specific target cells. Hormones do not initiate reactions but function as modulators of cellular and systemic responses. Most hormones are present in body fluids at all times, but in greater or lesser amounts depending on the needs of the body.

2. Hormones are divided into three categories: (a) amines and amino acids; (b) peptides, polypeptides, proteins, and glycoproteins; and (c) steroids. The first category, the amines, includes norepinephrine and epinephrine, which are derived from a single amino acid, and the thyroid hormones, which are derived from two iodinated tyrosine amino acid residues. The second category, the peptides, polypeptides, proteins, and glycoproteins, can be as small as to only contain three amino acids, and as large and complex as to consist of approximately 200 amino acids. The third category consists of the steroid hormones, which are derivatives of cholesterol.

3. The response of a target cell to a hormone varies with the number of receptors present and with the affinity of these receptors for hormone binding. The number of hormone receptors on a cell may be altered for any of several reasons. Antibodies may destroy or block the receptor proteins. Increased or decreased hormone levels often induce changes in the activity of the genes that regulate receptor synthesis. For example, decreased hormone levels often produce an increase in receptor numbers by means of a process called up-regulation; this increases the sensitivity of the body to existing hormone levels. Likewise, sustained levels of excess hormone often bring about a decrease in receptor numbers by down-regulation, producing a decrease in hormone sensitivity.

4. The intracellular signal system is termed the second messenger, and the hormone is considered the first messenger. The most widely distributed second messenger is cyclic adenosine monophosphate. Adenylate cyclase is functionally coupled to various cell surface receptors by the regulatory actions of G proteins. The second major cell surface receptor involving the binding of a hormone or neurotransmitter to a surface receptor acts directly to open an ion channel in the cell membrane. The influx of ions, then, serves as an intracellular signal to convey the hormonal message to the interior of the cell.

5. Hormones produced by the anterior pituitary control body growth and metabolism (GH), function of the thyroid gland (TSH), glucocorticoid hormone levels (ACTH), function of the gonads (FSH and LH), and breast growth and milk production (prolactin). Melanocyte-stimulating hormone, which is involved in the control of pigmentation of the skin, is produced by the pars intermedia of the pituitary gland.

6. The level of hormones in the body is regulated by negative feedback mechanisms. Sensors detect a change in the hormone level and adjust hormone secretion so that body levels are maintained within an appropriate range. When the sensors detect a decrease in hormone levels, they initiate changes that cause an increase in hormone production; when hormone levels rise above the set-point of the system, the sensors cause hormone production and release to decrease the level.

SECTION III: APPLYING YOUR KNOWLEDGE

Activity E

1. The nurse would expect a dual electron x-ray absorptiometry to be ordered because she knows that this test is used routinely for the diagnosis and monitoring of osteoporosis and metabolic bone diseases.

2. The nurse would expect an assessment of insulin function through a blood glucose level.

SECTION IV: PRACTICING FOR NCLEX

Activity F

1. a. *Rationale:* Neurotransmitters such as epinephrine can act as neurotransmitters or as hormones. The other answers are not correct.
2. b. *Rationale:* When hormones act locally on cells other than those that produced the hormone, the action is called paracrine. Hormones can also exert an autocrine action on the cells from which they were produced. The other terms are incorrect.
3. c. *Rationale:* Hormones that are synthesized by non–vesicle-mediated pathways include the glucocorticoids, androgens, estrogens, and mineralocorticoids—all steroids derived from cholesterol. The other answers are incorrect.
4. d. *Rationale:* Unbound adrenal and gonadal steroid hormones are conjugated in the liver, which renders them inactive, and then excreted in the bile or urine. Adrenal and gonadal steroid hormones are not excreted in the feces, cell metabolites, or lungs.
5. a. *Rationale:* The hypothalamus and pituitary (i.e., hypophysis) form a unit that exerts control over many functions of several endocrine glands as well as a wide range of other physiologic functions. These two structures are connected by blood flow in the hypophyseal portal system, which begins in the hypothalamus and drains into the anterior pituitary gland, and by the nerve axons that connect the supraoptic and paraventricular nuclei of the hypothalamus with the posterior pituitary gland. The other answers are not correct.
6. b. *Rationale:* The level of many of the hormones in the body is regulated by negative feedback mechanisms. The other answers are incorrect.
7. c. *Rationale:* Real progress in measuring plasma hormone levels came more than 40 years ago with the use of competitive binding and the development of radioimmunoassay methods. The other answers are incorrect.
8. d. *Rationale:* The advantages of a urine test include the relative ease of obtaining urine samples and the fact that blood sampling is not required. The other answers are not true.
9. a. *Rationale:* A suppression test may be useful to confirm this situation. The other answers are incorrect.
10. b. *Rationale:* Isotopic imaging includes radioactive scanning of the thyroid. The other answers are all examples of nonisotopic imaging.

CHAPTER 41 DISORDERS OF ENDOCRINE CONTROL OF GROWTH AND METABOLISM

SECTION II: ASSESSING YOUR UNDERSTANDING

Activity A

1. hypofunction, hyperfunction
2. Congenital
3. growth
4. insulin-like growth factors
5. Growth hormone
6. Constitutional short stature
7. Constitutional tall stature
8. gigantism
9. acromegaly
10. overstimulation
11. Precocious
12. Thyroid
13. metabolism, protein
14. metabolism
15. immunoassay
16. preventable mental retardation
17. Myxedema
18. Thyrotoxicosis
19. Graves
20. oxygen, metabolic
21. Thyroid storm
22. adrenal cortex
23. Aldosterone
24. glucocorticoid
25. Cortisol
26. Addison
27. Cushing syndrome

Activity B

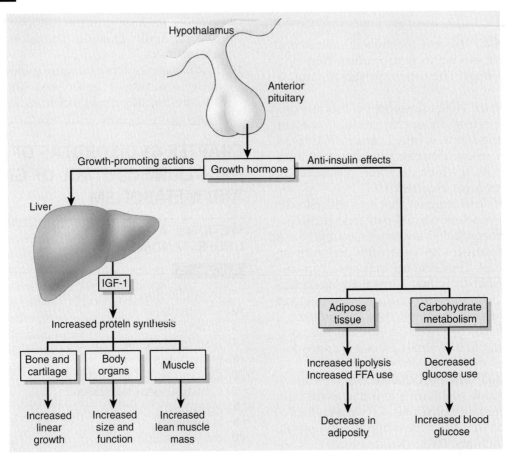

Activity C

1. i	**2.** j	**3.** d	**4.** e	**5.** b
6. g	**7.** f	**8.** c	**9.** a	**10.** h

Activity D

1. Primary defects in endocrine function originate in the target gland responsible for producing the hormone. In secondary disorders of endocrine function, the target gland is essentially normal, but its function is altered by defective levels of stimulating hormones or releasing factors from the pituitary system. A tertiary disorder results from hypothalamic dysfunction.

2. Hormones directly affected by hypopituitarism are ACTH, thyroid-stimulating hormone, growth hormone, the gonadotrophic hormones, and prolactin. Hypopituitarism is characterized by a decreased secretion of pituitary hormones, which affects many of the other endocrine systems by understimulation.

3. Growth hormone (GH) is necessary for growth and contributes to the regulation of metabolic functions. All aspects of cartilage growth are stimulated by GH; one of the most striking effects of GH is on linear bone growth, resulting from its action on the epiphyseal growth plates of long bones. The width of bone increases because of enhanced periosteal growth; visceral and endocrine organs, skeletal and cardiac muscle, skin, and connective tissue all undergo increased growth in response to GH. In many instances, the increased growth of visceral and endocrine organs is accompanied by enhanced functional capacity.

4. Growth hormone (GH) secretion is stimulated by hypoglycemia, fasting, starvation, increased blood levels of amino acids (particularly arginine), and stress conditions such as trauma, excitement, emotional stress, and heavy exercise. GH is inhibited by increased glucose levels, free fatty acid release, cortisol, and obesity. Impairment of secretion, leading

to growth retardation, is common in children with severe emotional deprivation.

5. The secretion of thyroid hormone is regulated by the hypothalamic-pituitary-thyroid feedback system. In this system, thyrotropin-releasing hormone (TRH) controls the release of thyroid-stimulating hormone (TSH) from the anterior pituitary gland. TSH increases the overall activity of the thyroid gland by increasing thyroglobulin breakdown and the release of thyroid hormone from follicles into the bloodstream, activating the iodide pump (by increasing Na^+/I symporter [NIS] activity), increasing the oxidation of iodide and the coupling of iodide to tyrosine, and increasing the number and size of the follicle cells. Increased levels of thyroid hormone act in the feedback inhibition of TRH or TSH.

6. The manifestations of the disorder are related largely to two factors: the hypometabolic state resulting from thyroid hormone deficiency, and myxedematous involvement of body tissues. The hypometabolic state associated with hypothyroidism is characterized by a gradual onset of weakness and fatigue, a tendency to gain weight despite a loss of appetite, and cold intolerance. As the condition progresses, the skin becomes dry and rough and acquires a pale yellowish cast, which primarily results from carotene deposition, and the hair becomes coarse and brittle. There can be loss of the lateral one- third of the eyebrows. Gastrointestinal motility is decreased, producing constipation, flatulence, and abdominal distention. Nervous system involvement is manifested in mental dullness, lethargy, and impaired memory.

7. Addison disease is a relatively rare disorder in which all layers of the adrenal cortex are destroyed. Autoimmune destruction is the most common cause. Because of a lack of glucocorticoids, the person with Addison disease has poor tolerance to stress. Hyperpigmentation results from elevated levels of ACTH. The skin looks bronzed or suntanned in exposed and unexposed areas, and the normal creases and pressure points tend to become especially dark. The gums and oral mucous membranes may become bluish-black. Mineralocorticoid deficiency causes increased urinary losses of sodium, chloride, and water, along with decreased excretion of potassium. The result is hyponatremia, loss of extracellular fluid, decreased cardiac output, and hyperkalemia.

8. The major manifestations of Cushing syndrome represent an exaggeration of the many actions of cortisol. Altered fat metabolism causes a peculiar deposition of fat characterized by a protruding abdomen; subclavicular fat pads or "buffalo hump" on the back; and a round, plethoric "moon face." There is muscle weakness, and the extremities are thin because of protein breakdown and muscle wasting.

SECTION III: APPLYING YOUR KNOWLEDGE

Activity E

1. "We are testing the baby for a disorder called congenital hypothyroidism. This means that the baby's thyroid gland is not functioning normally and is not producing thyroid hormone."
2. "Thyroid hormone is necessary for the brain to grow and develop. If the baby's thyroid gland is not working correctly, the doctor will order thyroid medicine for the baby. As long as the baby receives the medication as the doctor orders, the baby's brain will grow and develop just as it is supposed to."

SECTION IV: PRACTICING FOR NCLEX

Activity F

1. a. *Rationale:* When further information regarding pituitary function is required, combined hypothalamic-pituitary function tests are undertaken (although these are performed less often today). These tests consist mainly of hormone stimulation tests (e.g., rapid ACTH stimulation test) or suppression tests (e.g., growth hormone suppression test). The other answers are incorrect.
2. b. *Rationale:* The secretion of GH fluctuates over a 24-hour period, with peak levels occurring 1 to 4 hours after onset of sleep. The other answers are incorrect.
3. a, b, c. *Rationale:* In addition to its effects on growth, GH facilitates the rate of protein synthesis by all cells of the body, enhances fatty acid mobilization and increases the use of fatty acids for fuel, and maintains or increases blood glucose levels by decreasing the use of glucose for fuel. GH has an initial effect of increasing insulin levels. GH does not decrease the production of ACTH.
4. b. *Rationale:* When the production of excessive growth hormone occurs after the epiphyses of the long bones have closed, as in the

adult, the person cannot grow taller, but the soft tissues continue to grow. Enlargement of the small bones of the hands and feet and of the membranous bones of the face and skull results in a pronounced enlargement of the hands and feet, a broad and bulbous nose, a protruding lower jaw, and a slanting forehead. The other answers are incorrect.

5. c. *Rationale:* Persons with precocious puberty are usually tall for their age as children, but short as adults because of the early closure of the epiphyses. The other answers are incorrect.

6. d. *Rationale:* The assessment of thyroid autoantibodies (e.g., antithyroid peroxidase antibodies in Hashimoto thyroiditis) is important in the diagnostic work-up and consequent follow-up of thyroid patients.

7. a. *Rationale:* As a result of myxedematous fluid accumulation, the face takes on a characteristic puffy look, especially around the eyes. The tongue is enlarged, and the voice is hoarse and husky. The other answers are incorrect.

8. a, c, e. *Rationale:* Thyroid storm is manifested by a very high fever, extreme cardiovascular effects (i.e., tachycardia, congestive failure, angina), and severe central nervous system effects (i.e., agitation, restlessness, delirium). The mortality rate is high. Very low fever and bradycardia are not manifestations of a thyroid storm.

9. b. *Rationale:* Chronic suppression causes atrophy of the adrenal gland, and the abrupt withdrawal of drugs can cause acute adrenal insufficiency. The other answers are incorrect.

10. c. *Rationale:* In female infants, an increase in androgens is responsible for creating the virilization syndrome of ambiguous genitalia with an enlarged clitoris, fused labia, and urogenital sinus. The other answers are incorrect.

11. d. *Rationale:* Hydrocortisone is usually the drug of choice. The other answers are not drugs; they are naturally occurring steroids.

12. a, b, c, e. *Rationale:* If Addison disease is the underlying problem, exposure to even a minor illness or stress can precipitate nausea, vomiting, muscular weakness, hypotension, dehydration, and vascular collapse.

13. a. *Rationale:* The major manifestations of Cushing syndrome represent an exaggeration of the many actions of cortisol. Altered fat metabolism causes a peculiar deposition of fat characterized by a protruding abdomen;

subclavicular fat pads or "buffalo hump" on the back; and a round, plethoric "moon face." There is muscle weakness, and the extremities are thin because of protein breakdown and muscle wasting. The other answers are incorrect.

CHAPTER 42 DIABETES MELLITUS AND THE METABOLIC SYNDROME

SECTION II: ASSESSING YOUR UNDERSTANDING

Activity A

1. glucose
2. brain
3. hypoglycemia
4. glycogen
5. glycogenolysis
6. gluconeogenesis
7. 9, 4
8. proteins
9. fatty acids, proteins
10. glucose transporter
11. GLUT-4
12. Glucagon
13. glycogenolysis, gluconeogenesis
14. insulin
15. Diabetes
16. <100 mg/dL, 140 mg/dL
17. Type 1
18. idiopathic
19. Type 2
20. resistance
21. obesity, physical inactivity
22. obesity
23. Gestational
24. fasting
25. casual, 200
26. glycated hemoglobin
27. insulin
28. ketoacidosis
29. hyperosmolar hyperglycemic
30. Advanced glycation end products
31. diabetic nephropathy
32. Diabetic retinopathy
33. macrovascular disease

Activity B

1. d	2. c	3. f	4. e	5. h
6. a	7. j	8. i	9. b	10. g
11. k				

Activity C

- ↓ in insulin ↑ glucagon and gluconeogenesis
- ↑ blood glucose
- ↑ insulin release from beta cells
- ↓ glucagon
- removal of glucose from blood
- ↓ hepatic glucose production
- ↓ blood glucose

Activity D

1. The actions of insulin are threefold: (1) it promotes glucose uptake by target cells and provides for glucose storage as glycogen; (2) it prevents fat and glycogen breakdown; and (3) it inhibits gluconeogenesis and increases protein synthesis

2. The release of insulin from the pancreatic beta cells is regulated by blood glucose levels, increasing as blood glucose levels rise and decreasing when blood glucose levels decline. Blood glucose enters the beta cell by means of the glucose transporter; it is phosphorylated by an enzyme called glucokinase and metabolized to form the adenosine triphosphate (ATP) needed to close the potassium channels and depolarize the cell. Depolarization, in turn, results in opening of the calcium channels and insulin secretion.

3. The absolute lack of insulin in people with type 1 diabetes mellitus means that they are particularly susceptible to the development of ketoacidosis. One of the actions of insulin is the inhibition of lipolysis and release of free fatty acids (FFAs) from fat cells. In the absence of insulin, ketosis develops when these fatty acids are released from fat cells and converted to ketones in the liver.

4. Type 1A diabetes is thought to be an autoimmune disorder resulting from (1) a genetic predisposition; (2) an environmental triggering event, such as an infection; and (3) a T lymphocyte-mediated hypersensitivity reaction against some beta cell antigen. Much

evidence has focused on the inherited major histocompatibility (MHC) complex genes on chromosome 6. In addition to the MHC susceptibility genes for type 1 diabetes on chromosome 6, an insulin gene regulating beta cell replication and function has been identified on chromosome 11.

5. The metabolic abnormalities that lead to type 2 diabetes include (1) insulin resistance, (2) deranged secretion of insulin by the pancreatic beta cells, and (3) increased glucose production by the liver

6. Specific causes of beta cell dysfunction include (1) an initial decrease in the beta cell mass related to genetic or prenatal factors, (2) increased apoptosis and/or decreased beta cell regeneration, (3) beta cell exhaustion caused by long-standing insulin resistance, (4) glucotoxicity, (5) lipotoxicity, and (6) amyloid deposition, as well as other conditions that have the potential to reduce beta cell mass.

7. The manifestations of metabolic syndrome include obesity, high levels of plasma triglycerides and low levels of high-density lipoproteins (HDL), hypertension, systemic inflammation, abnormal fibrinolysis, abnormal function of the vascular endothelium, and macrovascular disease.

8. Insulin resistance and increased glucose production has several consequences: first, excessive and chronic elevation of FFAs can cause beta cell dysfunction (lipotoxicity); second, FFAs act at the level of the peripheral tissues to cause insulin resistance and glucose underutilization by inhibiting glucose uptake and glycogen storage; and, third, the accumulation of FFAs and triglycerides reduce hepatic insulin sensitivity, leading to increased hepatic glucose production and hyperglycemia, especially fasting plasma glucose levels. Thus, an increase in FFAs that occurs in obese individuals with a genetic predisposition to type 2 diabetes may eventually lead to beta cell dysfunction, increased insulin resistance, and greater hepatic glucose production.

9. The most commonly identified signs and symptoms of diabetes are referred to as the three polys: (1) polyuria (i.e., excessive urination); (2) polydipsia (i.e., excessive thirst); and (3) polyphagia (i.e., excessive hunger). These three symptoms are closely related to the hyperglycemia and glycosuria of diabetes.

10. Weight loss despite normal or increased appetite is a common occurrence in people with uncontrolled type 1 diabetes. First, loss of

body fluids results from osmotic diuresis. Second, body tissue is lost because the lack of insulin forces the body to use its fat stores and cellular proteins as sources of energy.

11. The technique of continuous subcutaneous insulin infusion involves the insertion of a small needle or plastic catheter into the subcutaneous tissue of the abdomen. Tubing from the catheter is connected to a syringe set into a small infusion pump worn on a belt or in a jacket pocket. The computer-operated pump then delivers one or more set basal amounts of insulin. In addition to the basal amount delivered by the pump, a bolus amount of insulin can be delivered when needed (e.g., before a meal) by pushing a button.

12. The three major metabolic derangements in DKA are hyperglycemia, ketosis, and metabolic acidosis. Hyperglycemia leads to osmotic diuresis, dehydration, and a critical loss of electrolytes. Serum potassium levels may be normal or elevated, despite total potassium depletion resulting from protracted polyuria and vomiting. Metabolic acidosis is caused by the excess ketoacids that require buffering by bicarbonate ions; this leads to a marked decrease in serum bicarbonate levels.

13. The chronic complications of diabetes include disorders of the microvasculature (i.e., neuropathies, nephropathies, and retinopathies); macrovascular complications (i.e., coronary artery, cerebral vascular, and peripheral vascular diseases), and foot ulcers. In the sorbitol pathway, glucose is transformed first to sorbitol and then to fructose. Although glucose is converted readily to sorbitol, the rate at which sorbitol can be converted to fructose and then metabolized is limited. Sorbitol is osmotically active, and it has been hypothesized that the presence of excess intracellular amounts may alter cell function in those tissues that use this pathway.

14. The peripheral neuropathies associated with chronic diabetes mellitus include thickening of the walls of the nutrient vessels that supply the nerve, leading to the assumption that vessel ischemia plays a major role in the development of neural changes. In addition, a segmental demyelinization process affects the Schwann cell. This demyelinization process is accompanied by a slowing of nerve conduction.

15. Various glomerular changes may occur in people with diabetic nephropathy, including capillary basement membrane thickening, diffuse glomerular sclerosis, and nodular glomerulosclerosis. Changes in the capillary basement membrane take the form of thickening of basement membranes along the length of the glomeruli. Diffuse glomerulosclerosis consists of thickening of the basement membrane and the mesangial matrix. Nodular glomerulosclerosis, Kimmelstiel-Wilson disease, is a form of glomerulosclerosis that involves the development of nodular lesions in the glomerular capillaries of the kidneys, causing impaired blood flow with progressive loss of kidney function and, eventually, renal failure. Changes in the basement membrane in diffuse glomerulosclerosis and Kimmelstiel-Wilson syndrome allow plasma proteins to escape in the urine, causing proteinuria and the development of hypoproteinemia, edema, and others signs of impaired kidney function.

SECTION III: APPLYING YOUR KNOWLEDGE

Activity E

1. Type 1A diabetes mellitus is thought to be a chronic autoimmune disease that has a genetic predisposition. Type 1A diabetes mellitus is characterized by a total lack of insulin, an elevation of blood glucose, and a breakdown of body fats and proteins. Type 1A diabetics are susceptible to the development of ketoacidosis. Type 1A diabetics require daily injections of exogenous insulin to control blood glucose levels and prevent ketosis.

2. Presently, there is no cure for diabetes mellitus. Research is being conducted into ways of preventing the disease, but none has yet been found.

SECTION IV: PRACTICING FOR NCLEX

Activity F

1. b. *Rationale:* Each islet is composed of beta cells that secrete insulin and amylin, alpha cells that secrete glucagon, and delta cells that secrete somatostatin. In addition, at least one other type of cell, the PP cell, is present in small numbers in the islets and secrets a hormone of uncertain function called pancreatic polypeptide.

2. a, b, c, e. *Rationale*: These hormones, along with glucagon, are sometimes called counter-regulatory hormones because they counteract the storage functions of insulin in regulating blood glucose levels during periods of fasting, exercise, and other situations that either limit glucose intake or deplete glucose stores. Mineralocorticoids are not considered counter-regulatory hormones.

3. c. *Rationale*: In predisposed persons, the prolonged elevation of glucocorticoid hormones can lead to hyperglycemia and the development of diabetes mellitus and starvation. These hormones stimulate gluconeogenesis by the liver, sometimes producing a 6- to 10-fold increase in hepatic glucose production. A prolonged increase in glucocorticoid hormones does not cause hepatomegaly, portal hypertension, or adrenal hyperplasia.

4. a. *Rationale*: Type 1A diabetes is thought to be an autoimmune disorder resulting from a genetic predisposition (i.e., diabetogenic genes); an environmental triggering event, such as an infection; and a T lymphocyte-mediated hypersensitivity reaction against some beta cell antigen. The other answers are incorrect.

5. a, c, d. *Rationale*: The metabolic abnormalities that lead to type 2 diabetes include (1) insulin resistance, (2) deranged secretion of insulin by the pancreatic beta cells, and (3) increased glucose production by the liver. The other answers are incorrect.

6. a. *Rationale*: Secondary diabetes can occur with pancreatic disease or the removal of pancreatic tissue and with endocrine diseases, such as acromegaly, Cushing syndrome, or pheochromocytoma. Endocrine disorders that produce hyperglycemia do so by increasing the hepatic production of glucose or decreasing the cellular use of glucose. Dwarfism, hepatomegaly, and pancreatic hyperplasia do not cause secondary diabetes.

7. b. *Rationale*: Diagnosis and careful medical management are essential because women with GDM are at higher risk for complications of pregnancy, mortality, and fetal abnormalities. Fetal abnormalities include macrosomia (i.e., large body size), hypoglycemia, hypocalcemia, polycythemia, and hyperbilirubinemia. Microsomia and hypercalcemia are not fetal abnormalities associated with GDM.

8. c. *Rationale*: The most commonly identified signs and symptoms of diabetes are referred to as the three polys: (1) polyuria (i.e., excessive urination), (2) polydipsia (i.e., excessive thirst), and (3) polyphagia (i.e., excessive hunger). Pheochromocytoma and polycythemia are not hallmark signs of diabetes mellitus.

9. 1-d, 2-c, 3-e, 4-b, 5-f, 6-a

10. d. *Rationale*: The definitive diagnosis of DKA consists of hyperglycemia (blood glucose levels >250 mg/dL), low bicarbonate (<15 mEq/L), and low pH (<7.3), with ketonemia (positive at 1:2 dilution) and moderate ketonuria. The other answers are not diagnostic for DKA.

11. a. *Rationale*: Alcohol decreases liver gluconeogenesis, and people with diabetes need to be cautioned about its potential for causing hypoglycemia, especially if alcohol is consumed in large amounts or on an empty stomach.

12. b. *Rationale*: The signs and symptoms of hypoglycemia can be divided into two categories: (1) those caused by altered cerebral function and (2) those related to activation of the autonomic nervous system. Because the brain relies on blood glucose as its main energy source, hypoglycemia produces behaviors related to altered cerebral function. Headache, difficulty in problem-solving, disturbed or altered behavior, coma, and seizures can occur. Muscle spasms are not one of the signs or symptoms of hypoglycemia.

13. c. *Rationale*: The Somogyi effect describes a cycle of insulin-induced posthypoglycemic episodes. In 1924, Joslin and associates noticed that hypoglycemia was associated with alternate episodes of hyperglycemia. The other answers are not correct.

14. d. *Rationale*: The loss of feeling, touch, and position sense increases the risk of falling. Impairment of temperature and pain sensation increases the risk of serious burns and injuries to the feet. Denervation of the small muscles of the foot result in clawing of the toes and displacement of the submetatarsal fat pad anteriorly. These changes, together with joint and connective tissue changes, alter the biomechanics of the foot, increasing plantar pressure and predisposing to development of foot trauma and ulcers. The other answers are incorrect.

15. a. *Rationale*: Diabetic nephropathy is the leading cause of chronic kidney disease, accounting for 40% of new cases. Also, diabetes is the leading cause of acquired blindness in the United States. The liver and pancreas are not organs that diabetes attacks.

16. a. *Rationale*: Multiple risk factors for macrovascular disease, including obesity, hypertension, hyperglycemia, hyperinsulinemia, hyperlipidemia, altered platelet function, endothelial dysfunction, systemic inflammation (as evidenced by increased C-reactive protein [CRP]), and elevated fibrinogen levels, frequently are found in people with diabetes. Hypotension, hypoinsulinemia, and decreased fibrinogen levels are not risk factors for macrovascular disease in diabetics.

17. b. *Rationale*: Foot problems have been reported as the most common complication leading to hospitalization among people with diabetes.

18. c. *Rationale*: Pyelonephritis and urinary tract infections are relatively common in persons with diabetes, and it has been suggested that these infections may bear some relation to the presence of a neurogenic bladder or nephrosclerotic changes in the kidneys. Urinary retention and urinary incontinence can both be the result of a neurogenic bladder. Nephrotic syndrome is not thought to be related to a neurogenic bladder in diabetics.

CHAPTER 43 STRUCTURE AND FUNCTION OF THE MALE GENITOURINARY SYSTEM

SECTION II: ASSESSING YOUR UNDERSTANDING

Activity A

1. genitourinary
2. antimüllerian hormone
3. Testosterone
4. inguinal canal
5. accessory organs
6. prostate
7. Spermatogenesis
8. Testosterone
9. protein synthesis
10. andropause

Activity B

1.

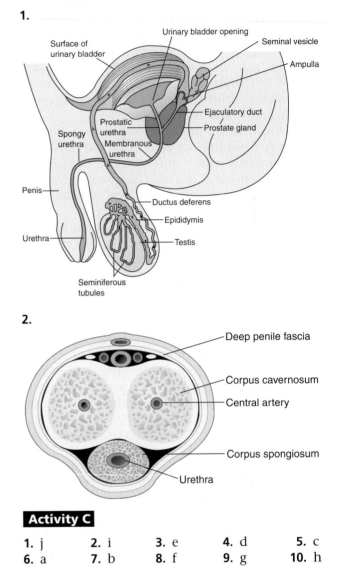

2.

Activity C

1. j	2. i	3. e	4. d	5. c
6. a	7. b	8. f	9. g	10. h

Activity D

1. At approximately 10 or 11 years of age, the adenohypophysis, or anterior pituitary, under the control of the hypothalamus begins to secrete the gonadotropins that stimulate testicular function and cause the interstitial cells of Leydig to begin producing testosterone. Approximately the same time, hormonal stimulation induces mitotic activity of the germ cells that develop in sperm. After cell maturation has begun, the testes begin to enlarge rapidly as the individual tubules grow. Full maturity and spermatogenesis usually are attained by 15 or 16 years of age.

2. In the first stage of spermatogenesis, small and unspecialized diploid germinal cells located immediately adjacent to the tubular wall, called the spermatogonia, undergo rapid mitotic division and provide a continuous source of new germinal cells. As these cells multiply, the more mature spermatogonia divide into two daughter cells, which grow and become the primary spermatocytes—the precursors of sperm. Over several weeks, large primary spermatocytes divide by a process called meiosis to form two smaller secondary spermatocytes. The spermatid elongates into a spermatozoon, or mature sperm cell, with a head and tail.

3. Among the undesired or harmful effects of supraphysiologic doses of androgens are acne, decreased testicular size, and azoospermia. These effects may persist for months after use of the agents has ceased. Because testosterone can be aromatized to estradiol in the peripheral tissues, androgens can also produce gynecomastia.

4. Erection involves the shunting of blood into the corpus cavernosum. It is controlled by the sympathetic, parasympathetic, and nonadrenergic–noncholinergic systems. Nitric oxide is the released locally as a mediator that produces relaxation of vascular smooth muscle. In the flaccid state, sympathetic discharge through α-adrenergic receptors maintains contraction of the arteries that supply the penis and vascular sinuses of the corpora cavernosa and corpus spongiosum. Parasympathetic stimulation produces erection by inhibiting sympathetic neurons that cause detumescence and by stimulating the release of nitric oxide to effect a rapid relaxation of the smooth muscle in the sinusoidal spaces of the corpus cavernosum.

SECTION III: APPLYING YOUR KNOWLEDGE

Activity E

1. Serum testosterone level, drawn at its peak, which is around 8 AM. If the initial total testosterone level is low, the diagnosis of hypogonadism should be confirmed with either a repeat measure of total testosterone or a measure of free (bioavailable) testosterone. Other tests include serum LH and FSH levels and seminal fluid analysis (SFA)

2. Secondary hypogonadism is related to either the pituitary gland or the hypothalamus. More

tests will be needed to determine what is causing this condition before treatment is determined.

SECTION IV: PRACTICING FOR NCLEX

Activity F

1. a. *Rationale*: Two systems maintain the temperature of the testes at a level consistent with sperm production. One is the pampiniform plexus of testicular veins that surround the testicular artery. This plexus absorbs heat from the arterial blood, cooling it as it enters the testes. The other is the cremaster muscle, which responds to decreases in testicular temperature by moving the testes closer to the body. The testicular artery and the tunica vaginalis are not used by the body to maintain optimal temperature in the testes for sperm production. The cremaster is a muscle, not a vein.

2. b. *Rationale*: Spermatozoa can be stored in the genital ducts for as long as 42 days and still maintain their fertility. The other answers are incorrect.

3. c. *Rationale*: Because sperm mobilization occurs at a pH of 6.0 to 6.5, the alkaline nature of the prostatic secretions is essential for successful fertilization of the ovum. The other answers are incorrect.

4. a, c. *Rationale*: The cylindrical body or shaft of the penis is composed of three masses of erectile tissue held together by fibrous strands and covered with a thin layer of skin. The two lateral masses of tissue are called the corpora cavernosa. The third, ventral mass is called the corpus spongiosum. All other answers are incorrect.

5. d. *Rationale*: The outer layer of the seminiferous tubules is made up of connective tissue and smooth muscle; the inner lining is composed of Sertoli cells, which are embedded with sperm in various stages of development. The other answers are incorrect.

6. a. *Rationale*: The function of the male reproductive system is under the negative feedback control of the hypothalamus and the anterior pituitary gonadotropic hormones, FSH and LH. Testosterone, AMG, and GH are not part of the negative feedback loop that regulates the male reproductive system.

7. a, b, d. *Rationale*: Among the undesired or harmful effects of supraphysiologic doses of androgens are acne, decreased testicular size,

and azoospermia. These effects may persist for months after use of the agents have ceased. Because testosterone can be aromatized to estradiol in the peripheral tissues, androgens can also produce gynecomastia (breast enlargement).

8. b. *Rationale*: Plasminogen activator, which converts plasminogen to plasmin, functions in the final detachment of mature spermatozoa from Sertoli cells. Prostate secretions, testosterone, and androgen-binding protein do not release mature spermatozoa from the Sertoli cells.

9. c. *Rationale*: Erectile dysfunction can be caused by disease or dysfunction of the brain, spinal cord, cavernous or pudendal nerves, or terminal nerve endings or receptors. The other answers do not cause erectile dysfunction.

10. d. *Rationale*: The term andropause has been used to describe an ill-defined collection of symptoms in aging men, typically those older than 50 years, who have a relative or absolute hypogonadism associated with aging. The other answers are incorrect.

CHAPTER 44 DISORDERS OF THE MALE GENITOURINARY SYSTEM

SECTION II: ASSESSING YOUR UNDERSTANDING

Activity A

1. Hypospadias, epispadias
2. Peyronie disease
3. Peyronie
4. parasympathetic, sympathetic
5. nitric oxide, arterial
6. Erectile dysfunction
7. cardiovascular, metabolic
8. Priapism
9. penile cancer
10. cryptorchidism
11. motility
12. Epididymitis
13. Prostatitis
14. acute bacterial prostatitis
15. prostate
16. chronic bacterial prostatitis
17. extraprostatic
18. prostate-specific antigen

Activity B

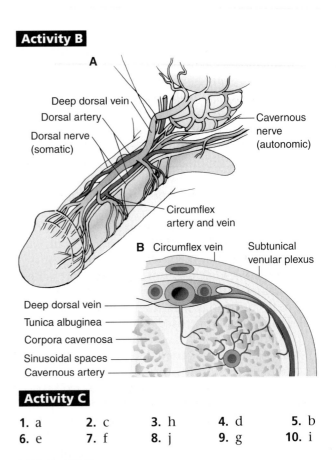

A

Deep dorsal vein
Dorsal artery
Dorsal nerve (somatic)
Cavernous nerve (autonomic)
Circumflex artery and vein

B Circumflex vein   Subtunical venular plexus

Deep dorsal vein
Tunica albuginea
Corpora cavernosa
Sinusoidal spaces
Cavernous artery

Activity C

1. a   2. c   3. h   4. d   5. b
6. e   7. f   8. j   9. g   10. i

Activity D

1. Neurogenic disorders, such as Parkinson disease, stroke, and cerebral trauma, often contribute to erectile dysfunction by decreasing libido or preventing the initiation of erection. In spinal cord injury, the extent of neural impairment depends on the level, location, and extent of the lesion. Hormonal causes of erectile dysfunction include a decrease in androgen levels owing to both primary and secondary hypogonadism. Common risk factors for generalized penile arterial insufficiency include hypertension, hyperlipidemia, cigarette smoking, diabetes mellitus, and pelvic irradiation.

2. Sildenafil (Viagra) is a selective inhibitor of phosphodiesterase type 5 (PDE-5), the enzyme that inactivates cyclic guanosine monophosphate (cGMP). This acts by facilitating corporeal smooth muscle relaxation in response to sexual stimulation.

3. Testicular torsion is a twisting of the spermatic cord that suspends the testis. Extravaginal torsion, which occurs almost exclusively in

neonates, is the less common form. It occurs when the testicle and the fascial tunicae that surround it rotate around the spermatic cord at a level well above the tunica vaginalis. The torsion probably occurs during fetal or neonatal descent of the testes before the tunica adheres to the scrotal wall. Intravaginal torsion is considerably more common than extravaginal torsion. It occurs when the testis rotates on the long axis in the tunica vaginalis. In most cases, congenital abnormalities of the tunica vaginalis or spermatic cord exist. The tunica vaginalis normally surrounds the testes and epididymis, allowing the testicle to rotate freely in the tunica. Patients usually present in severe distress within hours of onset and often have nausea, vomiting, and tachycardia. The affected testis is large and tender, with pain radiating to the inguinal area.

4. The clinical staging for testicular cancer is as follows: stage I, tumor confined to testes, epididymis, or spermatic cord; stage II, tumor spread to retroperitoneal lymph nodes below the diaphragm; and stage III, metastases outside the retroperitoneal nodes or above the diaphragm.

5. The anatomic location of the prostate at the bladder neck contributes to the pathophysiology and symptomatology of benign prostatic hyperplasia (BPH). The two prostatic components to the obstructive properties of BPH and development of lower urinary tract symptoms are dynamic and static. The static component of BPH is related to an increase in prostatic size; it gives rise to symptoms such as a weak urinary stream, postvoid dribbling, frequency of urination, and nocturia. The dynamic component of BPH is related to prostatic smooth muscle tone. α_1-Adrenergic receptors are the main receptors for the smooth muscle component of the prostate.

6. The diagnosis of prostate cancer is based on history and physical examination and confirmed through biopsy methods. Transrectal ultrasonography is used to guide a biopsy needle and document the exact location of the biopsied tissue. Radiologic examination of the bones of the skull, ribs, spine, and pelvis can be used to reveal metastases. Prostatic-specific antigen (PSA) levels are important in the staging and management of prostate cancer. In

untreated cases, the level of PSA correlates with the volume and stage of disease.

SECTION III: APPLYING YOUR KNOWLEDGE

Activity E

1. The cause of penile cancer is not known, although several risk factors are thought to be linked to this cancer.
2. Research data has shown that the most important prognostic indicator is the status of your lymph nodes. The more lymph nodes that are involved, the more advanced your cancer has become. It is important that you ask your physician what your prognosis is.

SECTION IV: PRACTICING FOR NCLEX

Activity F

1. a, c, e. *Rationale*: Factors that influence the timing of surgical repair include anesthetic risk, penile size, and the psychological effects of the surgery on the child. In mild cases, the surgery is done for cosmetic reasons only. In more severe cases, repair becomes essential for normal sexual functioning and to prevent the psychological sequelae of having malformed genitalia. Testicular involvement and presence of an abdominal hernia have no bearing on the timing of the surgery.
2. a. *Rationale*: Peyronie disease involves a localized and progressive fibrosis of unknown origin that affects the tunica albuginea (i.e., the tough, fibrous sheath that surrounds the corpora cavernosa) of the penis The disorder is characterized initially by an inflammatory process that results in dense fibrous plaque formation. The plaque usually is on the dorsal midline of the shaft, causing upward bowing of the shaft during erection. The other answers are incorrect.
3. b. *Rationale*: Priapism can occur at any age, in the newborn as well as other age groups. Sickle cell disease or neoplasms are the most common cause in boys between 5 and 10 years of age. Hemophilia and hypospadias are not linked to priapism in any age group.
4. c. *Rationale*: The treatment goals for the boys with cryptorchidism include measures to

enhance future fertility potential, placement of the gonad in a favorable place for cancer detection, and improved cosmetic appearance. The other answers are incorrect.

5. d. *Rationale*: Hydroceles are palpated as cystic masses that may attain massive proportions. With sufficient fluid, the mass may be mistaken for a solid tumor. Transillumination of the scrotum (i.e., shining a light through the scrotum to visualize its internal structures) or ultrasonography can help to determine whether the mass is solid or cystic and whether the testicle is normal. The other answers are incorrect.

6. a. *Rationale*: The most common acute scrotal disorder in the pediatric population is testicular torsion. The other answers are incorrect.

7. b. *Rationale*: Sexually transmitted acute epididymitis occurs mainly in young men without underlying genitourinary disease and is most commonly caused by *Chlamydia trachomatis* and *Neisseria gonorrhoeae*. *Candida albicans* and *Escherichia coli* are not the most common causes of epidiymitis in young men without underlying genitourinary disease.

8. a, b, c. *Rationale*: Signs of metastatic spread include swelling of the lower extremities, back pain, neck mass, cough, hemoptysis, or dizziness. Gynecomastia (breast enlargement) may result from human chorionic gonadotropin (hCG)-producing tumors and occurs in about 5% of men with germ cell tumors. The other answers are not signs of metastatic spread of a testicular cancer.

9. c. *Rationale*: The manifestations of acute bacterial prostatitis include fever and chills, malaise, myalgia, arthralgia, frequent and urgent urination, dysuria, and urethral discharge. Dull, aching pain often is present in the perineum, rectum, or sacrococcygeal region. The other answers are incorrect.

10. d. *Rationale*: The incidence of benign prostatic hyperplasia increases with advanced age and is highest in African Americans and lowest in native Japanese. The other answers are incorrect.

CHAPTER 45 CONCEPTS OF HEALTH AND DISEASE

SECTION II: ASSESSING YOUR UNDERSTANDING

Activity A

1. mons pubis
2. labia majora
3. labia minora
4. clitoris
5. vagina
6. uterus
7. broad, round, uterosacral, transverse
8. myometrium
9. endometrium
10. fallopian tube
11. estrogen, progesterone
12. follicle-stimulating hormone (FSH), luteinizing hormone (LH)
13. sex
14. fat tissue
15. anti-inflammatory
16. progesterone
17. endometrium
18. oocyte
19. corpus albicans, menstruation
20. human chorionic gonadotropin
21. endometrium
22. ferning
23. Menopause
24. urogenital atrophy
25. osteoporosis, cardiovascular
26. breasts
27. Estrogen
28. Progesterone

1.

2.

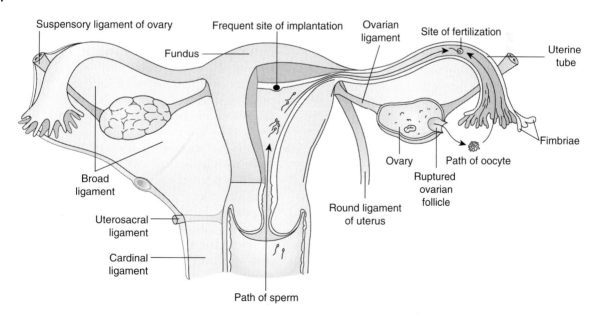

Activity C

1. f   **2.** j   **3.** c   **4.** h   **5.** a
6. g   **7.** i   **8.** b   **9.** d   **10.** e

Activity D

1. Vaginal tissue usually is moist, with a pH maintained within the bacteriostatic range of 3.8 to 4.2. Glycogen is fermented to lactic acid by the lactobacilli (i.e., Döderlein's bacilli) that are part of the normal vaginal flora, accounting for the mildly acid pH of vaginal fluid.
2. Evidence indicates that a certain minimal body weight (48 kg) and fat content (16%–24%) are necessary for menarche to occur and for the menstrual cycle to be maintained. This is supported by the observation of amenorrhea in women with anorexia nervosa, chronic disease, and malnutrition and in those who are long-distance runners. In women with anorexia nervosa, gonadotropin and estradiol secretion, including LH release and responsiveness to the hypothalamic gonadotropin-releasing hormone (GnRH), can revert to prepubertal levels.
3. Estrogens have additional cardioprotective actions, including direct antiatherosclerotic effects on the arterial wall (augmentation of vasodilating and antiplatelet aggregation factors such as nitric oxide and prostacyclin), vasodilation through endothelium-independent mechanisms, antioxidant activity, reduced levels of angiotensin-converting enzyme and renin, reduction of homocysteine levels, improved peripheral glucose metabolism with subsequent decreased circulating insulin levels, and direct effects on cardiac function.
4. Estrogens are necessary for normal female physical maturation. In concert with other hormones, estrogens provide for the reproductive processes of ovulation, implantation of the products of conception, pregnancy, parturition, and lactation by stimulating the development and maintaining the growth of the accessory organs. In the absence of androgens, estrogens stimulate the intrauterine development of the vagina, uterus, and uterine tubes from the embryonic müllerian system. They also stimulate the stromal development and ductal growth of the breasts at puberty. Estrogens are responsible for the accelerated pubertal skeletal growth phase and for closure of the epiphyses of the long bones; they contribute to the growth of axillary and pubic hair, and alter the distribution of body fat to produce the typical female body contours, including the accumulation of body fat around the hips and breasts. Larger quantities of estrogen stimulate pigmentation of the skin in the nipple, areolar, and genital regions.
5. Over the past four to five decades, hormone therapy (HT) became increasingly prescribed for postmenopausal women. Initially, HT was used only for symptom management and later for prevention of osteoporosis. During the 1990s, HT evolved to the status of replacement for a vital hormone lost because of an endocrine organ failure (menopause). It was routinely offered to all postmenopausal women based on mounting evidence of preventive benefits in numerous areas. During this time, data from observational studies demonstrated a 50% reduction in coronary artery disease (CAD) mortality rates in women using HT. Other demonstrated advantages of HT included a reduced risk of Alzheimer disease, decreased risk of colon cancer, less tooth loss, and lower incidence of macular degeneration. Unopposed estrogen can lead to the development of endometrial hyperplasia which, in some cases, can increase a woman's risk for endometrial cancer. The Women's Health Initiative study to investigate the potential effects of HT was stopped after 5.2 years of data analysis when it was found that the risk of breast cancer crossed the predetermined safety boundary and it was determined that the risks of HT outweighed its benefits. In addition to breast cancer risk, CAD, stroke, and venous thromboembolic disease were all increased. On the positive side, a reduction was noted in colorectal cancer and hip fractures among the women using HT.
6. During lactation, milk is secreted by alveolar cells, which are under the influence of the anterior pituitary hormone prolactin. Milk ejection from the ductile system occurs in response to the release of oxytocin from the posterior pituitary. The suckling of the infant provides the stimulus for milk ejection. Suckling produces feedback to the hypothalamus, stimulating the release of oxytocin from the posterior pituitary. Oxytocin causes contraction of the myoepithelial cells lining the alveoli and ejection of milk into the ductal system.

SECTION III: APPLYING YOUR KNOWLEDGE
Activity E

1. Several studies have been conducted to either confirm or refute the use of HT in post-menopausal women. Evidence-based practice now shows that HT can increase the risk of cardiovascular events, as well as increase the risk of breast cancer.
2. No research data show that HT can reverse the normal signs of aging in the female body.

SECTION IV: PRACTICING FOR NCLEX
Activity F

1. a. *Rationale*: The area between labia minora is called the vestibule. Located in the vestibule are the urethral and vaginal openings and Bartholin's lubricating glands. The other answers are incorrect.
2. b. *Rationale*: The glycogen is fermented to lactic acid by the lactobacilli (i.e., Döderlein's bacilli), which are part of the normal vaginal flora, accounting for the mildly acid pH of vaginal fluid. The other answers are incorrect.
3. c. *Rationale*: Anteriorly, the perimetrium is reflected over the bladder wall, forming the vesicouterine pouch; posteriorly, it extends to form the cul-de-sac, or pouch of Douglas. The other answers are incorrect.
4. d. *Rationale*: The end of the fallopian tube nearest the ovary forms a funnel-like opening with fringed, fingerlike projections called fimbriae, which pick up the ovum after its release into the peritoneal cavity after ovulation. The other answers are incorrect.
5. a. *Rationale*: After ovulation, the follicle becomes luteinized; as the corpus luteum, it produces estrogen and progesterone to support the endometrium until conception occurs or the cycle begins again. The other answers are incorrect.
6. b. *Rationale*: Although the mechanism is uncertain, progesterone increases basal body temperature and is responsible for the increase in body temperature that occurs with ovulation. The other answers are effects of estrogen.
7. c. *Rationale*: High levels of estrogen exert a negative feedback effect on FSH, inhibiting multiple follicular development and causing an increase in LH levels. The other answers are incorrect.
8. a, b, d. *Rationale*: Problems that can arise as a result of urogenital atrophy include vaginal dryness, urinary stress incontinence, urgency, nocturia, vaginitis, and urinary tract infection. URI, an upper respiratory infection, has nothing to do with menopause and urinary retention is not a problem that arises from menopause.
9. d. *Rationale*: The small bumps or projections on the areolar surface known as Montgomery's tubercles are sebaceous glands that keep the nipple area soft and elastic. The other answers are incorrect.
10. a. *Rationale*: Milk ejection from the ductile system occurs in response to the release of oxytocin from the posterior pituitary. The other answers are incorrect.

CHAPTER 46 DISORDERS OF THE FEMALE REPRODUCTIVE SYSTEM

SECTION II: ASSESSING YOUR UNDERSTANDING
Activity A

1. hair-bearing
2. vulva
3. Bartholin gland cyst
4. Chronic dermatitis
5. ecology
6. Vaginitis
7. bleeding
8. metaplasia
9. Cervical
10. cervicitis
11. Polyps
12. Human papillomavirus (HPV)
13. Endometriosis
14. Adenomyosis
15. Dilatation, curettage
16. leiomyomas
17. Pelvic inflammatory disease (PID)
18. Ectopic pregnancy
19. menstrual, fertility
20. Polycystic ovary
21. luteinizing hormone (LH)
22. Ovarian
23. ovulatory age
24. tumor suppressor
25. Rectocele
26. cardinal
27. uterine prolapse
28. amenorrhea
29. Galactorrhea

30. Mastitis
31. Fibroadenomas
32. Fibrocystic

33. Paget
34. Infertility

Activity B

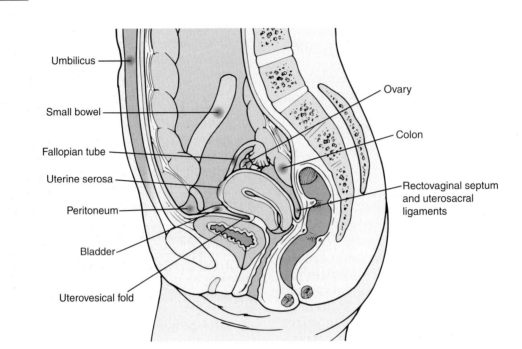

Umbilicus

Small bowel

Fallopian tube

Uterine serosa

Peritoneum

Bladder

Uterovesical fold

Ovary

Colon

Rectovaginal septum and uterosacral ligaments

Activity C

1.

1. i	**2.** h	**3.** c	**4.** b	**5.** d
6. f	**7.** e	**8.** j	**9.** a	**10.** g

2.

1. d	**2.** f	**3.** b	**4.** a	**5.** g
6. c	**7.** e			

Activity D

1. The prevention and treatment of vaginal infections depend on proper health habits and accurate diagnosis and treatment of ongoing infections. Measures to prevent infection include those that keep the genital area clean and dry, maintenance of normal vaginal flora and healthy vaginal mucosa, and avoidance of contact with organisms known to cause vaginal infections. Perfumed products, such as feminine deodorant sprays, douches, bath powders, soaps, and even toilet paper, can be irritating and may alter the normal vaginal flora. Tight clothing prevents the dissipation of body heat and evaporation of skin moisture and promotes favorable conditions for irritation and the growth of pathogens. Cotton un-

dergarments that can withstand hot water and bleach (a fungicide) may be preferable for women to prevent such infections.

2. A quadrivalent vaccine (Gardisil) to prevent infection with the HPV subtypes 6, 11, 16, and 18 was licensed by the US Food and Drug Administration (FDA) in June 2006. The vaccine targets the two strains of HPV (HPV 16 and 18), which are responsible for 70% of cervical cancer, and the two most common benign strains (HPV 6 and 11), which account for up to 90% of genital warts. The vaccine is targeted for females between the ages of 9 to 26 years, optimally before initiating sexual activity. Clinical studies provided to the FDA have confirmed that the vaccine appears safe and effective in inducing long-term immunity to HPV.

3. Diagnosis of cervical cancer requires pathologic confirmation. Papanicolaou smear results demonstrating squamous intraepithelial lesion (SIL) often require further evaluation by colposcopy during which a biopsy sample may be obtained from suspect areas and examined microscopically. An alternate diagnostic tool in areas where colposcopy is not readily available is a noninvasive photographic technique, in

which a cervicography camera is used to photograph the cervix. The projected cervicogram (a slide made from the film) is then sent for expert evaluation. In one study, the cervicogram was found to give a greater yield of cervical intraepithelial neoplasia (CIN) than Papanicolaou smear alone in patients with previous abnormal Papanicolaou smears.

4. The first theory, the regurgitation/implantation theory suggests that menstrual blood containing fragments of endometrium is forced upward through the fallopian tubes into the peritoneal cavity. Retrograde menstruation is not an uncommon phenomenon, and it is unknown why endometrial cells implant and grow in some women but not in others. A second theory, the metaplastic theory, proposes that dormant, immature cellular elements, spread over a wide area during embryonic development, persist into adult life and then differentiate into endometrial tissue. A third theory, the vascular/lymphatic theory, suggests that the endometrial tissue may metastasize through the lymphatics or vascular system. Genetic and immune factors also have been studied as contributing factors to the development of endometriosis.

5. The organisms ascend through the endocervical canal to the endometrial cavity, and then to the tubes and ovaries. The endocervical canal is slightly dilated during menstruation, allowing bacteria to gain entrance to the uterus and other pelvic structures. After entering the upper reproductive tract, the organisms multiply rapidly in the favorable environment of the sloughing endometrium and ascend to the fallopian tube.

6. There is also concern that women with PCOS who are anovulatory do not produce significant amounts of progesterone. This, in turn, may subject the uterine lining to an unopposed estrogen environment, which is a significant risk factor for development of endometrial cancer. Although an association with breast cancer and ovarian cancer has been reported, PCOS has not been conclusively shown to be an independent risk factor for either malignancy.

7. The uterus and the pelvic structures are maintained in proper position by the uterosacral, round, broad, and cardinal ligaments. The two cardinal ligaments maintain the cervix in its normal position. The uterosacral ligaments hold the uterus in a forward position and the broad ligaments suspend the uterus, fallopian

tubes, and ovaries in the pelvis. The vagina is encased in the semirigid structure of the strong supporting fascia. The muscular floor of the pelvis is a strong, slinglike structure that supports the uterus, vagina, urinary bladder, and rectum.

8. Dysfunctional menstrual cycles are related to alterations in the hormones that support normal cyclic endometrial changes. Estrogen deprivation causes retrogression of a previously built-up endometrium and bleeding. Such bleeding often is irregular in amount and duration, with the flow varying with the time and degree of estrogen stimulation and with the degree of estrogen withdrawal. A lack of progesterone can cause abnormal menstrual bleeding; in its absence, estrogen induces development of a much thicker endometrial layer with a richer blood supply. The absence of progesterone results from the failure of any of the developing ovarian follicles to mature to the point of ovulation, with the subsequent formation of the corpus luteum and production and secretion of progesterone.

9. Approximately 5% to 10% of all breast cancers are hereditary, with genetic mutations causing up to 80% of breast cancers in women under age 50. Two breast cancer susceptibility genes—BRCA1 on chromosome 17 and BRCA2 on chromosome 13—may account for most inherited forms of breast cancer. BRCA1 is known to be involved in tumor suppression. A woman with known mutations in BRCA1 has a lifetime risk of 60% to 85% for breast cancer and an increased risk of ovarian cancer. BRCA2 is another susceptibility gene that carries an elevated cancer risk similar to that with BRCA1

SECTION III: APPLYING YOUR KNOWLEDGE
Activity E

1. A colposcopy is the examination of the vagina and cervix with an optical magnifying instrument. It is usually done after a Papanicolaou smear shows abnormal cells.

2. A LEEP uses a thin, rigid, wire loop that is attached to a generator. It blends high-frequency, low-voltage current for cutting with a higher voltage current for coagulation. The wire loop allows the physician to remove the entire transformation zone of the cervix. This removes the entire lesion and provides a

specimen for further histologic evaluation. The procedure is done under local anesthesia in the physician's office at a lower cost than a cone biopsy, which is done in the hospital or out-patient surgery clinic.

SECTION IV: PRACTICING FOR NCLEX
Activity F

1. a. *Rationale*: Surgical treatment of a Bartholin cyst that has abscessed or blocks the entroitis is called marsupialization, a procedure that involves removal of a wedge of vulvar skin and the cyst wall. The other answers are incorrect.

2. b. *Rationale*: One-third to one-half of vulvar intraepithelial neoplasm (VIN) cases appear to be caused by the cancer-promoting potential of certain strains (subtypes 16 and 18) of HPV that are sexually transmitted and are associated with the type of vulvar cancer found in younger women. The other answers are not thought to be associated with vulvar cancer in younger women.

3. a, b, c. *Rationale*: In premenarchal girls, most vaginal infections have nonspecific causes, such as poor hygiene, intestinal parasites, or the presence of foreign bodies. Vaginal deodorants and tampons are not associated with vaginal infections in premenarchal girls.

4. c. *Rationale*: Blockage of the mucosal glands results in trapping of mucus in the deeper glands leading to the formation of dilated cysts within the cervix, called nabothian cysts. The other answers are incorrect.

5. d. *Rationale*: Risk factors for endometriosis may include early menarche; regular periods with shorter cycles (<27 days), longer duration (>7 days), or heavier flow; increased menstrual pain; and other first-degree relatives with the condition. Late menarche, light flow, and periods shorter than 7 days are not risk factors for endometriosis.

6. a. *Rationale*: Leiomyomas are asymptomatic approximately half of the time and may be discovered during a routine pelvic examination, or they may cause menorrhagia (excessive menstrual bleeding), anemia, urinary frequency, rectal pressure/constipation, abdominal distention, and, infrequently, pain. Diarrhea and urinary retention are not symptoms of leiomyomas.

7. b. *Rationale*: New-onset breakthrough bleeding in women who are on oral contraceptives or medroxyprogesterone contraceptive injection (Depo-Provera) has been associated with pelvic inflammatory disease (PID). The other forms of contraception have not been associated with PID.

8. c. *Rationale*: Diagnostic tests for ectopic pregnancy include a urine pregnancy test, ultrasonography, and β-human chorionic gonadotropin (hCG), the hormone produced by placental cells) levels. Serial β- hCG tests may detect lower-than-normal hCG production. Transvaginal ultrasound studies after 5 weeks' gestation may demonstrate an empty uterine cavity or presence of the gestational sac outside the uterus. In a comparison of various protocols for diagnosing ectopic pregnancy, ultrasound followed by serial hCG levels was found to yield the best results. The other answers are incorrect.

9. d. *Rationale*: Metformin, an insulin-sensitizing drug, used with or without ovulation-inducing medications, is emerging as an important component of polycystic ovary syndrome (PCOS) treatment. Dehydroepiandrosterone (DHEAS) is often found in the blood of women with PCOS; Methotrexate is used in ectopic pregnancies; Spironalactone, an antimineralocorticoid, is used in treating PCOS, not mineralocorticoids.

10. a, c, e. *Rationale*: Symptoms believed to have a strong correlation with ovarian cancer include abdominal or pelvic pain, increased abdominal size or bloating, and difficulty eating or feeling full quickly after ingesting food. Increased intestinal gas and an increased appetite are not highly correlated with ovarian cancer.

11. a. *Rationale*: A pessary can be inserted to hold the uterus in place and it may stave off surgical intervention in women who want to have children or in older women for whom the surgery may pose a significant health risk. The other answers are incorrect.

12. b. *Rationale*: Although analgesic agents, such as aspirin and acetaminophen, may relieve minor uterine cramping or low back pain, prostaglandin synthetase inhibitors (e.g., ibuprofen, naproxen, mefenamic acid, indomethacin) are more specific for dysmenorrhea and the treatment of choice, if contraception is not desired. Metformic acid is incorrect.

13. c. *Rationale*: Treatment for mastitis symptoms include application of heat or cold, excision, aspiration, mild analgesics, antibiotics, and a

supportive brassiere or breast binder. The other answers are incorrect.

14. d. *Rationale*: Diagnosis of fibrocystic changes is made by physical examination, mammography, ultrasonography, and biopsy (i.e., aspiration or tissue sample). Patient history and galactography are not used to diagnose fibrocystic changes in the breast.

15. a. *Rationale*: Postmenopausal women and women who have had a hysterectomy can perform the examination any day of the month. The other answers are incorrect.

16. b. *Rationale*: The specimen is best collected by masturbation into a sterile container after 3 days of abstinence. The other answers are incorrect.

17. c. *Rationale*: Between 12 and 24 hours after insemination, the ova are evaluated for signs of fertilization. If signs are present, the ova are returned to the incubator, and 48 to 72 hours after egg retrieval, the fertilized eggs are placed into the woman's uterus by means of a transcervical catheter. The other answers are incorrect.

CHAPTER 47 SEXUALLY TRANSMITTED INFECTIONS

SECTION II: ASSESSING YOUR UNDERSTANDING

Activity A

1. mucocutaneous
2. fetus or newborn
3. Genital warts
4. external genitalia
5. Genital herpes
6. neurotropic
7. type-2
8. primary genital herpes
9. Molluscum contagiosum
10. yeast
11. Trichomonads
12. Bacterial
13. Chlamydiae
14. fallopian tube
15. gonococcus
16. Syphilis

Activity B

1. j	2. h	3. a	4. d	5. g
6. f	7. i	8. b	9. e	10. c

Activity C

1. Risk factors for acquiring the human papillomavirus (HPV) include young age (<25 years), early age of first intercourse (<16 years), increasing numbers of sex partners, and having a male partner with multiple sex partners. HPV infection can occur with any type of vaginal or anal penetration and is common in men having sex with men and women having sex with women. Oral–genital and manual–genital contact are less likely means of spreading this infection.

2. Herpes simplex virus (HSV) is transmitted by contact with infectious lesions or secretions. Herpes simplex virus type-1 is transmitted by oral secretions, and infections frequently occur in childhood. Herpes simplex virus type-1 can be spread to the genital area by autoinoculation after poor handwashing or through oral–genital contact. Herpes simplex virus type-2 usually is transmitted by sexual contact but can be passed to an infant during childbirth if the virus is actively being shed from the genital tract. In genital herpes, the virus ascends through the peripheral nerves to the sacral dorsal root ganglia. The virus can remain dormant in the dorsal root ganglia, or it can reactivate, in which case the viral particles are transported back down the nerve root to the skin, where they multiply and cause a lesion to develop.

3. Reported risk factors for the overgrowth of *Candida albicans* include recent antibiotic therapy, which suppresses the normal protective bacterial flora; high hormone levels owing to pregnancy or the use of oral contraceptives, which cause an increase in vaginal glycogen stores; and uncontrolled diabetes mellitus or human immunodeficiency virus (HIV) infection, because they compromise the immune system.

4. Trichomoniasis is a risk factor for HIV transmission and infectivity in both men and women. In women, it increases the risk of tubal infertility and atypical pelvic inflammatory disease, and it is associated with adverse outcomes, such as premature birth in pregnant women. Trichomonads attach easily to mucous membrane. They can serve as vectors for the spread of other organisms, carrying pathogens attached to their surface into the fallopian tubes. In men, it is a common cause of nongonococcal urethritis and is a risk factor for infertility, altering sperm motility and viability.

It has also been associated with chronic prostatitis.

5. Men are more likely to be symptomatic than women. In men, the initial symptoms include urethral pain and a creamy yellow, sometimes bloody, discharge. The disorder may become chronic and affect the prostate, epididymis, and periurethral glands. Rectal infections are common in homosexual men. In women, recognizable symptoms include unusual genital or urinary discharge, dysuria, dyspareunia, pelvic pain or tenderness, unusual vaginal bleeding (including bleeding after intercourse), fever, and proctitis. Symptoms can occur or increase during or immediately after menses because the bacterium is an intracellular diplococcus that thrives in menstrual blood but cannot survive long outside the human body. There may be infections of the uterus and development of acute or chronic infection of the fallopian tubes, with ultimate scarring and sterility.

6. The clinical disease is divided into three stages: primary, secondary, and tertiary. Primary syphilis is characterized by the appearance of a chancre at the site of exposure. These lesions usually are painless and located at the site of sexual contact. The timing of the second stage of syphilis varies even more than that of the first, lasting from 1 week to 6 months. The symptoms of a rash, fever, sore throat, stomatitis, nausea, loss of appetite, and inflamed eyes may come and go for a year but usually last for 3 to 6 months. Secondary manifestations can include alopecia and genital condylomata latum. Condylomata latum are elevated, red-brown lesions that can ulcerate and produce a foul discharge. They are 2 to 3 cm in diameter, contain many spirochetes, and are highly infectious. Tertiary syphilis is a delayed response of the untreated disease. It can occur as long as 20 years after the initial infection. When syphilis does progress to the symptomatic tertiary stage, it commonly takes one of three forms: development of localized destructive lesions called *gummas*, development of cardiovascular lesions, or development of central nervous system lesions.

SECTION III: APPLYING YOUR KNOWLEDGE

Activity D

1. While taking the nursing history, you would find it important to note the following:

urethral itching, meatal erythema and tenderness, urethral discharge, history of sexual relations with someone being treated for a chlamydial infection, and history of recent conjunctivitis

2. The expected treatment for chlamydial infection includes pharmacologic treatment with either azithromycin or doxycycline, simultaneous treatment of both sexual partners, and abstinence from sexual activity to facilitate cure.

SECTION IV: PRACTICING FOR NCLEX

Activity E

1. a. *Rationale*: The incubation period for HPV-induced genital warts ranges from 6 weeks to 8 months, with a mean of 2 to 3 months. The other answers are incorrect.

2. a, c, e. *Rationale*: The initial symptoms of primary genital herpes infections include tingling, itching, and pain in the genital area, followed by eruption of small pustules and vesicles. Chancres and eczemalike lesions are not indicative of genital herpes.

3. b. *Rationale*: The antiviral drugs acyclovir, valacyclovir, and famciclovir have become the cornerstone for the treatment of genital herpes. The other drugs are not used in the treatment of genital herpes.

4. c. *Rationale*: Chancroid organisms have shown resistance to treatment with sulfamethoxazole alone and to tetracycline. The Centers for Disease Control and Prevention (CDC) recommends treatment with azithromycin, erythromycin, or ceftriaxone. The other answers are incorrect.

5. d. *Rationale*: An important characteristic of *Lymphogranuloma venereum* (LGV) is the early (1 to 4 weeks later) development of large, tender, and sometimes fluctuant inguinal lymph nodes called buboes.

6. a. *Rationale*: Antifungal agents, such as clotrimazole, miconazole, butaconazole, and terconazole, in various forms, are effective in treating candidiasis. These drugs, with the exception of terconazole, are available without prescription for use by women who have had a previously confirmed diagnosis of candidiasis.

7. b. *Rationale*: Trichomoniasis can cause a number of complications. It is a risk factor for HIV transmission and infectivity in both men and women. In women, it increases the risk of

tubal infertility and atypical pelvic inflammatory disease, and it is associated with adverse outcomes, such as premature birth, in pregnant women. The other answers are incorrect.

8. c. *Rationale*: The predominant symptom of bacterial vaginosis is a thin, grayish-white discharge that has a foul, fishy odor. The other answers are incorrect.

9. a, b, e. *Rationale*: A specimen should be collected from the appropriate site (i.e., endocervix, urethra, anal canal, or oropharynx), inoculated onto a suitable medium, and transported under appropriate conditions. The nasal passages and the exocervix are not sites that would be used for the collection of *Neisseria gonorrhoeae*.

10. d. *Rationale*: The syphilitic gumma is a peculiar, rubbery, necrotic lesion that is caused by noninflammatory tissue necrosis. Gummas can occur singly or multiply and vary in size from microscopic lesions to large, tumorous masses. They most commonly are found in the liver, testes, and bone. Chancres occur in primary syphilis. Chancroid is a sexually transmitted infection (STI). Gummies are candy.

CHAPTER 48 ORGANIZATION AND CONTROL OF NEURAL FUNCTION

SECTION II: ASSESSING YOUR UNDERSTANDING

Activity A

1. neurons
2. Schwann cells, neuroglial
3. body, dendrites, axons, synapses
4. Dendrites
5. anterograde, retrograde
6. Schwann, satellite
7. Satellite
8. myelin
9. nodes of Ranvier, saltatory conduction
10. oligodendrocytes
11. Glucose
12. action potentials
13. resting membrane potential
14. synapses
15. Chemical

16. synaptic cleft
17. depolarization, hyperpolarization
18. excitatory postsynaptic
19. neurotransmission
20. Neuromodulator
21. Neurotrophic
22. reticular activating system
23. pia mater
24. spinal nerves
25. paired segmental spinal nerves
26. plexuses
27. reflex
28. withdrawal
29. hindbrain, midbrain, forebrain
30. hypoglossal
31. vagus
32. spinal accessory nerve
33. glossopharyngeal nerve
34. vestibulocochlear nerve
35. facial nerve
36. abducens
37. trigeminal nerve
38. cerebellum
39. thalamus
40. gyrus, sulcus
41. basal ganglia
42. primary somatosensory cortex
43. meninges
44. CSF
45. autonomic nervous system.
46. parasympathetic nervous system

Activity B

1.

2.

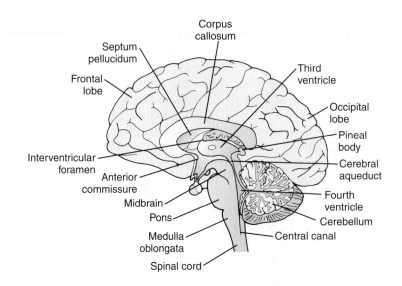

Corpus callosum
Septum pellucidum
Frontal lobe
Third ventricle
Occipital lobe
Pineal body
Cerebral aqueduct
Interventricular foramen
Anterior commissure
Midbrain
Pons
Medulla oblongata
Spinal cord
Fourth ventricle
Cerebellum
Central canal

Activity C

1.

1. f	**2.** h	**3.** e	**4.** b	**5.** d
6. c	**7.** a	**8.** j	**9.** g	**10.** i

2.

1. b	**2.** i	**3.** e	**4.** g	**5.** f
6. a	**7.** h	**8.** c	**9.** d	

Activity D

1. Myelin formation is essentially the same in both the peripheral nervous system (PNS) and central nervous system (CNS); both contain myelin basic protein and both involve the winding of plasma membranes around the nerve fiber. During the wrapping of myelin, the cytoplasm between two adjacent inner leaflets of the plasma membrane is expelled. The two adjacent inner leaflets and any remaining cytoplasm appear as a dark line called the "major dense line." Likewise, during the wrapping of the plasma membranes to form myelin, adjacent outer plasma membrane leaflets become opposed, creating the interperiod or minor dense line. Linking proteins, proteolipid protein (PLP) found only in the CNS and myelin protein zero (MPZ) found only in the PNS, help stabilize adjacent plasma membranes of the myelin sheath.

2. Nervous tissue has a high rate of metabolism. Although the brain comprises only 2% of the body's weight, it receives approximately 15% of the resting cardiac output and consumes 20% of its oxygen. Despite its substantial energy requirements, the brain cannot store oxygen or effectively engage in anaerobic metabolism. An interruption in the blood or oxygen supply to the brain rapidly leads to clinically observable signs and symptoms. Without oxygen, brain cells continue to function for approximately 10 seconds. Unconsciousness occurs almost simultaneously with cardiac arrest, and the death of brain cells begins within 4 to 6 minutes.

3. The local currents resulting from an excitatory postsynaptic potential (EPSP) (sometimes called a generator potential) are usually insufficient to reach threshold and cause depolarization of the axon's initial segment. However, if several EPSPs occur simultaneously, the area of depolarization can become sufficiently large and the currents at the initial segment can become sufficiently strong to exceed the threshold potential and initiate an action potential. This summation of depolarized areas is called "spatial summation." EPSPs also can summate and cause an action potential if they occur in rapid succession. This temporal aspect of the occurrence of two or more EPSPs is called "temporal summation." Inhibitory postsynaptic potentials (IPSPs) also can undergo spatial and temporal summation with each other and with EPSPs, reducing the effectiveness of the latter by a roughly algebraic summation. If the sum of EPSPs and IPSPs keeps the depolarization at the initial segment below threshold levels, no action potential occurs.

4. (1) They can be broken down into inactive substances by enzymes; (2) they can be taken back up into the presynaptic neuron in a process called "reuptake"; or (3) they can diffuse away into the intercellular fluid until its

concentration is too low to influence postsynaptic excitability.

5. The nervous system appears very early in embryonic development. At the beginning of week 3, the ectoderm begins to invaginate and migrates between the two layers, forming a third layer called the "mesoderm." Mesoderm along the entire midline of the embryo forms a specialized rod of embryonic tissue called the "notochord." The notochord and adjacent mesoderm provide the necessary induction signal for the overlying ectoderm to differentiate and form a thickened structure called the "neural plate." Within the neural plate an axial groove develops and sinks into the underlying mesoderm, allowing its walls to fuse across the top and form an ectodermal tube called the "neural tube." As the neural tube closes, ectodermal cells called "neural crest cells" migrate away from the dorsal surface of the neural tube to become the progenitors of the neurons and supporting cells of the peripheral nervous system. During development, the more rostral portions of the embryonic neural tube—approximately 10 segments—undergo extensive modification and enlargement to form the brain.

6. Four columns of afferent (sensory) neurons in the dorsal root ganglia directly innervate four corresponding columns of IA neurons in the dorsal horn. These columns are categorized as special and general afferents: special somatic afferent, general somatic afferent, special visceral afferent, and general visceral afferent. The ventral horn contains three longitudinal cell columns: general visceral efferent, pharyngeal efferent, and general somatic efferent. Each of these cell columns contains OA and efferent neurons. The OA neurons coordinate and integrate the function of the efferent motor neurons cells of its column.

7. Maintenance of a chemically stable environment is essential to the function of the brain. In most regions of the body, extracellular fluid undergoes small fluctuations in pH and concentrations of hormones, amino acids, and potassium ions during routine daily activities such as eating and exercising. If the brain were to undergo such fluctuations, the result would be uncontrolled neural activity, because some substances, such as amino acids, act as neurotransmitters, and ions, such as potassium, influence the threshold for neural firing. Two barriers, the blood–brain barrier and the CSF–brain barrier, provide the means for maintaining the stable chemical environment of the brain. Only water, carbon dioxide, and oxygen enter the brain with relative ease; the transport of other substances between the brain and the blood is slower and more controlled.

8. The blood–brain barrier prevents many drugs from entering the brain. Most highly water-soluble compounds are excluded from the brain, especially molecules with high ionic charge, such as many of the catecholamines. In contrast, many lipid-soluble molecules cross the lipid layers of the blood–brain barrier with ease. Some drugs, such as the antibiotic chloramphenicol, are highly lipid soluble and therefore enter the brain readily. Other medications have a low solubility in lipids and enter the brain slowly or not at all. Alcohol, nicotine, and heroin are very lipid soluble and rapidly enter the brain. Some substances that enter the capillary endothelium are converted by metabolic processes to a chemical form incapable of moving into the brain.

SECTION III: APPLYING YOUR KNOWLEDGE

Activity E

1. Your baby has a meningomyeloceles.
2. Most children with meningomyeloceles have clinical dysfunction in both the motor and sensory nerves of the lower extremities. Dysfunction usually extends to bowel and bladder control. The extent of the dysfunction cannot be assessed until the infant is born and can be better assessed.

SECTION IV: PRACTICING FOR NCLEX

Activity F

1. a. *Rationale*: The supporting cells, such as Schwann cells in the peripheral nervous system and the neuroglial cells in the central nervous system, protect the nervous system and provide metabolic support for the neurons. The other answers are incorrect.
2. b. *Rationale*: These membrane channels are guarded by voltage-dependent gates that open and close with changes in the membrane potential. The other answers are incorrect.
3. c. *Rationale*: The most common type of synapse is the chemical synapse. The other answers are incorrect.
4. d. *Rationale*: Neurotransmitters are synthesized in the cytoplasm of the axon terminal. The other answers are incorrect.

5. a. *Rationale:* Neuromodulator molecules react with presynaptic or postsynaptic receptors to alter the release of or response to neurotransmitters. The other answers are incorrect.

6. b. *Rationale:* With rare exceptions, peripheral nerves, including the cranial nerves, contain afferent and efferent processes of more than one of the four afferent and three efferent cell columns. This provides the basis for assessing the function of the any peripheral nerve. The other answers are incorrect.

7. c. *Rationale:* On the lateral sides of the spinal cord, extensions of the pia mater, the denticulate ligaments, attach the sides of the spinal cord to the bony walls of the spinal canal. Thus, the cord is suspended by both the denticulate ligaments and the segmental nerves. The posterior vertebra and vertebral blood vessels do not support the spinal cord.

8. d. *Rationale:* The myotatic or stretch reflex controls muscle tone and helps maintain posture. Specialized sensory nerve terminals in skeletal muscles and tendons relay information on muscle stretch and joint tension to the central nervous system. This information, which drives postural reflex mechanisms, also is relayed to the thalamus and the sensory cortex and is experienced as *proprioception*, the sense of body movement and position.

9. a. *Rationale:* The cerebellum compares what is actually happening with what is intended to happen. It then transmits the appropriate corrective signals back to the motor system, instructing it to increase or decrease the activity of the participating muscle groups so that smooth and accurate movements can be performed. Answer B describes the trigeminal nerve which exits the brainstem. Answer C describes the pons. Answer D describes midbrain.

10. b. *Rationale:* Parkinson disease, Huntington chorea, and some forms of cerebral palsy, among other dysfunctions involving the basal ganglia, result in a frequent or continuous release of abnormal postural or axial and proximal movement patterns. If damage to the basal ganglia is localized to one side, the movements occur on the opposite side of the body. The other answers are incorrect.

11. c. *Rationale:* Some drugs, such as the antibiotic chloramphenicol, are highly lipid soluble and therefore enter the brain readily. The other answers are incorrect.

12. c. *Rationale:* The sympathetic and parasympathetic nervous systems are continually active.

The effect of this continual or basal (baseline) activity is referred to as "tone."

13. d. *Rationale:* Dopamine, which is an intermediate compound in the synthesis of norepinephrine, also acts as a neurotransmitter. It is the principal inhibitory transmitter of internuncial neurons in the sympathetic ganglia. It also has vasodilator effects on renal, splanchnic, and coronary blood vessels when given intravenously and is sometimes used in the treatment of shock.

CHAPTER 49 SOMATOSENSORY FUNCTION, PAIN, AND HEADACHE

SECTION II: ASSESSING YOUR UNDERSTANDING

Activity A

1. somatosensory
2. General
3. Special
4. visceral
5. trigeminal
6. dermatome
7. discriminative
8. anterolateral
9. modalities
10. action potentials
11. acuity
12. tactile
13. Thermal
14. pain
15. sensory, perception
16. Neuropathic
17. neuromatrix
18. Nociceptive
19. C fibers
20. neospinothalamic
21. paleospinothalamic
22. periaqueductal gray
23. enkephalins, endorphins, dynorphins
24. threshold
25. Cutaneous
26. Deep somatic
27. warning
28. analgesic
29. hyperalgesia
30. Analgesia
31. Neuralgia
32. Cluster
33. tension-type
34. temporomandibular joint (TMJ)

Activity B

1.

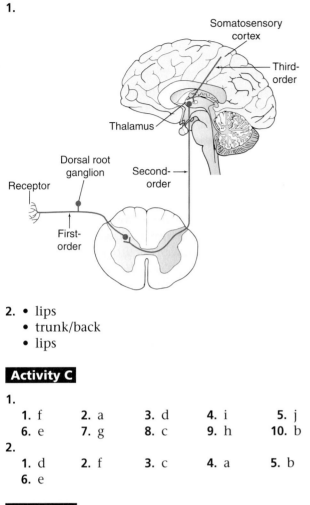

Somatosensory cortex

Third-order

Thalamus

Dorsal root ganglion

Second-order

Receptor

First-order

2. • lips
   • trunk/back
   • lips

Activity C

1.

1. f	**2.** a	**3.** d	**4.** i	**5.** j
6. e	**7.** g	**8.** c	**9.** h	**10.** b

2.

1. d	**2.** f	**3.** c	**4.** a	**5.** b
6. e				

Activity D

1. Sensory systems are organized in a serial succession of neurons consisting of first-order, second-order, and third-order neurons. First-order neurons transmit sensory information from the periphery to the central nervous system. Second-order neurons communicate with various reflex networks and sensory pathways in the spinal cord and travel directly to the thalamus. Third-order neurons relay information from the thalamus to the cerebral cortex. This organizing framework corresponds with the three primary levels of neural integration in the somatosensory system: the sensory units, which contain the sensory receptors; the ascending pathways; and the central processing centers in the thalamus and cerebral cortex.

2. These somatosensory receptors monitor four major types or modalities of sensation: discriminative touch, which is required to identify the size and shape of objects and their movement across the skin; temperature sensation; sense of movement of the limbs and joints of the body; and nociception, or pain.

3. A pinpoint pressed against the skin of the sole of the foot that results in a withdrawal reflex and a complaint of skin pain confirms the functional integrity of the afferent terminals in the skin, the entire pathway through the peripheral nerves of the foot, leg, and thigh to the sacral (S1) dorsal root ganglion, and through the dorsal root into the spinal cord segment. It confirms that the somatosensory input association cells receiving this information are functioning and that the reflex circuitry of the cord segments (L5 to S2) is functioning. In addition, the lower motor neurons of the L4 to S1 ventral horn can be considered operational, and their axons through the ventral roots, the mixed peripheral nerve, and the motor neuron to the muscles producing the withdrawal response can be considered intact and functional. The communication between the lower motor neuron and the muscle cells is functional, and these muscles have normal responsiveness and strength. Observation of a normal withdrawal reflex rules out peripheral nerve disease, disorders of the dorsal root and ganglion, diseases of the myoneural junction, and severe muscle diseases. Normal reflex function also indicates that many major descending central nervous system tract systems are functioning within normal limits. If the person is able to report the pinprick sensation and accurately identify its location, many ascending systems through much of the spinal cord and brain also are functioning normally, as are basic intellect and speech mechanisms.

4. According to the gate control theory, the internuncial neurons involved in the gating mechanism are activated by large-diameter, faster-propagating fibers that carry tactile information. The simultaneous firing of the large-diameter touch fibers has the potential for blocking the transmission of impulses from the small-diameter myelinated and unmyelinated pain fibers. Pain therapists have long known that pain intensity can be temporarily reduced during active tactile stimulation.

5. Referred pain is pain that is perceived at a site different from its point of origin, but innervated by the same spinal segment. It is hypothesized that visceral and somatic afferent neurons converge on the same dorsal horn

projection neurons. For this reason, it can be difficult for the brain to identify the original source of pain. Pain that originates in the abdominal or thoracic viscera is diffuse, poorly localized, and often perceived at a site far removed from the affected area.

6. Heat dilates blood vessels and increases local blood flow; it also can influence the transmission of pain impulses and increase collagen extensibility. An increase in local circulation can reduce the level of nociceptive stimulation by reducing local ischemia caused by muscle spasm or tension, increase the removal of metabolites and inflammatory mediators that act as nociceptive stimuli, and help to reduce swelling and relieve pressure on local nociceptive endings. It also may trigger the release of endogenous opioids. Heat also alters the viscosity of collagen fibers in ligaments, tendons, and joint structures so that they are more easily extended and can be stretched further before the nociceptive endings are stimulated.

7. Phantom limb pain often begins as sensations of tingling, heat and cold, or heaviness, followed by burning, cramping, or shooting pain. It may disappear spontaneously or persist for many years. Several theories have been proposed as to the causes of phantom pain. One theory is that the end of a regenerating nerve becomes trapped in the scar tissue of the amputation site. It is known that when a peripheral nerve is cut, the scar tissue that forms becomes a barrier to regenerating outgrowth of the axon. The growing axon often becomes trapped in the scar tissue, forming a tangled growth of small-diameter axons, including primary nociceptive afferents and sympathetic efferents. It has been proposed that these afferents show increased sensitivity to innocuous mechanical stimuli and to sympathetic activity and circulating catecholamines. A related theory moves the source of phantom limb pain to the spinal cord, suggesting that the pain is caused by the spontaneous firing of spinal cord neurons that have lost their normal sensory input from the body. In one hypothesis, the pain is caused by changes in the flow of signals through somatosensory areas of the brain.

8. Migraine without aura is a pulsatile, throbbing, unilateral headache that typically lasts 1 to 2 days and is aggravated by routine physical activity. The headache is accompanied by nausea and vomiting, which often is disabling, and sensitivity to light and sound. Visual disturbances commonly occur and consist of visual hallucinations, such as stars, sparks, and flashes of light. Migraine with aura has similar symptoms, but with the addition of reversible visual symptoms including positive features (e.g., flickering lights spots, or lines) and/or negative features (loss of vision); fully reversible sensory symptoms including positive features (feeling or pins or needles) or negative features (numbness); and fully reversible speech disturbance.

9. Activation of the trigeminal sensory fibers can lead to the release of neuropeptides, causing painful neurogenic inflammation within the meningeal vasculature characterized by plasma protein extravasation, vasodilation, and mast cell degranulation. Another possible mechanism implicates neurogenic vasodilation of meningeal blood vessels as a key component of the inflammatory processes that occur during migraine. Activation of trigeminal sensory fibers evokes a neurogenic dural vasodilation mediated by calcitonin gene-related peptide. It also has been observed that calcitonin gene-related peptide level is elevated during migraine.

SECTION III: APPLYING YOUR KNOWLEDGE

Activity E

1. It is difficult to assess pain and discomfort in someone suffering with dementia. In our facility we use *The Assessment for Discomfort in Dementia Protocol* as it has been shown to improve pain management in this population.
2. Acetaminophen is the drug of choice to manage this patient's discomfort. You can also place ice on the cast at the point of fracture for 20 minutes, each hour, to help reduce the discomfort.

SECTION IV: PRACTICING FOR NCLEX

Activity F

1. 1-e, 2-a, 3-g, 4-b, 5-c, 6-h, 7-d, 8-f
2. 1-c, 2-g, 3-i, 4-d, 5-h, 6-a, 7-f, 8-j, 9-b, 10-k, 11-e
3. a. *Rationale:* Clinically, neurologic assessment of somatosensory function can be done by testing the integrity of spinal segmental nerves. The other answers are incorrect.
4. b. *Rationale:* Stimuli used include pressure from a sharp object, strong electric current to the skin, or application of heat or cold of

approximately 10°C above or below normal skin temperature. The other answers are incorrect.

5. c. *Rationale:* The amino acid glutamate is a major excitatory neurotransmitter released from the central nerve endings of the nociceptive neurons. The other answers are incorrect.

6. d. *Rationale:* The paleospinothalamic tract is a slower-conducting, multisynaptic tract concerned with the diffuse, dull, aching, and unpleasant sensations that commonly are associated with chronic and visceral pain. The other answers are incorrect.

7. 1-c, 2-d, 3-f, 4-g, 5-e, 6-b, 7-a

8. a, c. *Rationale:* Assessment includes such things as the nature, severity, location, and radiation of the pain. Spinal reflex involvement and spinal tract involvement are not assessed when assessing pain.

9. a. *Rationale:* Part of the reluctance of health care workers to provide adequate relief for acute pain has been fear of addiction. However, addiction to opioid medications is thought to be virtually nonexistent when these drugs are prescribed for acute pain. The other answers are not the major concern.

10. b. *Rationale:* The World Health Organization has created an analgesic ladder for cancer pain that assists clinicians in choosing the appropriate analgesic. The other answers are incorrect.

11. a, b, c. *Rationale:* The ideal analgesic would be effective, nonaddictive, and inexpensive. In addition, it would produce minimal adverse effects and not affect the person's level of consciousness.

12. c. *Rationale:* Surgery for severe, intractable pain of peripheral or central origin has met with some success. It can be used to remove the cause or block the transmission of intractable pain from phantom limb pain, severe neuralgia, inoperable cancer of certain types, and causalgia. The other answers are incorrect.

13. d. *Rationale:* Primary hyperalgesia describes pain sensitivity that occurs directly in damaged tissues. The other answers are incorrect.

14. 1-d, 2-b, 3-a, 4-c

15. a. *Rationale:* Treatment of phantom limb pain is accomplished by the use of sympathetic blocks, transcutaneous electrical nerve stimulation (TENS) of the large myelinated afferents innervating the area, hypnosis, and relaxation training.

16. b. *Rationale:* Based on clinical trials, first-line agents include acetylsalicylic acid, combinations of acetaminophen, acetylsalicylic acid, caffeine, and nonsteroidal anti-inflammatory drugs (NSAIDs) (e.g., naproxen sodium, ibuprofen), serotonin (5-HT$_1$) receptor agonists (e.g., sumatriptan, naratriptan, rizatriptan, zolmitriptan), ergotamine derivatives (e.g., dihydroergotamine), and antiemetic medications (e.g., ondansetron, metoclopramide). Morphine, tramadol, and syrup of ipecac are not first-line drugs in the treatment of migraine.

17. c. *Rationale:* Cluster headache is a type of primary neurovascular headache that typically includes severe, unrelenting, unilateral pain located, in order of decreasing frequency, in the orbital, retro-orbital, temporal, supraorbital, and infraorbital region. The other answers are incorrect.

18. d. *Rationale:* With children 3 to 8 years of age, scales with faces of actual children or cartoon faces can be used to obtain a report of pain. The other pain rating scales are inappropriate in this age group.

19. a. *Rationale:* The overriding principle in all pediatric pain management is to treat each child's pain on an individual basis and to match the analgesic agent with the cause and the level of pain. The other answers are incorrect.

CHAPTER 50 DISORDERS OF MOTOR FUNCTION

SECTION II: ASSESSING YOUR UNDERSTANDING

Activity A

1. Motor function
2. spinal cord
3. polysynaptic
4. posture
5. cortex
6. motor
7. cerebellum, basal ganglia
8. circuits
9. muscle spindles
10. Golgi tendon organs
11. peripheral
12. motor
13. atrophy
14. muscle tone
15. Upper motor neuron (UMN)
16. Hyporeflexia

17. lower motor neuron disorders, peripheral, myopathies
18. dystrophy
19. fibrillations
20. Duchenne
21. neuromuscular junction
22. acetylcholine
23. Myasthenia gravis
24. spinal cord, cranial nerve
25. peripheral nerve
26. Mononeuropathies
27. Polyneuropathies
28. herniated disk
29. cerebellar
30. basal ganglia
31. tremor
32. Parkinson
33. bradykinesia
34. Amyotrophic lateral sclerosis
35. Multiple sclerosis (MS)
36. demyelination
37. spinal cord injury (SCI)
38. loss
39. Tetraplegia
40. Paraplegia
41. vasovagal
42. Orthostatic
43. deep venous thrombosis

Activity B

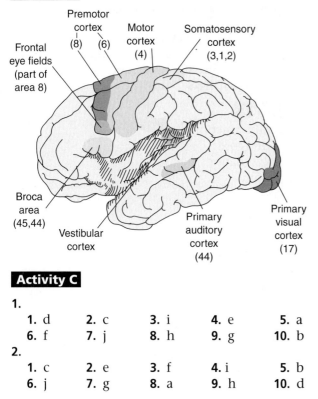

Premotor cortex (8) (6)
Motor cortex (4)
Somatosensory cortex (3,1,2)
Frontal eye fields (part of area 8)
Broca area (45,44)
Vestibular cortex
Primary auditory cortex (44)
Primary visual cortex (17)

Activity C

1.

| 1. d | 2. c | 3. i | 4. e | 5. a |
| 6. f | 7. j | 8. h | 9. g | 10. b |

2.

| 1. c | 2. e | 3. f | 4. i | 5. b |
| 6. j | 7. g | 8. a | 9. h | 10. d |

Activity D

1.

2 → 5 → 4 → 3 → 1

Activity E

1. The lowest level of the hierarchy occurs at the spinal cord, which contains the basic reflex circuitry needed to coordinate the function of the motor units involved in the planned movement. Above the spinal cord is the brain stem, and above the brain stem is the cerebellum and basal ganglia, structures that modulate the actions of the brain stem systems. Overseeing these supraspinal structures are the motor centers in the cerebral cortex. The highest level of function, which occurs at the level of the frontal cortex, is concerned with the purpose and planning of the motor movement. The efficiency of movement depends on input from sensory systems that operate in parallel with the motor systems.

2. The motor neuron and the group of muscle fibers it innervates in a muscle is called a "motor unit." When the motor neuron develops an action potential, all of the muscle fibers in the motor unit it innervates develop action potentials, causing them to contract simultaneously. Thus, a motor neuron and the muscle fibers it innervates function as a single unit—the basic unit of motor control. Each motor neuron undergoes multiple branching, making it possible for a single motor neuron to innervate a few to thousands of muscle fibers. In general, large muscles—those containing hundreds or thousands of muscle fibers and providing gross motor movement—have large motor units (LMUs). This sharply contrasts with those that control the hand, tongue, and eye movements, for which the motor units are small and permit very precise control.

3. The muscle spindles consist of a group of specialized miniature skeletal muscle fibers called intrafusal fibers that are encased in a connective tissue capsule and attached to the extrafusal fibers of a skeletal muscle. In the center of the receptor area, a large sensory neuron spirals around the intrafusal fiber forming the so-called primary or annulospiral ending. The intrafusal muscle fibers function as stretch receptors. When a skeletal muscle is

stretched, the spindle and its intrafusal fibers are stretched, resulting in increased firing of their afferent nerve fibers. Segmental branches make connections, along with other branches, that pass directly to the anterior gray matter of the spinal cord and establish monosynaptic contact with each of the lower motor neurons (LMNs) that have motor units in the muscle containing the spindle receptor. This produces an opposing muscle contraction. Another segmental branch of the same afferent neuron innervates an internuncial neuron that is inhibitory to motor units of antagonistic muscle groups. This disynaptic inhibitory pathway is the basis for the reciprocal activity of agonist and antagonist muscles (i.e., when an agonist muscle is stretched, the antagonists relax).

4. Coordination of muscle movement requires that four areas of the nervous system function in an integrated manner—the motor system for muscle strength, the cerebellar system for rhythmic movement and steady posture, the vestibular system for posture and balance, and the sensory system for position sense.

5. Duchenne muscular dystrophy (DMD) is caused by mutations in a gene located on the short arm of the X chromosome that codes for a protein called dystrophin. Dystrophin is a large cytoplasmic protein located on the inner surface of the sarcolemma or muscle fiber membrane. The dystrophin molecules are concentrated over the Z-bands of the muscle, where they form a strong link between the actin filaments of the intracellular contractile apparatus and the extracellular connective tissue matrix. Abnormalities in the dystrophin-associated protein complex compromise sarcolemma integrity, particularly with sustained contractions. This disruption in integrity may be responsible for the observed increased fragility of dystrophic muscle, excessive influx of calcium ions, and release of soluble muscle enzymes, such as creatine kinase into the serum. The degenerative process in DMD consists of a relentless necrosis of muscle fibers, accompanied by a continuous process of repair and regeneration, and progressive fibrosis.

6. Segmental demyelination occurs when there is a disorder of the Schwann cell (as in Guillain-Barré syndrome) or damage to the myelin sheath (e.g., sensory neuropathies), without a primary abnormality of the axon. It typically affects some Schwann cells while sparing others. Axonal degeneration is caused by primary injury to a neuronal cell body or its axon. Damage to the axon may be caused by either a focal event occurring at some point along the length of the nerve (e.g., trauma or ischemia) or a more generalized abnormality affecting the neuronal cell body (neuropathy).

7. Carpal tunnel syndrome can be caused by a variety of conditions that produce a reduction in the capacity of the carpal tunnel (i.e., bony or ligament changes) or an increase in the volume of the tunnel contents (i.e., inflammation of the tendons, synovial swelling, or tumors). Carpal tunnel syndrome is an example of a compression-type mononeuropathy that is relatively common. It is caused by compression of the median nerve as it travels with the flexor tendons through a canal made by the carpal bones and transverse carpal ligament

8. Guillain-Barré syndrome is an acute immune-mediated polyneuropathy that is characterized by rapidly progressive limb weakness and loss of tendon reflexes. The disorder is marked by progressive ascending muscle weakness of the limbs, producing a symmetric flaccid paralysis. Symptoms of paresthesia and numbness often accompany the loss of motor function. Paralysis may progress to involve the respiratory muscles. Autonomic nervous system involvement that causes postural hypotension, arrhythmias, facial flushing, abnormalities of sweating, and urinary retention is common. Pain is another common feature.

9. The primary brain abnormality found in all persons with Parkinson disease is degeneration of the nigrostriatal dopamine neurons. On microscopic examination, there is loss of pigmented substantia nigra neurons. Some residual nerve cells are atrophic, and a few contain *Lewy bodies*, which are visualized as spherical, eosinophilic cytoplasmic inclusions. Although the cause of Parkinson disease is still unknown, it is widely believed that most cases are caused by an interaction of environmental and genetic factors. Over the past several decades, several pathologic processes (e.g., oxidative stress, apoptosis, and mitochondrial disorders) that might lead to degeneration have been identified. One theory is that the auto-oxidation of catecholamines,

such as dopamine, during melanin synthesis injures neurons in the substantia nigra. Increasing evidence suggests that the development of Parkinson disease may be related to oxidative metabolites of this process and the inability of neurons to render these products harmless.

10. The death of lower motor neurons leads to denervation, with subsequent shrinkage of musculature and muscle fiber atrophy. It is this fiber atrophy, called amyotrophy, which appears in the name of the disease. The loss of nerve fibers in lateral columns of the white matter of the spinal cord, along with fibrillary gliosis, imparts a firmness or sclerosis to this central nervous system (CNS) tissue; the term lateral sclerosis designates these changes.

11. The primary neurologic injury occurs at the time of mechanical injury and is irreversible. It is characterized by small hemorrhages in the gray matter of the cord, followed by edematous changes in the white matter that lead to necrosis of neural tissue. This type of pathology results from the forces of compression, stretch, and shear associated with fracture or compression of the spinal vertebrae, dislocation of vertebrae, and contusions owing to jarring of the cord in the spinal canal. Secondary injuries follow the primary injury and promote the spread of injury. Although there is considerable debate about the pathogenesis of secondary injuries, the tissue destruction that occurs ends in progressive neurologic damage. After a spinal cord injury, several pathologic mechanisms come into play, including vascular damage, neuronal injury that leads to loss of reflexes below the level of injury, and release of vasoactive agents and cellular enzymes.

SECTION III: APPLYING YOUR KNOWLEDGE

Activity F

1. "The medicine that we are giving your husband is methylprednisolone, a short-acting corticosteroid. In a case of spinal cord injury, the drug is thought to enhance the generation of impulses down the spinal cord and improve the blood flow around the site of the injury."

2. • Bed rest with log rolling only
   • Continuous pulse oximetry
   • Vital signs hourly until stable
   • Methylprednisolone intravenously (IV)
   • Monitor for gastric bleeding; venous thrombosis and steroid myopathy

SECTION IV: PRACTICING FOR NCLEX

Activity G

1. a. *Rationale:* The highest level of function, which occurs at the level of the frontal cortex, is concerned with the purpose and planning of the motor movement. The other answers are incorrect.

2. 1-b, 2-a, 3-d, 4-c

3. b. *Rationale:* The anatomic basis of a reflex consists of an afferent neuron, which synapses either directly with an effector neuron that innervates a muscle or with an interneuron that synapses with an effector neuron.

4. a, b, c, e. *Rationale:* These signs and symptoms include changes in muscle characteristics (strength, bulk, and tone), spinal reflex activity, and motor coordination. Muscle innervation is incorrect.

5. c. *Rationale:* The postural muscles of hip and shoulder are usually the first to be affected. The other answers are incorrect.

6. d. *Rationale:* The aminoglycoside antibiotics (e.g., gentamicin) can produce a clinical disturbance similar to botulism by preventing the release of acetylcholine from nerve endings. These drugs are particularly dangerous in persons with preexisting disturbances of neuromuscular transmission, such as myasthenia gravis. The other answers are incorrect.

7. a. *Rationale:* Myasthenia crisis occurs when muscle weakness becomes sufficiently severe to compromise ventilation to the extent that ventilatory support and airway protection are needed. The other answers are incorrect.

8. b. *Rationale:* Carpal tunnel syndrome is an example of a compression-type mononeuropathy that is relatively common. The other answers are not mononeuropathies.

9. c. *Rationale:* The straight-leg test is an important diagnostic maneuver for a herniated disk in the lumbar area. The other answers are incorrect.

10. 1-a, 2-b, 3-c

11. d. *Rationale:* The function of the striatum also involves local cholinergic interneurons and their destruction is thought to be related to the choreiform movements of Huntington disease, another basal ganglia-related syndrome. The other answers do not involve the cholinergic interneurons of the striatum.

12. a. *Rationale:* In Parkinson disease, also known as idiopathic parkinsonism, dopamine depletion results from degeneration of the

dopamine nigrostriatal system. The other answers are incorrect.

13. b. *Rationale:* The most common clinical presentation is slowly progressive weakness and atrophy in distal muscles of one upper extremity. The other answers do not describe the clinical presentation of amyotrophic lateral sclerosis (ALS).

14. c. *Rationale:* A large percentage of patients with multiple sclerosis (MS) have elevated immunoglobulin G (IgG) levels, and some have oligoclonal patterns (i.e., discrete electrophoretic bands) even with normal IgG levels.

15. d. *Rationale:* A functional C7 injury allows full elbow flexion and extension, wrist plantar flexion, and some finger control. At the C8 level, finger flexion is added. The other answers are incorrect.

16. a. *Rationale:* Cord injuries involving C1 to C3 result in a lack of respiratory effort, and affected patients require assisted ventilation. The other answers involve injuries further down the spinal column.

17. a, c, e. *Rationale:* Autonomic dysreflexia is characterized by vasospasm, hypertension ranging from mild (20 mm Hg above baseline) to severe (as high as 240/120 mm Hg or higher), skin pallor, and gooseflesh associated with the piloerector response. Fever and vasoconstriction are not manifestations of autonomic dysreflexia.

18. b. *Rationale:* Although the enteric nervous system innervation of the bowel remains intact, without the defecation reflex, peristaltic movements are ineffective in evacuating stool. The other answers are incorrect.

CHAPTER 51 DISORDERS OF THE BRAIN FUNCTION

SECTION II: ASSESSING YOUR UNDERSTANDING

Activity A

1. brain's
2. 20
3. hypoxia
4. focal, global
5. sodium
6. Laminar necrosis
7. amino acids, proteases
8. intracranial
9. herniation
10. edema
11. vasogenic
12. Cytotoxic
13. primary, cerebral hypoxia
14. Epidural hematomas
15. tear
16. Consciousness
17. brain
18. vegetative
19. autoregulation
20. carbon dioxide, hydrogen ion, oxygen
21. Stroke
22. Ischemic, hemorrhagic
23. ministroke, angina
24. Thrombi
25. Lacunar
26. embolic
27. hemorrhage
28. cerebral artery
29. cerebral aneurysm
30. Arteriovenous
31. Encephalitis
32. Vomiting
33. chemotherapy
34. seizure
35. Simple partial
36. Complex partial
37. muscle contractions
38. Tonic-clonic
39. status epilepticus

Activity B

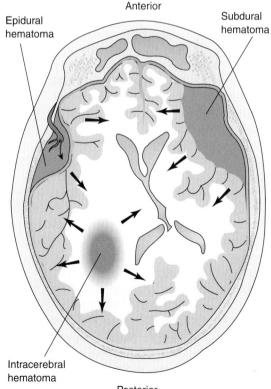

Activity C

1. f   **2.** g   **3.** d   **4.** j   **5.** b
6. c   **7.** e   **8.** h   **9.** a   **10.** i

Activity D

1.

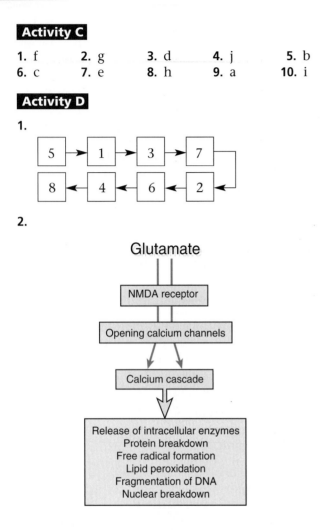

2.

Glutamate

NMDA receptor

Opening calcium channels

Calcium cascade

Release of intracellular enzymes
Protein breakdown
Free radical formation
Lipid peroxidation
Fragmentation of DNA
Nuclear breakdown

Activity E

1. Global ischemia occurs at a time when blood flow is inadequate to meet the metabolic needs of the entire brain. The result is a spectrum of neurologic disorders reflecting global brain dysfunction. Unconsciousness occurs within seconds of severe global ischemia, such as that resulting from complete cessation of blood flow, as in cardiac arrest, or with marked decrease in blood flow, as in serious cardiac arrhythmias. If cerebral circulation is restored immediately, consciousness is regained quickly. However, if blood flow is not promptly restored, severe pathologic changes take place. Energy sources, glucose, and glycogen, are exhausted in 2 to 4 minutes, and cellular adenosine triphosphate (ATP) stores are depleted in 4 to 5 minutes. When ischemia is sufficiently severe or prolonged, infarction or death of all the cellular elements of the brain occurs. Even if blood flow is restored, if ischemic thresholds for injury were exceeded, then permanent cell death ensues.

2. Watershed infarcts are concentrated in anatomically vulnerable border zones between the overlapping territories supplied by the major cerebral arteries, notably the middle, anterior, and posterior cerebral arteries. The overlapping territory at the distal ends of these vessels forms extremely vulnerable areas in terms of global ischemia, called "watershed zones." During events such as severe hypotension, these distal territories undergo a profound lowering of blood flow, predisposing to focal ischemia and infarction of brain tissues. Therefore, global ischemia can result in focal infarcts that occur in the border zones between major vascular territories.

3. During prolonged ischemia, the glutamate transport mechanisms become immobilized, causing extracellular glutamate to accumulate. Additionally, intracellular glutamate is released from the damaged cells. This glutamate excess then drives the uncontrolled opening of N-methyl-D-aspartate (NMDA) receptor-operated channels producing an increase in intracellular calcium. Excess intracellular calcium leads to a series of calcium-mediated processes called the calcium cascade, including the release of intracellular enzymes that cause protein breakdown, free radical formation, lipid peroxidation, fragmentation of DNA, mitochondrial injury, nuclear breakdown, and eventually cell death.

4. Although recovery usually takes place within 24 hours, mild symptoms, such as headache, irritability, insomnia, and poor concentration and memory, may persist for months. The memory loss usually includes an interval of time preceding the accident (retrograde amnesia) and following the injury (anterograde amnesia).

5. Global brain injury, whether caused by head trauma, stroke, or other pathologies, is manifested by alterations in sensory, motor, and cognitive function and by changes in the level of consciousness. In contrast to focal injury, which causes focal neurologic deficits without altered consciousness, global injury nearly always results in altered levels of consciousness ranging from inattention to stupor or coma. Severe injury

that seriously compromises brain function can result in brain death.

6. (1) Arousal and wakefulness, and (2) content and cognition. The content and cognition aspects of consciousness are determined by a functioning cerebral cortex. Arousal and wakefulness requires the concurrent functioning of both cerebral hemispheres and an intact RAS in the brainstem. The earliest signs of diminution in level of consciousness are inattention, mild confusion, disorientation, and blunted responsiveness. With further deterioration, the delirious person becomes markedly inattentive and variably lethargic or agitated. The person may become obtunded and respond only to vigorous or noxious stimuli.

7. A bilateral loss of the pupillary light response is indicative of lesions of the brain stem. A unilateral loss of the pupillary light response may be caused by a lesion of the optic or oculomotor pathways. The oculocephalic reflex (doll's-head eye movement) can be used to determine whether the brain stem centers for eye movement are intact and the oculovestibular may be used to elicit nystagmus.

8. During the evolution of a stroke, there usually is a central core of dead or dying cells, surrounded by an ischemic band or area of minimally perfused cells called the "penumbra." Brain cells of the penumbra receive marginal blood flow, and their metabolic activities are impaired; although the area undergoes an "electrical failure," the structural integrity of the brain cells is maintained. Whether the cells of the penumbra continue to survive depends on the successful timely return of adequate circulation, the volume of toxic products released by the neighboring dying cells, the degree of cerebral edema, and alterations in local blood flow. If the toxic products result in additional death of cells in the penumbra, the core of dead or dying tissue enlarges, and the volume of surrounding ischemic tissue increases.

9. First, blood is shunted from the high-pressure arterial system to the low-pressure venous system without the buffering advantage of the capillary network. The draining venous channels are exposed to high levels of pressure, predisposing them to rupture and hemorrhage. Second, the elevated arterial and venous pressures divert blood away from the surrounding tissue, impairing tissue perfusion.

10. Seizures can be caused by alterations in cell membrane permeability or distribution of ions across the neuronal cell membranes. Another cause may be decreased inhibition of cortical or thalamic neuronal activity or structural changes that alter the excitability of neurons. Neurotransmitter imbalances, such as an acetylcholine excess or γ-aminobutyric acid (GABA, an inhibitory neurotransmitter) deficiency, have been proposed as causes. Certain epilepsy syndromes have been linked to specific genetic mutations causing ion channel defects.

SECTION III: APPLYING YOUR KNOWLEDGE

Activity F

1.
Family history of stroke
- history of hypertension
- history of smoking
- history of diabetes mellitus
- history of sickle cell disease
- history of hyperlipidemia
- history of atrial fibrillation
- weight
- alcohol and drug use
- hormone replacement therapy
- oral contraceptive use
- activity level

2. Administration of tissue-type plasminogen activator (tPA) to be given within 3 hours of onset
- Administration of neuroprotective drugs
- Hypothermia treatment

SECTION IV: PRACTICING FOR NCLEX

Activity G

1. 1-g, 2-c, 3-a, 4-f, 5-b, 6-e, 7-d
2. 1-e, 2-a, 3-b. 4-g, 5-c, 6-d, 7-f
3. a, b, d, e. *Rationale:* The direct brain injuries include diffuse axonal injury and the focal lesions of laceration, contusion, and hemorrhage. Hypoxic brain injury is considered a secondary type of injury.
4. a. *Rationale:* In contrast to focal injury, which causes focal neurologic deficits without altered consciousness, global injury nearly always results in altered levels of consciousness ranging from inattention to stupor or coma.

The other answers are manifestations of different types of brain injury, not a global injury.

5. b. *Rationale:* Decorticate (flexion) posturing is characterized by flexion of the arms, wrists, and fingers, with abduction of the upper extremities, internal rotation, and plantar flexion of the lower extremities. Decerebrate and extensor posturing are the same thing and are incorrect. Diencephalon posturing does not exist, so it is incorrect.

6. c. *Rationale:* Clinical examination must disclose at least the absence of responsiveness, brain stem reflexes, and respiratory effort. Brain death is a clinical diagnosis, and a repeat evaluation at least 6 hours later is recommended. An ECG is not assessed in an examination for brain death.

7. a, c, e. *Rationale:* The criteria for diagnosis of vegetative state include the absence of awareness of self and environment and an inability to interact with others; the absence of sustained or reproducible voluntary behavioral responses; lack of language comprehension; sufficiently preserved hypothalamic and brain stem function to maintain life; bowel and bladder incontinence; and variably preserved cranial nerve (e.g., pupillary, gag) and spinal cord reflexes. People in a persistent vegetative state can open their eyes and have sufficient hypothalamic function to maintain life.

8. d. *Rationale:* If blood pressure falls below 60 mm Hg, cerebral blood flow becomes severely compromised and, if it rises above the upper limit of autoregulation, blood flow increases rapidly and overstretches the cerebral vessels. The other answers are incorrect.

9. a. *Rationale:* The diagnosis of subarachnoid hemorrhage and intracranial aneurysms is made by clinical presentation, computed tomographic (CT) scan, lumbar puncture, and angiography. Magnetic resonance imaging (MRI) is not necessary for the diagnosis of subarachnoid hemorrhage and intracranial aneurysm. Loss of cranial nerve reflexes is not diagnostic of subarachnoid hemorrhage and intracranial aneurysm and neither is venography.

10. b. *Rationale:* Two assessment techniques can help determine whether meningeal irritation is present. Kernig's sign is resistance to extension of the knee while the person is lying with the hip flexed at a right angle. Brudzinski sign is elicited when flexion of the neck induces flexion of the hip and knee. The other answers are incorrect.

11. c. *Rationale:* Intracranial tumors give rise to focal disturbances in brain function and increased intracranial pressure (ICP). Focal disturbances occur because of brain compression, tumor infiltration, disturbances in blood flow, and brain edema. Blood pressure, either increased or decreased, is not a manifestation of a brain tumor.

12. 1-f, 2-e, 3-d, 4-a, 5-b, 6-c

13. d. *Rationale:* The most common surgery consists of removal of the amygdala and an anterior part of the hippocampus and entorhinal cortex, as well as a small part of the temporal pole, leaving the lateral temporal neocortex intact. Only a portion of the hippocampus and entorhinal cortex, and temporal pole are removed.

14. a. *Rationale:* Treatment consists of appropriate life-support measures. Medications are given to control seizure activity. Intravenously (IV) administered diazepam or lorazepam is considered first-line therapy for the condition. Lorazepam is not given intramuscularly (IM) in status epilepticus. Cyclobenzaprine and cyproheptadine are not used to treat status epilepticus.

CHAPTER 52 SLEEP AND SLEEP DISORDERS

SECTION II: ASSESSING YOUR UNDERSTANDING

Activity A

1. Wakefulness, sleep
2. growth, repair
3. reticular formation
4. Electroencephalogram (EEG)
5. Non-REM
6. REM
7. REM
8. Melatonin
9. sleep history
10. dyssomnias
11. synchronization
12. Jet lag
13. advanced sleep phase syndrome
14. Insomnia
15. hygiene
16. Periodic limb movement disorder
17. 10 seconds
18. Nightmares
19. Elderly

Activity B

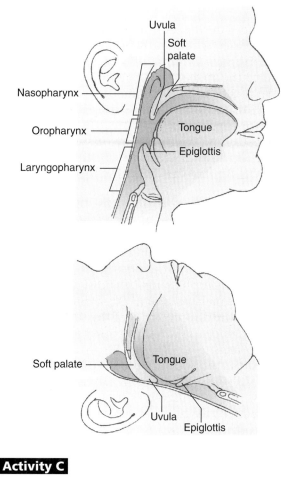

Uvula
Soft palate
Nasopharynx
Oropharynx
Laryngopharynx
Tongue
Epiglottis

Soft palate
Tongue
Uvula
Epiglottis

Activity C

1. j	**2.** a	**3.** i	**4.** f	**5.** g
6. d	**7.** e	**8.** b	**9.** h	**10.** c

Activity D

1. The sleep–wake cycle normally consists of a synchronous pattern of wakefulness and sleep. Wakefulness is a state of being aware of the environment—of receiving and responding to information arriving from all the senses, placing that information into memory, and recalling and integrating present experiences with previously stored memories. During wakefulness, both the thalamocortical loop and brain stem centers are active. A full repertoire of motor movements is made possible by corticospinal circuits that travel through the brain stem. Sleep represents a period of diminished consciousness from which a person can be aroused by sensory or other stimuli. It occurs in stages during which the brain remains active, but does not effectively process sensory information.

2. Stage 1 consists of low-voltage, mixed-frequency EEG activity. It occurs at sleep onset and is a brief transitional stage between wakefulness and true sleep. Stage 1 serves as a transitional stage for repeated sleep cycles throughout the night. Stage 2 is a deeper sleep during which EEG activity is interrupted by sleep spindles consisting of bursts of high frequency (12–14 Hz) waves. Stages 3 and 4 represent deep sleep and are dominated by high-voltage, low frequency waves. Stage 3 usually lasts only a few minutes and is transitional to stage 4, which lasts for approximately 20–40 minutes. During deep sleep, the muscles of the body relax and posture is adjusted intermittently. Heart rate and blood pressure decrease and gastrointestinal activity is slowed. An incrementally larger stimulus is required for arousal from slow-wave sleep.

3. External sensory input is inhibited in REM sleep, whereas internal sensory circuits such as those of the auditory and visual systems are aroused. During this time, the brain can replay previous memories but cannot acquire new sensory information. At the same time, motor systems that control body movements are inhibited. There is a loss of muscle movement and muscle tone. There also are changes in autonomic nervous system–controlled functions during REM sleep—blood pressure, heart rate, and respirations increase and fluctuate and temperature regulation is lost. Cerebral blood flow and metabolic rate decrease. Sleep-related penile erection occurs during this stage of sleep.

4. (1) Dyssomnias, which are disorders of initiating and maintaining sleep and disorders of excessive sleepiness; (2) parasomnias, which are not responsible for disturbing the sleep–wake cycle but are undesirable phenomena that occur primarily during sleep; (3) sleep disorders associated with other medical or psychiatric disorders; and (4) proposed sleep disorders, such as pregnancy-induced sleep disruptions.

5. A typical sleep study, or *polysomnography*, involves use of the EEG, electro-oculogram (EOG), electromyogram (EMG), electrocardiogram (ECG), breathing movements, and pulse oximetry. The EOG records eye movements. Because the eye is like a small battery with the retina negative to the cornea, an electrode placed on the skin near the eye records changes in voltage as the eye rotates in its socket. The EMG records the electrical activity from muscle movement. It is recorded from

the surface of the skin. It typically is recorded from under the chin because muscles in this area of the body show very dramatic changes associated with the sleep cycle. The ECG is used to measure the heart rate and detect cardiac dysrhythmias. The pulse oximeter (ear or finger) measures arterial oxygen saturation.

6. Chronic insomnia often is related to medical or psychiatric disorders. Factors such as pain, immobility, and hormonal changes associated with pregnancy or menopause also can cause insomnia. Interrupted sleep can accompany other sleep disorders, such as restless legs syndrome and sleep apnea. Many health problems worsen during the night. Heart failure, respiratory disease, and gastroesophageal reflux can cause frequent awakening during the night. Mood and anxiety disorders are the most frequent cause of insomnia in persons with psychiatric diagnoses. A number of drugs can lead to poor-quality sleep. Drugs commonly related to insomnia are caffeine, nicotine, stimulating antidepressants, alcohol, and recreational drugs. Although alcohol initially may induce sleep, it often causes disrupted and fragmented sleep. Sleep also is disrupted in persons undergoing alcohol or sleep medication withdrawal.

7. The National Institute of Health defines RLS as (1) an urge to move the limbs with or without sensations, (2) worsening at rest; (3) improving with activity; and (4) worsening in the evening or night.

8. A critical pathophysiologic feature of obstructive sleep apnea is sleep-related collapse of the upper airway at the level of the pharynx. All skeletal muscles, except the diaphragm, undergo a decrease in tone during sleep. This loss of muscle tone is most pronounced during REM sleep. The loss of muscle tone in the upper airways predisposes to airway obstruction as the negative airway pressure produced by contraction of the diaphragm brings the vocal cords together, collapses the pharyngeal wall, and sucks the tongue back into the throat.

SECTION III: APPLYING YOUR KNOWLEDGE

Activity E

1. Apnea is defined as cessation of airflow through the nose and mouth for 10 seconds or longer. The apneic periods typically last for 15–120 seconds, and some persons may have as many as 100 apneic periods per night. A

critical feature of obstructive sleep apnea is sleep-related collapse of the upper airway at the level of the pharynx and is most pronounced during REM sleep.

2. You correctly respond that the average number of apnea-hypopnea periods per hour is called the apnea-hypopnea index (AHI). An AHI of 5 or greater in combination with reports of excessive daytime sleepiness is indicative of sleep apnea.

3. Continuous positive airway pressure (CPAP)

SECTION IV: PRACTICING FOR NCLEX

Activity F

1. a. *Rationale:* During REM sleep, the brain can replay previous memories, but cannot acquire new sensory information. The other answers are incorrect.

2. b. *Rationale:* The pineal gland synthesizes and releases melatonin at night, a rhythm that is under the direct control of the suprachiasmatic nucleus (SCN). The other answers are incorrect.

3. c. *Rationale:* The multiple sleep latency test (MSLT) is used to evaluate daytime sleepiness. This test usually is completed the morning after a diagnostic sleep study. An average adult requires 10 or more minutes to fall asleep. An MSLT result of less than 5 minutes is considered abnormal.

4. d. *Rationale:* Diagnosis of RLS is based on a history of (1) a compelling urge to move the legs, usually associated with paresthesias; (2) motor restlessness, as seen by activities such as pacing, tossing and turning in bed, or rubbing the legs; (3) symptoms that become worse at rest and are relieved by activity; and (4) symptoms that are worse in the evening or at night.

5. 1-d, 2-b, 3-c, 4-a, 5-f, 6-e

6. a. *Rationale:* During a typical episode, the sleepwalker appears dazed and relatively unresponsive to the communication efforts of others. The other answers are incorrect.

7. a, b, c. *Rationale:* In a typical episode, the child sits up abruptly in bed, appears frightened, and demonstrates signs of extreme anxiety, including dilated pupils, excessive perspiration, rapid breathing, and tachycardia. Children with sleep terrors typically do not scream on awakening or refuse to sleep in their own bed.

8. b. *Rationale:* Many medications have stimulating effects and interfere with sleep. These

include some of the antidepressants, decongestants, bronchodilators, corticosteroids, and some antihypertensives. The other medications are not linked to sleep disturbances.

9. c. *Rationale:* Persons with Alzheimer disease often have increased periods of nighttime awakening and daytime napping. The other diseases are not associated with increased periods of nighttime awakening and daytime sleeping.

10. a. *Rationale:* The actigraph is a compact device that is worn on the wrist and is used most often in conjunction with a sleep diary. The other answers are not correct.

CHAPTER 53 DISORDERS OF THOUGHT, MOOD, AND MEMORY

SECTION II: ASSESSING YOUR UNDERSTANDING

Activity A

1. biologic, psychosocial
2. chlorpromazine
3. alterations
4. frontal
5. association
6. prefrontal
7. hallucinations, delusional
8. Release, ictal
9. Delusions
10. neurotransmitter, receptor
11. Antidepressants
12. Schizophrenia
13. emotion
14. Dysthymia
15. Kindling
16. decreased, increased
17. abuse, dependence
18. Memory
19. dementia
20. Alzheimer
21. neuritic (senile) plaques, neurofibrillary tangles
22. tau
23. chronic debilitation
24. cholinesterase inhibitors
25. Vascular
26. frontotemporal dementia
27. prion
28. Wernicke
29. Huntington
30. gamma-aminobutyric acid (GABA), GABA receptors

Activity B

1.

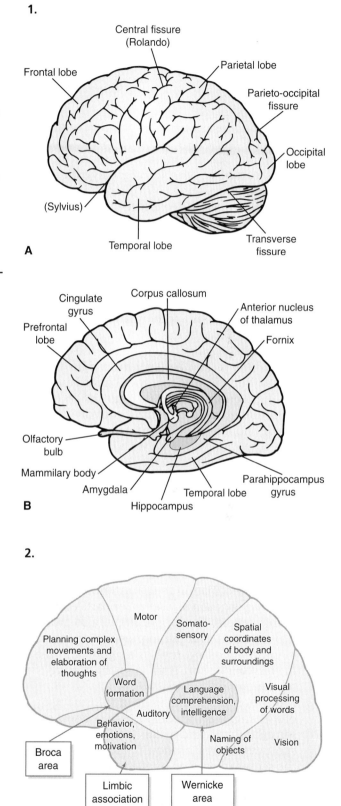

2.

Activity C

1.

1. b	**2.** j	**3.** d	**4.** i	**5.** e
6. g	**7.** f	**8.** a	**9.** h	**10.** c

2.

1. e	**2.** j	**3.** d	**4.** a	**5.** f
6. g	**7.** b	**8.** h	**9.** c	**10.** i

Activity D

1. Studies of twins have shown a 45% concordance for schizophrenia among monozygotic twins, compared with 15% for dizygotic twins or other siblings. With bipolar depression, there is an 80% concordance in monozygotic twins, compared with 10% for siblings. In monozygotic twins living apart, the concordance rate for affective disorders is 40% to 60%. Even the concordance rates among siblings for these two disorders are suggestive of a genetic influence because schizophrenia has approximately a 1% incidence and depression a 5% incidence among the general population. Although the evidence for a genetic basis for mental illness is compelling, the fact that the concordance among monozygotic twins is not 100% indicates that other factors may be involved in the development of a mental illness.

2. The hippocampus, along with its adjacent temporal and parietal lobe structures, has numerous indirect connections with many portions of the cerebral cortex and other parts of the limbic system. The hippocampus plays a major role in the encoding, consolidation, and retrieval of memories. Almost all types of sensory information activate some part of the hippocampus. In turn, the hippocampus distributes information to the anterior thalamus, hypothalamus, and other parts of the limbic system. The hippocampus also groups and schematizes input in preparation for memory encoding. It plays a significant role in converting short-term memory to long-term memory.

3. Perception is the final stage of information processing. It is the conscious awareness of sensory stimuli and results in behavioral responses to that sensation. Information from the senses is received by the thalamus, and then projected to the somatosensory cortex and prefrontal association area. The prefrontal association area keeps track of where information has been stored in long-term memory, and is responsible for retrieving and then integrating memories with sensory input for decision making.

4. The substances generally agreed to be neurotransmitters and that are implicated in mental illness include acetylcholine, the biogenic amines (dopamine, epinephrine, norepinephrine, and serotonin), and amino acids (gamma-aminobutyric acid, glutamate, glycine, and aspartate).

5. Monoamine oxidase inhibitors increase the concentration of serotonin and norepinephrine by reducing the degradation of these neurotransmitters by monoamine oxidase. The tricyclic antidepressants block the reuptake of serotonin and norepinephrine by the presynaptic membrane, whereas the serotonin reuptake inhibitors inhibit the reuptake of serotonin. The atypical antidepressants affect serotonergic and noradrenergic neurotransmission.

6. The psychopathology of schizophrenia can be organized into positive and negative symptoms. Positive symptoms are those that reflect the presence of abnormal behaviors and include incomprehensible speech, delusions, hallucinations, and grossly disorganized or catatonic behavior. Alterations in speech patterns can include using invented words, derailment, tangentiality, incoherence, or word salad. Frequently, persons with schizophrenia lose the ability to appropriately sort and interpret incoming stimuli, which impairs the ability to respond to the environment. An enhancement or a blunting of the senses is very common in the early stages of schizophrenia. The negative symptoms of schizophrenia reflect the absence of normal social and interpersonal behaviors and include alogia, avolition, apathy, affective flattening, inappropriate affect, and anhedonia. Some persons with schizophrenia have a blunted response to pain.

7. There is an enlargement of the lateral and third ventricles; a reduction of frontal, temporal, and whole brain volumes; and diminished neuronal content in both the thalamus and hippocampus. At the cellular anatomic level, there is an increased density of dopamine receptor sites, particularly in the basal ganglia.

8. Major depressive disorder is characterized by depressed mood, anhedonia, feelings of worthlessness or excessive guilt, decreased concentration, psychomotor agitation or retardation, insomnia or hypersomnia, decreased libido, and change.

9. Depression has various subclassifications distinguished by symptom patterns. Depression with melancholic features is characterized by depression that is worse in the morning, insomnia with early morning awakening, anorexia with significant weight loss, psychomotor retardation or agitation, excessive or inappropriate guilt, loss of interest in activity, inability to respond to pleasurable stimuli, and a complete loss of capacity for joy. The symptoms of atypical depression are opposite that of melancholic depression; it is characterized by a depression that becomes worse as the day progresses, overeating, and hypersomnia. Depression with psychotic features involves the presence of delusions or hallucinations that may or may not be mood congruent. The classification of depression with catatonic features is applied when symptoms include excessive mobility or motoric immobility, extreme negativism, repetitive speech, and peculiar voluntary movements.

10. The biogenic amine hypothesis suggests that decreased levels of these neurotransmitters in the synaptic cleft, due either to decreased presynaptic release or decreased postsynaptic sensitivity, is the underlying pathology in depression. The hypothesis is derived from the fact that drugs that depleted brain serotonin and norepinephrine caused depression, and drugs that increased brain levels of norepinephrine and serotonin decreased depression.

11. Persons with panic disorder typically have attacks characterized by neurologic symptoms (dizziness or lightheadedness, paresthesias, fainting), cardiac symptoms (tachycardia, chest pain and palpitations), respiratory symptoms (shortness of breath, feeling of smothering or choking), sweating, nausea or abdominal distress, and psychological symptoms (feelings of impending doom, fear of dying, a sense of unreality). Panic attacks must be distinguished from acute cardiac disease.

12. Although age is the greatest risk, additional factors have been identified as adding to the risks for developing Alzheimer disease. These include head trauma, inflammatory factors, and oxidative stress. Education has been identified as a protective factor; with suggestions that education can increase synaptic density. Other studies have looked at exercise as a possible protective factor in maintaining hippocampal health.

SECTION III: APPLYING YOUR KNOWLEDGE

Activity E

1. The nurse should convey the following major points about Alzheimer disease to this family:
   - Alzheimer disease is a physiologic dementia that is progressive and occurs most often in middle or late life.
   - The pathophysiologic aspects of Alzheimer disease involve neuropathologic and neurotransmitter changes. It is characterized by cortical atrophy and loss of neurons, particularly in the parietal and temporal lobes.
   - It is likely that Alzheimer disease is caused by several factors that interact differently in different persons.
   - Alzheimer-type dementia follows an insidious and progressive course, with an average survival of 8 to 10 years after diagnosis.
   - The hallmark symptoms are loss of short-term memory and a denial of such memory loss, with eventual disorientation, impaired abstract thinking, apraxia, and changes in personality and affect.
   - In the initial stage, clients with Alzheimer disease forget where things are placed, get lost easily, and have trouble remembering appointments and performing novel tasks.
   - In the moderate stage, which may last several years, there is a more global impairment of cognitive functioning. During this stage, there are changes in higher cortical functioning needed for language, spatial relationships, and problem solving.
   - Severe Alzheimer disease is characterized by a loss of ability to respond to the environment. Individuals in this stage require total care and spend most of their time bedridden.
   - There is no curative treatment for Alzheimer dementia. Drugs are used primarily to slow the progression and to control depression, agitation, or sleep disorders. Two major goals of care are maintaining the person's socialization and providing support for the family.
   - It is important for the nurse to provide information for support groups in the area.

SECTION IV: PRACTICING FOR NCLEX

Activity F

1. a. *Rationale:* This antipsychiatry attitude, coupled with the advent of psychopharmacology,

laid the foundations for the deinstitutional-ization of the mentally ill and the move to community psychiatry. The other answers are incorrect.

2. b. *Rationale:* It is highly likely that mental ill-nesses are polygenic and multifactorial rather than simply inherited through transmission of a classic disordered dominant or recessive Mendelian trait.

3. a, b, d, e. *Rationale:* The substances generally agreed to be neurotransmitters and that are implicated in mental illness include acetyl-choline, the biogenic amines (dopamine, epi-nephrine, norepinephrine, and serotonin), and amino acids (gamma-aminobutyric acid, glutamate, glycine, and aspartate). Succinyl-choline is a depolarizing neuromuscular blocker.

4. c. *Rationale:* It is the function of the pre-frontal areas to keep track of many bits of in-formation simultaneously and then to recall this information as needed for subsequent intellectual tasks. The other answers are incorrect.

5. d. *Rationale:* Information from the senses is received by the thalamus, and then pro-jected to the somatosensory cortex and pre-frontal association area. The hypothalamus oversees temperature, sleep-rest, etc. Broca's area forms words. The amygdale processes emotion.

6. a. *Rationale:* During the process, new or reac-tivated pathways transmit neural circuits, sometimes called memory traces, through the brain. The other answers are incorrect.

7. b. *Rationale:* Ictal hallucinations are produced by abnormal neuronal discharges. Visual hal-lucinations are not from abnormal neuronal discharges. Emotional hallucinations are un-known. Release hallucinations occur at times when a normal sensory input is blocked and, as a replacement, stored images are experi-enced.

8. c. *Rationale:* Interestingly, delusions have been associated with conditions that produce sensory deprivation, such as hearing loss. The other answers have not been associated with delusions.

9. d. *Rationale:* Monoamine oxidase inhibitors (e.g., phenelzine [Nardil], tranylcypromine [Parnate]) increase the concentration of sero-tonin and norepinephrine by reducing the degradation of these neurotransmitters by monoamine oxidase. Valium is a sedative and antianxiety agent. Halcion is a hypnotic agent. Paxil is a serotonin reuptake inhibitor.

10. a. *Rationale:* An enhancement or a blunting of the senses is very common in the early stages of schizophrenia. Sounds may be experienced as louder and more intrusive; colors may be brighter and sharper. The other answers are later signs or symptoms of schizophrenia.

11. 1-d, 2-e, 3-c, 4-a, 5-b

12. b. *Rationale:* The severity of manic symptoms runs the gamut from a condition called cy-clothymia, in which mood fluctuates be-tween mild elation and depression to severe delusional mania. Mania is the overall term for mood fluctuations between mild elation and depression. Specifier has nothing to do with bipolar disorder. Kindling is a hypothe-sized phenomenon in which a stressor creates an electrophysiologic vulnerability to future stressful events by causing long-lasting changes in neuronal function.

13. c. *Rationale:* Lithium and several anticonvul-sant agents are used in the treatment of bipo-lar depression. Valium is a sedative and antianxiety agent. Flexeril is a muscle relax-ant. Restoril is a hypnotic agent.

14. d. *Rationale:* Neurophysiologic studies suggest that the attacks may result from an abnor-mally sensitive "fear network" that is centered in the amygdala and involves interactions with the hippocampus and prefrontal cortex. The thymus has nothing to do with the "fear network."

15. a. *Rationale:* Although the neurophysiology of OCD remains under investigation, the gen-eral anatomic model suggests dysfunction of prefrontal cortex and structures of the basal ganglia, particularly the caudate nucleus and globus pallidus. The frontal cortex and the amygdale are not believed to be involved in the neurophysiology of OCD.

16. b. *Rationale:* Habitual use of drugs, including alcohol, is believed to induce adaptations in brain systems that alter the normal dopamine pathways and increase dopamine transmis-sion. The other answers are incorrect.

17. c. *Rationale:* Confabulation (i.e., recitation of imaginary experiences to fill in gaps in memory) is probably the most distinctive feature of the disease.

18. a, b, c. *Rationale:* Depression and personality changes are the most common early psychological manifestations. Memory loss is often accompanied by impulsive behavior, moodiness, antisocial behavior, and a tendency toward emotional outbursts. Mania and heightened sensory awareness are not components of Huntington disease.

CHAPTER 54 DISORDERS OF VISUAL FUNCTION

SECTION II: ASSESSING YOUR UNDERSTANDING

Activity A

1. eyeball
2. sclera
3. palpebrae
4. levator palpebrae superioris, orbicularis oculi
5. Blepharitis
6. Seborrheic
7. anterior blepharitis
8. Posterior
9. conjunctivitis
10. Hyperacute
11. cornea
12. Keratitis
13. keratitis
14. ophthalmicus
15. iris
16. uveitis
17. pupils
18. Glaucoma
19. degenerative
20. Congenital
21. astigmatism
22. Accommodation
23. cataract
24. retina
25. color-blind
26. Retinitis pigmentosa
27. Macular
28. Retinoblastomas
29. visual field
30. inferior recti, lateral recti, obliques
31. Conjugate
32. Saccadic
33. Strabismus
34. Amblyopia

Activity B

1.

2.

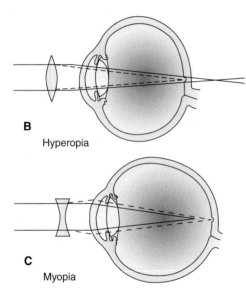

A

Normal focal length

B

Hyperopia

C

Myopia

3.

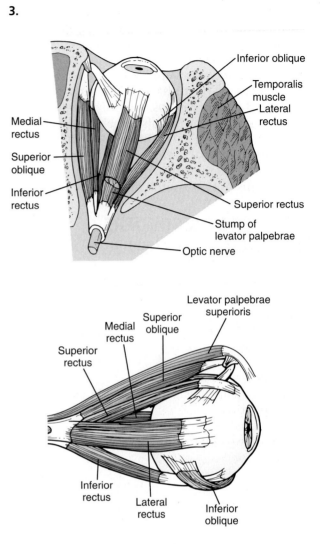

Inferior oblique

Temporalis muscle

Lateral rectus

Medial rectus

Superior oblique

Inferior rectus

Superior rectus

Stump of levator palpebrae

Optic nerve

Levator palpebrae superioris

Superior oblique

Medial rectus

Superior rectus

Inferior rectus

Lateral rectus

Inferior oblique

Activity C

1.

1. e	**2.** f	**3.** g	**4.** a	**5.** j
6. c	**7.** d	**8.** b	**9.** i	**10.** h

2.

1. f	**2.** c	**3.** g	**4.** b	**5.** a
6. e	**7.** j	**8.** d	**9.** i	**10.** h

Activity D

1. The lacrimal system includes the major lacrimal gland; it produces the tears; the puncta; canaliculi; the tear sac, which collect the tears; and the nasolacrimal duct, which empties the tears into the nasal cavity. Tears contain approximately 98% water; 1.5% sodium chloride; and small amounts of potassium, albumin, and glucose. The function of tears is to provide a smooth optical surface by abolishing minute surface irregularities. Tears also wet and protect the delicate surface of the cornea and conjunctiva. They flush and remove irritating substances and microorganisms, and provide the cornea with necessary nutrient substances. Tears also contain lysozymes and immunoglobulins A, G, and E, which synergistically act to protect against infection.

2. Chronic bacterial conjunctivitis is most commonly caused by *Staphylococcus* species, although other bacteria may be involved. It is often associated with blepharitis and bacterial colonization of eyelid margins. The symptoms of chronic bacterial conjunctivitis vary and can include itching, burning, foreign body sensation, and morning eyelash crusting. Other symptoms include flaky debris and erythema along the lid margins, eyelash loss,

and eye redness. Some people with chronic bacterial conjunctivitis also have recurrent styes and chalazia of the lid margins.

3. Trauma that causes abrasions of the cornea can be extremely painful, but, if minor, the abrasions usually heal in a few days. The epithelial layer can regenerate, and small defects heal without scarring. If the stroma is damaged, healing occurs more slowly, and the danger of infection is increased. Injuries to Bowman membrane and the stromal layer heal with scar formation and permanent opacification. Opacities of the cornea impair the transmission of light. A minor scar can severely distort vision because it disturbs the refractive surface.

4. Primary epithelial infections are the optical counterpart of labial herpes with similar immunologic and pathologic features as well as a similar time course. During childhood, mild primary herpes simplex virus infection may go unnoticed. After the initial primary infection, the virus may persist in a quiescent or latent state that remains in the trigeminal ganglion and possibly in the cornea without causing signs of infection.

5. Acanthamoeba keratitis is a rare but serious and sight-threatening complication caused by wearing soft contact lenses, particularly when they are worn overnight beyond doctor-recommended periods or when poor disinfection techniques are used. It also may occur in non–contact lens wearers after exposure to contaminated water or soil. It is characterized by pain that is disproportionate to the clinical manifestations, redness of the eye, and photophobia.

6. Changes in pupil size are controlled by contraction or relaxation of the sphincter and radial muscles of the iris. The pupillary reflex, which controls the size of the pupillary opening, is controlled by the autonomic nervous system, with the parasympathetic nervous system producing pupillary constriction or miosis, and the sympathetic nervous system producing pupillary dilation or mydriasis. The sphincter muscle that produces pupillary constriction is innervated by postganglionic parasympathetic neurons of the ciliary ganglion and other scattered ganglion cells between the scleral and choroid layers. The pupillary reflex is controlled by a region in the midbrain called the pretectum.

7. Glaucoma usually results from congenital or acquired lesions of the anterior segment of the eye that mechanically obstruct aqueous outflow. Primary glaucoma occurs without evidence of preexisting ocular or systemic disease. Secondary glaucoma can result from inflammatory processes that affect the eye, from tumors, or from blood cells of trauma-produced hemorrhage that obstruct the outflow of aqueous humor.

8. The term presbyopia refers to decrease in accommodation that occurs because of aging. The lens consists of transparent fibers arranged in concentric layers, of which the external layers are the newest and softest. No loss of lens fibers occurs with aging; instead, additional fibers are added to the outermost portion of the lens. As the lens ages, it thickens, and its fibers become less elastic, so that the range of focus or accommodation is diminished to the point where reading glasses become necessary for near vision.

9. Hemorrhage can be preretinal, intraretinal, or subretinal. Preretinal hemorrhages occur between the retina and the vitreous. These hemorrhages are usually large because the blood vessels are only loosely restricted; they may be associated with a subarachnoid or subdural hemorrhage and are usually regarded as a serious manifestation of the disorder. They usually reabsorb without complications unless they penetrate into the vitreous. Intraretinal hemorrhages occur because of abnormalities of the retinal vessels, diseases of the blood, increased pressure in the retinal vessels, or vitreous traction on the vessels. Systemic causes include diabetes mellitus, hypertension, and blood dyscrasias. Subretinal hemorrhages are those that develop between the choroid and pigment layer of the retina. A common cause of subretinal hemorrhage is neovascularization. Photocoagulation may be used to treat microaneurysms and neovascularization.

10. Proliferative diabetic retinopathy represents a more severe retinal change than background retinopathy. It is characterized by formation of new fragile blood vessels (i.e., neovascularization) at the disk and elsewhere in the retina. These vessels grow in front of the retina, along the posterior surface of the vitreous or into the vitreous. They threaten vision in two ways. First, because they are abnormal, they often bleed easily, leaking blood into the vitreous cavity and decreasing visual acuity. Second, the blood vessels attach firmly to the retinal surface and posterior surface of the vitreous, such that normal movement of the vitreous may exert a pull on the retina, causing

retinal detachment and progressive blindness.

11. Persistently elevated blood pressure results in the compensatory thickening of arteriolar walls, which effectively reduces capillary perfusion pressure. With severe uncontrolled hypertension, there is disruption of the blood-retinal barrier, necrosis of smooth muscle and endothelial cells, exudation of blood and lipids, and retinal ischemia. These changes are manifested in the retina by microaneurysms, intraretinal hemorrhages, hard exudates, and cotton-wool spots.

SECTION III: APPLYING YOUR KNOWLEDGE

Activity E

1. The nurse would expect the doctor to order an ophthalmoscopic exam under anesthesia by an ophthalmologist. CT or MRI scans are used to evaluate the extent of intraocular disease and extraocular spread.
2. Treatment options for retinoblastoma are laser thermotherapy, cryotherapy, chemotherapy, and nucleation.

SECTION IV: PRACTICING FOR NCLEX

Activity F

1. a. *Rationale:* Neurologic causes of eyelid weakness include damage to the innervating cranial nerves or to the nerve's central nuclei in the midbrain and the caudal pons. The other answers have nothing to do with the central nuclei of the oculomotor and the facial nerve.
2. b. *Rationale:* The symptoms include tearing and discharge, pain, swelling, and tenderness. The other answers are incorrect.
3. c. *Rationale:* Infection should be suspected when conjunctivitis develops 48 hours after birth. The other answers are not correct.
4. c. *Rationale:* The treatment of herpes simplex virus (HSV) keratitis focuses on eliminating viral replication within the cornea while minimizing the damaging effects of the inflammatory process. The other answers are not goals in the treatment of HSV keratitis.
5. b, c, d. *Rationale:* The low rejection rate is due to several factors: the cornea is avascular, including lymphatics, thereby limiting perfusion by immune elements; major histocompatibility complexes (class II) are virtually absent in the cornea; antigen-presenting cells are not present in great numbers; the cornea secretes immunosuppressive factors; and corneal cells secrete substances (e.g., Fas ligand) that protect against apoptosis, thereby minimizing inflammation. The other answers are incorrect.
6. d. *Rationale:* Miotic drugs (e.g., pilocarpine), which are used in the treatment of angle-closure glaucoma (to be discussed), produce pupil constriction and, in that manner, facilitate aqueous humor circulation. The other answers are classes of drugs that do not affect papillary constriction.
7. a. *Rationale:* Primary open-angle glaucoma usually occurs because of an abnormality of the trabecular meshwork that controls the flow of aqueous humor into the canal of Schlemm. The other answers are incorrect.
8. 1-d, 2-b, 3-a, 4-c, 5-e
9. b. *Rationale:* Age-related cataracts, which are the most common type, are characterized by increasingly blurred vision and visual distortion. The other answers are incorrect.
10. c. *Rationale:* With the loss of gel structure, fine fibers, membranes, and cellular debris develop. When this occurs, floaters (images) can often be noticed because these substances move within the vitreous cavity during head movement. Blind spots, meshlike structures, and red spots are not seen during head movement with a loss of the gel structure of the vitreous humor.
11. d. *Rationale:* Neovascularization occurs in many conditions that impair retinal blood flow, including stasis because of hyperviscosity of blood or decreased flow, vascular occlusion, sickle cell disease, sarcoidosis, diabetes mellitus, and retinopathy of prematurity. The other answers are incorrect.
12. a. *Rationale:* Nonexudative age-related macular degeneration is characterized by various degrees of atrophy and degeneration of the outer retina, Bruch membrane, and choriocapillary layer of the choroid. It does not involve leakage of blood or serum; hence, it is called dry age-related macular degeneration. The other answers are characterizations of the "wet" form of macular degeneration.
13. b. *Rationale:* Crude analysis of visual stimulation at reflex levels, such as eye- and head-orienting responses to bright moving lights, pupillary reflexes, and blinking at sudden bright lights, may be retained even though vision has been lost. The other answers are incorrect.

14. c. *Rationale:* Paralytic strabismus is uncommon in children, but accounts for nearly all cases of adult strabismus. It can be caused by infiltrative processes, including Graves disease, myasthenia gravis, stroke, and direct optical trauma. The other diseases have nothing to do with adult strabismus.

15. b. *Rationale:* The reversibility of amblyopia depends on the maturity of the visual system at the time of onset and the duration of the abnormal experience. The other answers are incorrect.

CHAPTER 55 DISORDERS OF HEARING AND VESTIBULAR FUNCTION

SECTION II: ASSESSING YOUR UNDERSTANDING

Activity A

1. ear
2. cerumen

3. Otitis externa
4. temporal
5. eustachian
6. abnormally patent
7. Otitis media
8. Acute otitis media
9. Otosclerosis
10. cochlea
11. Wernicke area
12. Sensorineural
13. bacterial meningitis
14. cranial nerve VIII
15. cytomegalovirus
16. vestibular
17. vertigo
18. Motion sickness
19. paroxysmal positional
20. vestibular neuronitis
21. Ménière
22. cerebellum

Activity B

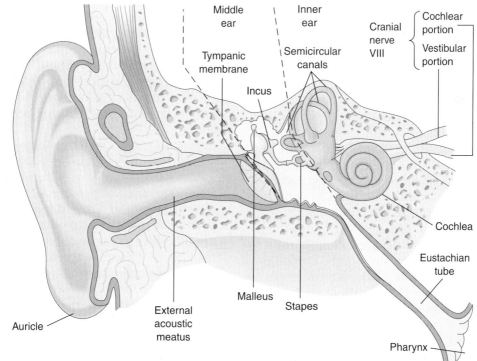

Activity C

1. j	**2.** h	**3.** e	**4.** c	**5.** i
6. a	**7.** g	**8.** d	**9.** b	**10.** f

Activity D

1. The eustachian tube serves three basic functions: (a) ventilation of the middle ear, along with equalization of middle ear and ambient pressures; (b) protection of the middle ear from unwanted nasopharyngeal sound waves and secretions; and (c) drainage of middle ear secretions into the nasopharynx.

2. Hearing loss, which is a common complication of otitis media, is usually conductive and temporary based on the duration of the effusion. Hearing loss that is associated with fluid collection usually resolves when the effusion clears. Permanent hearing loss may occur as the result of damage to the tympanic membrane or other middle ear structures. Cases of sensorineural hearing loss are rare. Persistent and episodic conductive hearing loss in children may impair their cognitive, linguistic, and emotional development.

3. During active bone resorption, the bone structure appears spongy and softer than normal. The resorbed bone is replaced by an overgrowth of new, hard, sclerotic bone. The process is slowly progressive, involving more areas of the temporal bone, especially in front of and posterior to the stapes footplate. As it invades the footplate, the pathologic bone increasingly immobilizes the stapes, reducing the transmission of sound. Pressure of otosclerotic bone on middle ear structures or the vestibulocochlear nerve (cranial nerve VIII) may contribute to the development of tinnitus, sensorineural hearing loss, and vertigo.

4. A number of causes and conditions have been associated with subjective tinnitus. Intermittent periods of mild, high-pitched tinnitus lasting for several minutes are common in normal-hearing persons. Impacted cerumen is a benign cause of tinnitus, which resolves after the earwax is removed. Medications such as aspirin and stimulants such as nicotine and caffeine can cause transient tinnitus. Conditions associated with more persistent tinnitus include noise-induced hearing loss, presbycusis (sensorineural hearing loss that occurs with aging), hypertension, atherosclerosis, head injury, and cochlear or labyrinthine infection or inflammation.

5. Conductive hearing loss occurs when auditory stimuli are not adequately transmitted through the auditory canal, tympanic membrane, middle ear, or ossicle chain to the inner ear. Temporary hearing loss can occur as the result of impacted cerumen in the outer ear or fluid in the middle ear. Foreign bodies, including pieces of cotton and insects, may impair hearing. More permanent causes of hearing loss are thickening or damage of the tympanic membrane or involvement of the bony structures (ossicles and oval window) of the middle ear due to otosclerosis or Paget disease.

6. The hair cells in both utricular and saccular maculae are embedded in a flattened gelatinous mass, the otolithic membrane, which is studded with tiny stones called otoliths. Although they are small, the density of the otoliths increases the membrane's weight and its resistance to change in motion. When the head is tilted, the gelatinous mass shifts its position because of the pull of the gravitational field, bending the stereocilia of the macular hair cells. Although each hair cell becomes more or less excitable depending on the direction in which the cilia are bending, the hair cells are oriented in all directions, making these sense organs sensitive to static or changing head position in relation to the gravitational field. In a condition called benign positional vertigo (to be discussed), the otoliths become dislodged from their gelatinous base, causing positional vertigo.

7. Caloric testing involves elevating the head 30 degrees and irrigating each external auditory canal separately with 30 to 50 mL of ice water. The resulting changes in temperature, which are conducted through the petrous portion of the temporal bone, set up convection currents in the endolymph that mimic the effects of angular acceleration. In an unconscious person with a functional brain stem and intact oculovestibular reflexes, the eyes exhibit a jerk nystagmus lasting 2 to 3 minutes, with the slow component toward the irrigated ear followed by rapid movement away from the ear. With impairment of brain stem function, the response becomes perverted and eventually disappears.

SECTION III: APPLYING YOUR KNOWLEDGE

Activity E

1. When talking about ototoxicity, aminoglycosides, antimalarial drugs, chemotherapeutic drugs, loop diuretics, and salicylates would be discussed.

SECTION IV: PRACTICING FOR NCLEX

Activity F

1. a. *Rationale:* The most common bacterial pathogens are gram-negative rods (*Pseudomonas aeruginosa, Proteus* spp.) and fungi (*Aspergillus*) that grow in the presence of excess moisture. The other answers are not fungi.
2. a. *Rationale:* The abnormally patent tube does not close or does not close completely. In infants and children with an abnormally patent tube, air and secretions are often pumped into the eustachian tube during crying and nose blowing. Cerumen and saliva are not let into the eustachian tube.
3. a, b, d. *Rationale:* Risk factors include premature birth, male gender, ethnicity (Native American, Inuit), family history of recurrent otitis media, presence of siblings in the household, genetic syndromes, and low socioeconomic status. Being an only child and being a female are not risk factors for AOM.
4. c. *Rationale:* Because much of the conductive hearing loss associated with otosclerosis is caused by stapedial fixation, surgical treatment involves stapedectomy with stapedial reconstruction using the patient's own stapes or stapedial prosthesis. The other answers are incorrect.
5. d. *Rationale:* The scala vestibuli and scala media are separated from each other by the vestibular membrane, also known as Reissner membrane. The other answers are incorrect.
6. a. *Rationale:* In some vascular disorders, sounds generated by turbulent blood flow (e.g., arterial bruits or venous hums) are conducted to the auditory system. Vascular disorders typically produce a pulsatile form of tinnitus. The other answers are incorrect.
7. b. *Rationale:* More permanent causes of hearing loss are thickening or damage of the tympanic membrane or involvement of the bony structures (ossicles and oval window) of the middle ear due to otosclerosis or Paget disease. Huntington, Alzheimer, and Parkinson diseases are not associated with conductive hearing loss.
8. c. *Rationale:* Acoustic neuromas are benign Schwann cell tumors affecting cranial nerve VIII. The other answers are incorrect.
9. d. *Rationale:* Tuning forks are used to differentiate conductive and sensorineural hearing loss. AudioScope, audiometer, and tone analysis do not differentiate between conductive and sensorineural hearing loss.
10. a. *Rationale:* Genetic causes are probably responsible for as much as 50% of sensorineural hearing loss in children. The other diseases are not the correct answer.
11. b. *Rationale:* The disorder first reduces the ability to understand speech and, later, the ability to detect, identify, and localize sounds.

CHAPTER 56 STRUCTURE AND FUNCTION OF THE MUSCULOSKELETAL SYSTEM

SECTION II: ASSESSING YOUR UNDERSTANDING

Activity A

1. muscles, tendons, ligaments
2. calcium, blood
3. axial, appendicular
4. Compact
5. Bones
6. periosteum
7. marrow
8. nutritional arteries
9. connective, calcium
10. osteoprogenitor
11. Osteoclasts
12. Elastic
13. Fibrocartilage
14. Hyaline
15. Calcitonin
16. Tendons
17. Ligaments
18. Synarthroses
19. Synovial
20. bursae

Activity B

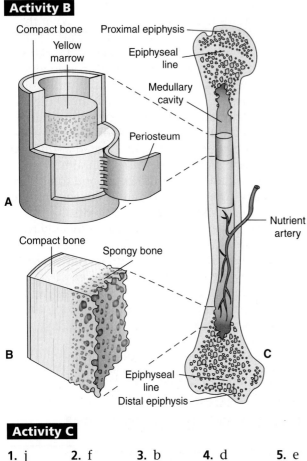

Compact bone
Yellow marrow
Proximal epiphysis
Epiphyseal line
Medullary cavity
Periosteum
A
Nutrient artery
Compact bone
Spongy bone
B
C
Epiphyseal line
Distal epiphysis

Activity C

1. j	**2.** f	**3.** b	**4.** d	**5.** e
6. i	**7.** a	**8.** c	**9.** g	**10.** h

Activity D

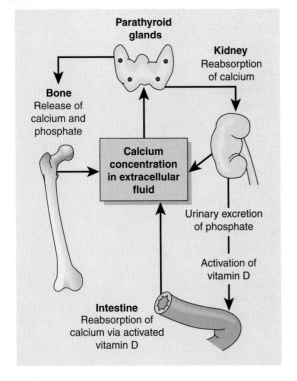

Parathyroid glands

Kidney
Reabsorption of calcium

Bone
Release of calcium and phosphate

Calcium concentration in extracellular fluid

Urinary excretion of phosphate

Activation of vitamin D

Intestine
Reabsorption of calcium via activated vitamin D

Activity E

1. A typical long bone has a shaft, or diaphysis, and two ends, called epiphyses. Long bones are usually narrow in the midportion and broad at the ends so that the weight they bear can be distributed over a wider surface. The shaft of a long bone is formed mainly of compact bone roughly hollowed out to form a marrow-filled medullary canal. The ends of long bones are covered with articular cartilage.

2. Red bone marrow contains developing red blood cells and is the site of blood cell formation. Yellow bone marrow is composed largely of adipose cells. At birth, nearly all marrow is red and hematopoietically active. As the need for red blood cell production decreases during postnatal growth, red marrow is gradually replaced with yellow bone marrow in most of the bones. In the adult, red marrow persists in the vertebrae, ribs, sternum, and ilia.

3. The intercellular matrix is composed of two types of substances—organic matter and inorganic salts. The organic matter, including bone cells, blood vessels, and nerves, constitutes approximately one-third of the dry weight of bone; the inorganic salts make up the other two-thirds. The organic matter consists primarily of collagen fibers embedded in an amorphous ground substance. The inorganic matter consists of hydroxyapatite, an insoluble macrocrystalline structure of calcium phosphate salts, and small amounts of calcium carbonate and calcium fluoride.

4. Both connective tissue types consist of living cells, nonliving intercellular fibers, and an amorphous (shapeless) ground substance. The tissue cells are responsible for secreting and maintaining the intercellular substances in which they are housed. However, cartilage consists of more extracellular substance than bone, and fibers are embedded in a firm gel rather a calcified cement substance. Hence, cartilage has the flexibility of a firm plastic material rather than the rigid characteristics of bone.

5. Parathyroid hormone (PTH) maintains serum calcium levels by initiation of calcium release from bone, by conservation of calcium by the kidney, by enhanced intestinal absorption of calcium through activation of vitamin D, and by reduction of serum phosphate levels. PTH also increases the movement of calcium and phosphate from bone into the extracellular fluid.

6. The most potent of the vitamin D metabolites is 1,25-$(OH)_2D_3$. This metabolite increases intestinal absorption of calcium and promotes the actions of parathyroid hormone on resorption of calcium and phosphate from bone. Bone resorption by the osteoclasts is increased, and bone formation by the osteoblasts is decreased; there is also an increase in acid phosphatase and a decrease in alkaline phosphatase. Intestinal absorption and bone resorption increase the amount of calcium and phosphorus available to the mineralizing surface of the bone.

SECTION III: APPLYING YOUR KNOWLEDGE

Activity F

1. "Tendonitis occurs because of overuse of the tendon, which causes inflammation of the tendon."
2. "Some tendons are enclosed in sheaths so that they slide inside the sheath and are cushioned by synovial fluid. Other tendons are not encased in a sheath. All tendons attach muscles to bone and do not stretch very much."

SECTION IV: PRACTICING FOR NCLEX

Activity G

1. a. *Rationale:* The metaphysis is composed of bony trabeculae that have cores of cartilage. The other answers are incorrect.
2. b. *Rationale:* Yellow bone marrow is composed largely of adipose cells. Hematopoietic cells are in red bone marrow. Cancellous cells are in spongy bone. Osteogenic cells line the latticelike pattern that forms bone marrow.
3. c. *Rationale:* Lamellar bone is composed largely of cylindrical units called osteons or haversian systems. Hematopoietic cells, spicules, and macrocrystalline cells do not comprise lamellar bone.
4. d. *Rationale:* Fibrocartilage is found in the intervertebral disks, in areas where tendons are connected to bone, and in the symphysis pubis. The other answers are incorrect.
5. a, b, c. *Rationale:* Parathyroid hormone maintains serum calcium levels by initiation of calcium release from bone, conservation of calcium by the kidney, enhanced intestinal absorption of calcium through activation of vitamin D, and reduction of serum phosphate levels.

6. a. *Rationale:* The most potent of the vitamin D metabolites is 1,25-$(OH)_2D_3$. This metabolite increases intestinal absorption of calcium and promotes the actions of parathyroid hormone on resorption of calcium and phosphate from bone. None of the other answers are correct.
7. b. *Rationale:* Synchondroses are joints in which bones are connected by hyaline cartilage and have limited motion. The other answers are incorrect.
8. c. *Rationale:* Diarthrodial joints are the joints most frequently affected by rheumatic disorders. The other types of joint are not the ones most frequently affected by rheumatic disorders.
9. d. *Rationale:* The tendons and ligaments of the joint capsule are sensitive to position and movement, particularly stretching and twisting. The other answers are incorrect.
10. a. *Rationale:* These sacs, called bursae, contain synovial fluid. Their purpose is to prevent friction on a tendon. Bursae do not prevent injury to a joint, nor do they cushion joints. They also do not prevent friction on a ligament.

CHAPTER 57 DISORDERS OF MUSCULOSKELETAL FUNCTION: TRAUMA, INFECTION, AND NEOPLASMS

SECTION II: ASSESSING YOUR UNDERSTANDING

Activity A

1. musculoskeletal
2. falls
3. Soft tissue
4. strain
5. sprain
6. dislocation
7. Loose
8. Rotator cuff
9. rotational
10. Dislocations
11. sudden injury, pathologic
12. pathologic
13. fracture
14. Traction
15. Fracture blisters
16. thromboemboli
17. fat embolism
18. Tuberculosis

19. Osteonecrosis
20. osteosarcoma
21. Benign
22. chondroma
23. Chondrosarcoma

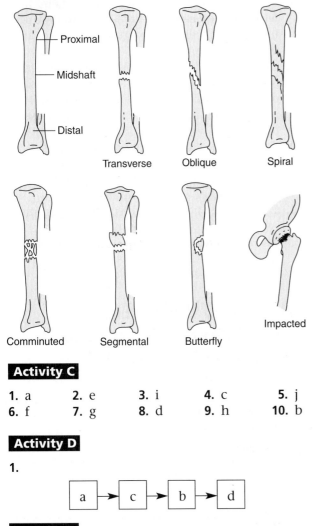

Transverse   Oblique   Spiral

Comminuted   Segmental   Butterfly   Impacted

Activity C

1. a	**2.** e	**3.** i	**4.** c	**5.** j
6. f	**7.** g	**8.** d	**9.** h	**10.** b

Activity D

1.

a → c → b → d

Activity E

1. Any joint can be sprained, but the ankle joint is most commonly involved, especially in fast-moving injuries in which an ankle or knee can be suddenly twisted. Most ankle sprains occur in the lateral ankle when the foot is turned inward under a person, forcing the ankle into inversion beyond the structural limits. Other common sites of sprain are the knee (the collateral ligament and anterior cruciate ligament) and elbow (the ulnar side). As with a strain, the soft tissue injury that occurs with a sprain is not evident on the radiograph. Wrist sprains most often occur with a fall on an outstretched hand.

2. If properly treated, injuries usually heal with the restoration of the original tensile strength. Repair is accomplished by fibroblasts from the inner tendon sheath or, if the tendon has no sheath, from the loose connective tissue that surrounds the tendon. Capillaries infiltrate the injured area during the initial healing process and supply the fibroblasts with the materials they need to produce large amounts of collagen. Formation of the long collagen bundles occurs within the first 2 weeks and, although tensile strength increases steadily thereafter, it is not sufficient to permit strong tendon pulls for 6 to 8 weeks. The danger is that muscle contraction will pull the injured ends apart, causing the tendon to heal in the lengthened position. Another danger is that adhesions will develop in areas where tendons pass through fibrous channels, such as in the distal palm of the hands, rendering the tendon useless.

3. Motion of the arm involves the coordinated movement of muscles of the rotator cuff (supraspinous, teres minor, infraspinatus, and subscapularis) and their musculotendinous attachments. These muscles are separated from the overlying coracoacromial arch by two bursae, the subdeltoid and subcoracoid. These two bursae, sometimes referred to as the subacromial bursa, often communicate and are affected by lesions of the rotator cuff. Rotator cuff injuries and impingement disorders can result from a number of causes, including excessive use, a direct blow, or stretch injury, usually involving throwing or swinging, as with baseball pitchers or tennis players. Overuse and degenerative disorders have a slower onset and are seen in older persons with minor or no trauma. The tendons of the rotator cuff fuse together near their insertions into the tuberosites of the humerus to form the musculotendinous cuff.

4. A hip fracture is generally a fracture of the proximal femur. Such fractures are commonly categorized according to the anatomic site in which they occur. Femoral-neck fractures are located in the area distal to the femoral head but proximal to the greater and lesser trochanters and are considered intracapsular, because they are located within the capsule of the hip joint. Intertrochanteric fractures occur in the metaphyseal region between the greater and lesser trochanter. Subtrochanteric fractures are those that occur just below the greater trochanter. Femoral-neck and intertrochanteric fractures account for more

than 90% of hip fractures, occurring in approximately equal proportions.

5. The compartment syndrome has been described as a condition of increased pressure within a limited space (e.g., abdominal and limb compartments) that compromises the circulation and function of the tissues within the space. The muscles and nerves of an extremity are enclosed in a tough, inelastic fascial envelope called a muscle compartment. If the pressure in the compartment is sufficiently high, tissue circulation is compromised, causing death of nerve and muscle cells. Permanent loss of function may occur. The amount of pressure required to produce a compartment syndrome depends on many factors, including the duration of the pressure elevation, the metabolic rate of the tissues, vascular tone, and local blood pressure. Compartment syndrome can result from a decrease in compartment size, an increase in the volume of its contents, or a combination of the two factors.

6. Osteomyelitis after trauma or bone surgery usually is associated with persistent or recurrent fevers, increased pain at the operative or trauma site, and poor incisional healing, which often is accompanied by continued wound drainage and wound separation. Prosthetic joint infections often present with joint pain, fever, and cutaneous drainage.

7. The pathologic features of bone necrosis are the same, regardless of cause. The lesion site is related to the vessels involved. There is necrosis of cancellous bone and marrow. The cortex usually is not involved because of collateral blood flow. In subchondral necrosis, a triangular or wedge-shaped segment of tissue that has the subchondral bone plate as its base and the center of the epiphysis as its apex, undergoes necrosis. When medullary infarcts occur in fatty bone marrow, the death of bone cells causes calcium release and necrosis of fat cells, with the formation of free fatty acids. Released calcium forms an insoluble "soap" with free fatty acids. Because bone lacks mechanisms for resolving the infarct, the lesions remain for life.

8. The three major manifestations of bone tumors are pain, presence of a mass, and impairment of function. Pain is a feature common to almost all malignant tumors, but may or may not occur with benign tumors. A mass or hard lump may be the first sign of a bone tumor. A malignant tumor is suspected when a painful mass exists that is enlarging or eroding the cortex of the bone. The ease of discovery of a mass depends on the location of the tumor; a small lump arising on the surface of the tibia is easy to detect, whereas a tumor that is deep in the medial portion of the thigh may grow to a considerable size before it is noticed. Benign and malignant tumors can cause the bone to erode to the point at which it cannot withstand the strain of ordinary use. In such cases, even a small amount of bone stress or trauma precipitates a pathologic fracture. A tumor may produce pressure on a peripheral nerve, causing decreased sensation, numbness, a limp, or limitation of movement.

9. Metastatic lesions are seen most often in the spine, femur, pelvis, ribs, sternum, proximal humerus, and skull, and are less common in anatomic sites that are further removed from the trunk of the body that are secondary tumors. Tumors that frequently spread to the skeletal system are those of the breast, lung, prostate, kidney, and thyroid, although any cancer can ultimately involve the skeleton. More than 85% of bone metastases result from primary lesions in the breast, lung, or prostate.

SECTION III: APPLYING YOUR KNOWLEDGE

Activity F

1. Magnetic resonance imaging (MRI) of the injured knee
2. Knee is place in removable knee immobilizer and isometric quadriceps exercises
3. An arthroscopic meniscectomy may be performed if there is recurrent or persistent locking, recurrent fluid build-up in the knee, or disabling pain.

SECTION IV: PRACTICING FOR NCLEX

Activity G

1. a. *Rationale:* Overuse injuries have been described as chronic injuries, including stress fractures that result from constant high levels of physiologic stress without sufficient recovery time. They commonly occur in the elbow ("Little League elbow" or "tennis elbow") and in tissue where tendons attach to the bone, such as the heel, knee, and shoulder. The other answers are incorrect.
2. 1-g, 2-d, 3-b, 4-f, 5-c, 6-a, 7-e
3. b, c, d. *Rationale:* Conservative treatment with anti-inflammatory agents, corticosteroid

injections, and physical therapy often is undertaken. A period of rest is followed by a customized exercise and rehabilitation program to improve strength, flexibility, and endurance. Pain medicine and anesthetic injections are not usually prescribed for conservative treatment of a shoulder or rotator cuff injury.

4. b. *Rationale:* Hip dislocation is an emergency. In the dislocated position, great tension is placed on the blood supply to the femoral head and avascular necrosis can result. Pain caused by a dislocated knee is not considered an emergency. The longer the hip is dislocated, the more time it takes to heal and remain in place, but this is not an emergency, and dislocation of the hip does not interrupt the blood supply to the femoral head.

5. b. *Rationale:* Various growth factors, such as bone morphologic protein (BMP), are thought to induce bone formation and repair bone defects. The other choices listed are not used to induce healing in fractures.

6. b, c, d. *Rationale:* A thorough history includes the mechanism, time, and place of the injury; first recognition of symptoms; and any treatment initiated. It is unimportant if anyone else in the family is susceptible to fractures. It is also unimportant what the patient has eaten. If surgery were indicated, then it would be important to find out *if* the patient had eaten.

7. 1-a, 2-c, 3-b

8. c. *Rationale:* The main clinical features of fat emboli syndrome (FES) are respiratory failure, cerebral dysfunction, and skin and mucosal petechiae. Cerebral manifestations include encephalopathy, seizures, and focal neurologic deficits unrelated to head injury. The other answers are incorrect.

9. d. *Rationale:* Intravenous therapy is usually needed for up to 6 weeks. Initial antibiotic therapy is followed by surgery to remove foreign bodies (e.g., metal plates, screws) or sequestra and by long-term antibiotic therapy. The other answers are incorrect.

10. a. *Rationale:* Any bone, joint, or bursae can be affected, but the spine is the most common site, followed by the knees and hips. The ankles and shoulders are not common sites for tuberculosis to be found.

11. b. *Rationale:* Besides fracture, the most common causes of bone necrosis are idiopathic (i.e., those of unknown cause) and prior steroid therapy. Vessel injury, radiation therapy, and embolism can cause osteonecrosis, but prior steroid therapy is the most common cause other than fracture.

12. c. *Rationale:* The primary clinical feature of osteosarcoma is deep localized pain with nighttime awakening and swelling in the affected bone. In osteosarcoma the pain is worse at night. There may be erythema in the overlaying skin, but that is not the primary clinical feature of the disease. Osteosarcoma does not cause soreness in the nearest joint; it may impede range of motion.

13. a, c, e. *Rationale:* The primary goals in treatment of metastatic bone disease are to prevent pathologic fractures and promote survival with maximum functioning, allowing the person to maintain as much mobility and pain control as possible. Cure of the disease and preventing bone segment ischemia are not primary goals of treatment in metastatic bone disease.

CHAPTER 58 DISORDERS OF MUSCULOSKELETAL FUNCTION: DEVELOPMENTAL AND METABOLIC DISORDERS

SECTION II: ASSESSING YOUR UNDERSTANDING

Activity A

1. Skeletal
2. epiphyseal growth plate
3. hypermobility, torsional
4. Blount
5. polydactyly
6. type I collagen
7. dysplasia
8. clubfoot
9. avascular necrosis
10. Osgood-Schlatter
11. osteoprogenitor
12. Osteopenia
13. Osteoporosis
14. Postmenopausal
15. Secondary
16. Osteomalacia
17. renal rickets
18. calcification
19. turnover
20. Paget

Activity B

1. h   **2.** b   **3.** c   **4.** e   **5.** a
6. j   **7.** i   **8.** g   **9.** d   **10.** f

Activity C

1. Epiphyseal separation can occur in children as the result of trauma. The separation usually occurs in the zone of the mature enlarged cartilage cells, which is the weakest part of the growth plate. The blood vessels that nourish the epiphysis pass through the growth plate. These vessels are ruptured when the growth plate separates. This can cause cessation of growth and a shortened extremity. The growth plate also is sensitive to nutritional and metabolic changes. Scurvy (i.e., vitamin C deficiency) impairs the formation of the organic matrix of bone, causing slowing of growth at the epiphyseal plate and cessation of diaphyseal growth. In rickets (i.e., vitamin D deficiency), calcification of the newly developed bone on the metaphyseal side of the growth plate is impaired. Thyroid and growth hormones are required for normal growth. Alterations in these and other hormones can also affect growth.

2. Toeing-in because of adduction of the forefoot usually is the result of the fetal position maintained *in utero*. It can occur in one foot or both feet. The forefoot commonly is adducted and gives the foot a kidney-shaped appearance, whereas the hind foot is normal. It can be caused by torsion in the foot, lower leg, or entire leg. Toeing-out, a common problem in children, is caused by external femoral torsion. This occurs when the femur can be externally rotated to approximately 90 degrees but internally rotated only to a neutral position or slightly beyond. Because the femoral torsion persists when a child habitually sleeps in the prone position, an external tibial torsion also may develop. If external tibial torsion is present, the feet point lateral to the midline of the medial plane. External tibial torsion rarely causes toeing-out; it only intensifies the condition.

3. The disorder, osteogenesis imperfecta, is characterized by thin and poorly developed bones that are susceptible to multiple fractures. Children with this disorder have short limbs and a soft, thin cranium with bifrontal prominences that give a triangular appearance to the face. Other problems associated with defective connective tissue synthesis include thin skin, blue or gray sclera, abnormal tooth development, hypotonic muscles, loose-jointedness, scoliosis, and a tendency toward hernia formation. Hearing loss owing to otosclerosis of the tiny bones in the middle ear is common in affected adults.

4. Congenital scoliosis can be divided into failures of formation and failures of segmentation. Failures of formation include the absence of a portion of the vertebra, such as hemivertebra (absence of a whole side of the vertebra) and wedge vertebra (missing only a portion of the vertebra). Failure of segmentation is the absence of the normal separations between the vertebrae. The child may have other anomalies and neurologic complications if the spine is involved. Neuromuscular scoliosis develops from neuropathic or myopathic diseases. It is seen with cerebral palsy, myelodysplasia, and poliomyelitis. There is often a long, "C"-shaped curve from the cervical to the sacral region. In children with cerebral palsy, severe deformity may make treatment difficult. Myopathic neuromuscular scoliosis develops with Duchenne muscular dystrophy and usually is not severe. Idiopathic scoliosis is a structural spinal curvature for which no cause has been established. It occurs in healthy, neurologically normal children.

5. The sequence of bone resorption and bone formation begins with osteoclastic resorption of existing bone, during which the organic (protein matrix) and the inorganic (mineral) components are removed. The sequence proceeds to the formation of new bone by osteoblasts. In the adult, the length of one sequence (i.e., bone resorption and formation) is approximately 4 months. Ideally, the replaced bone should equal the absorbed bone. If it does not, there is a net loss of bone. In the elderly, for example, bone resorption and formation no longer are perfectly coupled, and bone mass is lost.

6. The pathogenesis of osteoporosis involves an imbalance between bone resorption and formation such that bone resorption exceeds bone formation. Exercise may prevent or delay the onset of osteoporosis by increasing peak bone mineral density during periods of growth. Poor nutrition or an age-related decrease in intestinal absorption of calcium because of deficient activation of vitamin D may contribute to the development of osteoporosis, particularly in the elderly. Postmenopausal osteoporosis, which is caused by an estrogen deficiency, is manifested by a loss of cancellous bone and a predisposition to fractures of

the vertebrae and distal radius. The loss of bone mass is greatest during early menopause when estrogen levels are withdrawing.

7. Osteoporotic changes occur in the diaphysis and metaphysis of bone. In severe osteoporosis, the bones begin to resemble the fragile structure of a fine porcelain vase. There is loss of trabeculae from cancellous bone and thinning of the cortex to such an extent that minimal stress causes fractures. The changes that occur with osteoporosis have been explained by two distinct disease processes: postmenopausal and senile osteoporosis. In postmenopausal women, the increase in osteoclastic activity affects mainly bones or portions of bone that have increased surface area, such as the cancellous compartment of the vertebral bodies. The osteoporotic trabeculae become thinned and lose their interconnections, leading to microfractures and eventual vertebral collapse. In senile osteoporosis, the osteoporotic cortex is thinned by subperiosteal and endosteal resorption and the haversian systems are widened. Hip fractures, which are seen later in life, are more commonly associated with senile osteoporosis.

SECTION III: APPLYING YOUR KNOWLEDGE

Activity D

1. Drugs include nonsteroidal or other anti-inflammatory agents, and biphosphonates and calcitonin to manage pain and prevent further spread of the disease and neurologic defects

SECTION IV: PRACTICING FOR NCLEX

Activity E

1. a. *Rationale:* Patellar subluxation can result in patellofemoral malalignment with patellar subluxation or dislocation and pain. The other answers are incorrect.
2. b. *Rationale:* Genu varum can cause gait awkwardness and increased risk for sprains and fractures. Uncorrected genu valgum can cause subluxation and recurrent dislocation of the patella, with a predisposition to chondromalacia and joint pain and fatigue. The other answers are incorrect.
3. a, c, e. *Rationale:* The clinical manifestations of osteogenesis imperfecta include a spectrum of disorders marked by extreme skeletal fragility. Four major subtypes of the disorder have been identified. The disorder is characterized by thin and poorly developed bones, which are susceptible to multiple fractures. Children with osteogenesis imperfecta have short limbs and a soft, thin cranium with bifrontal prominences that give a triangular appearance to the face. Other problems associated with defective connective tissue synthesis include thin skin, blue or gray sclera, abnormal tooth development, hypotonic muscles, loose-jointedness, scoliosis, and a tendency toward hernia formation. There are neither thick bones in the lower extremities nor thick skin in osteogenesis imperfecta.
4. c. *Rationale:* The correction of clubfoot is maintained by full-time wear of a Denis Browne splint for 3 months and part-time night and nap wear for approximately 2 to 3 years. The other answers are incorrect.
5. a, b, c. *Rationale:* Treatment of Legg-Calvé-Perthes disease involves periods of rest, use of assistive devices for walking, non–weight-bearing and abduction braces to keep the legs separated in abduction with mild internal rotation. The Atlanta Scottish Rite brace, which does not extend below the knee, is the most widely used orthosis because it provides containment while allowing free knee motion and ambulation without crutches or external support. Weight-bearing braces and adduction braces are not used in the treatment of Legg-Calvé-Perthes disease.
6. d. *Rationale:* Osgood-Schlatter disease is characterized by pain in the front of the knee that is associated with inflammation and thickening of the patellar tendon. The pain usually is associated with specific activities, such as kneeling, running, bicycle riding, or stair climbing. There are swelling, tenderness, and increased prominence of the tibial tubercle. The symptoms usually are self-limiting. The other answers are incorrect.
7. a. *Rationale:* Scoliosis usually is first noticed because of the deformity it causes. A high shoulder, prominent hip, or projecting scapula may be noticed by a parent or seen in a school-based screening program A child with scoliosis can stand straight, does not feel pain, and can walk straight, so these answers are incorrect.

8. b. *Rationale:* The clinical method of choice for bone mineral density (BMD) studies is dual-energy x-ray absorptiometry (DXA) of the spine and hip. The other answers will not diagnose osteoporosis.

9. c. *Rationale:* The elderly with intestinal malabsorption also may benefit from vitamin D. The least expensive and most effective long-term treatment is a diet rich in vitamin D (i.e., fish, dairy products, and margarine) along with careful exposure to the midday sun. The other answers are incorrect.

10. d. *Rationale:* As with osteomalacia in the adult, rickets can result from kidney failure; malabsorptive syndromes, such as celiac disease and cystic fibrosis; and medications, such as anticonvulsants, which cause target organ resistance to vitamin D, and aluminum-containing antacids, which bind phosphorous and prevent its absorption. The other drugs are not used to treat rickets.

CHAPTER 59 DISORDERS OF MUSCULOSKELETAL FUNCTION: RHEUMATIC DISORDERS

SECTION II: ASSESSING YOUR UNDERSTANDING

Activity A

1. rheumatoid arthritis
2. T cell-mediated
3. chronic inflammatory
4. scleroderma
5. Ankylosing spondylitis
6. arthropathies
7. Reiter syndrome
8. enteropathic
9. Osteoarthritis
10. wear and tear
11. Gout
12. Juvenile idiopathic arthritis
13. systemic lapis erythematosus
14. dermatomyositis
15. Arthritis
16. Osteoarthritis
17. Polymyalgia rheumatica

Activity B

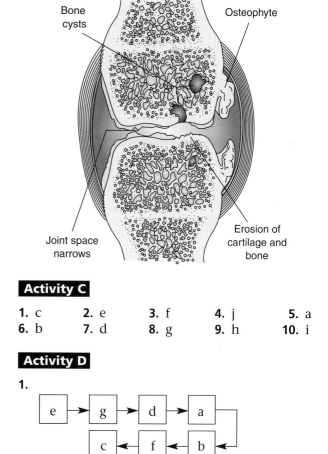

Bone cysts

Osteophyte

Joint space narrows

Erosion of cartilage and bone

Activity C

1. c	**2.** e	**3.** f	**4.** j	**5.** a
6. b	**7.** d	**8.** g	**9.** h	**10.** i

Activity D

1.

e → g → d → a
c ← f ← b ←

Activity E

1. The pathogenesis of rheumatoid arthritis (RA) can be viewed as an aberrant immune response that leads to synovial inflammation and destruction of the joint architecture. It has been suggested that the disease is initiated by the activation of helper T cells, release of cytokines, and antibody formation. Approximately 70%–80% of those with the disease have a substance called the *rheumatoid factor (RF)*, which is an autologous (self-produced) antibody (Ig RF) that reacts with a fragment of immunoglobulin G (IgG) to form immune complexes. Immune complexes (IgG RF + IgG) and complement components are found in the synovium, synovial fluid, and extrarticular lesions of persons with RA.

2. At the cellular level, neutrophils, macrophages, and lymphocytes are attracted to the area. The neutrophils and macrophages phagocytize the immune complexes and, in the process, release lysosomal enzymes capable of causing destructive changes in the joint cartilage. The inflammatory response that follows attracts additional inflammatory cells, setting into motion a chain of events that perpetuates the condition. As the inflammatory process progresses, the synovial cells and subsynovial tissues undergo reactive hyperplasia. Vasodilation and increased blood flow cause warmth and redness. The joint swelling that occurs is the result of the increased capillary permeability that accompanies the inflammatory process.

3. Arthralgias and arthritis are among the most commonly occurring early symptoms of systemic lupus erythematosus (SLE). The polyarthritis of SLE initially can be confused with other forms of arthritis, especially rheumatoid arthritis (RA), because of the symmetric arthropathy. Flexion contractures, hyperextension of the interphalangeal joint, and subluxation of the carpometacarpal joint contribute to the deformity and subsequent loss of function in the hands. Other musculoskeletal manifestations of SLE include tenosynovitis, rupture of the intrapatellar and Achilles tendons, and avascular necrosis, frequently of the femoral head.

4. The joint changes associated with osteoarthritis, which include a progressive loss of articular cartilage and synovitis, result from the inflammation caused when cartilage attempts to repair itself, creating osteophytes or spurs. These changes are accompanied by joint pain, stiffness, limitation of motion, and, in some cases, by joint instability and deformity.

5. The pathogenesis of gout resides in an elevation of the serum uric acid levels. Uric acid (UA) is the end product of purine (adenine and guanine from DNA and RNA) metabolism. UA elevation and the subsequent development of gout can result from overproduction of purines, decreased salvage of free purine bases, augmented breakdown of nucleic acids because of increased cell turnover, or decreased urinary excretion of UA. Primary gout, which constitutes 90% of cases, may be a consequence of enzyme defects that result in an overproduction of UA; inadequate elimination of UA by the kidney; or a combination of the two. In secondary gout, the hyperuricemia may be caused by increased breakdown in the production of nucleic acids, as occurs with rapid tumor cell lysis during treatment for lymphoma or leukemia. Other cases of secondary gout result from chronic renal disease.

SECTION III: APPLYING YOUR KNOWLEDGE

Activity F

1. Juvenile idiopathic arthritis (JIA) can be regarded not as a single disease, but as a category of diseases with three principal types of onset: (1) systemic onset disease, (2) pauciarticular arthritis, and (3) polyarticular disease.
2. You would expect blood work for rheumatoid factor and a complete metabolic panel along with a complete blood count (CBC) to be ordered.

SECTION IV: PRACTICING FOR NCLEX

Activity G

1. c, e, d, i, f, g, a, h, b. *Rationale:* The role of the autoimmune process in the joint destruction of rheumatoid arthritis (RA) remains obscure. At the cellular level, neutrophils, macrophages, and lymphocytes are attracted to the area. The neutrophils and macrophages phagocytize the immune complexes and, in the process, release lysosomal enzymes capable of causing destructive changes in the joint cartilage. The inflammatory response that follows attracts additional inflammatory cells, setting into motion a chain of events that perpetuates the condition. As the inflammatory process continues, the synovial cells and subsynovial tissues undergo reactive hyperplasia. Vasodilation and increased blood flow cause warmth and redness. The joint swelling that occurs is the result of the increased capillary permeability that accompanies the inflammatory process.
2. a. *Rationale:* Arthralgias and arthritis are among the most commonly occurring early symptoms of systemic lupus erythematosus (SLE)

(SLE). The other answers are symptoms of SLE in differing stages of the disease.

3. c, d. *Rationale:* Almost all persons with scleroderma develop polyarthritis and Raynaud phenomenon, a vascular disorder characterized by reversible vasospasm of the arteries supplying the fingers. Dumping syndrome, chronic diarrhea, and chronic vasoconstriction are not diseases developed by people with scleroderma.

4. b. *Rationale:* Corticosteroids are the mainstay of treatment for polymyositis and dermatomyositis. The other drug types are not the treatment of choice for polymyositis and dermatomyositis.

5. c. *Rationale:* The pain, which becomes worse when resting, particularly when lying in bed, initially may be blamed on muscle strain or spasm from physical activity. The other answers are incorrect.

6. d. *Rationale:* Reiter syndrome was the first rheumatic disease to be recognized in association with human immunodeficiency virus (HIV) infection. Symptoms of arthritis may precede any overt signs of HIV disease. The other sexually transmitted diseases (STDs) have not been associated with Reiter syndrome.

7. a. *Rationale:* The biologic response modifiers, specifically the tumor necrosis factor (TNF) inhibitors (e.g., etanercept, infliximab, and adalimumab) have been found to be beneficial in controlling arthritis, as well as psoriasis in patients with psoriatic arthritis. The other drugs have not been found to be beneficial in psoriatic arthritis.

8. a, c, e. *Rationale:* The joint changes associated with osteoarthritis, which include a progressive loss of articular cartilage and synovitis, result from the inflammation caused when cartilage attempts to repair itself, creating osteophytes or spurs. These changes are accompanied by joint pain, stiffness, limitation of motion, and, in some cases, by joint instability and deformity. The other answers are incorrect.

9. b. *Rationale:* A definitive diagnosis of gout can be made only when monosodium urate crystals are found in the synovial fluid or in tissue sections of tophaceous deposits. The other answers are not diagnostic of gout.

10. c. *Rationale:* In terms of medications, the selection of drugs used in the treatment of arthritic disorders and their dosages may need to be considered when prescribing for the elderly. For example, the nonsteroidal anti-inflammatory drugs (NSAIDs) may be less well tolerated by the elderly, and their side effects are more likely to be serious. In addition to bleeding from the gastrointestinal tract and renal insufficiency, there may be cognitive dysfunction, manifested by forgetfulness, inability to concentrate, sleeplessness, paranoid ideation, and depression. Malaise, lethargy, and mania are not side effects of NSAIDs.

CHAPTER 60 STRUCTURE AND FUNCTION OF THE SKIN

SECTION II: ASSESSING YOUR UNDERSTANDING

Activity A

1. integumentum
2. thickness
3. epidermis
4. stratum corneum
5. Keratinocytes
6. Melanocytes
7. eumelanin
8. Langerhans
9. basal lamina
10. epidermis
11. dermis
12. papillary
13. Eccrine
14. Apocrine
15. keratinized
16. keratinized
17. blister
18. callus
19. Corns
20. xerosis

Activity B

1.

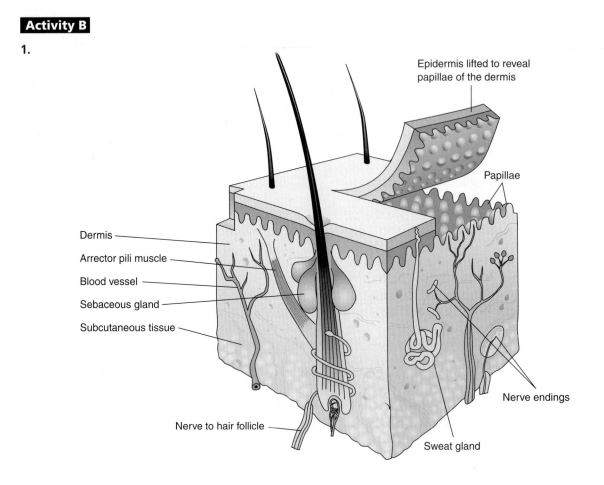

Epidermis lifted to reveal papillae of the dermis

Papillae

Dermis

Arrector pili muscle

Blood vessel

Sebaceous gland

Subcutaneous tissue

Nerve endings

Nerve to hair follicle

Sweat gland

2.

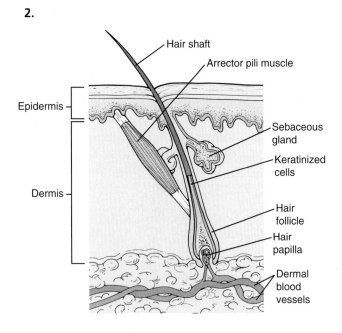

Hair shaft

Arrector pili muscle

Epidermis

Sebaceous gland

Keratinized cells

Dermis

Hair follicle

Hair papilla

Dermal blood vessels

Activity C

1. d	**2.** j	**3.** i	**4.** c	**5.** a
6. h	**7.** f	**8.** g	**9.** b	**10.** e

Activity D

1. The skin serves several other vital functions, including somatosensory function, temperature regulation, and vitamin D synthesis. The skin is richly innervated with pain, temperature, and touch receptors. Skin receptors relay the numerous qualities of touch, such as pressure, sharpness, dullness, and pleasure to the central nervous system for localization and fine discrimination. The rate at which heat is dissipated from the body is determined by constriction or dilation of the arterioles that supply blood to the skin and through evaporation of moisture and sweat from the skin surface. Vitamin D_3, the most important of these, is formed in the skin as the result of irradiation of 7-dehydrocholesterol, a substance normally found in the skin, by ultraviolet rays from the sun.

2. The epidermis is composed of stratified squamous keratinized epithelium, which, when viewed under the microscope, is seen to consist of five distinct layers, or strata, that represent a progressive differentiation or maturation of the keratinocytes: the stratum germinativum, or basal layer; the stratum spinosum; the stratum granulosum; the stratum lucidum; and the stratum corneum.

3. The ability to synthesize melanin depends on the ability of the melanocytes to produce an enzyme called *tyrosinase*, which converts the amino acid tyrosine to a precursor of melanin. A genetic lack of this enzyme results in a clinical condition called *albinism*. Persons with this disorder lack pigmentation in the skin, hair, and iris of the eye.

4. Dark-skinned and light-skinned people have approximately the same number of melanocytes, but the production and packaging of pigment differ. In dark-skinned people, *larger* melanin-containing melanosomes are produced and transferred individually to the keratinocyte; whereas, in light-skinned people, *smaller* melanosomes are produced and then packaged together in a membrane before being transferred to the keratinocyte. Although the number of melanosomes in dark and white skin is the same, black skin produces more melanin and produces it faster than white skin.

5. The sebaceous glands are located over the entire skin surface except for the palms, soles, and sides of the feet. They are part of the *pilosebaceous unit*. They secrete a mixture of lipids, including triglycerides, cholesterol, and wax. This mixture is called *sebum*; it lubricates hair and skin. Sebum is not the same as the surface lipid film. Sebum prevents undue evaporation of moisture from the stratum corneum during cold weather and helps to conserve body heat. Sebum production is under the control of genetic and hormonal influences.

6. It is generally agreed that itch is a sensation that originates in free nerve endings in the skin, is carried by small myelinated type C nerve fibers to the dorsal horn of the spinal cord, and is then transmitted to the somatosensory cortex via the spinothalamic tract, differing from the pain pathways.

SECTION III: APPLYING YOUR KNOWLEDGE

Activity E

1. Skin color is determined by the melanin produced by the melanocytes. Black skin produces more melanin and produces it faster than white skin. Because of their skin color, dark-skinned persons are better protected against skin cancer, premature wrinkling, and aging of the skin that occurs with sun exposure. Dry or "ashy" skin also can be a problem for people with dark skin. It often is uncomfortable, and it also is easily noticed because it gives the skin an ashen or grayish appearance. The darker pigmentation can make skin pallor, cyanosis, and erythema more difficult to observe. Changes in skin color, in particular hypo- and hyperpigmentation, often accompany disorders of dark skin and are very important signs to observe when diagnosing skin conditions.

SECTION IV: PRACTICING FOR NCLEX

Activity F

1. a. *Rationale:* The skin also serves as an immunologic barrier. The Langerhans cells detect foreign antigens, playing an important part in allergic skin conditions and skin graft rejections. The other cell types are not part of the immunologic barrier.

2. 1-c, 2-b, 3-a, 4-d

3. b. *Rationale:* The basement membrane is also a major site of immunoglobulin and complement deposition in skin disease. The other answers are incorrect.

4. c. *Rationale:* The reticular dermis (pars reticularis) is the thicker area of the dermis and forms the bulk of the dermal layer. The other three answers are part of the reticular dermis but it is not characterized by them.

5. a, c, e. *Rational:* Because the eccrine glands and deep hair follicles extend to this layer and several skin diseases involve the subcutaneous tissue, the subcutaneous tissue may be considered part of the skin. The keratinocytes and the Merkel cells are not part of the subcutaneous tissue.

6. d. *Rationale:* This mixture is called sebum; it lubricates hair and skin. Sweat comes from sweat glands. Chalasia is an abnormal relaxation or the cardiac sphincter of the stomach. Cerumen is found in the ear.

7. a. *Rationale:* The nearly transparent nail plate provides a useful window for viewing the amount of oxygen in the blood, providing a view of the color of the blood in the dermal vessels. The other answers are incorrect.

8. b. *Rationale:* When a blister occurs, histologically, there is degeneration of the epidermal cells and a disruption of the intercellular junctions that causes the layers of the skin to separate. Lichenifications are thickened areas of the skin. Petechiae are pinpoint rashes on the skin. A pressure ulcer is sometimes referred to as a "bed sore" and is caused by continuous pressure on a bony prominence.

9. c. *Rationale:* Given these new findings, it has been postulated that itch exists both locally and centrally, that, in addition to localized itch, an "itch center" exists in the somatosensory cortex. The other answers are incorrect.

10. d. *Rationale:* Moisturizing agents are the cornerstone of treatment for dry skin. These agents exert their effects by repairing the skin barrier, increasing the water content of the skin, reducing transepidermal water loss, and restoring the lipid barrier's ability to attract, hold, and redistribute water. The other answers are incorrect.

CHAPTER 61 DISORDERS OF SKIN INTEGRITY AND FUNCTION

SECTION II: ASSESSING YOUR UNDERSTANDING

Activity A

1. Primary
2. melanin
3. Albinism
4. Fungi
5. Candidiasis
6. bacterial
7. Impetigo
8. Cellulitis
9. Verrucae plantaris, verrucae palmaris
10. zoster
11. Acne
12. Sebum
13. comedones, blackheads, whiteheads
14. Inflammatory
15. dermatoses
16. Allergic contact
17. nummular
18. urticaria
19. Topical, systemic
20. Papulosquamous
21. Lichen planus
22. repeated
23. scabies
24. UVB rays
25. photosensitive
26. Sunburn
27. Burns
28. Burn
29. ischemic
30. *dysplastic nevus*
31. melanocytes
32. melanoma
33. Basal cell carcinoma
34. Squamous cell carcinomas
35. birthmarks
36. Hemangiomas
37. Port-wine stains
38. Irritant diaper dermatitis
39. Prickly heat
40. Cradle cap

Activity B

1.

1. b	2. e	3. a	4. g	5. f
6. h	7. d	8. c	9. j	10. i

2.

1. h	2. a	3. j	4. e	5. d
6. g	7. b	8. f	9. c	10. i

Activity C

1. The most common type of albinism is recessively inherited oculocutaneous albinism, in which there are a normal number of melanocytes, but they lack tyrosinase, the enzyme needed for synthesis of melanin. Individuals have pale or pink skin, white or yellow hair, and light-colored or sometimes pink eyes. Persons with albinism have ocular problems, such as extreme sensitivity to light, refractive errors, lack of stereopsis, and nystagmus.

2. The fungi that cause superficial mycoses live on the dead keratinized cells of the epidermis. They emit an enzyme that enables them to digest keratin, which results in superficial skin scaling, nail disintegration, or hair breakage, depending on the location of the infection. Deeper reactions involving vesicles, erythema, and infiltration are caused by the inflammation that results from exotoxins liberated by the fungus. Fungi also are capable of producing an allergic or immune response.

3. The two common types of tinea capitis are primary (noninflammatory) and secondary (inflammatory). The infection is spread most often among household members who share combs and brushes on which the spores are shed and remain viable for long periods. Depending on the invading fungus, the lesions of the noninflammatory type can vary from grayish, round, hairless patches to balding spots, with or without black dots on the head. The individual usually is asymptomatic, although pruritus may exist. The inflammatory type of tinea capitis is caused by virulent strains. The onset is rapid, and inflamed lesions usually are localized to one area of the head. The inflammation is believed to be a delayed hypersensitivity reaction to the invading fungus. The initial lesion consists of a pustular, scaly, round patch with broken hairs. A secondary bacterial infection is common and it may lead to a painful, circumscribed, boggy, and indurated lesion called a kerion.

4. Preexisting wounds (e.g., ulcers, erosions) and tinea pedis are often portals of entry. Legs are the most common sites, followed by the hands and pinnas of the ears, but cellulitis may be seen on many body parts. The lesion consists of an expanding red, swollen, tender plaque with an indefinite border, covering a small to wide area. Cellulitis is frequently accompanied by fever, erythema, heat, edema, and pain. Cellulitis often involves the lymph system and, once compromised, repeat infections may impair lymphatic drainage, leading to chronically swollen legs, and eventually dermal fibrosis and lymphedema.

5. The recurrent lesions of HSV-1 usually begin with a burning or tingling sensation. Umbilicated vesicles and erythema follow and progress to pustules, ulcers, and crusts before healing. Lesions are most common on the lips, face, mouth, nasal septum, and nose. When a lesion is active, HSV-1 is shed and there is risk of transmitting the virus to others. Pain is common, and healing takes place within 10–14 days. Precipitating factors may be stress, menses, or injury. In particular, UVB exposure seems to be a frequent trigger for recurrence. Individuals who are immunocompromised may have severe attacks.

6. (1) Increased sebum production, (2) increased proliferation of the keratinizing epidermal cells that form the sebaceous cells, (3) the colonization and proliferation of *Propionibacterium acnes*, and (4) inflammation

7. Atopic dermatitis (atopic eczema) is an itchy, inflammatory skin disorder that is characterized by poorly defined erythema with edema, vesicles, and weeping at the acute stage and skin thickening (lichenification) in the chronic stage. The infantile form of atopic dermatitis is characterized by vesicle formation, oozing, and crusting with excoriations. The skin of the cheeks may be paler, with extra creases under the eyes. Adolescents and adults usually have dry, red patches affecting the face, neck, and upper trunk, but without the thickening and discrete demarcation associated with psoriasis. The bends of the elbows and knees are usually involved. In chronic cases, the skin is dry, leathery, and lichenified.

8. It is thought that activated T lymphocytes (mainly CD4 helper cells) produce chemical messengers that stimulate abnormal growth of keratinocytes and dermal blood vessels. Accompanying inflammatory changes are caused by infiltration of neutrophils and monocytes. Skin trauma (i.e., prepsoriasis) is a common precipitating factor in people predisposed to psoriasis. The reaction of the skin to an original trauma of any type is called the *Köebner reaction*. Stress, infections, trauma, xerosis, and use of medications, such as angiotensin-converting enzyme inhibitors, β-adrenergic blocking drugs, lithium, and the antimalarial agent, hydroxychloroquine (Plaquenil), may precipitate or exacerbate the condition.

9. A mite, *Sarcoptes scabiei*, which burrows into the epidermis, causes scabies. After a female mite is impregnated, she burrows into the skin and lays two to three eggs each day for 4 or 5 weeks. The eggs hatch after 3–4 days, and the larvae migrate to the skin surface. At this point, they burrow into the skin only for food or protection. The larvae molt and become nymphs; they molt once more to become adults. After the new adult females are impregnated, the cycle is repeated. Small vesicles may cover the burrows. Pruritus is common and may result from the burrows, the fecal material of the mite, or both. Excoriations may develop from scratching, leaving the host vulnerable to secondary bacterial infections and severe skin lesions if left untreated.

10. Skin damage induced by UVB is believed to be caused by the generation of reactive oxygen species and by damage to melanin. Cellular proteins and DNA are primarily damaged because of their abundance and ability to absorb UV radiation. Both UVA and UVB also deplete Langerhans cells and immune cells. It is believed that these effects prevent immune cells from detecting and removing sun-damaged cells with malignant potential.

11. A patient should (a) wear a wide-brimmed hat, (b) cover up in the sun, (c) seek shade, (d) wear wrap-around sunglasses, and (e) avoid the sun during the hours of 10 AM to 4 PM, while using a broad spectrum sunscreen with an SPF of 15 or higher. It is also important to avoid sun tanning booths, perform a self-assessment of the skin every month, and obtain a professional skin examination every year.

12. The massive loss of skin tissue not only predisposes to attack by microorganisms that are present in the environment but it allows for the massive loss of body fluids and their contents, it interferes with temperature regulation, it challenges the immune system, and it imposes excessive demands on the metabolic and reparative processes that are needed to restore the body's interface with the environment.

13. Basal cell carcinoma usually is a nonmetastasizing tumor that extends wide and deep if left untreated. Nodular ulcerative basal cell carcinoma is the most common, accounting for 60% of all basal cell carcinoma. It has a nodulocystic structure that begins as a small, flesh-colored or pink, smooth, translucent nodule that enlarges over time. Telangiectatic vessels frequently are seen beneath the surface. Over the years, a central depression forms that progress to an ulcer surrounded by the original shiny, waxy border. The second most common form is superficial basal cell carcinoma, which is seen most often on the chest or back. It begins as a flat, nonpalpable, erythematous plaque. The red, scaly areas slowly enlarge, with nodular borders and telangiectatic bases. This type of skin cancer is difficult to diagnose because it mimics other dermatologic problems.

SECTION III: APPLYING YOUR KNOWLEDGE

Activity D

1. Attack by microorganisms in the environment; massive loss of body fluids; interferes with temperature regulation; imposes excessive demands on the metabolic system; and challenges the immune system

2. Hemodynamic instability owing to fluid loss; smoke inhalation and postburn lung injury; hypermetabolism, characterized by increased oxygen consumption, increased glucose use, and protein and fat wasting; impaired function of the kidneys; hypovolemic shock and impaired organ perfusion; and sepsis

SECTION IV: PRACTICING FOR NCLEX

Activity E

1. 1-a, 2-c, 3-b
2. a. *Rationale:* Treatment of fungal infections usually follows diagnosis confirmed by KOH preparation or culture. The other answers are incorrect.
3. 1-b, 2-a, 3-f, 4-g, 5-e, 6-d, 7-c
4. b. *Rationale:* Benzoyl peroxide is a topical agent that has both antibacterial and comedolytic properties. It is the topical agent most effective in reducing *P. acnes*. The other topical agents do not act both as comedolytic and antibacterial agents.
5. a, c, e. *Rationale:* Prominent symptoms include eyes that are itchy, burning, or dry; a gritty or foreign sensation; and erythema and swelling of the eyelid. Heat sensitivity and telangiectasia occur later in the disease and are not considered prominent symptoms.
6. c. *Rationale:* The lesions of allergic contact dermatitis range from a mild erythema with edema to vesicles or large bullae. The other answers are incorrect.
7. d. *Rationale:* In persons with black skin, pigmentation may be lost from lichenified skin. The other answers do not occur in people with black skins who have eczema.
8. a. *Rationale:* Intravenous immunoglobulin may hasten the healing response of the skin. Broad-spectrum antibiotics and corticosteroids may be given but they do not hasten the healing response of the skin. Diflucan is given for vaginal candidiasis.
9. b. *Rationale:* In psoriasis vulgaris, the primary lesions are sharply demarcated thick red plaques with a silvery scale that vary in size and shape. The other answers are incorrect.
10. c. *Rationale:* Most persons with lichen planus who have skin lesions also have oral lesions, appearing as milky white lacework on the buccal mucosa or tongue. The other answers are incorrect.

11. d. *Rationale:* Oral ivermectin, a broad-spectrum antiparasitic agent, has been used for treatment-resistant scabies. The other drugs are not used for treatment-resistant scabies.

12. b. *Rationale:* Methods for preventing pressure ulcers include frequent position change, meticulous skin care, and frequent and careful observation to detect early signs of skin breakdown. The other answers are incorrect.

13. c. *Rationale:* Another form of nevi, the dysplastic nevus, is important because of its capacity to transform to malignant melanoma. The other answers are incorrect.

14. d. *Rationale:* Other risk factors include a family history of malignant melanoma, presence of marked freckling on the upper back, history of three or more blistering sunburns before 20 years of age, and presence of actinic keratoses. The other answers are incorrect.

15. a. *Rationale:* The most important treatment goal for basal cell carcinoma is complete elimination of the lesion. Also important is the maintenance of function and optimal cosmetic effect. Curettage with electrodesiccation, surgical excision, irradiation, laser, cryosurgery and chemosurgery are effective in removing all cancerous cells. The other answers are incorrect.

16. b. *Rationale:* In black-skinned persons, the lesions may appear as hyperpigmented nodules and occur more frequently on non–sun-exposed areas. The other answers do not describe squamous cell carcinoma in black-skinned people.

17. c. *Rationale:* Hemangiomas of infancy typically undergo an early period of proliferation during which they enlarge, followed by a period of slow involution where the growth is reversed until complete resolution. Surgical excision, laser surgery, and chemotherapy are not used for hemagiomas of infancy.

18. d. *Rationale:* Immunization is accomplished by live-virus injection. Rubella vaccination has close to 100% immunity response in immunized children. The other answers are incorrect.

19. a. *Rationale:* Lentigines can be removed surgically (cryotherapy, laser therapy, liquid nitrogen). Topical creams and lotions containing adapalene, tertinoin, have been used. The other answers are incorrect.